Thieme

The Glioma Book

Michael E. Sughrue, MD
Associate Professor
Department of Neurosurgery
Prince of Wales Private Hospital
Randwick, NSW, Australia

345 illustrations

Thieme
New York • Stuttgart • Delhi • Rio de Janeiro

Library of Congress Cataloging-in-Publication Data

Names: Sughrue, Michael E., author.
Title: The glioma book / Michael E. Sughrue.
Description: New York : Thieme, [2020] | Includes bibliographical references and index.
Identifiers: LCCN 2019027673| ISBN 9781626234444 (hardback) | ISBN 9781626234451 (ebook)
Subjects: | MESH: Glioma–surgery | Cerebrum–surgery | Neurosurgical Procedures–methods
Classification: LCC RD594 | NLM WL 307 | DDC 617.4/81–dc23
LC record available at https://lccn.loc.gov/2019027673

Thieme Publishers New York
333 Seventh Avenue, New York, NY 10001 USA
+1 800 782 3488, customerservice@thieme.com

Thieme Publishers Stuttgart
Rüdigerstrasse 14, 70469 Stuttgart, Germany
+49 [0]711 8931 421, customerservice@thieme.de

Thieme Publishers Delhi
A-12, Second Floor, Sector-2, Noida-201301
Uttar Pradesh, India
+91 120 45 566 00, customerservice@thieme.in

Thieme Revinter Publicações Ltda.
Rua do Matoso, 170 – Tijuca
Rio de Janeiro RJ 20270-135 - Brasil
+55 21 2563-9702
www.thiemerevinter.com.br

Cover design: Thieme Publishing Group
Typesetting by DiTech Process Solutions

Printed in the United States of America by King Printing Co., Inc.
5 4 3 2

ISBN 978-1-62623-444-4

Also available as an e-book:
eISBN 978-1-62623-445-1

Important note: Medicine is an ever-changing science undergoing continual development. Research and clinical experience are continually expanding our knowledge, in particular our knowledge of proper treatment and drug therapy. Insofar as this book mentions any dosage or application, readers may rest assured that the authors, editors, and publishers have made every effort to ensure that such references are in accordance with **the state of knowledge at the time of production of the book.**

Nevertheless, this does not involve, imply, or express any guarantee or responsibility on the part of the publishers in respect to any dosage instructions and forms of applications stated in the book. **Every user is requested to examine carefully** the manufacturers' leaflets accompanying each drug and to check, if necessary in consultation with a physician or specialist, whether the dosage schedules mentioned therein or the contraindications stated by the manufacturers differ from the statements made in the present book. Such examination is particularly important with drugs that are either rarely used or have been newly released on the market. Every dosage schedule or every form of application used is entirely at the user's own risk and responsibility. The authors and publishers request every user to report to the publishers any discrepancies or inaccuracies noticed. If errors in this work are found after publication, errata will be posted at www.thieme.com on the product description page.

Some of the product names, patents, and registered designs referred to in this book are in fact registered trademarks or proprietary names even though specific reference to this fact is not always made in the text. Therefore, the appearance of a name without designation as proprietary is not to be construed as a representation by the publisher that it is in the public domain.

FSC
www.fsc.org
100%
Paper from well-managed forests
FSC® C103101

Contents

Preface

It is uncommon that an author spends two years writing a book with the fervent hope that it will be rendered obsolete in short order, but that is the goal of this book. In this book, I summarize my current approach and experience with glioma surgery, which numbers about 1,000 surgeries at the time of writing. However, unlike most books in our field which aim to be a "How I Do It" tome from the master, this book aims more to be provocative, with the hope of generating a new field of thought in glioma surgery.

This book is built around the idea that we can achieve better outcomes in glioma patients by updating our models of how the cerebrum works by thinking about glioma surgery in terms of large-scale brain networks, and by realizing that regardless of how we perform a glioma surgery, we are cutting around or across the parts of networks whether we are aware of it or not. A few key principles/biases which are fundamental to this book and its philosophy are outlined below.

Concept 1: Our surgical models of the cerebrum are embarrassingly outdated

A quick look at images of the functional anatomy of the brain with a critical eye reveals the limitations of the anatomic models locating function in the human brain used to teach people how to avoid problems in the cerebrum. Broca and Wernicke have been dead for over a century, yet we have not updated their language model very much. Wernicke's area is defined imprecisely and can span a part of the STG or most of the left temporal lobe depending on the artist. Most of the brain is considered non-eloquent, implying it doesn't do anything. The subcortex is mostly ignored.

Most surgeons have caused a neurologic deficit that they couldn't immediately explain. I would suggest that this results from using bad models of the brain. A better model involves more specific localization of functions, acknowledges that functionally connected areas are usually physically connected and that this is essential for them to work together, and incorporates the whole brain into its world view: the so-called non-eloquent areas are not there to soak up CSF.

A large part of this book is dedicated to making more updated models of the brain relevant to neurosurgery and explaining how to utilize them.

Concept 2: The brain is a big data problem

Cadaveric dissection has been a hobby of neurosurgeons for decades, and it has taken us far, particularly at the base of the skull. Cerebral dissection, especially white matter dissection, has also provided some useful insights. However, it is clear that gross anatomic knowledge has had a more profound impact at the skull base than in the cerebrum. The explanation is obvious: it is easier to explain skull base anatomy with the naked eye than it is to explain the cerebrum. In other words, the visual appearance of the third nerve is more representative of its true structure and function to the required level of detail for good decision making in surgery, than the visual appearance of the cut cerebral hemisphere. The cerebrum is made up of a staggering collection of interconnections, leading to individual uniqueness, complexity on a massive scale, and crossing of connections, which makes the idea of sorting all this out with the naked eye absurd.

Computer science has created the possibility of working out the brain connections on a level of detail never before possible, and it is obvious that this is the only way our surgeries in the cerebrum will become more rational and safer. This book doubles down on big data and begins what I hope will be a long process of working out the details of how to make better decisions in surgery.

Concept 3: Glioma surgery is not curative, but it is helpful

It is important to be honest with patients about what we are providing and not providing by taking out the tumor. Having said this, it is hard to argue that we are doing the patient a favor by leaving a large amount of non-radiosensitive tumor in their brain and hoping it works. The data lies with common sense and with the experience of those of us who have been doing aggressive surgery on gliomas for some time. In short, cytoreduction is helpful even if the patient is not cured. There are several points in this book where I argue for this principle, but it is hard to read a book about glioma surgery without the basic idea that it is important and worth improving on.

Glioma surgery can be frustrating as even a great operation can lead to clinical failure. There have been few ideas in neurosurgery which have been as persistently resisted as the idea that it is helpful to cytoreduce a glioma. Thus, while it is important to be honest with ourselves and the patients about our limitations, it is equally important to recognize how bad this disease really is, acknowledge the limitations of just throwing chemotherapy and/or radiation at an unresected tumor, and appreciate the fact that many patients have a totally different view of risk than we do.

Concept 4: There is no such thing as an "inoperable" glioma

It is worth a quick mention that numerous previous structural brain diseases have been given this term, "inoperable," including myelomeningoceles, petroclival meningiomas, foramen magnum meningiomas, basilar aneurysms and many more. The result in all these cases was gradual improvement in surgical techniques due to technological advances, refinement of surgical technique, questioning and rethinking "conventional wisdom," bravery, and most importantly persistence and humility. In all these cases, this term was obviously misplaced in retrospect, and while none of them are desirable diagnoses, they are not uniformly fatal by anyone's current mindset.

Difficult gliomas have not been a serious topic of study as many people have quit seriously considering ways to try to improve the outcomes for these patients. As a result, their bad outcome becomes a self-fulfilling prophesy, and progress stops.

The key argument of this book is not that I have slain these monsters—in some cases, far from it. It is the idea that technology, especially connectomic imaging, provides insights which can help us crack these nuts and put these tumors into play. In many ways, connectomics is to the cerebrum what the microscope was to the skull base: it shows us things we hadn't known were there previously.

A preemptive attribution of credit

It's a bit impossible to outline a conceptual framework without unintentionally appropriating a concept that another first brought to your mind. Certainly, that is the case with this book: some of the ideas are my own, but without doubt this book contains the ideas of others. In lieu of trying to attribute all of them to their authors one by one, I think it might be best to describe three of the most influential.

First is Eddie Chang, who was my co-resident at UCSF. Eddie doesn't even focus on glioma surgery anymore; however, during our training together, he raised some of the best questions about the disease that I have ever had posed to me, many of which I am still addressing. For example, once when we were closing a glioma he noted to me, "Just because it is not curable, doesn't mean you have a license to do sloppy work." This influence is obvious.

Hughes Duffau never trained me, but I would be dishonest if I didn't acknowledge the significant influence his ideas had on my own. The concept that we are operating on networks and not cortical areas is obviously his, and his methods of subcortical dissection are also liberally described in this book. Clearly, much of this book involves extension of these ideas (the use of DTIs being an obvious difference). Nevertheless, I would unlikely be as interested in these networks had he not pointed this idea out to me.

Finally, probably no one taught me more about how to operate on gliomas than Charlie Teo. He will likely recognize the technique sections as many of them are ones I learned from him. However, more importantly, I learned courage from him, as he showed me time and again that things were achievable that I had never thought were possible. Even if the system I propose in this book is not his identically, his ideas that we should be continuing to improve our techniques, and that the patient views this as a battle for their life as opposed to an exercise in eventual failure, are ones which have guided my own ever since.

Michael E. Sughrue, MD

List of Videos

Part I

Foundations

I

1 Why Better Glioma Surgery Matters

1.1 Introduction

In my experience as a trainee and as a practicing brain tumor surgeon, I have found that there are few topics about which more people have more strongly held views about than treating patients with gliomas, especially glioblastoma. I personally have met few neurosurgeons with a 100% spinal practice who hold strong views about whether aneurysms should be clipped or coiled, of whether craniopharyngiomas should be removed through the nose or a craniotomy. But many have an opinion (often negative) on whether or not a glioblastoma patient should get an operation.

Gliomas are unquestionably a bad disease, and the patients are often sympathetic victims, who in many cases slowly lose their battle despite our treatments. So it shouldn't be surprising that people have come to strong conclusions about this disease. It can't be cured, and surgery inevitably eventually fails in a large number of cases. Glioblastoma has an amazing ability to humble us by growing back a few weeks after the most technically excellent resection, which is a deflating experience even to a glioma surgeon.

1.2 Where has Nihilism Taken Us with this Disease?

My personal opinion is that by giving up on aggressively treating these patients that our field has collectively made the grim outcome a self-fulfilling prophecy.[1] I have heard glioma surgery described as "easy" in comparison with skull base surgery, and it is often a case done occasionally by neurosurgeons who spend most of their time in the lab. A common method is to do the case with loupes and a headlight, the patient asleep, and the methodology is to suck the center of the "tumor" and not enter "eloquent" cortex. Basically, it is felt that because a cure cannot be obtained, that it is not as important to be technically excellent at doing it.

As a result, I regularly see many patients who have had no surgery or completely inadequate surgery. I see patients who have been told they have an "inoperable" tumor, when in reality; their tumor is located in a simple area and can be removed with minimal risk, provided the surgeon uses a good technique based on sound principles. Even worse, I often see patients where the surgical plan transgresses the worst possible trajectory in route to a subtotal resection, the worst of both worlds. Finally, I have seen all of the above occur at otherwise technically excellent neurosurgical centers (four examples of cases which were done at high quality academic neurosurgical programs are provided in ▸ Fig. 1.1), which can only occur from the view that it is not critical that we do glioma surgery at a technically excellent level.

This technical standard would never be accepted as the community standard for acoustic neuroma, which is a much less common disease and one where other treatments and repeat surgery are much more able to bail the patient out of a bad situation. The only conclusion is that we as a community do not believe that glioma surgery is important and that we should strive to refine our techniques until they are excellent, and that we should demand similar results from our peers.

1.3 My Own Contrary View

While glioma surgery cannot obtain a complete resection and cure, it does not necessarily follow that there aren't good reasons to work towards excellence. Most notably is the repeated observation that improved resection improves overall survival for both low and high grade[1,2,3,4,5] glioma. Many studies demonstrate a survival advantage for aggressive resection of low-grade gliomas which can be as substantial as 10 years compared to doing only a minimal amount of resection or a biopsy.[1,2,3,4,5] By viewing outcomes with the binary view that our results are "cure or nothing," we often deny patients a survival benefit that treating brain mets (a far less emotionally laden topic for most neurosurgeons) has never approached.

Further, even in the case of glioblastoma, when the survival benefit is less mathematically profound, logic and experience tell us that surgery provides these patients their best chance with a bad problem. I have yet to meet anyone alive and doing well 4 years after diagnosis with a biopsy and radiation but have met several individuals alive thanks to surgery. Cytoreduction probably improves the probability of efficacy of any radiation or chemotherapy, and it's hard to expect a single drug to kill billions of cancer cells in a disease known for its ability to develop resistance and which hides behind the blood brain barrier. Thus, surgery gives the patient a chance, which is all most of these patients really ever ask from us.

Until a drug exists that can wipe the entire tumor out, permanently, without cytoreduction, this is the treatment paradigm most likely to end in a good result for them. I personally am skeptical that any of the present adjuvant treatments being studied will be able to tackle the entire disease without surgical cytoreduction and think the eventual treatment outcomes for GBM will be the result of incremental improvements gained by the statistical improbability of a cancer cell evading a series of effective treatments. Surgery's role will be to drastically change that probability by providing a non-probabilistic treatment prior to exposing the cancer cells to your drug.

As well, the fear of surgery is usually grounded in the idea that you might make the patient worse, and that this risk is undertaken for an unclear benefit. I would answer that by pointing out that the belief in the idea that leaving a large cancer in the brain at initial diagnosis as a method for providing a good quality of life requires one to not remain in contact with these patients. Patients with tumors invading speech, motor, or other critical areas generally have a terrible quality of life, and controlling the tumor can preserve these functions. Many patients treated aggressively can remain neurologically normal with an excellent quality of life which lasts as long as tumor remains under control. Further, the worry about incurring neurologic risk has never slowed the development of skull base meningioma or acoustic neuroma surgery, two benign tumors for which the mandate to try to save the patient is nowhere near as acute. If we take glioma surgery as seriously as we take meningioma surgery, this risk inevitably falls, as any surgery done badly is dangerous and unwarranted. When you view the goal of surgery is the effort to save neurologic function that the tumor is trying to take, the justification for taking calculated risks is obvious.

1.4 The Foundations of this System and the Organization of this Book

I would propose that the gap between what can be achieved in glioma surgery with our existing knowledge, technology, and techniques, and the present way glioma surgery is frequently performed, is the recognition of some truths about infiltrating WHO grade II-IV gliomas (hereafter referred to as "gliomas"), and building from these truths towards a simple repeatable system for addressing these truths in an organized and systematic way. We will start by outlining these truths in the following paragraphs and providing the tools for dealing with them in the rest of the book.

1.5 The Hard Truths of Glioma Surgery

1.5.1 Gliomas Infiltrate and Mix with the Functional Brain

A look at histopathologic images of glioma specimens demonstrate that tumor cells grow between neurons.[6] While this feature is not uniformly present throughout the tumor, for example there are not viable neurons in the necrotic center of glioblastoma or in densely packed areas of tumor, until proven otherwise, it is best to assume that viable neurons are present in at least the boundary of the tumor, and often can be located throughout the tumor, especially in some types of low-grade tumors with a more infiltrative than proliferative phenotype.

Thus, it is important to recognize that in a glioma case, you are basically removing a large piece of brain.[6] The idea that you can "stay in the tumor," and avoid problems is generally misguided, and I have seen lead to avoidable problems and inadequate surgeries. While a highly dense area of tumor cells might displace functional brain, and be marginally "quiet," in general it's best to assume that there are probably neurons in the tissue you are removing and to adjust your thinking appropriately.

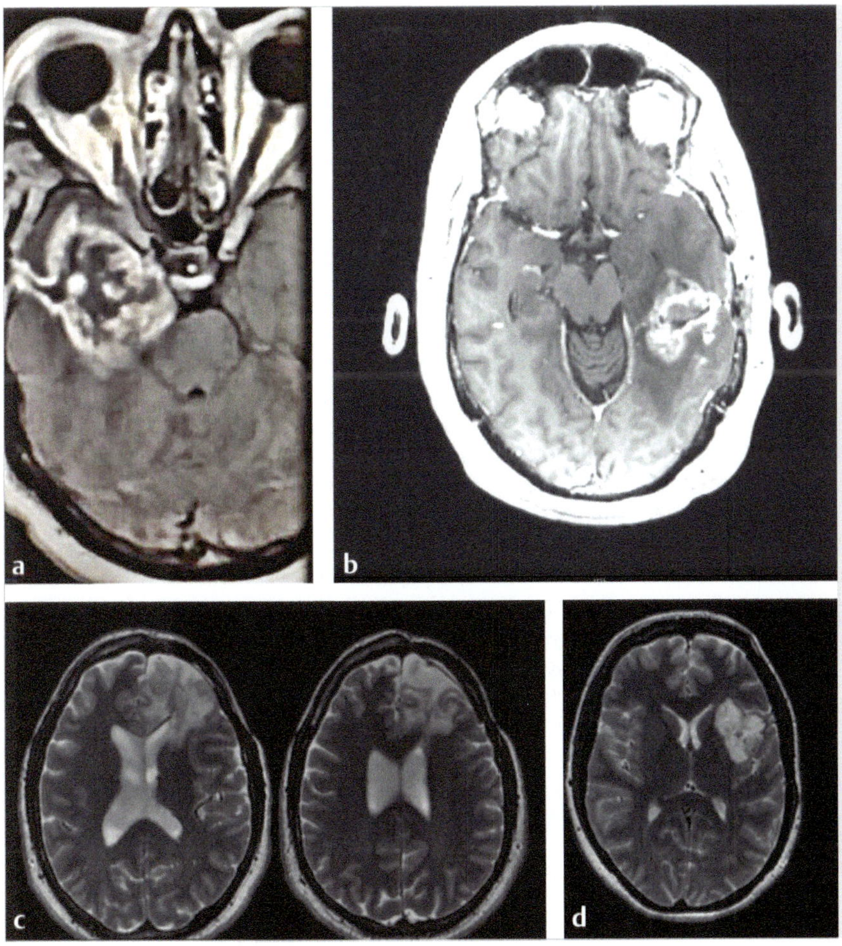

Fig. 1.1 (**a-d**) Four examples of inadequate glioma resections performed at respected academic neurosurgical centers. These are provided as proof that we still have much to improve upon with glioma operations.

1.5.2 The Tumor Has No Boundaries

The idea that you can remain "within the tumor" is further challenged by the well-known observation that these tumors have unclear boundaries (especially with low-grade tumors), with cells usually extending beyond the radiographic boundaries seen on the preoperative MRI.[7] In my experience, trying to stop when you stop seeing abnormal tissue is a recipe for disappointment when viewing your postoperative imaging.

When you remove a glioma, you are not removing a tumor, you are removing a province. By that, I mean that anatomic resection is the secret to technical excellence. For example, you can be certain there is not a residual tumor in the temporal tip in a temporal glioma case, when you continue the resection until you see an empty middle fossa and cleared tentorial edge.

1.5.3 The Brain Organization of Glioma Patients is Unpredictable

The degree of re-organization I personally have seen in glioma patients is sometimes astounding. I have found speech and semantic areas in entirely different gyri or even lobes. There are cases in this book where we were able to remove major parts of the motor and sensory strips as well as Broca's area without deficits. Additionally, major white matter tracts can often rewire to new brain areas. Usually, this is in the patient's favor, as function generally moves out of the tumor, but this is not always the case, and at a minimum, it takes a deep understanding of networks and a flexible interpretation of brain function to make sense of what you are finding.

The long and short is that no tumor or part of a tumor is operable or inoperable until you map it and see how the brain is organized.

1.5.4 The Anatomy is Unclear

Once you have cut the cortical surface, the subcortical brain is a big white blob with few landmarks, through which a patient's soul and cognition are running. Faced with such complexity, most neurosurgeons have resigned themselves either to doing surgery without paying a lot of attention to this or not going in there. I have heard many neurosurgeons claim at courses and meetings that the grey matter is what is important and that the white matter doesn't matter that much. The absurdity of that statement is clear when we note that these regions constitute the same neurons, and cutting them has similar consequences, and that is even ignoring many of the issues about which type of injury (white vs. grey matter) recovers better.

In short, this book is an effort to try to put landmarks and anatomy where previously we have not considered them. The extreme complexity of cerebral organization is not an excuse to ignore it on your way into the brain, especially as technology and neuroscience have progressed to where we can begin to ask and answer some of these questions and put an ordered view to what seems to be impenetrable complexity.

1.6 The Foundation of this Book and its System

This book is centered around the idea that 1) almost all glioma patients would be better off with less of the tumor if it was possible, even if that benefit is only a little, 2) almost all gliomas can be at least mostly or completely removed with acceptable results using awake mapping techniques centered around a more detailed understanding of brain networks and how they work. In other words, we should be taking these tumors out, and there is some method (which we may not yet know) by which any glioma can be removed, at least mostly, with a result that is acceptable given the patient's starting point.

This book is a summary of preliminary work towards making that second statement reality. At its core, it is an effort to provide a better understanding of the cerebrum and how it works, specifically from the standpoint of surgical anatomy. It is based on the idea that we can work out a basic set of macro-connectomic networks that explain the core essential aspects of how higher brain functions work and to perform surgery that minimizes the damage to these networks while optimizing tumor resection. These are the essential truths of glioma surgery which will continue to be true even if robotic or laser surgery begins to displace traditional surgical techniques.

At its periphery, it is a summary of many years of my experience working in such a paradigm where I have offered surgery (which is usually accepted) to all patients with glioma regardless of location, and have performed awake surgery for gliomas in unconventional locations such as the thalamus, the corpus callosum, and the right frontal lobe, among others, with the goal of preserving functions beyond speech and motor (the traditional intraoperative brain mapping functions). This has led to a personal experience with over 600 awake-brain surgeries at the time of this writing. Many of these observations can only be the result of mistakes, or challenges, and the aim is to provide insight into what is possible, and what is ill advised. In all likelihood, much of this information will be obsolete in the future (similar to pictures of brain surgery done with fingers in classical neurosurgery texts); however, even technically obsolete work carries foundational truths and ways of thinking that outlive their application. Note all the people who still read and find insights from Cushing's meningioma text, well after meningioma surgery has radically changed to its present form.

References

[1] Han SJ, Sughrue ME. The rise and fall of "biopsy and radiate": a history of surgical nihilism in glioma treatment. Neurosurg Clin N Am. 2012; 23(2):207–214, vii

[2] Capelle L, Fontaine D, Mandonnet E, et al. French Réseau d'Étude des Gliomes. Spontaneous and therapeutic prognostic factors in adult hemispheric World Health Organization Grade II gliomas: a series of 1097 cases: clinical article. J Neurosurg. 2013; 118(6):1157–1168

[3] Jakola AS, Myrmel KS, Kloster R, et al. Comparison of a strategy favoring early surgical resection vs a strategy favoring watchful waiting in low-grade gliomas. JAMA. 2012; 308(18):1881–1888

[4] Keles GE, Lamborn KR, Berger MS. Low-grade hemispheric gliomas in adults: a critical review of extent of resection as a factor influencing outcome. J Neurosurg. 2001; 95(5):735–745

[5] Smith JS, Chang EF, Lamborn KR, et al. Role of extent of resection in the long-term outcome of low-grade hemispheric gliomas. J Clin Oncol. 2008; 26 (8):1338–1345

[6] Acioly MA, Cunha AM, Parise M, Rodrigues E, Tovar-Moll F. Recruitment of Contralateral Supplementary Motor Area in Functional Recovery Following Medial Frontal Lobe Surgery: An fMRI Case Study. J Neurol Surg A Cent Eur Neurosurg. 2015; 76(6):508–512

[7] Kelly PJ, Daumas-Duport C, Kispert DB, Kall BA, Scheithauer BW, Illig JJ. Imaging-based stereotaxic serial biopsies in untreated intracranial glial neoplasms. J Neurosurg. 1987; 66(6):865–874

2 Sughrue's Three Laws of Glioma Surgery

2.1 Introduction

Giving a set of principles an eponymous name named after yourself is fraught with danger as inevitably someone will point out that you are not the first person to note this (usually claiming that they noted it a long time ago or that this is an obvious point). I am doing it anyway, despite knowing that almost certainly many others have noted these things for the sole reason I have never heard anyone point out these issues in a clearer way prior to my own observations, and plus giving principles a name like this makes the idea memorable.

Sughrue's three laws are based on principles which I teach my trainees that I have repeatedly found to be true statements in our quest to aggressively remove gliomas while avoiding complications. More accurately, I have found that the violation of these rules repeatedly has been the root cause of my disappointing outcomes. Thus, knowing the three laws does not make one a great glioma surgeon, but sticking to these rules will reduce one's failure rate substantially.

2.2 Sughrue's First Law

2.2.1 Never Take an Artery Unless You Are Certain Where It's Going and That Place is about to Become a Big Hole

Time and time again during my learning curve, I have been taught this lesson, as it is the bus taking you to the school of hard knocks. Arterial injuries are front and center of many of the most epic failures in glioma surgery, as injury to even a small artery in the wrong location can lead to a disastrous result and undo hours of careful work, or lose the battle before you have really started. In fact, I have come to believe that no matter how the initial outcome is, that most things will ultimately be ok if the postoperative DWI scan shows no infarcts.

Why are arterial injuries so bad? In addition to the injury of both white and grey matter, an additional explanation is that they damage a much bigger area of the brain than you can possibly injure with suction in the same amount of time (▶ Fig. 2.1). As a thought experiment, consider the amount of time needed to remove the entire putamen with suction versus the amount of time needed to bipolar a lenticulostriate artery closed. Simply put, injuring an artery is a much faster way to damage more brain than the patient can compensate, and thus it can happen before you know it. You have a lot more time to realize your angle is off and you are in a bad area when direct damage is the mechanism of injury.

In addition, by damaging a large area of the brain, you have destroyed the soil for future reorganization and recovery. A way I explain this concept to patients is that if the cable line is cut to your house, you can watch TV at a neighbor's house given enough time to walk over there; however, if someone nukes the whole neighborhood, then TV watching is unlikely to happen anywhere.

What about venous injury? Well, it is never worth destroying anatomy for no reason, the risk of venous sacrifice and its relation to venous infarction has been greatly overstated in our literature in my opinion. With the exception of the midline bridging veins near the superior sagittal sinus, I have yet to see anything resembling a venous ischemic event in a case not involving a fixed blade brain retractor, and I personally ceased dealing with these complications when I ceased using retractors. The need to use brain retractors in any situation in glioma surgery is unclear to me, so while preserving veins is probably a good way to reduce the risk of postoperative hydrocephalus, I do not think that people should fear that taking a vein will lead to disastrous outcomes as I have not found this to be true. Remember that the veins most at risk in glioma surgery are the ones draining the brain which is being removed. For example, you do not need the Vein of Labbe if the temporal lobe is being removed.

One might take the above discussion to mean that in order to save brain arteries we should stay as far from them as possible, but this is not a realistic approach in most cases. Removing a glioma means removing a part of the brain, and some arteries will have to be sacrificed selectively, and thus dealing with the arteries appropriately is inevitably a part of technically excellent glioma surgery. Instead, I advocate a strategy which goes right at the arteries and actively finds them and separates them from the tumor as early as reasonably possible. Again this doesn't mean we should go after all arteries, as some, like the lenticulostriates are best left alone; but it instead means that a cowardly approach is usually a bad one which either leaves an untenable amount of tumor, or just sucks out tumor slowly and hopes for the best (i.e., that they won't be injured).

2.2.2 How to Deal with the Involved Arteries

Method One: Avoid Injuring Them

This is an obvious piece of advice, which is harder to execute in practice. The easiest arterial hole to repair is the one you don't create. Bleeding is inevitable in glioma cases, as is the need to stop bleeding numerous times during the case. I suspect that many surgeons probably aren't aware at the time that the bleeding they are stopping is from a critical artery as they are doing it. Thus it may not dawn on many people why they got a bad outcome from a particular case, especially if the infarct is relatively small (but critically located).

While it is possible to perform glioma surgery without a microscope, it is also possible to perform it with the naked eye, and there is essentially no way in which it is better to have less light and magnification. Many neurosurgeons believed in the past that loupes and a headlight were adequate visualization for pineal and aneurysm surgery, an idea which has since generally been dismissed as substandard practice. Today, the same arguments are still put forward for glioma surgery as if they are valid, namely that there is no anatomy to see in these cases. Yet when Drake brought the microscope into his basilar apex aneurysm surgeries, he suddenly saw the perforators and preserved them, making an inoperable problem treatable. It is amazing to me that people maintain the cognitively dissonant argument that certain gliomas are "inoperable" yet you don't need to see any specific details like small vessels and subtle sulcal borders, which allow many of these tumors to be removed. It is shocking that we cling to 19th century technology so tightly.

I do not allow my residents to use loupes in these cases, as I believe that the use of loupes to remove a glioma encourages surgeons to attempt things that they would do better with better visualization and light provided by a microscope (or other similar visualization tools), and provides this confidence in the absence of being able to see the critical arterial anatomy (or basal ganglia anatomy, or sulcal anatomy, etc.) that could doom the case if you are not aware of it. Thus, while people can do glioma surgery without the microscope, I have yet to hear a coherent reason how it is better done with loupes, or how a microscope make the surgery worse. If it were your brain, you would probably want your surgeon to have the best available visualization, and that most certainly is not loupe based technology.

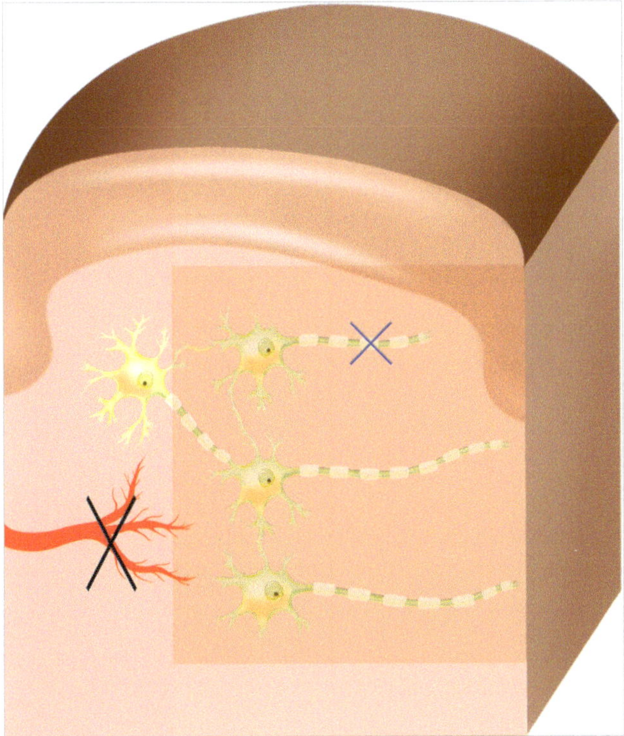

Fig. 2.1 Artistic schematic demonstrating the relative damage caused by a pure injury to a part of the brain versus an injury to an artery. Note that the injury to the brain only disconnected and injures the brain immediately in the area, while the artery injury can damage areas quite far from the area where it occurs, and is thus more extensive.

For similar reasons, I do not use ultrasonic aspirators in these cases. Beyond just cost considerations, these devices were not developed for intra-axial brain tumor surgery, and it is exceedingly rare that these tumors have a fibrous character where a powered aspiration device is really necessary. Some have argued that it is faster to use an ultrasonic aspirator, and I would counter that an osteotome and mallet would also speed up the resection; however, neither approach, in my opinion, is appropriately delicate enough for intraaxial brain surgery. The reason why conventional suction is generally safer, in my opinion, than ultrasonic aspirators, is that while both devices can and will put holes in arteries, I have found that conventional suction leaves holes which are smaller and easier to seal with bipolar spot welding techniques (described below) or other methods which preserve artery patency. I think this is because usually, the hole comes from the avulsion of a small side branching artery, which is manageable. Aspirator holes are often larger and harder to fix without occluding the artery (▶ Fig. 2.2). Of course, with loupes, you may not really see any of these differences.

Method Two: Know the Vessel Anatomy and Work It into Your Planning

As stated above, you have to sacrifice some arteries to remove a glioma as you are removing a piece of the brain. However, it is

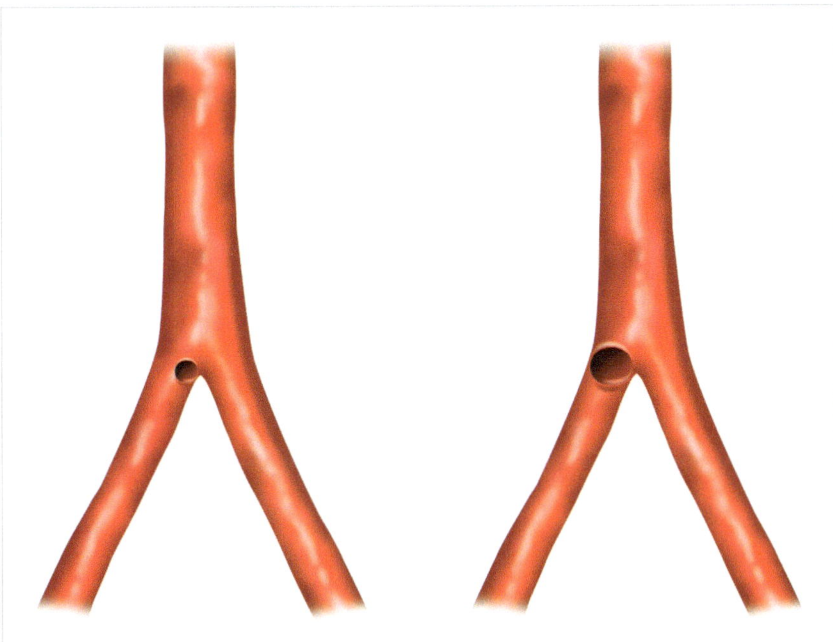

Fig. 2.2 Artistic schematic demonstrating the relative difference between the typical extent of artery injuries caused by ultrasonic aspirators versus those caused by conventional suction. While both devices can injure arteries, in my experience suctions can partially avulse small branches, or tear branch points, which can be fixed, often preserving the parent artery, while ultrasonic aspirators often leave larger holes which cannot be fixed.

always best to delay this sacrifice until you are certain of the vessels identity as a vessel supplying soon to be removed brain. You want to avoid sacrificing an artery that is supplying an important part of the brain beyond what you plan to remove. However, as you gain experience, it becomes easier to recognize which vessels pose some risk for being an en passage artery, meaning it is supplying brain which you do not plan to remove, and which ones almost certainly are not going to a different part of the brain. It speeds up the resection significantly when you do not fixate on the identity of anterior temporal MCA branches when the plan is for temporal lobectomy. It is more important when you realize you are dealing with an en passage situation ahead of time, and behave appropriately.

Common En Passage Situations (▶ Fig. 2.3)

Midline frontal lobe: As the resection proceeds inwards towards the cingulate gyrus and corpus callosum, you begin to encounter more ACA branches, eventually reaching the ACA trunk. It is impossible the remove the corpus callosum, cingulate gyrus, or midline frontal lobe without addressing these branches safely. The majority of these branches are internal frontal branches, which are supplying the brain which you are going to remove; however, there are critical en passage branches, namely the callosomarginal artery, which are feeding the motor strip and SMA regions among others, which much be preserved. Here, it is critical to follow the rule that you should follow an artery to its target before taking it.

Frontal or parietal operculum: Removing an opercular tumor successfully is synonymous with safely working around the en passage arteries exiting the Sylvian fissure.

Insula: Accessing the insula requires working past the MCA branches which overlie it. Thus, most of the large arteries encountered are en passage arteries. Sacrificing the circumflex branches which supply the insula is critical for preserving the integrity of the numerous en passage vessels at risk in these cases.

Back of the Sylvian fissure: Dealing with tumors involving the supramarginal gyrus or superior temporal gyrus brings you to critical en passage arteries, including the branch I call the artery of death (described below).

Medial temporal lobe: Removing the uncus or parahippocampal gyrus puts arteries such as the anterior choroidal and PCA at risk, as they are supply blood to structures beyond the resection boundaries.

Arteries generally not en passage: 1) Vessels at the anterior temporal pole during temporal lobectomy, 2) Vessels at the anterior frontal pole during frontal lobectomy, 3) Vessels in the middle frontal gyrus (you are at the end artery by then), 4) Vessels at the occipitotemporal junction (you are at the end artery by then), 5) Vessels encountered in the medial parietal lobe (those vessels supply local brain), 6) PCA branches during an occipital lobectomy.

This list is not exhaustive and other situations can occur. The key is to always look at the T2 images ahead of time (▶ Fig. 2.4) and get a sense of where the en passage arteries are in relation to the tumor. There are numerous ways to address these arteries and to get them out of the tumor, or at least not injure them. Removing brain in a subpial manner keeps a boundary which helps you identify the vessel and save it. Certainly, this is the standard method for complication avoidance in the medial temporal lobe. Additionally, while it is usually necessary to provide some counter traction to remove a tumor, knowing that an en passage artery is there probably should change your willingness to be aggressive in an area. In more difficult situations, such as high-grade glioma caked on the vessel, meningioma type surgical techniques, such as finding the vessel with a Doppler and serially dividing tumor next to the vessel may be necessary. In rare situations, it may be impossible to get the vessel out of the tumor with any technique.

Method 3: Avoid Manipulating High-Risk Arteries

Technically any artery can enter vasospasm, dissect, or tear when you manipulate it surgically; however, experience (my own and numerous other surgeons) has taught us that certain

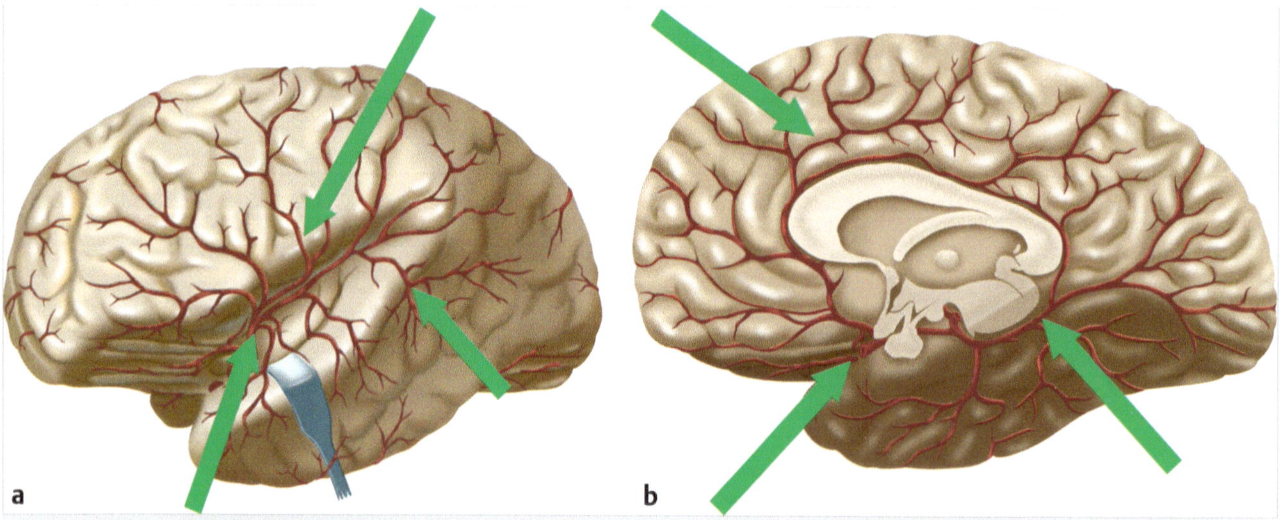

Fig. 2.3 Artistic depiction of en passage arteries commonly involved in glioma operations. Common sites include the ACA branches in the frontal midline, the anterior choroidal and PCA near the uncus, the frontal operculum, the back of the Sylvian fissure, and the insula. Note that this is not an exhaustive list, but demonstrates the arteries I am most often concerned about.

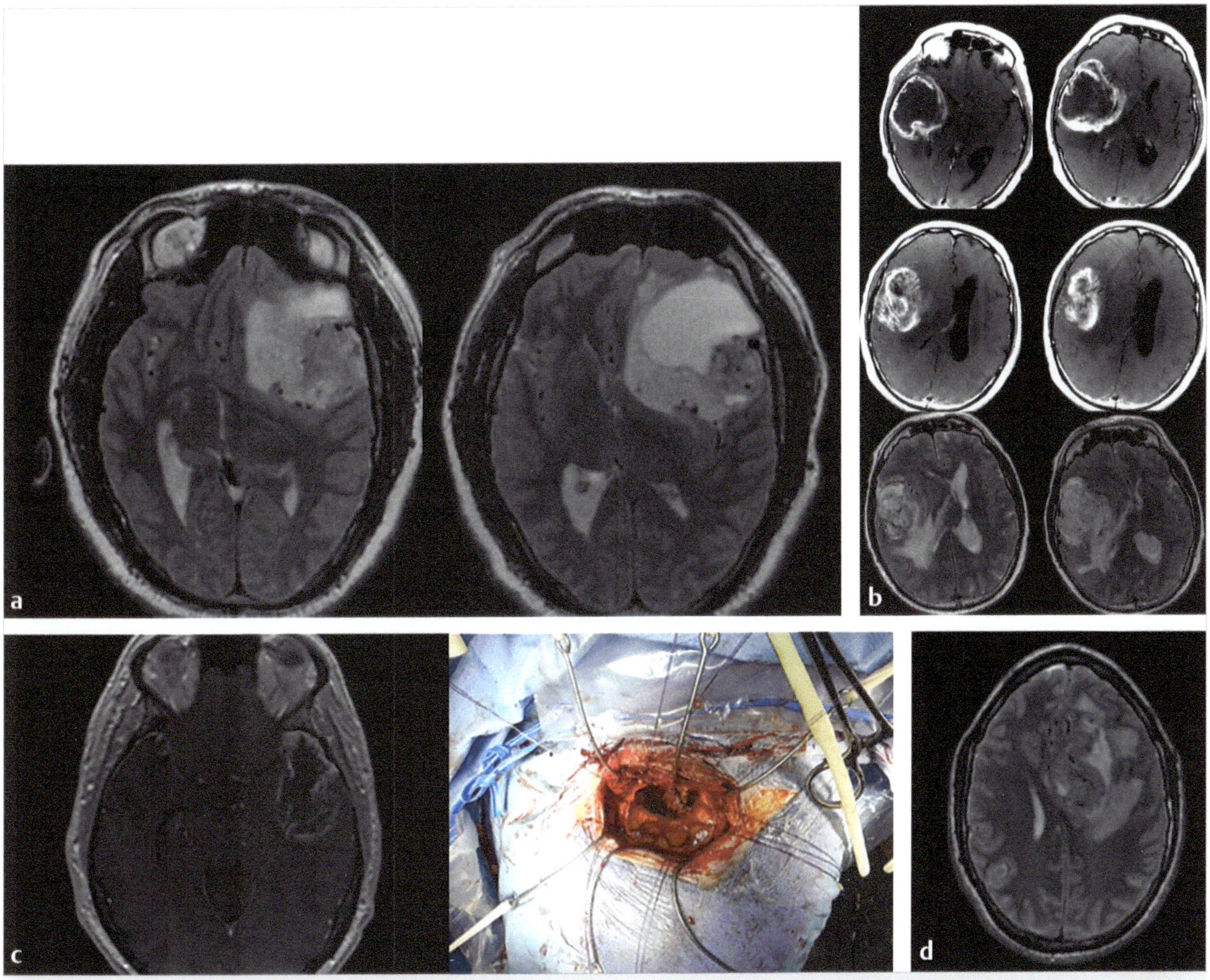

Fig. 2.4 MRI images of arteries encased in gliomas: (a) T2 images of this GBM demonstrate the trunks and branches of the MCA which are clearly in the tumor in multiple places. (b) T1 post-contrast and T2 images of a temporal perisylvian GBM also encasing numerous MCA branches. (c) This is an intraoperative photo following resection of the GBM in the corresponding MRI. You can see tumor was densely caked on the MCA and needed to be left behind. (d) This midline GBM has encased multiple ACA branches.

arteries are far more likely to cause disaster than others. In these cases, it is generally wise to leave these arteries alone, or at least to handle them with great care.

Lenticulostriate arteries (▶ Fig. 2.5): These small branches of the proximal MCA supply critical structures such as the basal ganglia and internal capsule. Numerous surgeons have found that these arteries are particularly prone to cause a stroke when we try to remove tumor from them. Also, if you are encountering them in a glioma surgery, then there is a high chance you are in the basal ganglia, which seldom has a tumor in it, in my experience. As I emphasize at numerous points in this book, basal ganglia tissue looks and feels like glioma, and it is easy to continue into it unless you are always vigilant with considering the possibility that what looks like tumor may be basal ganglia. Thus, if you are seeing lenticulostriate arteries, you probably should rethink what you are doing there.

Anterior choroidal artery (▶ Fig. 2.6): This tiny artery runs on the medial surface of the uncus and can undo an otherwise excellent resection of the temporal lobe by causing permanent injury to the internal capsule. Subpialization of the medial temporal structures is critical to avoid this, but if the pia is disrupted, then you should strongly consider stopping, especially with high grade gliomas and especially if the patient has previously had radiotherapy.

Optic nerve vasculature: This issue is seldom encountered in glioma surgery, but I have seen it occur a few times, and have seen surgeons get into trouble with optic nerve vascular injury in glioma cases. In short, the optic nerve has a tenuous blood supply, and loss of this blood supply can cause blindness. Avoid cautery when working on the posterior inferior frontal lobe, even when working subpially, as this can conduct through to the optic nerve and injury its blood supply.

"Artery of death" (▶ Fig. 2.7): This is my name for the posterior temporal branch exiting the back of the Sylvian fissure and supplying the posterior temporal lobe. I have been haunted by this artery many times, notably by its ability to occlude or spasm right in front of me from even minimal manipulation. While it is always bad to occlude this artery, in speech mapping cases,

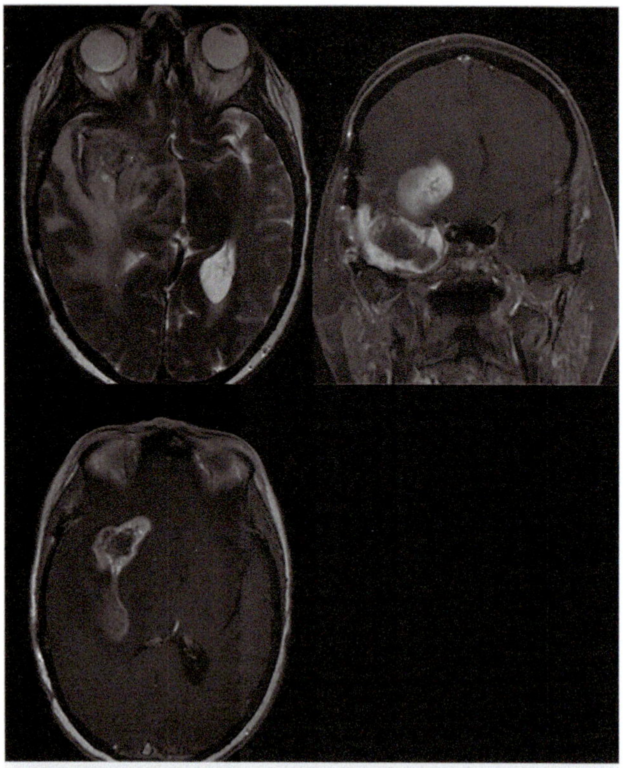

Fig. 2.5 Three views of a recurrent GBM which involves the lenticulostriate arteries. The T2 images show tumor directly posterosuperior to the M1 segment, and these small arteries running through it. It is wise to not attempt to remove this part of the tumor.

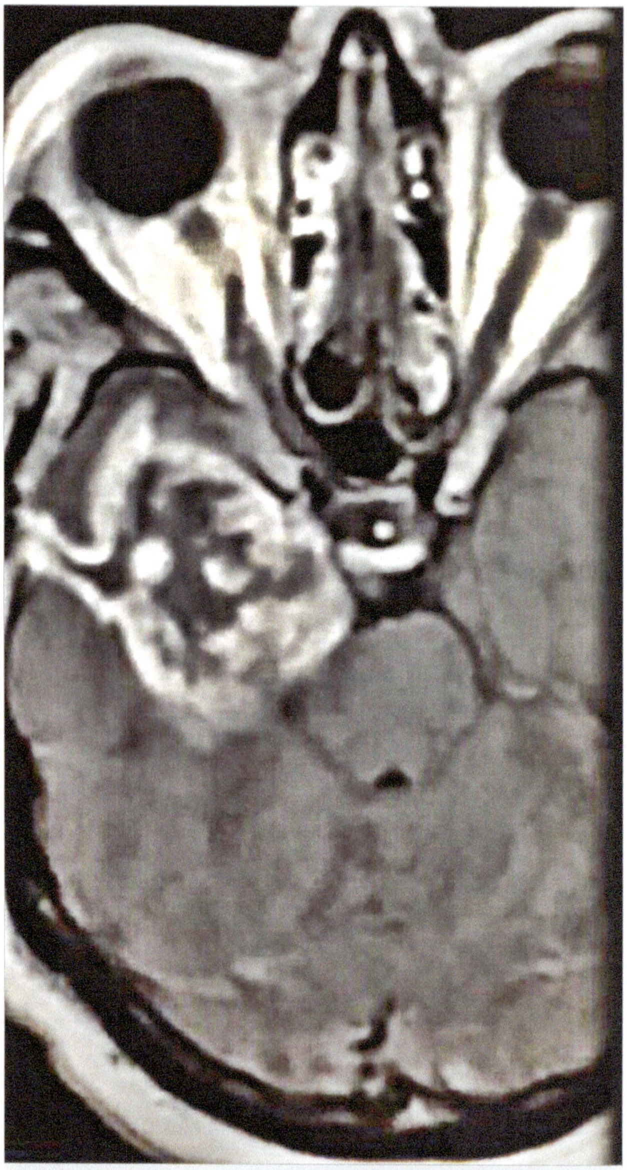

Fig. 2.6 This image demonstrates a GBM which has massively expanded the uncus, putting the anterior choroidal artery at risk.

particularly on the left side, the infarct can densely involve the language areas and end the mapping before you have really got a chance to get started. I have seen this infarct end in ultimately in good long term speech recovery, but presently do everything in my power to touch this artery as little as possible.

Method 4: Minimize Risk in High-Risk Situations

While a vessel can be injured in any situation where you are operating near it, there are situations that are predictably higher risk than others, and which should change your threshold for when to stop trying to get that part of the tumor out.

High-grade glioma that is encasing arteries: It is possible to safely remove high-grade glioma from arteries in most cases; however, these tumors are capable of invading arterial adventitia or at least being firmly adherent to them. Thus, removing the tumor in some situation can seriously damage these arteries, and force you to try to seal the hole in the middle of a bleeding tumor mass, which is difficult and dangerous. Interestingly, these tumors are particularly adherent in areas of necrosis, so care with peeling necrosis material off of arteries is strongly advised, especially given the relatively small benefit gained by removing dead tumor tissue.

Tumor in the Sylvian fissure: As noted previously, removing tumors which straddle the Sylvian fissure involves risk to the en passage branches of the MCA (▶ Fig. 2.4). In their worst form, high-grade gliomas can invade MCA branches or even the M1. You need to approach these cases ready for a battle, one that you may need to retreat from.

Tumors enlarging the uncus: This radiographic finding (▶ Fig. 2.6) puts numerous vessels at risk, but most critically the anterior choroidal artery. This is especially true for recurrent high- grade gliomas where the pia doesn't necessarily need to be disrupted for the artery to lose patency, sometimes in a delayed fashion. I have learned from experience to be very cautious in this situations, and will only attempt complete removal of the uncus when it is clearly easy.

Post-radiation cases: Radiotherapy weakens vascular walls and makes them more prone to surgical injury. In some cases, vessels encased in tumor rely on the tumor for support of their damaged wall and trying to get tumor off it, particularly fibrous tumor, can leave you with a defective vessel wall which is difficult or impossible to repair. Radiotherapy is not a contraindication for trying to get tumor off arteries, but it certainly makes me think twice.

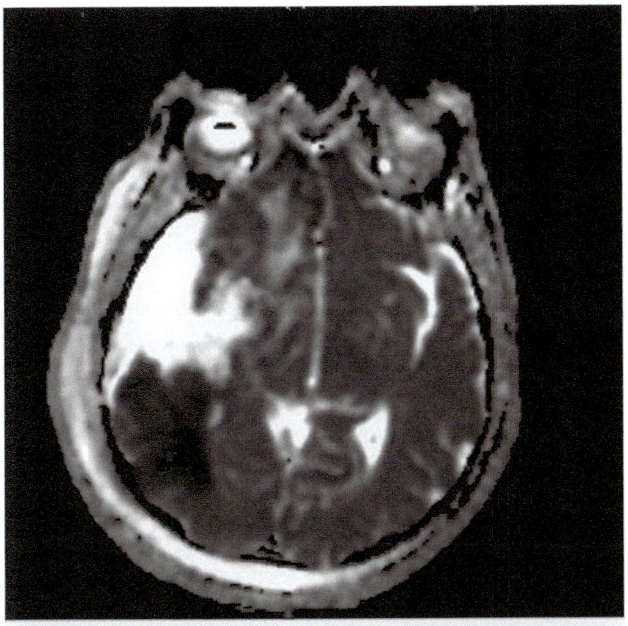

Fig. 2.7 This post-op ADC image demonstrates the infarct pattern caused by manipulation of the "artery of death" (aka the posterior temporal branch of the MCA). This infarct pattern extensively injures the posterior temporal lobe, damaging much of the semantic network, which especially on the left, can be devastating.

Method 5: Stop Bleeding Responsibly

If done correctly, stopping bleeding in gliomas often takes as long as the resection, and in many ways, stopping bleeding in a way which maintains blood flow to critical areas is as important to the long-term outcome of the case as competently mapping the brain. Unlike meningiomas, there is no way to finish off the tumor's blood supply to eliminate the bleeding, and you can expect that the resection cavity in a glioma case will take much longer to obtain hemostasis in compared to most other tumor cases as there is always some residual tumor at the edge (or at least hypervascular brain)

Even if you are an excellent glioma surgeon, you are going to encounter bleeding during tumor removal, often substantial, and if you are overly concerned with this then you will make decisions that are ultimately not in anyone's best interest. I have met many surgeons who are so afraid of a small amount of bleeding that they defeat themselves to not see red. It's important to develop a Zen attitude towards bleeding, and instead of trying to make the field always look perfect at all points of the case, aim for making the end result perfect. In other words, if you stop to address every bleeder, you are doing it wrong, and if your surgical field looks like the battle of Stalingrad you are also doing it wrong. It is very unlikely anyone is going to die in the hands of a competent anesthesiologist from glioma grade bleeding. Remember that most anesthesiologists are trained to manage aortic injury level bleeding and neurosurgical bleeding below the caliber of the internal carotid or vertebral artery rarely approaches this. Thus, if your bipolar device never shuts off during the case because you are trying to stop every bleeder as you go, then you are really doing it wrong,

Responsible hemostasis involves maintaining a field where you can still see what you are doing, but at the same time acknowledging that the only necessary time to have a perfectly dry field is when it is time to close the dura, but that it is always necessary to maintain blood flow to parts of the brain you wish to remain working after you leave the OR.

Techniques for Responsible Hemostasis

Technique 1: Pack off bleeding areas until you can see them clearly

One of the most important pieces of advice I was ever given is to let things bleed until you have enough exposure to see what you are cauterizing and have a clear plan how to stop it. This is especially true with the Sylvian fissure, where you can expect to have at least one arterial bleeder in every insular glioma case, but it is true in most cases. Not all of these need to be stopped with bipolar cautery, as many of them, and most venous bleeding will stop by simply packing the area off with a hemostatic material (I am a big fan of Nu-Knit personally) and working somewhere else. This is especially true when making the division cut (explained at length in the rest of the book) during brain mapping, during which we are working (and thus causing bleeding) usually in a deep hole, and the patient has a fixed time period where they will cooperate with the mapping. It's often best to come back to the work of hemostasis later when your view of the area will be better (as a part of the brain has been removed), and you will have a better idea what vessels you are hemostasis and where it needs to be stopped. You may also find it has stopped and you need to do nothing at all. Probably the best hemostatic method in glioma surgery is taking the tumor out and I repeat to my trainees that there is no glory in hemostasing tumor.

The wrong approach is to fire up the bipolar and burn everything as you go, as you may end up finding out later that this was not what you wanted to do. Another wrong approach is to let blood pool up from multiple areas making the whole field unworkable.

Technique 2: Spot-welding arteries

In some cases, you will have to get an artery to stop bleeding. It is always necessary to have enough of the artery visualized to see what you are doing, so if this is not completely possible at the stage of the operation when the bleeding starts, you should pack it off and come back to it after enough dissection allows you to see it.

Before cauterizing an artery, it is important to get a mental plan of what probably needs to happen. This plan involves thinking importantly about what artery you are probably dealing with and how this artery is likely running in three-dimensional space. In an ideal world, you will be able to trace the artery to its target and confirm its identity, but this is not always possible, and in most cases, it's best to assume that an artery is important until proven otherwise. When this is not possible, sometimes a brief thought about the situation leads you to realize that the bleeding artery is almost certainly supplying brain which is going to be removed (for example a vessel at the frontal pole during a frontal lobectomy), and this insight can free you up to aggressively sacrifice the artery and move on.

If you need to stop bleeding from an artery which you cannot sacrifice, or when you aren't sure yet, spot-welding the artery is

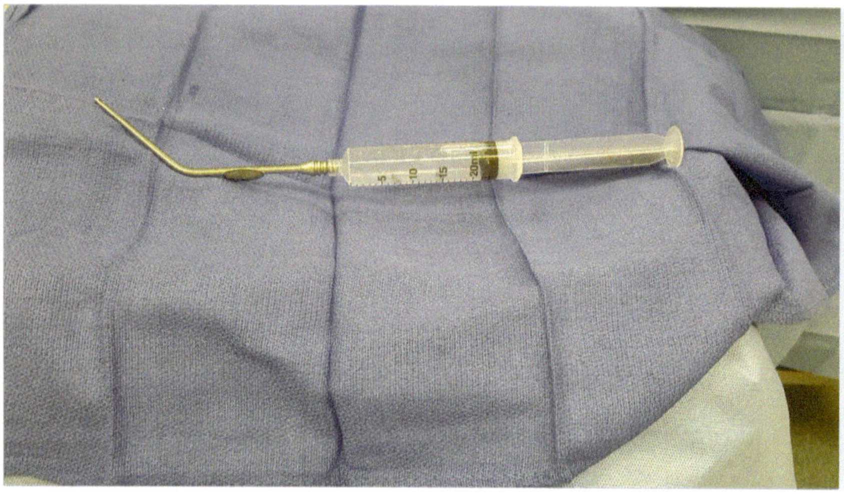

Fig. 2.8 This picture depicts the most helpful micro-irrigation device that I have encountered to date. By putting a suction device on a syringe (with the thumb hole covered), you can retract and irrigate at the same time, which significantly improves your ability to find bleeding sources.

a technique which allows you to get primary hemostasis and usually maintain the patency of medium to large arteries by fusing the arterial wall closed with a small tined bipolar applied to a small diameter of the wall. Admittedly, while smaller arteries can be spot-welded as well, they cannot be as reliably saved, and given the risk with some of these smaller arteries, then it is usually better to avoid these situations. I am aware that some people are capable of primarily repairing these vessels, and I wish them the best of luck with their efforts to repair small MCA branches caked in glioma. Personally, I have found spot-welding to be a reliable method which is quick and highly effective in my hands.

The first step in spot-welding an artery is to clearly visualize the hole and know its relationship to the rest of the artery. Irrigation is critical, and I have found a long, rigid irrigation device (I use a micro suction attached to a syringe with bone wax over the hole) to be far superior to simply irrigating externally with an angiocath (or other similar setups) in terms of allowing me to retract other structures out of the way and use my irrigating device as a search device (▸ Fig. 2.8). Also, it is very important to let the bleeding occur so you can see for certain where it is coming from. This means removing packing, which may be allowing blood to ooze around it which obscuring the hole. It may also mean removing some tumor which is in the way. Once you approach the hole, a good rule of thumb I have been told for where you place your suction is wherever it catches about 95% of the blood, as this allows you enough blood clearance to see what you are doing without the suction tip completely blocking the hole (▸ Fig. 2.9).

Arteries can be injured in countless ways, but in general, the overwhelming majority of holes created by conventional suction, bipolar tines, or microdissectors come in two forms depicted in ▸ Fig. 2.10. The first, and more common involves the partial or complete avulsion of a small, weak side branch off the main trunk. The solution here is to grab a small amount of adventitia from both sides of the hole and pinch them together until the bleeding stops and the artery looks patent. This may require a few adjustments until you get it right, at which point a 1 sec cautery burst usually will seal the artery. The second form involves a tear at a symmetric division of two arteries of equal size and is trickier to deal with, as you will need to maintain patency of both vessels, one of which is usually partially torn at its origin at the axilla of the bifurcation. I have found that by using the bipolars to bunch up some tissue from the axilla of the bifurcation onto the hole, I can often get this to fuse to the hole and not shrink the lumen of the vessels. Obviously, none of this is possible without the microscope.

I keep gel foam squares soaked in an anti-spasm agent (presently I use verapamil) on the field and apply this to the vessel immediately following any significant degree of manipulation. I probably do this 10 times per case. I am not certain this works, but I believe it does because I have seen arteries spasm and unspasm in front of me until the microscope with verapamil, and I cannot see how doing this is harmful.

Technique 3: Muscle

Some holes are too large to fix with spot-welding and occur in vessels which cannot be sacrificed. Often placing some hemostatic material to be left in is enough to wall off the artery, as it's hard to compress an artery until it closes off. Be careful when declaring an artery stopped by this method, as it is possible to wall off an artery where you do not see the blood collecting because it is bleeding into an unseen space. However, most of the time if it looks stopped, it is ok to assume it is.

In rare cases, a critical artery cannot be spot-welded, and is bleeding too much to be packed with Surgicel or Nu-Knit to achieve an acceptable seal which the patient can be sent out of OR with. When all else fails, a small piece of temporalis muscle harvested, gently crushed (to concentrate tissue factors to promote hemostasis), and held over an artery for about 8 minutes is capable of achieving a seal on a large hole in the internal carotid or vertebral artery while maintaining patency. So, there is always a way to save the vessel.

Method 6: Keep the Blood Pressure Up

As a trainee, I was taught that post-operative tumor craniotomies needed to have normal range blood pressure to prevent post-operative cavity hemorrhages. Experience has taught me that within some limits, an elevated blood pressure is good for the first 24–48 hours. We routinely keep the MAP above 90 mmHg, even tolerating some systolic hypertension, in patients who have required more than trivial work on arteries to remove the tumor, and subjectively I have seen this improve neurologic function in some patients as we are driving the

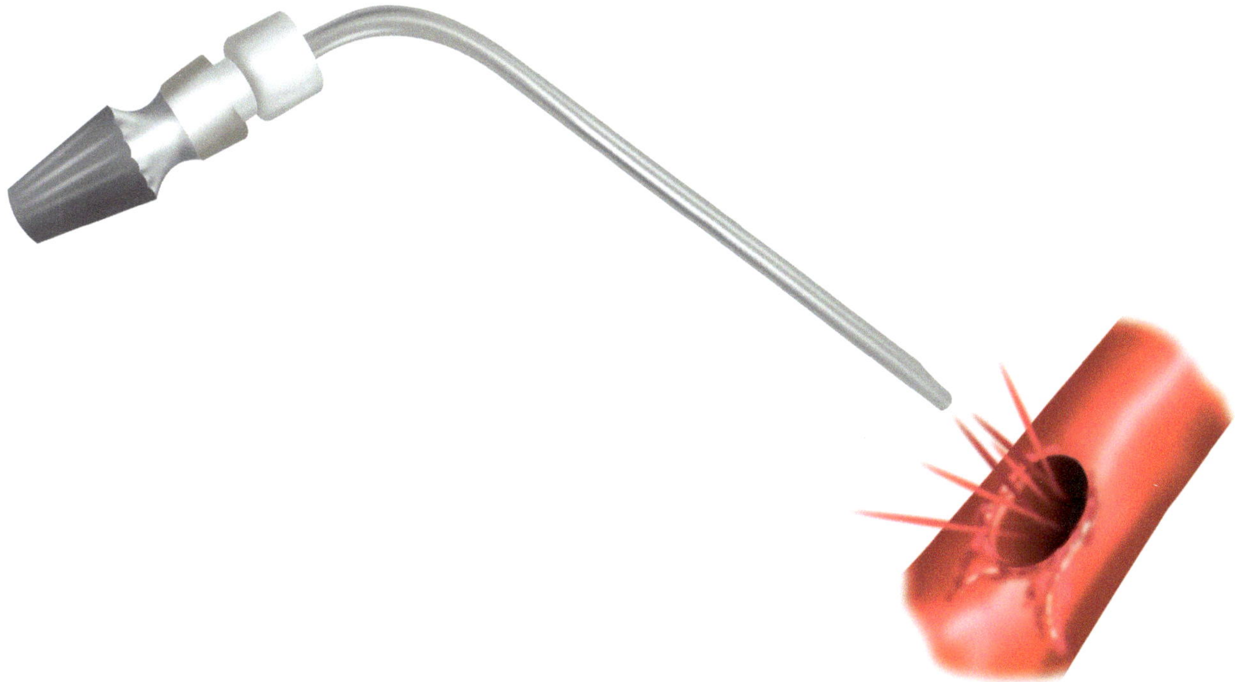

Fig. 2.9 This schematic demonstrates the proper position for placing a suction when attempting to find a bleeding source. The instinct of a beginner is to try to get the suction over the hole in the artery so the bleeding stops; however, this technique is incorrect, because it obscures the site of the hole. The correct method is to hover over the hole so that ~90% of the bleeding is captured, but that enough of a stream remains visible so that the hole can be identified.

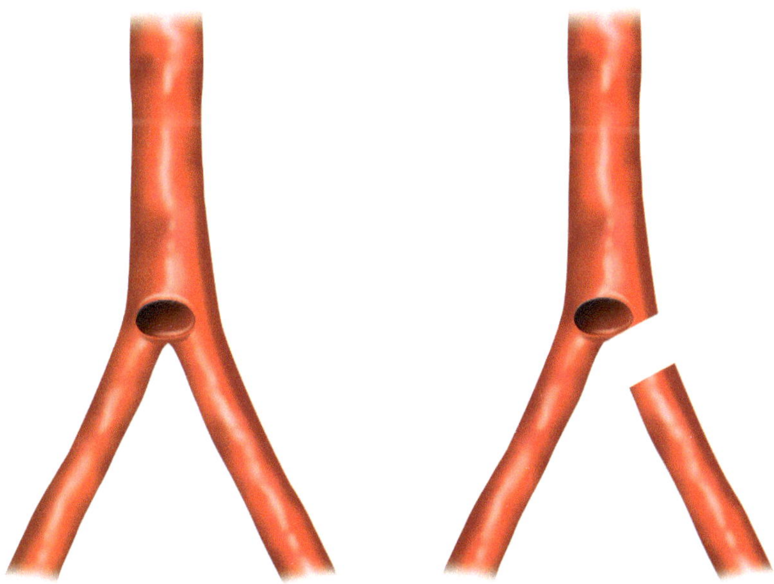

Fig. 2.10 Schematic demonstrating the two most patterns of holes in arteries. One form involves a tear at an arterial bifurcation, with the blood leaking from a tear at the axilla of this bifurcation. The other involves a partial or complete avulsion of a small branch off the main trunk of a larger artery. Obviously, the latter injury is harder to fix.

pressure upward. While this does not mean we drive systolic pressures over 220 mmHg, I do believe that some hypertension is a good thing, and can maintain vessel patency, minimize vasospasm, and maintain some marginally ischemic brain until collaterals can form. Obviously, this is a hard fact to prove, yet I have never had a resection cavity hemorrhage from hypertension from doing this, so I currently believe aggressive maintenance of normal tension is unnecessary.

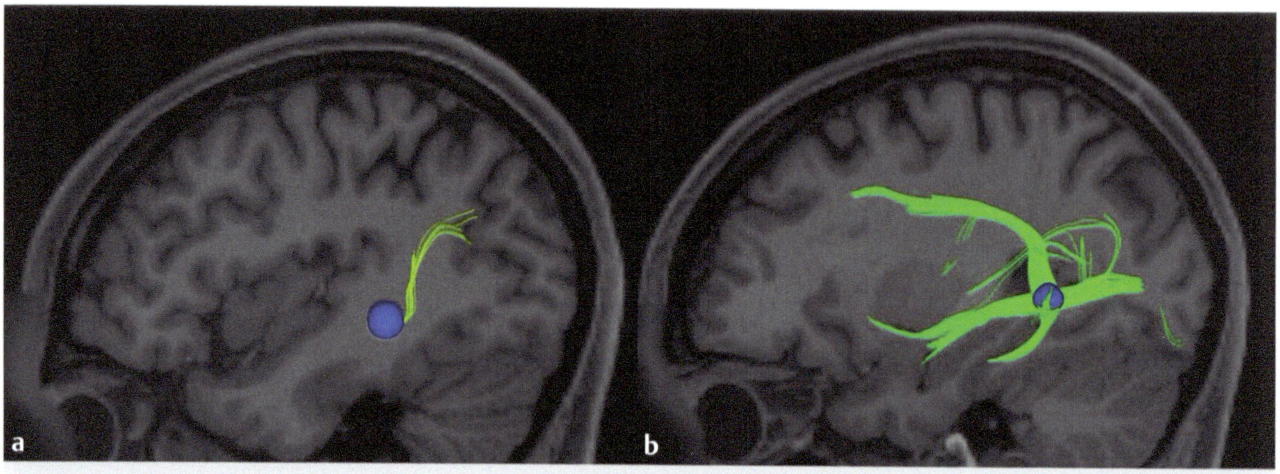

Fig. 2.11 These two DSI images compare of the extent of disconnection caused by similarly sized lesions in the (**a**) posterolateral temporal cortex versus (**b**) in the white matter deep to the same gyrus. Note much more extensive areas affected by the white matter lesion.

2.3 Sughrue's Second Law

2.3.1 If You Respect the Patient, Respect their White Matter

This section will be relatively shorter than the previous discussion about the first law and arteries: White matter anatomy and its preservation is the topic of much of the rest of the book, and this chapter will just introduce some key points which the later chapters will obsess over at length.

For a long time, neurosurgeons ignored white matter anatomy or at least viewed it as an esoteric topic. Most still do. Cortical anatomy has been taught to us as the defining principle underlying organization of the cerebrum. For example, much ink has been spilled describing how to find "Broca's Area" and "Wernicke's area", with far less effort expended about how to figure out how those two areas talk to each other and how their products lead to observable cognitive functions. I was taught during my training that brain mapping meant mapping the cortex at which point the patient was put to sleep for the tumor work.

My experience with glioma surgery is that those that ignore white matter do so at their own peril. While we cannot see white matter tracts during surgery as organized bundles of fibers in the way we can see the optic nerve or a trunk of the brachial plexus as discrete structures, they are still there and often are much larger structures than either the optic nerve or the brachial plexus. The connection of neural structures to relevant other structures is the foundational principle of how the nervous system works, and it is irrational to believe that we can cut connections between cortices but yet they can maintain their functions. Two examples familiar to neurosurgeons are the consequences of injuring the spinal cord or cutting the optic nerve. Yet there have been only limited efforts to put the analogous correlates of white matter disconnection into mainstream thought for other functions such as speech, or other higher brain functions.

Alternately, I have seen those who are proponents of white matter anatomy and its application in neurosurgery. Mainly the efforts have been to avoid injury to the tracts, and this is followed by impressive techniques of numerous flavors showing ways to stay out of the tracts on the way to deep tumors. Certainly, this represents a quantum leap in thinking, but the limitation is that we cannot always avoid tangling with the tracts and still address difficult gliomas. Most cases I have seen presented are methods for removing tumors where avoiding the SLF or motor fibers is possible, but my experience of sitting in a great number of talks is that there is a lot less interest in dealing with cases where this is not possible, and where the tracts are clearly involved in the tumor. Perhaps people do not operate on these cases because they are less fulfilling, or do not show them because they are less able to brag about a dirty stalemate than a dashing blowout victory. Either way, these are the types of cases which present to tumor surgeons, and if we want to have a system for surgery which makes the chip shots easy, then we need to have a system that can accommodate the monsters.

While injury to either grey or white matter essential to a critical function like speech is undesirable, I would argue that white matter injury is much worse, particularly with regards to the injury of large fiber tracts. Damage to deeper which matter affects a more diverse group of brain structures than a more peripherally placed lesion. ▶ Fig. 2.11 demonstrates the effect of identical sizes lesions in the precentral gyrus and the white matter tracts just deep to it. In another example, it is well known that putting the same size lesion in the posterior limb of the internal capsule is more devastating than that lesion would be in the motor cortex, in large part because the density of neurons essential for motor tasks is greater.

Further, while no one presently fully understands the mechanism of re-organization as a means by which patients recover from brain injuries, very few people are attributing it to a white matter process, and most people feel that it is most likely cortically mediated. As another anecdotal example, most neurosurgeons have noted a better chance of recovery with damage from motor strip lesions (mostly cortical injuries) than with spinal cord lesions (almost all white matter injuries). Or alternately, most neurosurgeons are well aware of the optic nerve's ability to recover from insults as an example of the limited ability of white matter to heal. Part of this is biologic differences between white and grey matter, part of it is related to severity of the injury, but I believe that in part, this results from the wider spread cortical areas which are taken off-line with white matter tract injury, as this reduces the ability for nearby cortices (which are also disconnected) to take over the lost function, as they are not connected to the target aspects of the network. Regardless of the mechanism, white matter injuries are not only more dense and severe, by in my experience they are more permanent.

All intra-axial tumor surgeries involve cutting some white matter, and this does not always lead to observable neurologic problems, but sometimes it does. In many cases, if we choose to remove a part of a tumor this might require cutting tracts infiltrated by tumors, some of which may be important, yet leaving the tumor there is not a realistic way to prevent their injury. And presently there is no way to see these tracts, and know where they are going or what they are doing. How do we deal with this issue?

2.3.2 Methods for Intelligently Managing the White Matter

Method 1: Awake Brain Mapping Which Continues into the Subcortex

Brain mapping that stops at the cortex is not really functional preservation surgery, in my opinion, it is an academic exercise. There is no point in knowing that a gyrus is essential for speech function if you then go on to disconnect it from its partner structures needed to create speech (▶ Fig. 2.12). Using awake techniques which continue until the white matter tracts of interest allow you to continuously define white matter from a functional perspective and to define appropriate boundaries in the otherwise featureless amorphous blob of the subcortical structures.

Method 2: Diffusion Tensor Tractography

During the middle ages, the city of Venice withstood repeated attempts by outside rulers to forcefully incorporate it into their empires and persisted as an independent nation until defeated by Napoleon in the early 1800s. The principle reason for this is the Venetian Lagoon, a complex set of waterways that surround the city, and would cause ships to misnavigate due to lack of familiarity and to wreck, thus preventing a successful amphibious landing. Presently, there are wooden stakes in the waterway which show water taxis how to navigate these waters safely.

In this analogy, the central core of the white matter is the Venetian Lagoon: a complex and treacherous set of waterways, with few landmarks to prevent one from wrecking. Diffusion tensor imaging (DTI) is that stake in the water. You still could wreck your boat, but at least you have some idea about where to travel to avoid this.

DTIs have their limits. Two such limits are that edema or even T2 changes from tumor can seriously impair their accuracy (think about how a technique based on the movement patterns of extracellular water can be affected by a disease which drastically increases the amount of extracellular water), and the use of the dominant Eigenvector to determine the direction of tracts in a voxel, which eliminates the possibility of two or more directions, and thus eliminates the ability to see small crossing fibers. Diffusion spectrum imaging (DSI) gets around some of the crossing fiber issues (which is why the anatomic studies in this book are made using DSI), but its acquisition length and the lack of commercially available programs to navigate this reduce its day to day appeal.

Despite these limits, white matter imaging platforms, like DTI, allow us to see the brain for what it really is, a complex set of connections, and allow us to reduce the complexity of the human cerebrum to a manageable dataset able to probe some meaningful questions, such as, "Where is the superior longitudinal fasciculus?" ▶ Fig. 2.13 shows a case which warns us ahead of time of the challenges involved in removing a small tumor. However helpful DTIs are, they cannot and should not replace awake surgery: they lack the millimetric accuracy needed to fly blind without functional feedback, they are subject to the same effect of intraoperative brain shift that image guidance is well known to suffer from. But more critically, anatomy does not

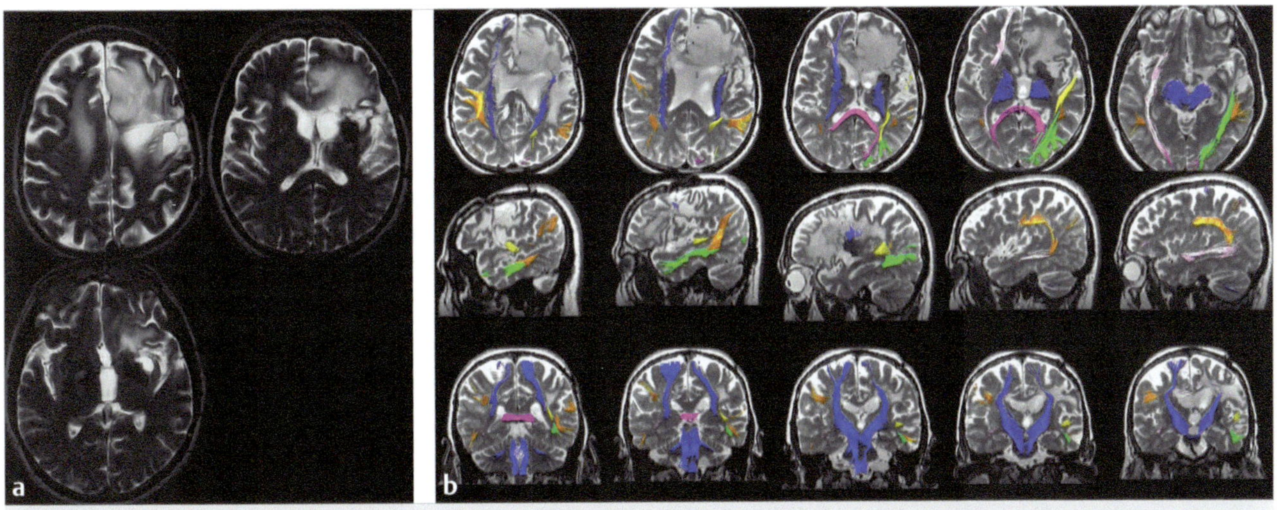

Fig. 2.12 This MRI (**a**) and DTI (**b**) demonstrate the unfortunate case of a patient who underwent surgery at another facility several years prior to presenting to us. Note that the trajectory taken crosses through the usual positions of the SLF and IFOF. His speech had never recovered to usable function years later.

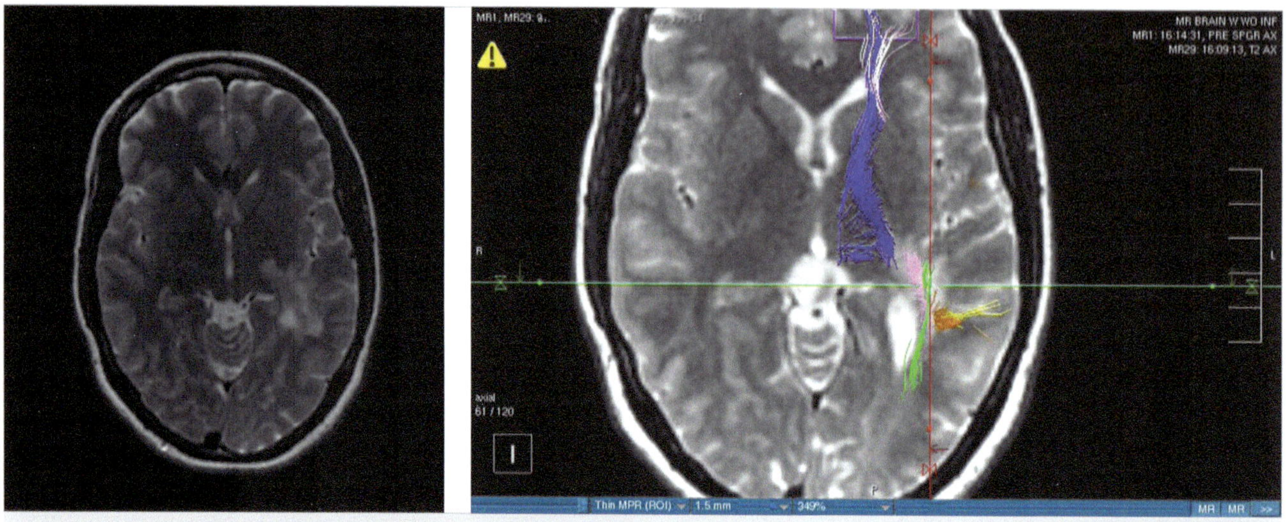

Fig. 2.13 This MRI (**a**) demonstrates a small glioma of the posterior left temporal lobe. In a book full of descriptions of removing basal ganglia, thalamic, butterfly and other bad gliomas, it should be surprising to note that this is a tumor which I consider largely inoperable (I attempted to but couldn't get anything out). Note that it is nestled into the junctional white matter near the crossing point of SLF and IFOF (among other tracts). A tumor (**b**) following this many tracts which is this small has little to gain and much to lose, making the tradeoff for gross total resection of this low grade tumor unwise.

perfectly line up with function in the cerebrum, and it is unclear how one can really know what part of a tract is essential for the task you are trying to save if you are not testing the tract in an awake patient. Just knowing that a tract connects two parts of the brain does not mean any of those areas are essential for the task tested. But paired with other techniques, they give you a mental image of what you are operating on, and a new ability to think about the white matter not as a large blob without definitive features, but as an understandable network of functions with real anatomy, is a radical departure indeed.

2.4 Sughrue's Third Law

2.4.1 If You Are Not Shocked at What You Have Just Done, You Have Just Done a Biopsy

Gliomas are big tumors in general, and the MRI usually leads you to believe that the tumor is smaller than it really is, and thus you have done more than you really have. This law could be applied to most brain tumors, but it is especially true for gliomas, for which complete resection requires removing a very large piece of the brain. It is probably true that the infiltrative nature of gliomas allow these tumors to reach an impressive size before causing symptoms which bring the patient to medical attention. Either way, if the hole is not impressive, then there is almost certainly gross tumor left, and especially in the case of high-grade tumors, there will be less room to tolerate the brain swelling that occurs after surgery, which is particularly bad when a glioma is only partially resected.

The Dual Nature of Gliomas?

For many years, neurosurgeons have felt they had a firm grasp on this problem. For example, a grade 2 oligodendroglioma was a ball of cells with unclear borders and cell migration into the brain. The greatest argument against that being a full picture of reality is simple observation: the tumor looks a lot like the brain and can have functional tissue within it. We know from histopathology that while some areas of the tumor are wall to wall cancer cells, that it is not rare to see tumor cells between normal neurons in other parts of the same specimen.

Certainly, there are areas where the tumor cell density is high, and that removing that part is removing mostly tumor, in other places, this is not true. Thus, gliomas are a tumor of dual nature, both tumor and brain/tumor. In most cases, it is best to think of them as the latter, as brain with tumor cells in it, but it is important to know that at times, even when it seems like it is difficult or dangerous to do so, that you can go for it sometimes, especially in the center.

The issue of diffuse borders in gliomas is a well-known problem and has been discussed as long as people have been removing them. Perhaps one day we will have a technological solution which truly deals with this issue, but until that is truly validated, my approach is to perform what is best described as an anatomic-functional resection. This means that I create a plan to remove anatomy until I encounter one of two boundaries.

Anatomic boundaries: These structures, which provide a visual cue that you have not left tumor, include the falx, the tentorium, the middle fossa floor, the orbital roof, a ventricle, or a sulcal boundary. There is zero chance you have left tumor in the medial frontal pole if you have cleared off the orbit and the falx, meaning that there is no frontal pole remaining.

Functional boundaries: These boundaries are defined using DTIs and awake brain mapping, and tell us that even if there is tumor left behind, that it is unwise to remove more brain to get more cytoreduction.

Am I advocating for removing "normal brain" outside of the "tumor?" The question in diffuse gliomas is absurd. There is no such thing as the "tumor" and no such thing as "normal brain" next to it in any form that we as humans can distinguish using the tools available to us. Everyone reading this knows this as these tumors most commonly recur on the margins (around 70% of Glioblastoma (GBM) recurrences), suggesting that we are primarily experiencing marginal failures, and not primarily distant spread. It is better to think of a glioma brain as a series of postal codes, with different densities of criminals. Good police work should focus on the high crime neighborhoods, but to neglect lesser crime neighborhoods without reason is to avoid the benefit of reducing the overall crime rate. Our goal is always to leave the patient with as few cancer cells as we can possibly achieve for them without making unacceptable functional trades. We know that there are cancer cells in the radiographical negative margins of these tumors, why not take them if we can determine that there is no major consequence to doing so. The logic that was for years used to dismiss glioma surgery as pointless is the same logic that dictates that trying to do just a lesionectomy is inconsistent with the nature of the disease.

Further, we know now that the T2 signal around the enhancement of a GBM is mostly tumor tissue and not edema. This should not be surprising to anyone who has thought about it. If a T2 bright, non-enhancing low-grade glioma has a focus which transforms to GBM, does the low grade tumor that was there previously just turn into edema? Of course, it doesn't, it's still a tumor, it's just not the worst part.

The concept of "staying in the tumor" has led many of us to perform resections which are not consistent with either neuroscientific principles (i.e., brain that is not connected to other relevant brain doesn't do anything) or oncologic principles (i.e., tumors with infiltrative features on their borders should be removed with margins when possible). ▶ Fig. 2.14 shows three examples of this concept. In all three examples, a lesionectomy was performed, of varying quality. In all three cases, a rim of "normal brain" was left which after the surgery was disconnected from the brain. But we know that almost certainly this is not truly "normal" brain, there is almost certainly a fair number of cancer cells there, and the thin lip of brain has been disconnected from its normal targets, and is very unlikely to contribute meaningfully to neuro-psychological function (this lip of brain is almost certainly not helping to write a follow-up to War and Peace). If the patient recurs in this lip of disconnected brain, what possible justification is there for why it was left behind. At least if a patient recurs in brain left behind to save speech or motor or some other function, then a logical tradeoff in the patient's best interest was made. Unless we think in terms of connectivity, then we cannot make rational decisions about what stays and what goes.

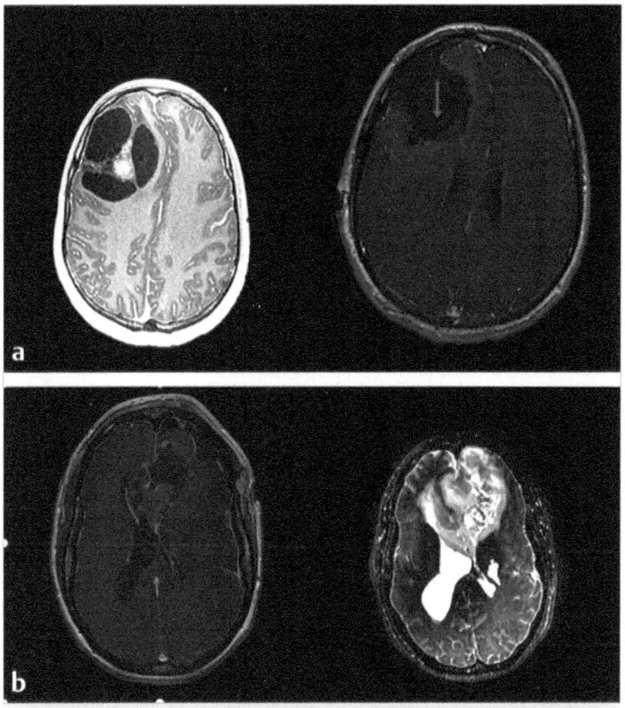

Fig. 2.14 Leaving a "road to nowhere" is a term I use to describe to complete a resection which leaves brain which is largely or completely disconnected from the rest of the brain. These images demonstrate three cases of leaving "roads to nowhere": (**a**) demonstrates a case I performed as a trainee, of a cystic low grade glioma which was completely resected. The included postop image demonstrates that while the tumor has been completely resected, the small rim of brain left at the anterior frontal pole is a "road to nowhere" because its normal connections have been severed posteriorly and it cannot conduct across a huge hole (*red arrow*). (**b**) This case demonstrates one of my first attempts at resecting an butterfly glioma. While the resection could have been worse, note that not only is the anterior-medial frontal tip a "road to nowhere" but that I have disconnected the genu of the corpus callosum on both sides but left it in (partially because I was afraid to push this any further, and the idea of widely opening both frontal horns was something I was not aware I needed to do to ensure complete removal; remember I did not have a book to teach me how to take out the callosum). There is nothing inherently dangerous with leaving a "road to nowhere," it just doesn't make a lot of sense. It is unfortunate when a patient recurs in a disconnected lip of nonfunctioning brain, so in my estimation, if you are going to render it nonfunctional, you might as well gain the benefit of removing whatever tumor cells are in it.

Of course, the rational application of principles means that there is always a line when judgment needs to overrule principle. For example, while resecting a small glioma of the right temporal pole, I do not continue to resect posteriorly until I encounter the visual system in the occipital lobe, every case is tailored to the goals of the surgery, with the idea that we are resecting an area as much as tolerated, and some margin taken around the tumor probably reduces the post-operative tumor burden. However, the idea that you are resecting a discrete tumor and microdissecting it from the normal brain like it is a meningioma is pure fantasy and we know this. Our goal always is the leave the patient in the best shape possible with the least number of tumor cells possible. Margins work in every other type of solid tissue cancer surgery, so it is unclear why glioma is so unique and can violate principles so well understood in every other discipline. An end stage GBM is a T4N0M0 tumor after all; however, we usually meet it as a T3N0M0 and satisfactory margins are usually impossible to take acceptably.

What About When There are No Good Anatomic or Functional Boundaries

The concept of resecting until you see the falx, or performing a temporal lobectomy when possible is easy to grasp, even the insula has anatomic boundaries to define your resection if you know where to look for them. However, there are situations when there are not clear boundaries to tell you when to stop prior to encountering trouble. One good example are motor strip tumors, where the resection could go on for some time before reaching an anatomic boundary, and you are always surrounded by a functional brain, so there are no clear functional boundaries. However, it is safe to say that resection of a motor strip glioma probably shouldn't continue until it is unquestionable that you have gone too far. The thalamus is another example of a similar problem.

When lacking a better option, visual cues are often the only thing to go by. Glioma tissue has been long felt to be hard to distinguish from normal, especially low-grade tumors; however, to a trained eye, the densest concentration of tumor tissue is usually obvious. The features listed below were first elaborated long ago by Yasargil, and are demonstrated in accompanying videos. Even with difficult tumors, some anatomic and functional boundaries can be established in almost all cases but in cases when a lesionectomy is the best we can reasonably hope for, these features are often all you have to guide you in many places.

The Four Classic Features of Glioma Tissue

1. Color: Dense areas of glioma are grey or at least glassy white
2. Response to cautery: Because of the higher water content, glioma tissue bubbles when cauterized as opposed to normal brain which tends to char
3. Response to suctioning: Glioma tissue tends to suction up in sheets as opposed to normal brain which does not pull into sheets as easily
4. Sound: Because of its higher water content, glioma tissue sounds like snot when it goes up the suction.

What About Image Guidance?

Image guidance is an invaluable tool which I use every case to plan the smallest possible craniotomy for that case, to locate the likely position of white matter tracts, and to reorient myself occasionally. However, if you use it as a volumetric guide to be know when you have cleared out what you think you have, then you will probably wonder why there is so much tumor left on the scan.

What About Intraoperative MRI, 5-ALA?

The use of intraoperative MRI is based on the concept that a lesionectomy represents the best possible resection of a glioma you can do, and that it's worth $10 million dollars, using inferior instruments, and adding large amounts of surgical time to do better lesionectomies. What it can't do is find microscopic disease, which would make it an actually helpful tool. Until such time when it can find microscopic disease, I would argue that if an intraoperative MRI tells me there is a tumor in a place which I have mapped and know it is the speech network, then it is unclear how this has helped the situation, as I am not going to remove it. In other words, using my approach, I can't see how this technique will show me something left that is resectable, at least often enough to justify the immense institutional headache these devices create.

The concept of fluorescent tumor finding probes, like 5-ALA, is conceptually appealing; however, presently to my knowledge it is unclear how many cells in the brain are actually necessary to make something light up. Presently, the best available data tells us it helps surgeons do better lesionectomies of the enhancing part of a GBM, but I am not certain if it will actually alter the technique I currently use. Needless to say, such adjuncts are interesting, but I think a certain degree of skepticism is necessary before determining its true role in glioma surgery.

3 Surface and Gross Anatomy of the Cerebrum

3.1 Introduction

The contents of this chapter have been extensively covered by numerous authors, including Rhoton. This chapter is included not to redo this work, but to provide a reference, to point out a few features of sulcal, gyral, and structural anatomy which is not usually covered in other work, but which I think is helpful to glioma surgery, and most importantly to demonstrate how to practically apply this anatomy to precisely remove these tumors. In general, I have tried to make this section shorter and more practically focused than other similar chapters; however, I highly recommend supplementing this reading with more fundamental texts if the content of this brief overview is not entirely familiar to you.

3.2 Why Study Gross Cerebral Anatomy in the Image Guidance Era?

Besides the obvious possibility that the image guidance might be inaccurate, and the fact that the tool is only as useful as the brain interpreting it, it is critical to have a sense of what anatomy exactly needs to be removed, and what potential functional consequences there are for doing so. By infiltrating and expanding brain structures, gliomas can radically alter the appearance and organization of the brain. They often distort the anatomy to such an extent as to completely obscure their origin and exact anatomy at first glance. For example, it is not at all rare to see a glioma which at first glance appears to be a motor region tumor, but in fact is a parietal glioma, which has so distorted and expanded, the anatomy that it has pushed its way into the expected location of the motor strip. A good example of such a situation is the sizeable GBM in ▶ Fig. 3.1. A quick glance at the contrasted images in ▶ Fig. 3.1 might lead you to conclude that this tumor is beginning in the back of the temporal lobe and is invading the basal ganglia and internal capsule. However, looking at the T2 images (which are better at defining sulcal anatomy), this tumor seems to be arising from the angular gyrus which is massively expanded. The precentral and postcentral gyri are both pushed forward and not heavily involved. Most critically, the basal ganglia and internal capsule are also pushed anteriorly (as we would expect an enlarged angular gyrus to do). Based on this, we were able to get an excellent resection of this tumor leaving the patient only with the homonymous hemianopsia he entered with. As should be obvious, careful observation of the preoperative images can radically alter your expectations.

Additionally, as I repeatedly point out in this book, the functional organization of the cerebral cortex is not entirely predictable based on the anatomy, but at the same time, it is not random. Even more than inter-individual variability, the presence of a glioma, especially oligodendroglioma but any glioma, can cause the functional anatomy of the brain to reorganize sometimes drastically; however, you should not expect to find the primary motor function at the occipital pole. Thus, while we need to clear our mind of the poison of exact anatomic expectations in the neocortex, knowing gyri and sulci gives us a reasonable framework to start with.

Finally, in a paradigm like this, where resection continues until encountering an anatomic or functional boundary, sulci are godsends. They provide an orienting landmark, and in some cases following a sulci can help keep you from crossing into the brain where you do not wish to be. Sulci show you where unseen vessels may be lie, give you a boundary to perform subpial dissection, and as long as you remain above the bottom of the sulci, you generally are not into the deep white matter

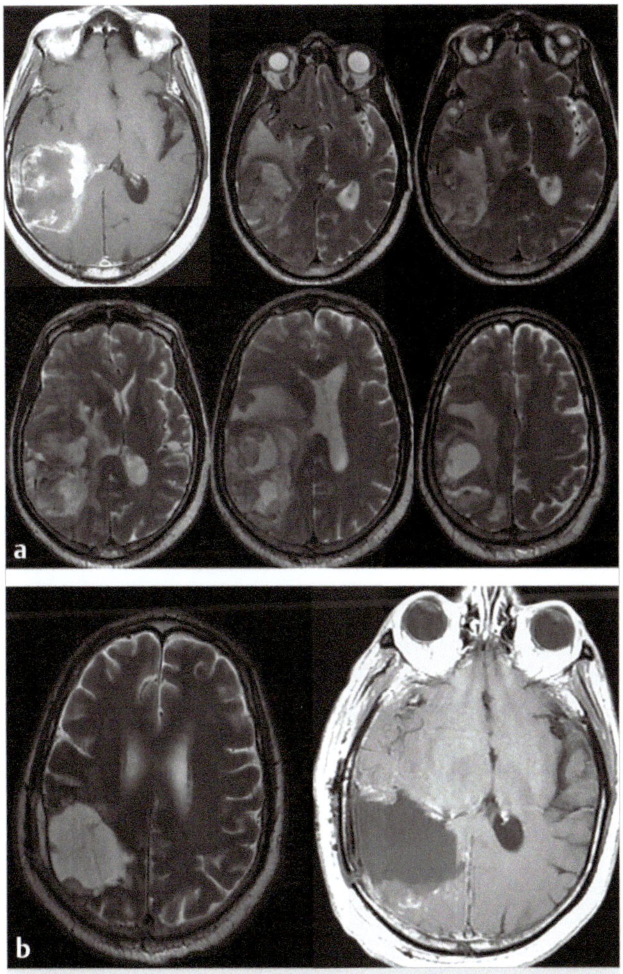

Fig. 3.1 Preoperative (**a**) and post-operative (**b**) images of a large GBM of the parietal lobe. At first glance, it may appear that this tumor involves the basal ganglia or internal capsule as the tumors anterior border is located in the usual location of these structures. Closer examination of the T2 images, however, indicates that it does not involve these structures, as they are pushed forward, and this tumor was able to be completely removed without any noticeable deficit. This case highlights the critical importance of carefully examining the involved structures on the preoperative images, and not going just on a rough idea that a tumor is located in a bad location.

tracts. Similarly, knowing the relationship of the brain to the ventricles, the basal ganglia, and other critical deep structures is essential for keeping out of trouble.

The bottom line is that the cerebrum does not have a lot of landmarks, and you need to be prepared to use whatever landmarks you have available.

3.3 Anatomy of Cerebral Sulci and Gyri

When providing a list of gyri and sulci and some descriptions, it's best to start with some general observations and disclaimers. First, the term gyrus is best viewed as a concept which describes the basic direction and anatomic pattern of a strip of cortex that is usually identifiable in most brains. Thus, some gyri are more consistent and uniformly coherent than others, and to not understand the limits of the term is to try to force uniformity on anatomy which is frequently quite variable. For example, most people mapping the motor strip for the first time are surprised to find that motor function seldom maps to a single continuous strip of the brain, as the precentral gyrus is often interrupted by variable numbers of small sulci.

Another critical general observation is that almost all sulci point at a ventricle. The only exception to this is the sulci outlining limbic cortices of the medial hemispheric surface which instead parallel the corpus callosum. This is especially important when we begin to discuss the division phase of subcortical mapping in future chapters. In this phase, our plan is to continue mapping the patient until the cut is completely past the white matter tract at risk, and thus the tumor specimen has been made non-eloquent. Entering the ventricle is often the way to assure that you are past it as there is no way the tract runs through the ventricle. In many such cases, the true danger occurs once the dissection proceeds beyond the depth of the sulci, as the large fiber tracts are there, and there are often no landmarks. While one guide to preventing getting lost in the brain is functional mapping, keeping your cut parallel to the sulci is another guide to quickly getting into the oriented safety of the ventricle.

You might be surprised when I say that it is a good idea to enter the ventricle, as we are all taught not to do this. Certainly, this maneuver increases the risks of needing a shunt, and you should not do this for no reason; however, it is easier to place a shunt than to fix an incomplete resection, and it is much easier to place a shunt, than to rehabilitate someone whose brain you got lost in because you didn't want to use the ventricular anatomy as a landmark.

What follows then are some basic descriptions of the gyral and sulcal patterns of various lobes, with general rules given whenever possible.

3.4 Surface Anatomy of the Frontal Lobe

The human frontal lobe is massive, as anyone who has resected a frontal lobe likely has observed. Its lateral surface is best known and is dominated by three large anterior to posterior gyri (superior, middle and inferior frontal gyri) which all about the precentral gyrus in a perpendicular manner on their posterior edge. These are divided by the superior and inferior frontal sulci.

When attempting to orient myself to the anatomy of any image in this region (▶ Fig. 3.2), I always find the superior frontal sulcus first, as this knowledge is critical for determining where the precentral gyrus (i.e., the motor strip) is, where the supplementary motor area is likely to be, and for figuring out which frontal gyrus is which. Numerous other gyri can be sorted out using deduction based on this fact.

The superior frontal sulcus is deep, usually continuous, and intersects the precentral sulcus at a right angle (which is what makes it so helpful to figuring what is what). Its continuation into the pre-central gyrus indents that gyrus in what's known as the hand knob (but which cannot be blindly considered to be hand motor cortex, especially in glioma patients).

In contrast, the inferior frontal sulcus is always interrupted, and always partially indents the inferior frontal gyrus to form the triangularis portion of that gyrus. The junction of the inferior frontal sulcus with the precentral gyrus provides another

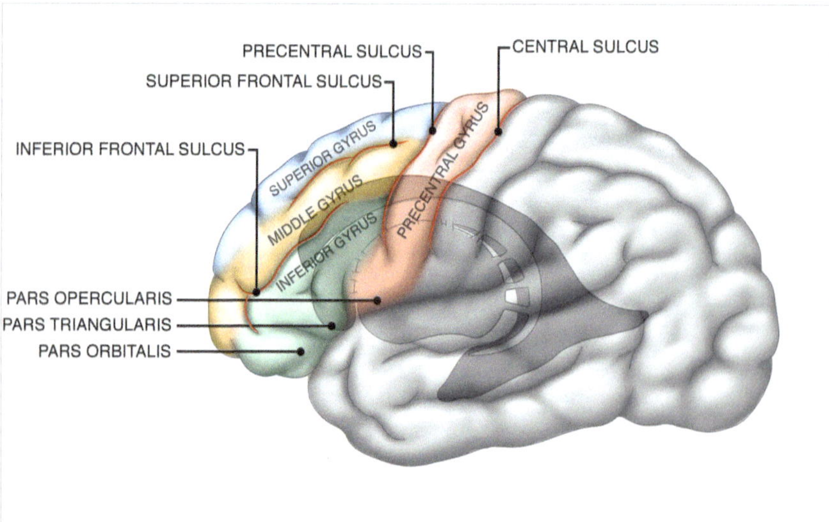

Fig. 3.2 Schematic demonstrating the lateral surface anatomy of the frontal lobe, and the gyri and sulci.

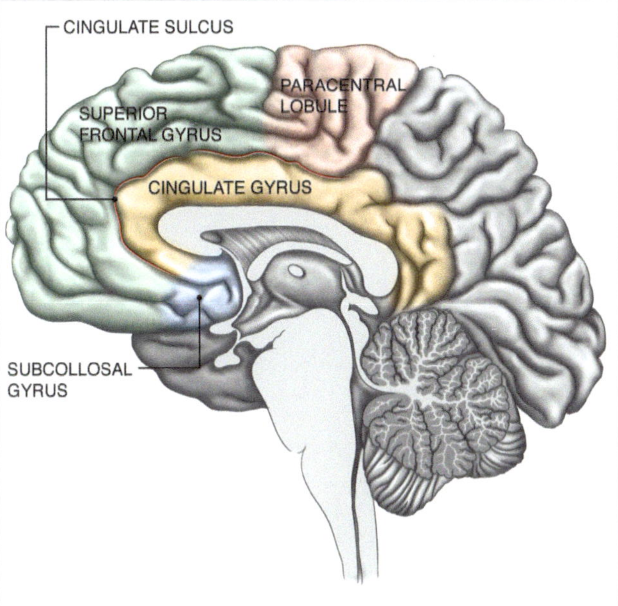

Fig. 3.3 Schematic demonstrating the medial surface anatomy of the frontal lobe, and the gyri and sulci.

cortical landmark. Inferior to this point, the precentral gyrus in normal people is usually face motor cortex (which can be sacrificed in many cases), and usually is operculum which overlies the insula. The inferior frontal gyrus has its three well known divisions: pars orbitalis, pars triangularis and pars opercularis.

The medial surface of the frontal lobe (▸ Fig. 3.3) is dominated by the medial border of the superior frontal gyrus which extends from the motor regions around to the orbital floor in a c-shaped fashion. The cingulate sulcus (one of the most useful sulcal landmarks in my opinion) separates the cingulate gyrus from the superior frontal gyrus. The cingulate gyrus parallels the corpus callosum and is separated from it by the callosal sulcus. Once it continues under the rostrum of the corpus callosum, there are three small gyri which overlie structures of the basal forebrain such as the septal nuclei and nucleus basalis.

The orbitofrontal surface of the frontal lobe is generally delineated by an H-shaped sulcus that divides the orbitofrontal cortex into four. The olfactory tract separates these gyri from the gyrus rectus which is medial to the tract. The posterior aspects of these cortices blend into the anterior perforated substance in the proximity of the optic nerve, and this is the location of the basal forebrain, and caudate nucleus. I have not spent much time describing these gyri in much detail because personally, I have not found them to be surgically very useful, and I think of the orbitofrontal cortex as a unit.

3.4.1 Functional Considerations

Care should be taken to not firmly link specific places in the cortex with specific functions; however, in this chapter I will make some basic comments on the specific location of various functions, and a more nuanced view will follow in subsequent chapters (▸ Fig. 3.4).

The frontal lobe has been considered mostly non-eloquent by neurosurgeons for some time; most of whom I suspect has not spent a great deal of time talking to family members of patients with frontal lobe injuries. The frontal lobe is highly eloquent, it is just highly complex, the problems its loss causes are less obvious that other parts of the brain, its regions likely have some degree of redundancy, and we understand very little about how it works or how to study it.

Textbooks on frontal lobe function divide the frontal lobe into three basic areas: Motor (the motor strip), Premotor (areas just in frontal of the motor strip involved in motor planning), and Prefrontal (all the thinking, motivation, judgment and emotional regulation parts in front of premotor areas), and for our purposes this is useful.

Prefrontal cortices can be further subdivided by functions conventionally attributed to them. The dorsolateral prefrontal cortex (DLPC) (i.e., the lateral convexity) has a complex relationship with working memory and concentration that is not well understood. The exact location the regions which make up the DLPC proper is hard to nail down from fMRI data; however, the posterior middle frontal gyrus just in front of the premotor areas is a common place this function localizes to. The medial structures, the medial superior frontal gyrus and especially the cingulate gyrus, contain brain networks involved in motivation and attention. The orbitofrontal cortices are involved in emotion and emotional regulation (i.e., the problems we see after bifrontal contusions which are classically an orbitofrontal injury).

Premotor cortices constitute a complex network which we will discuss in more detail in subsequent chapters. The supplementary motor area classically is located in the medial bank superior frontal gyrus just in front of the precentral gyrus. Its general vicinity can be estimated by locating the part of the superior frontal gyrus which joins with the precentral gyrus. The other premotor areas are located laterally just anterior to the motor strip, in the posterior edges of the middle and inferior frontal gyri, and this network has a highly variable anatomy.

Broca's area is classically defined as the inferior frontal gyrus just anterior to the motor strip. To give this site any more significance other than it is the premotor area which plans movement for the face, tongue, palate, and larynx is to misunderstand the role of this site in the speech network. As with any other cortical site, the site which causes speech arrest with cortical stimulation can reorganize and move to other parts of the brain, and thus it is sometimes located in the canonical Broca's are, but it can be many other places. One thing that is usually true is that it is the premotor area for the face, and usually finding facial movements will help you locate the speech arrest site which is generally anterior to the face motor area (logical, no?).

3.4.2 Important Distinctions in Frontal Glioma Anatomy

In every area of the brain, distortions of sulcal anatomy can make it challenging to determine where a tumor is really centered and what it really involves. Sometimes, this is academic, and other times it is easy. In each section of this chapter, there are examples of situations where the distinction is often challenging and the difference between two gyri make a big deal.

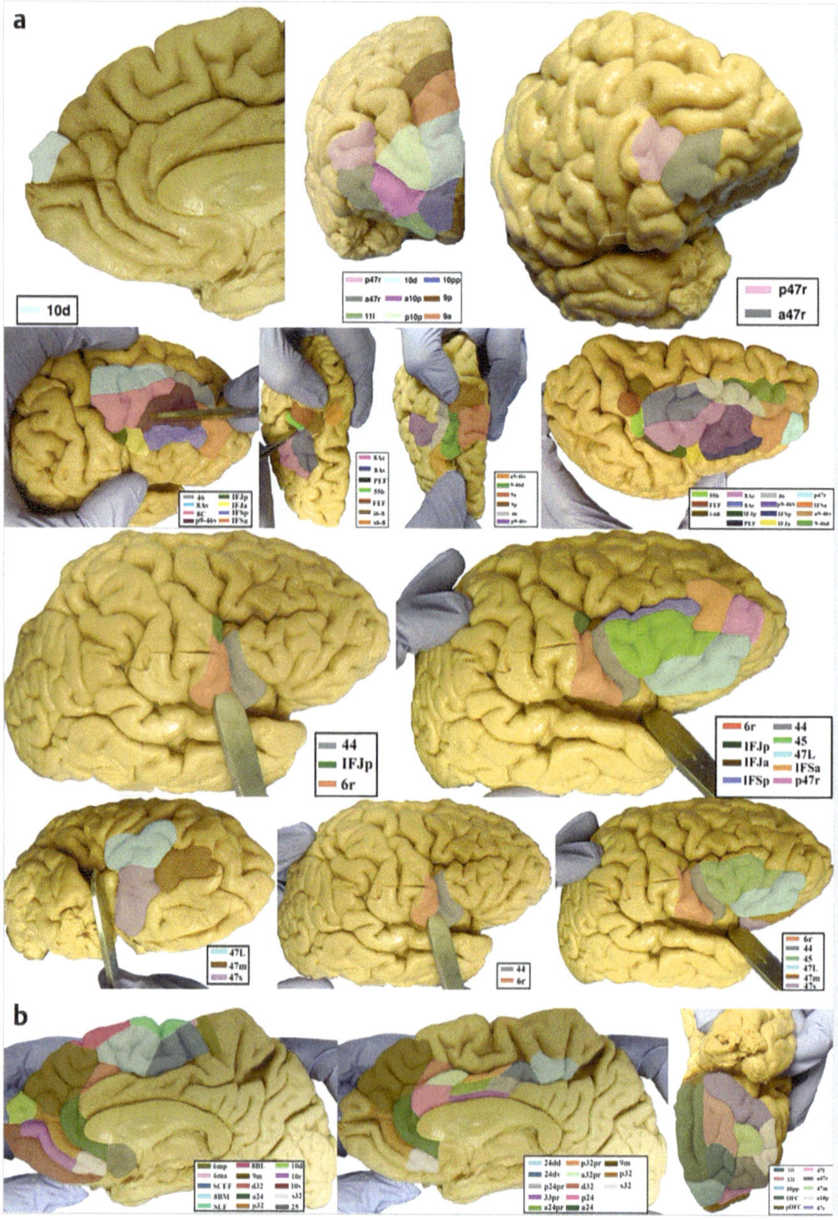

Fig. 3.4 Schematic demonstrating the cortical location linked to various neurologic functions within the frontal lobe.

The most common scenario are tumors of the posterior frontal lobe where the decision needs to be made whether this tumor involves the motor strip, sensory strip, premotor areas, etc. As described above, the key is locate the superior frontal sulcus and use this to define the precentral sulcus, which may be smashed (▶ Fig. 3.5, ▶ Fig. 3.6) and may be displaced remarkably posterior. Knowing whether you are dealing with a motor strip or premotor tumor can make a significant difference in your mapping strategy and plan.

The other common situation with frontal gliomas is differentiating whether the tumor arises from the superior frontal gyrus, the cingulate gyrus, or both. Experience has taught me a great deal of respect for the cingulate gyrus, especially if it is uninvolved with glioma, and I spend a fair bit of time sorting out this distinction. The exact status of the corpus callosum should also be studied, as many cingulate tumors will herniate under the falx and mimic a butterfly tumor when they really aren't. The last thing you want to do is to drift into the contralateral cingulate gyrus thinking somehow they are contiguous; this is easy to do when the tumor is bloody and the contralateral pia is abnormal. The key is to study the coronal images closely, as the axials can be confusing especially in giant medial frontal tumors. Three examples are provided in ▶ Fig. 3.7, ▶ Fig. 3.8, ▶ Fig. 3.9.

3.5 Surface Anatomy of the Central Sulcus Region

The motor strip and sensory strips can be confusing to people who expect them to look like a Netter drawing, as they are not always continuous structures, and they do not always look like the textbooks. As stated numerous times, the superior frontal sulcus is the best starting point when working this out as it reliably defines the pre-central sulcus, which can be used to work out the other sulcal boundaries.

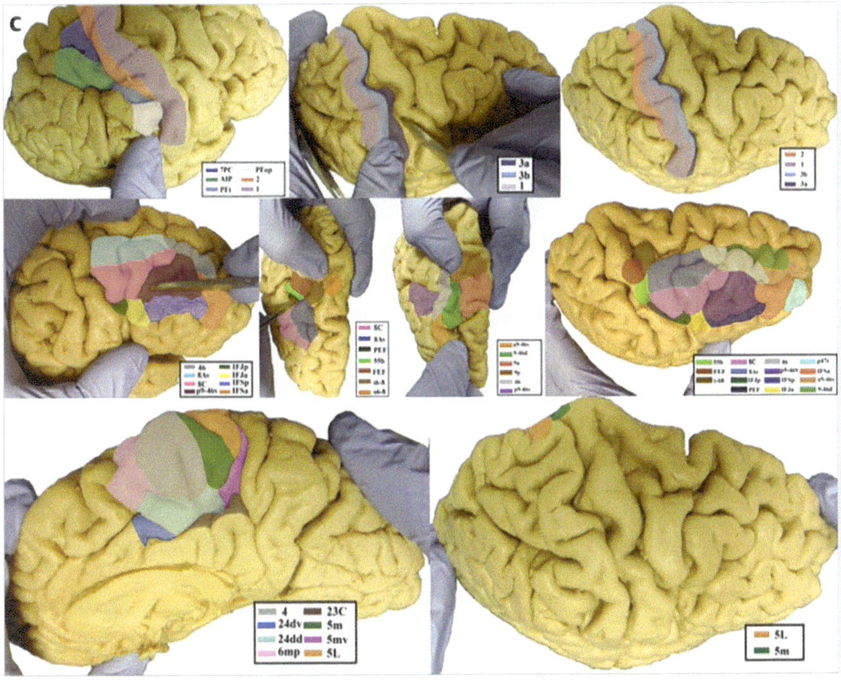

Fig 3.4 *(Continued)*

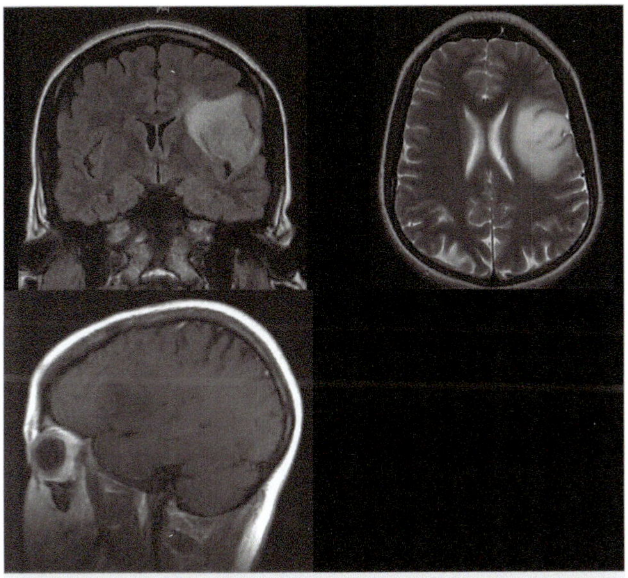

Fig. 3.5 Images from a glioma located within the inferior frontal gyrus.

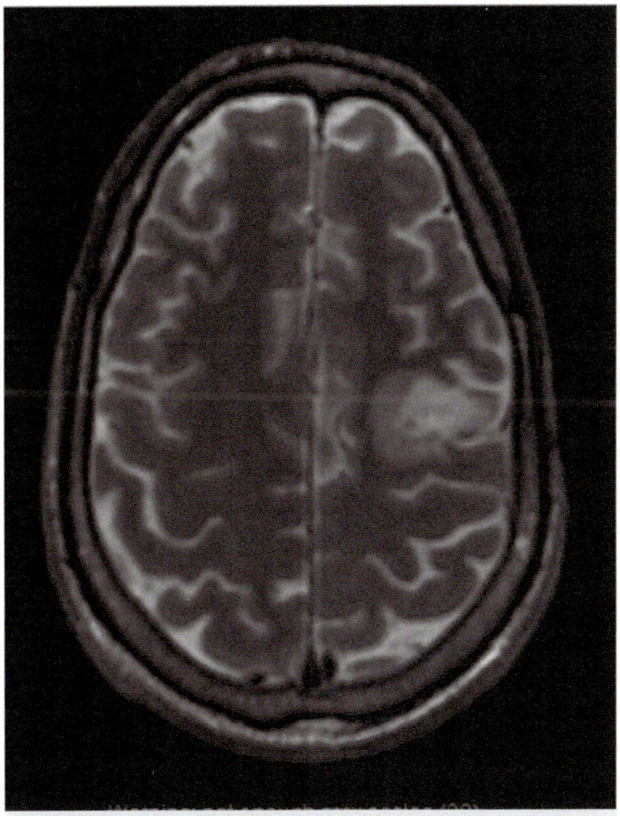

Fig. 3.6 Images from a glioma located within the middle frontal gyrus.

The precental sulcus and the central sulcus can be differentiated from each other at surgery or on sagittal images by the fact that the central sulcus never intersects the Sylvian fissure and the precentral always does (▶ Fig. 3.2). The central sulcus instead terminates in an operculum, the subcentral gyrus.

The postcentral sulcus shares some similarities with the precentral sulcus in that it is intersected at a right angle by the deep intraparietal sulcus.

Medially (▶ Fig. 3.3), the precentral and postcentral gyri are fused into the paracentral lobule. A ramus of the cingulate sulcus rises top define the posterior border and is called the marginal sulcus.

3.5.1 Important Distinctions in Central Sulcus Anatomy

While some tumors do involve the precentral and the postcentral gyrus, most involve one or neither (i.e., they look like they are in the area where the gyri are supposed to be; however, the

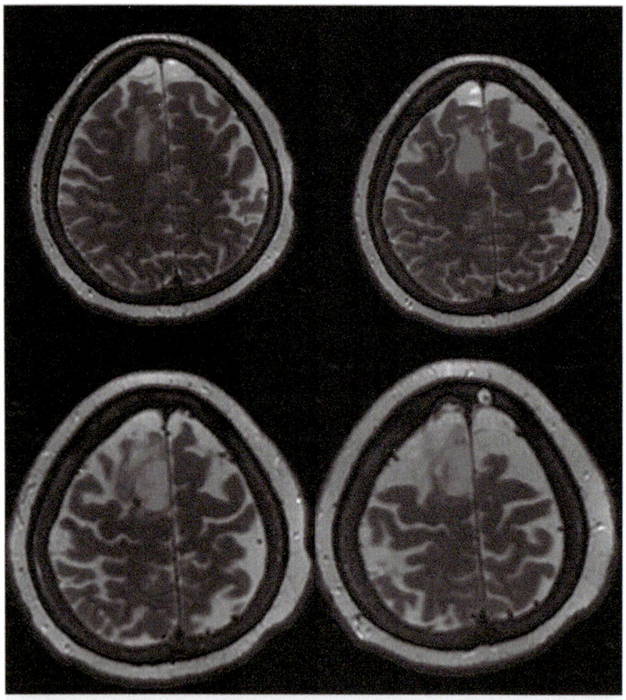

Fig. 3.7 Images from a glioma located within the superior frontal gyrus.

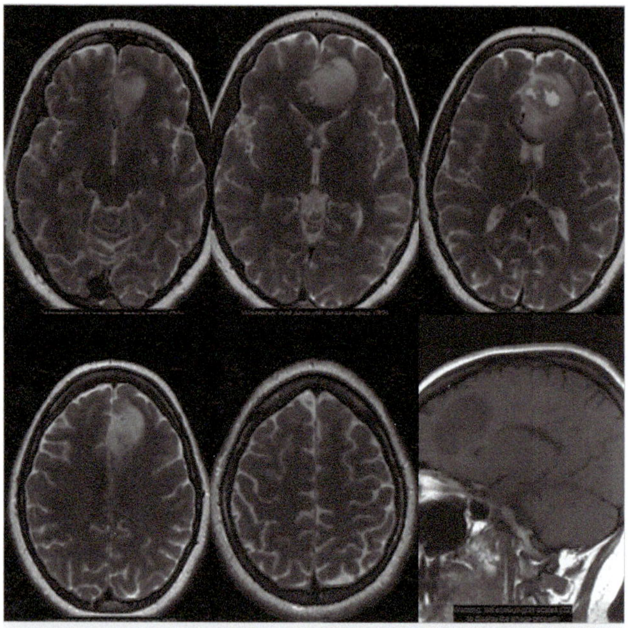

Fig. 3.8 Images from a glioma located within the anterior cingulate gyrus.

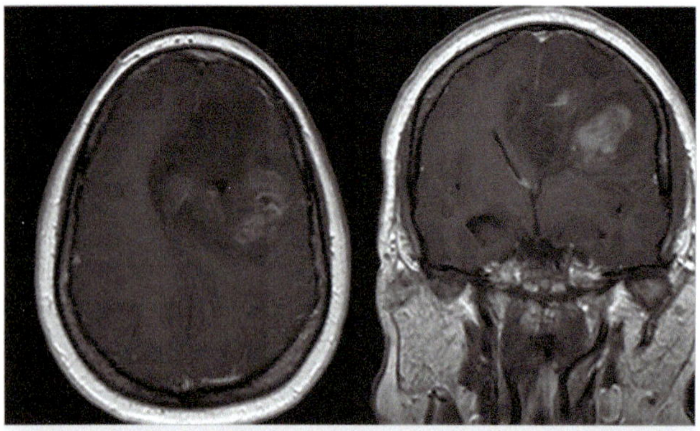

Fig. 3.9 Images from a massive glioma located within the cingulate gyrus. At first glance, this tumor looks like it crosses midline and it is a large frontal glioma. The coronal makes it clear that this is focused in the cingulate as there is overlying frontal lobe between the tumor and the surface. The part crossing the midline is merely herniating underneath the falx.

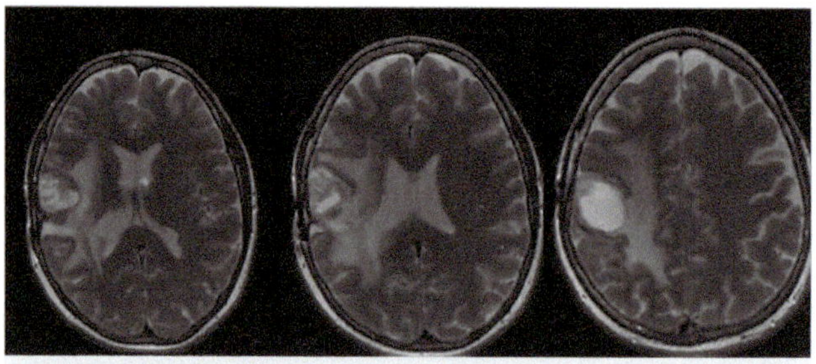

Fig. 3.10 Images from a glioma located within the lower sensory strip. The exact location of the tumor can be figured by first finding the right sulcal angle in the superior frontal lobe which helps to locate the precentral gyrus. Often, this is easier on the normal side which can be helpful for locating compressed gyri and distorted sulci.

real gyri is pushed forward. Using the superior frontal sulcus, the intraparietal sulcus, and the relation of sulci to the Sylvian fissure, it is usually possible to know ahead of time which gyrus is actually involved. One example is seen in ▶ Fig. 3.10.

3.6 Surface Anatomy of the Temporal Lobe

The most notable features of the lateral temporal lobe are the three horizontal gyri: the superior, middle and inferior temporal gyri, which are divided by the superior and inferior temporal sulci. A few critical observations are seen in ▶ Fig. 3.11. The inferior temporal gyrus is much lower than anatomic drawings usually portray it; most of it is hidden on the temporal floor. Thus when you open up even a large traditional craniotomy for temporal lobectomy, you generally are not looking at the inferior temporal gyrus (unless you remove a fair bit of squamous bone).

Second, the superior temporal gyrus is an operculum along its entire length, meaning that its deep surface is covered by Sylvian fissure arachnoid and removing it does not expose the temporal lobe white matter, it exposes the insula. The insula extends inferior to about the top of the middle temporal gyrus, and the middle temporal gyrus overlies the temporal horn and is the initial access point for most forays into the temporal lobe parenchyma.

The gyral pattern inferior surface of the temporal lobe (▶ Fig. 3.12) is also quite helpful for reorienting one's self at times. The inferior temporal gyrus extends onto the inferior

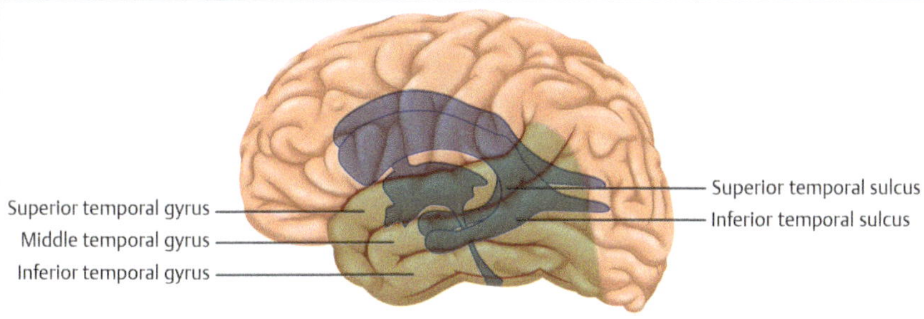

Fig. 3.11 Schematic demonstrating the lateral surface anatomy of the temporal lobe, and the gyri and sulci.

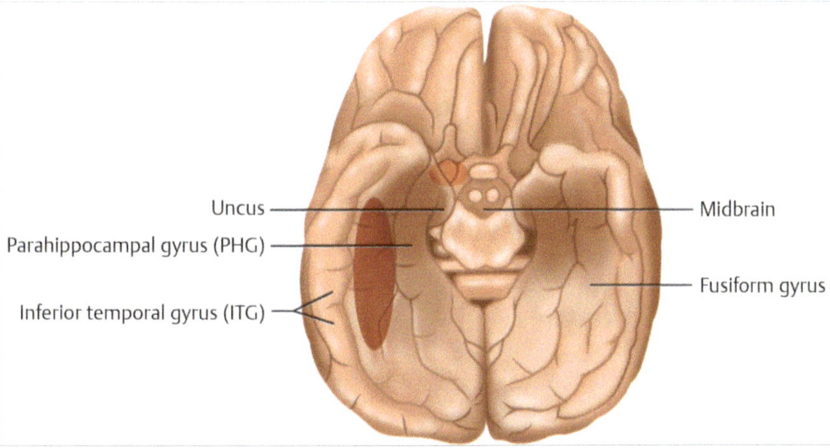

Fig. 3.12 Schematic demonstrating the inferior surface anatomy of the temporal lobe, and the gyri and sulci.

surface and comprises its lateral portion. The bulk of the inferior temporal lobe surface is made up of the fusiform gyrus which is separated from the inferior temporal gyrus by the occipitotemporal sulcus. As expected from its bounding sulcus, the fusiform gyrus extends well posteriorly into the inferior occipital lobe. Its medial sulcus, the collateral sulcus separates it from the parahippocampal gyrus.

3.6.1 The Medial Temporal Lobe

The medial anatomy of the temporal lobe is probably the most critical anatomy to master if you wish to do excellent glioma surgery. Gliomas have a high propensity to involve these structures, and often massively expand them. Thus, if you do not know this anatomy very well, it is quite easy to end up leaving most of the tumor. Additionally, the medial temporal lobe is a place where disasters can happen if you get lost, which explains the high rate of even experienced tumor surgeons who do not try to tackle tumor in these parts, though unfamiliarity with well-known anatomy is hardly a reason to leave tumor behind. Finally, knowing the medial temporal lobe is the key to knowing the insular anatomy, as these structures are intimately related and tumors often span both structures.

The structure which is best to ground your understanding of medial temporal lobe relationships is the hippocampus. This is a long structure which sits in the temporal horn, and thus is deep to the middle temporal gyrus. Note from ▶ Fig. 3.13, that the tip of the hippocampus does not come anywhere near the temporal tip, but instead is somewhat behind the coronal plane of the clivus. The uncus is anterior, superior, and deep (a phrase beaten into my residents heads) to this tip. The uncus comes to a point and that point faces away from you at surgery from the lateral approaches (which is almost all glioma approaches. It has superior and inferior small limiting sulci which can be noticed with experience, and seeing these sulci tell you when you have completely removed the uncus.

The parahippocampal gyrus sits underneath somewhat medial to the hippocampus. The hippocampus actually overlies the fusiform gyrus instead. Thus, when resecting the medial temporal structures which herniate over the tentorial edge, as you proceed from anterior to posterior, the structure you encounter as you subpially remove this tissue posterior to the uncus is the parahippocampal gyrus not the hippocampus. This is a key point in maintaining orientation, and was lost on me for at least my first 100 temporal lobectomies.

▶ Fig. 3.14 displays probably the most set important anatomic relationships in glioma surgery, which is the coronal relationship of the hippocampus to its neighboring structures. Note that the superior temporal gyrus overlies the insula, while the middle temporal gyrus primarily overlies the temporal parenchyma and temporal horn. The hippocampus, and especially the roof of the temporal horn sits directly inferior to the basal ganglia. The uncus, which is anterior, superior, and deep to the hippocampus sits inferior to the optic tract and internal capsule. When people ask me how I know when to stop during an insular glioma, I tell them to make the depth of the resection parallel to the depth of the hippocampus, which will roughly define the basal ganglia depth. When a patient with a giant uncus or hippocampal glioma comes in unable to walk, or hemiplegic, I am relatively sure this will improve as this is due to superior compression of the descending motor fibers, which generally recover after surgical removal of a hippocampal mass.

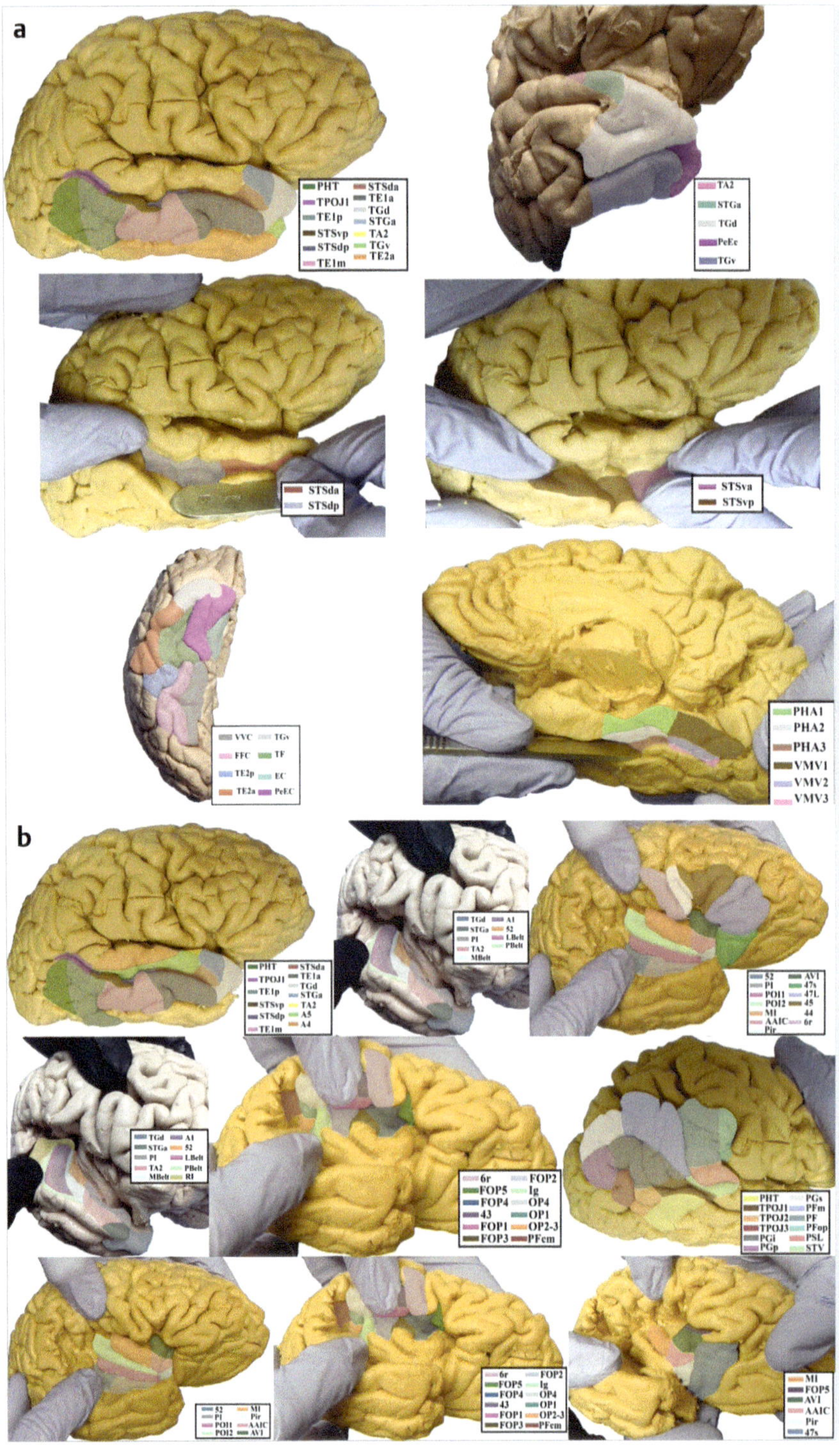

Fig. 3.13 Schematic demonstrating the cortical location linked to various neurologic functions within the temporal lobe.

3.6.2 The Posterior Temporal Lobe and the Temporoparietoocipital Junction

The Temporoparietoocipital junction (TPO junction for short) is one of the most complex and high risk areas of the human brain to operate in. Its nonlinear overlying gyri converge with the shallow posterior insula and overlie numerous large white matter tracts at their crossing points. This is also the easiest place to inadvertently enter the posterior limb of the internal capsule as the back of this area is exposed to the temporal stem due to its medial to lateral orientation. Thus it's easy to get lost and easy to wreak havoc.

There is no way to make TPO junctional anatomy simple, but I will try to explain its relations in the way I think about it, in relation to the atrium of the lateral ventricle (▶ Fig. 3.15). I choose to explain it in reference to the atrium as the anterior wall of the atrium contains most of the most important structures in this region, the lateral walls of the atrium contain the white matter tracts, and the gyral anatomy should be viewed in terms of the underlying structures.

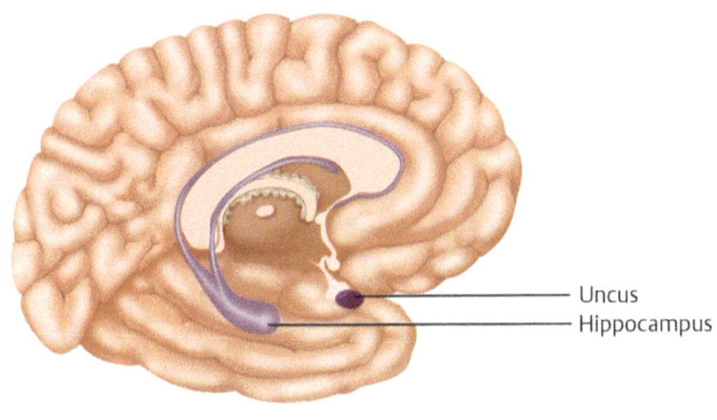

Fig. 3.14 Schematic demonstrating the anatomic relationships of the medial of the temporal lobe

The atrium as we know well is a triangular structure which points posteriorly at the occipital pole. Much of its posterior wall is made up of the splenium of the corpus callosum, a fact which is critical for removing posterior butterfly gliomas. The temporal horn which enters it contains the junction of the hippocampus and fornix, thus making the fusiform gyrus its floor. The optic radiations, superior longitudinal fasciculus, and inferior frontal-occipital fasciculus make up its lateral wall with the optic radiations comprising its immediate ependymal surface.

The anterior wall of the atrium contains a number of critical structures. The majority of this wall is made up of thalamus. The lateral extent of this wall is a complex structure where the posterior temporal gyri join to the white matter at the posterior edge of the insula. Deep to this, we find the posterior portion of the posterior limb of the internal capsule where it is most vulnerable. Slightly anterior to this is the putamen. The optic radiations and auditory radiations are escaping the thalamic geniculate nuclei near this point also.

As we move superficially, we see the surface structures which roughly overly the junctional anatomy. People have a tendency to confuse the angular and supramarginal gyrus so its key to understand them clearly. As the Sylvian fissure reaches its posterior extent, it indents a parietotemporal gyrus which is the supramarginal gyrus. Thus, the supramarginal gyrus is in part a continuation of the superior temporal gyrus, and it principally a posteriorly located opercular cortex. The superior temporal sulcus, running underneath the superior temporal gyrus, hooks posterosuperiorly behind the supramarginal gyrus and indents the angular gyrus. The angular gyrus is partially a continuation of the middle temporal gyrus, so not surprisingly it overlies the atrium the same way the middle temporal gyrus overlies the temporal horn anteriorly.

Heschl's gyrus lies within the Sylvian fissure on the upper surface of the supramarginal gyrus' temporal side. Its posterior end points at the atrium at its depth.

The supramarginal and angular gyri are c-shaped, so their limiting sulci are similarly c-shaped, which can be confusing to the uninitiated when removing portions of these gyri near the back of the insula and the TPO junction. Both of these sulci are roughly funnel shaped, and point inferomedially towards the back of the insula. This last point cannot be stressed enough as it is a common route of spread for these tumors, and it can be quite confusing to the uninitiated.

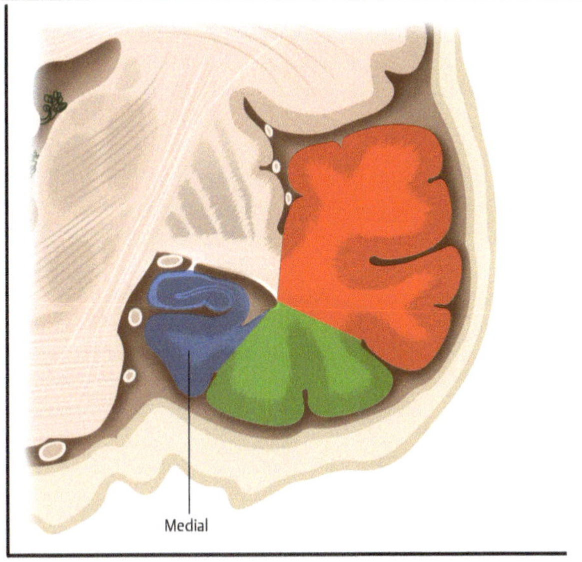

Fig. 3.15 Schematic demonstrating a coronal section through the temporal lobe demonstrating the relationship between the medial temporal structures and the central core.

3.6.3 Functional Considerations of the Temporal Lobe

Much of the temporal lobe is well known to be removable without severe neurologic problems. The specific functions of the amygdala and hippocampus in memory and emotion are well known to most readers, and I will not dwell on this.

Most of the neurologic function of the temporal lobe is located posteriorly near the TPO junction and the posterior Sylvian fissure (▶ Fig. 3.16). The left side in most patients contains the so-called Wernicke's area, which roughly surrounds the primary auditory cortex in Heschl's gyrus. One only needs to perform a search for the term "Wernicke's area" to see the extreme imprecision and variability with which this area is defined in anatomic drawings.

A better way to think of the lateral surface of the posterior temporal lobe is as the semantic network. Semantic memory is a collection of known facts about the world, such as the name of objects, the function of tools, the meaning of nonverbal expressions, and on the right side, probably the visual appearance of various objects as necessary to define one object as distinct from another. Thus the semantic network is as a library of varying extent which roughly extends outward from Heschl's gyrus, involving the MTG, the STG, and in most people into the supramarginal gyrus, and even the angular gyrus. This library which may cover a 1–3 discrete areas of the superior temporal gyrus, or which may extend over much of the superior and middle temporal gyrus. Destruction of the entire semantic network, will cause problems with comprehension; however, anything short of this usually causes expressive speech problems, anomia, or both. The idea that there is a small discrete area of cortex which can be damaged to cause pure receptive aphasia is neurosurgical fantasy which will cause one to approach brain mapping wrong. I have never caused this problem resecting a glioma. Stop thinking about it, as it is not the way the brain works.

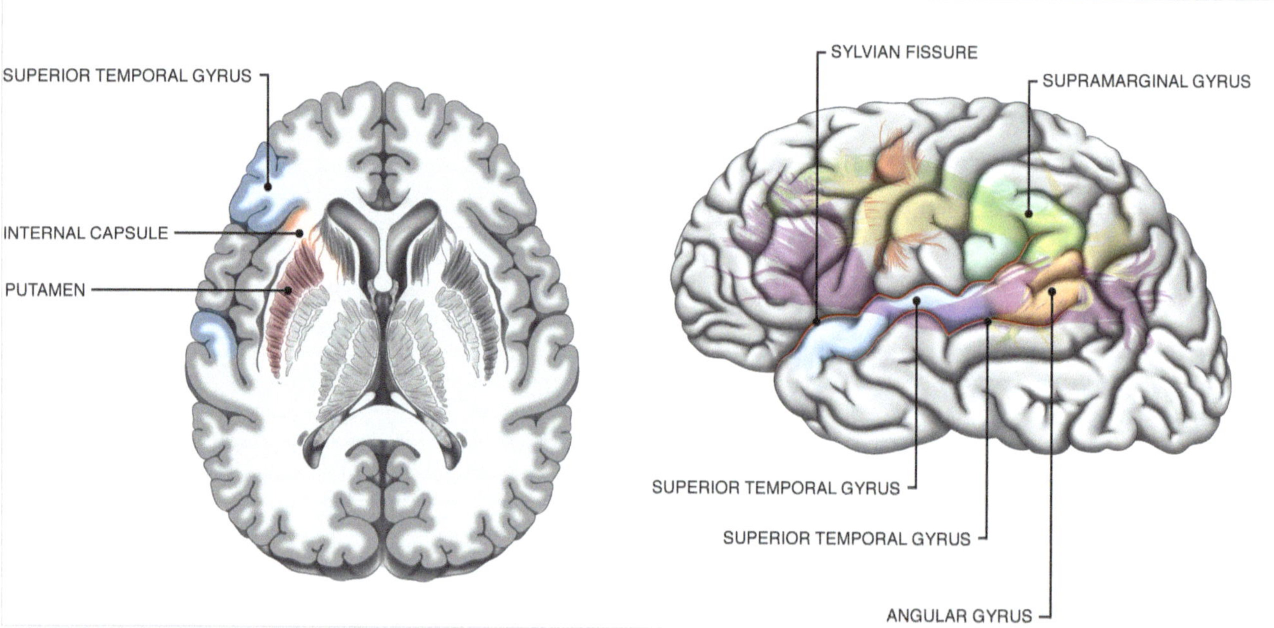

Fig. 3.16 Schematic demonstrating the anatomic relationships of various structures within the temporo-parieto-occipital (TPO) junction

Much more on these issues follows in subsequent chapters.

3.6.4 Important Distinctions in Temporal Lobe Glioma Anatomy

Misinterpreting the exact anatomy of a glioma in the temporal lobe is one of the most common pitfalls I have seen in failed surgical efforts in glioma surgery. Specific areas of the temporal lobe can be greatly enlarged and distorted which can give the false impression that there is tumor in a part of the brain where there is not. Failure to persist in your resection until validated by the identification of clear anatomic boundaries is a common reason why a large amount of tumor is missed in some cases.

A common mistake is to misjudge the exact position of the Sylvian fissure in cases expanding the lateral temporal lobe. The fissure can be pushed upward by pure tumor bulk (▸ Fig. 3.17) or the superior temporal gyrus can be distorted by tumor involvement. Careful attention to this detail, and observation of the position of the superficial middle cerebral vein can combat this common issue.

Involvement of the fusiform gyrus (▸ Fig. 3.18) can be difficult to distinguish from hippocampal involvement, and they often occur together making this a moot point. However, fusiform gyrus tumors tend to extend preferentially posteriorly along the inferior longitudinal fasciculus, whereas hippocampal tumors follow the fornix or the cingulum. By noting this minor detail, you can focus your efforts on the appropriate direction of anatomic extension.

Hippocampal gliomas are common (▸ Fig. 3.19) and often misinterpreted. The hippocampus can be massive, and often compresses the descending motor fibers superiorly. A study of the coronal images is often helpful at determining the exact location of the deep structures. The tumor tends to extend along the fornix or parahippocampal gyrus or both. Some very enlarged fornices can give the untrained eye the impression that there is invasion of the thalamus or internal capsule, as seen in ▸ Fig. 3.19), but awareness of the tumors nature as a hippocampal glioma, and not a TPO junctional glioma makes this pattern more obvious.

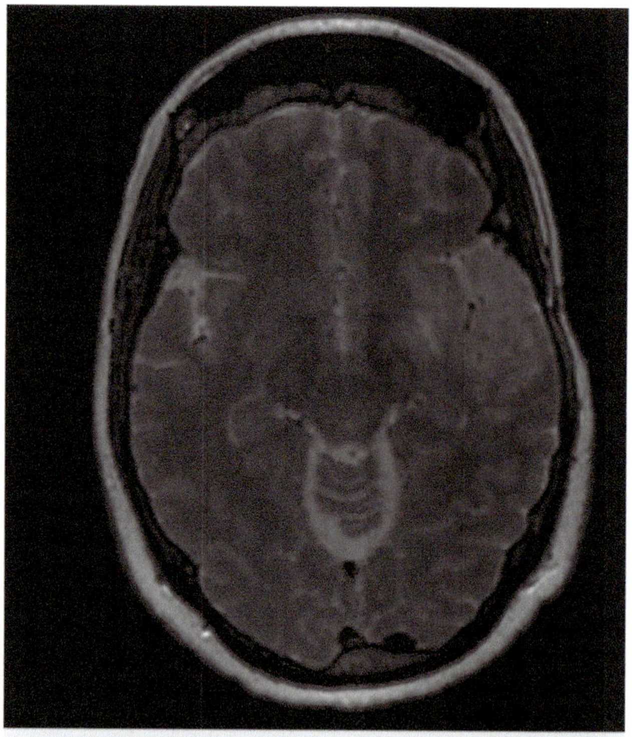

Fig. 3.17 Images from a glioma located within the superior temporal gyrus.

Tumors at the TPO junction are far more complex. Because of the complex anatomy of the supramarginal gyrus, and the narrow depth of the insula at this posterior limit, it can be quite hard

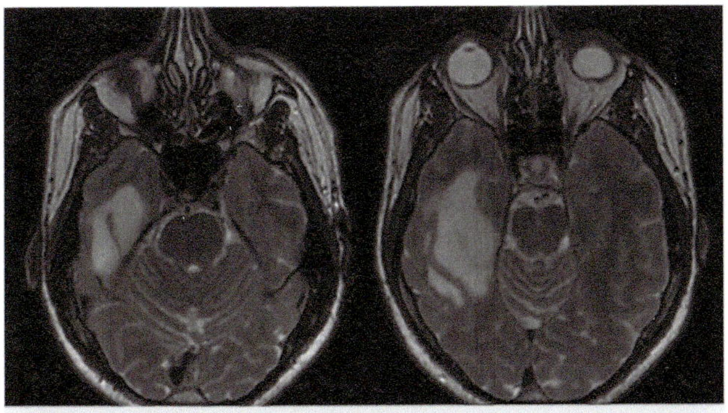

Fig. 3.18 Images from a glioma located within the fusiform gyrus of the inferior temporal surface.

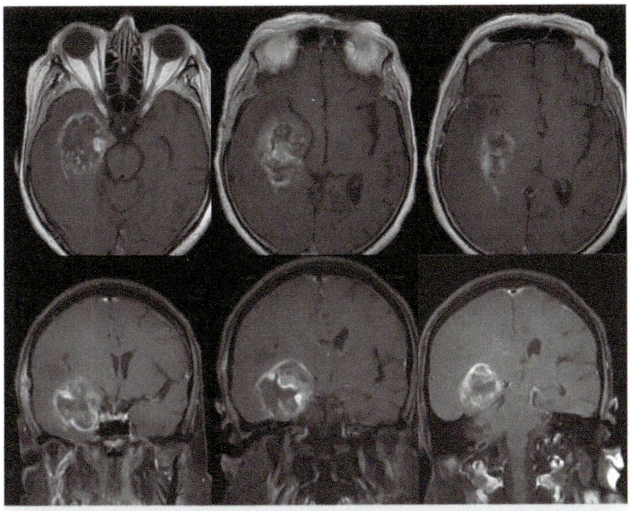

Fig. 3.20 Images from a glioma of the hippocampus and temporal lobe. This tumor appears to involve the internal capsule or basal ganglia on the upper axial images; however, careful examination of the coronal images demonstrates that it is merely pushing them upward, and likely fills the atrium as opposed to invading the deep brain.

to tell which lobe these tumors arise from. This is discussed in more detail after discussing the insula and parietal lobe.

3.7 Anatomy of the Insula

The insula is a roughly triangular lobe which is covered by brain. It is commonly thought to be somewhat rectangular, but this is probably an incorrect way of thinking about it, because the inferior limb of the insula gently curves superiorly and posteriorly to meet up with the posterior limb of the superior border.

The insula is thus roughly a right triangle with (a) a superior limb heading anterior to posterior under the IFG, the motor and sensory cortices and the upper SMG, (b) an anterior limb running downward into the limen insula down to the M1-M2 bend, and (c) an inferior limb (the hypotenuse) which runs under the SMG and STG to join the anterior-inferior, and posterior-superior corners of this triangle.

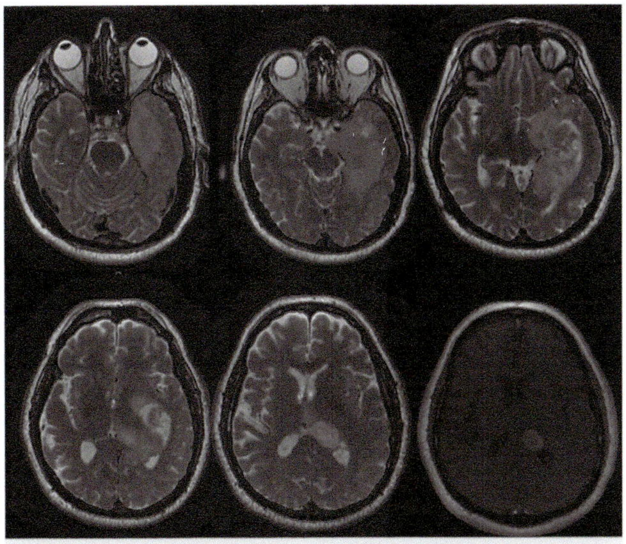

Fig. 3.19 Images from a glioma located within the hippocampus. The hippocampus is markedly expanded and there is a small area of enhancing tumor behind the thalamus. Careful examination demonstrates that this is tumor involvement of the fornix tracking behind the thalamus.

There are numerous long and short gyri which all point at the Sylvian valecula; however, I am skeptical these can be identified in any surgery where you have a legitimate reason to be working in the insula, as they are usually distorted (▶ Fig. 3.20). The more helpful anatomic landmark is the circular sulcus, which surrounds the insula on all sides and its critical to visualize if you wish to ensure an excellent insular resection.

Deep to the insula is the putamen, which itself lies superior to the temporal horn, a key landmark for staying out of it.

The insula lies at the bottom of the Sylvian fissure, and this fissure becomes less deep as you follow it from anterior to posterior. At the back, the deep portions of the supramarginal gyrus dive inward towards the back of the insula, making navigating this area quite challenging.

3.8 Surface Anatomy of the Parietal Lobe

The lateral surface of the parietal lobe (▶ Fig. 3.21) is made up of the superior parietal lobule and the inferior parietal lobule. The latter is made up of the supramarginal gyrus (SMG) and the angular gyrus. Both of these gyri are the c-shaped continuation of the STG and MTG respectively. It is critical to note, however, that the SMG is entirely anterior to the angular gyrus. These two lobules are separated by the intraparietal sulcus, which intersects the post-central sulcus at a right angle (similar to the superior frontal sulcus) (▶ Fig. 3.22).

The SMG is a conical gyrus with its point angling anteromedially towards the back of the insula. The Angular gyrus is similarly organized with its apex pointing at the STG (a preview of its white matter connections). A final observation is that the superior limb of the SMG heads anterior to blend into the sensory strip.

The medial bank of the parietal lobe contains the superior parietal lobule and the small subparietal gyrus below it, which make up the anterior portion of the medial parietal lobe, and the precuneus, which makes up the posterior half of this lobe. The precuneus is separated from the cuneus by the parietooccipital sulcus, which defines the boundary between the parietal and occipital lobes. The posterior segment of the cingulate gyrus runs around the splenium in the inferomedial parietal lobe on its way to the parahippocampal gyrus. This posterior bend is termed the isthmus (▶ Fig. 3.23).

3.8.1 Functional Considerations of the Parietal Lobe

The parietal lobe is classically associated with spatiotemporal functioning. This is largely due to the observation that injury to the parietal lobe causes neglect, and due to the large number of observations in monkeys and humans indicating activation of parietal neurons with orienting and navigational tasks. I will argue throughout this book that while these are clearly functions of the parietal lobe, that the parietal lobe is far more complex and essential to higher brain function that spatiotemporal function alone (▶ Fig. 3.24).

The SMG is part of the semantic network and as such, lies in the center of a number of functional networks, notably speech, praxis, and neglect. Together, with the angular gyrus, the inferior parietal lobule represents a structure not present in monkeys, highlighting its unique role in higher brain function (▶ Fig. 3.25).

The superior parietal lobule and the banks of the intraparietal sulcus, contain higher processing centers for spatial orientation. One simple explanation of their function is as a converter of visual information into a code usable by the motor planning areas. The precuneus contains higher visual processing areas involved in the dorsal visual processing stream.

The retrosplenial cingulate gyrus and the nearby parietal lobe contain the posterior components of the default mode network (▶ Fig. 3.26).

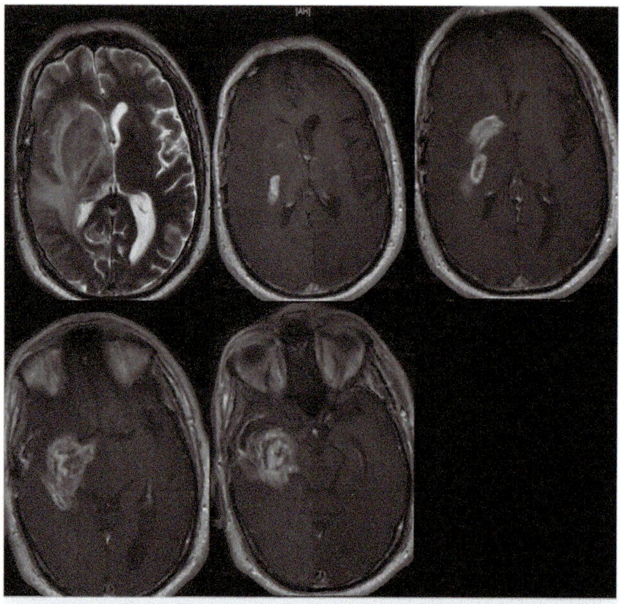

Fig. 3.21 Images from a glioma of the temporal lobe which has true involvement of the deeper structures above.

3.8.2 Important Distinctions in Parietal Lobe Glioma Anatomy

Despite the presence of only 6 named gyri in the entire lobe, it can be quite challenging to distinguish one parietal lobe glioma from another. This is especially true in the inferior parietal lobule. One such challenging example is seen in ▶ Fig. 3.27. This large GBM is located in the inferior parietal lobule as indicated by the fact that it is lateral to the intraparietal sulcus. However, it is somewhat too anterior to be obviously located in the angular gyrus, but the preserved sulcal c-shaped boundary suggests that it is not purely in the SMG. ▶ Fig. 3.28 demonstrates a tumor more obviously in the SMG, but its deep location raises the question if this is truly an SMG tumor, or arising from the periventricular white matter.

A more obvious angular gyrus tumor is provided in ▶ Fig. 3.29.

Posterior cingulate tumors can occur in isolation or as part of a parietal tumor, but either way they are easy to mistake for a medial parietal glioma. ▶ Fig. 3.30 demonstrates a posterior cingulate glioma which highlights the importance of studying sulcal boundaries especially on multiple imaging planes. Here the sagittal cut gives away that this is a posterior cingulate tumor.

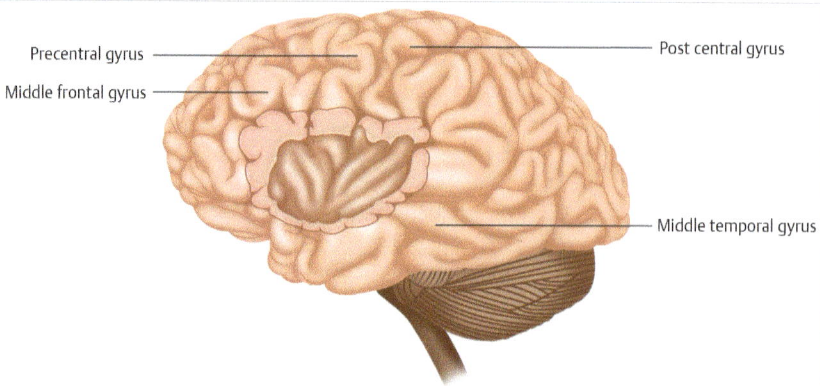

Fig. 3.22 Schematic demonstrating the gross anatomy of the insular surface

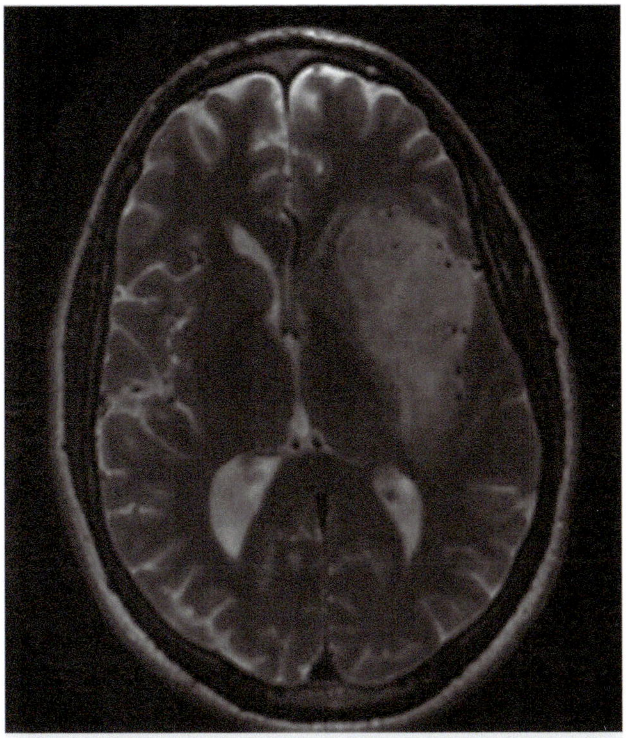

Fig. 3.23 Images from a glioma located within the insula.

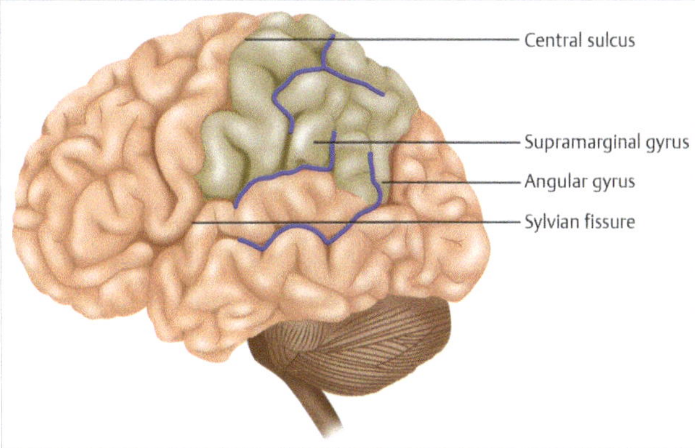

Fig. 3.24 Schematic demonstrating the lateral surface anatomy of the parietal lobe, and the gyri and sulci.

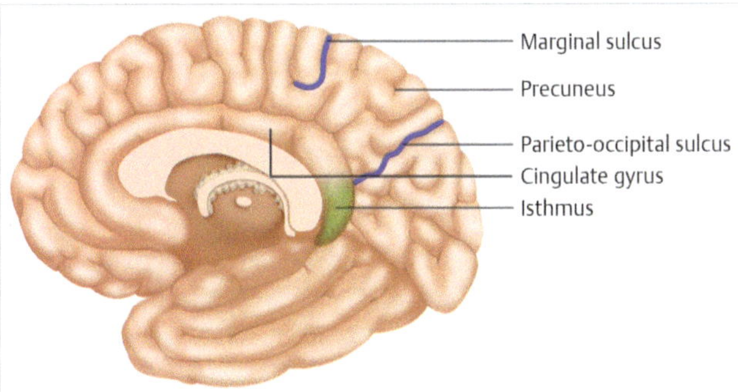

Fig. 3.25 Schematic demonstrating the medial surface anatomy of the parietal lobe, and the gyri and sulci.

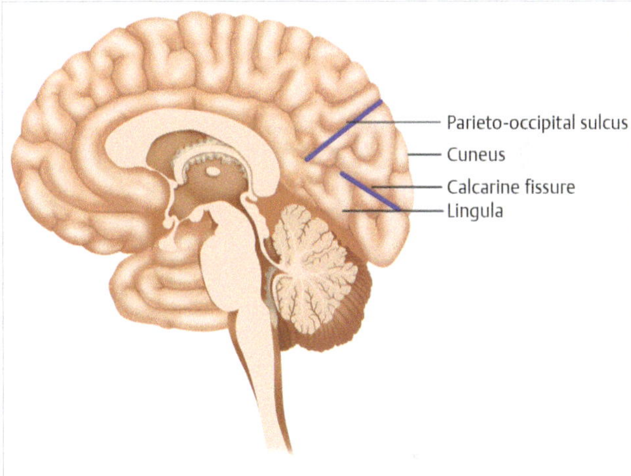

Fig. 3.26 Schematic demonstrating the cortical location linked to various neurologic functions within the parietal lobe.

3.9 Surface Anatomy of the Occipital Lobe

This is a short section, as the occipital lobe has simple surface anatomy, because much of it is inconsistent, and this does not lend itself to detailed descriptions.

The occipital lobe (▶ Fig. 3.31) is a three-sided pyramid pointing posterior and inferior towards the torcula. The lateral surface has inconsistent gyral anatomy and is best thought of as a single unit. The inferior surface contains continuations of the inferior temporal and fusiform gyri. The medial surface is made up of the cuneus and the lingula which straddle the calcarine fissure. The lingula extends medial towards the isthmus of the posterior cingulate, which it joins to enter the parahippocampal gyrus. The cuneus in contrast, is a structure contained within the occipital lobe.

The only other noteworthy surface landmark in the occipital lobe is the pre-occipital notch, which consistently indents the inferolateral occipital surface. This notch causes a consistent deflection of the ILF and IFOF.

3.9.1 Functional Considerations

The occipital lobe is almost entirely dedicated to visual processing. It is notable that this processing is known to proceed in two "streams": the dorsal "where" pathway and the ventral "what" pathway. The dorsal pathway proceeds superiorly to the upper border of the precuneus, and carries information about object position. The ventral pathway proceeds along the inferolateral occipital lobe where it eventually joins with the occipital temporal regions and carries information about object identity (▶ Fig. 3.32).

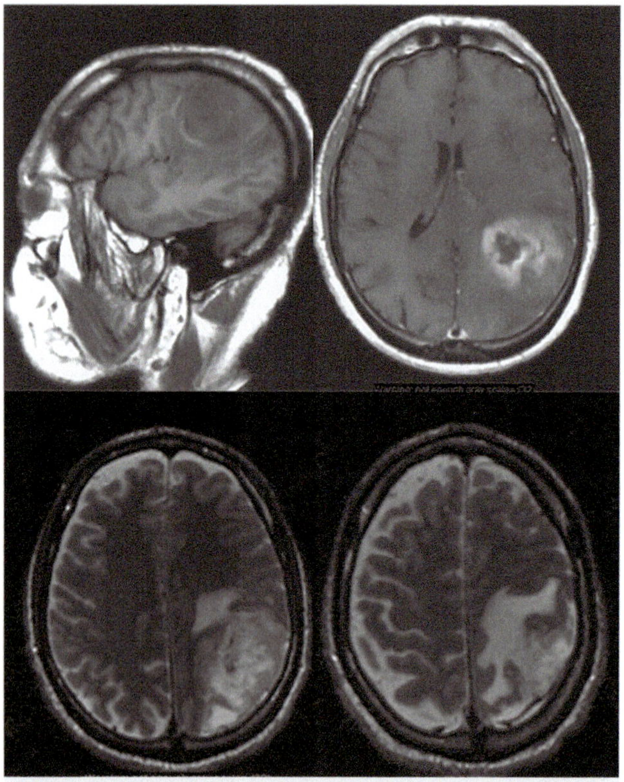

Fig. 3.27 Images from a glioma located within the inferior parietal lobule, probably from the superior portion of the supramarginal gyrus.

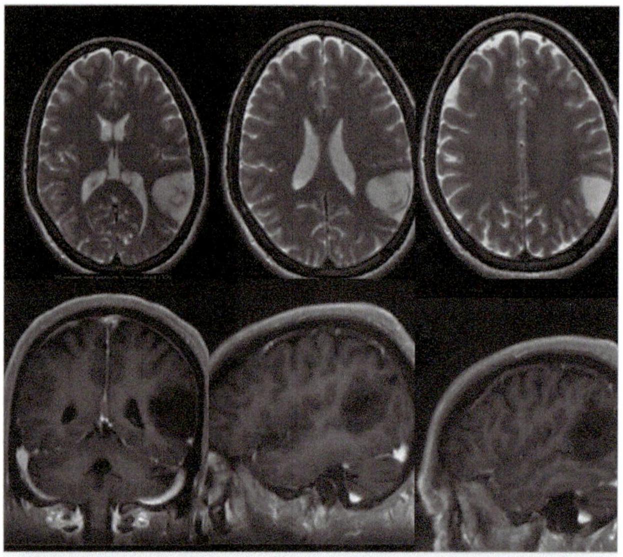

Fig. 3.29 Images from a glioma located within the angular gyrus.

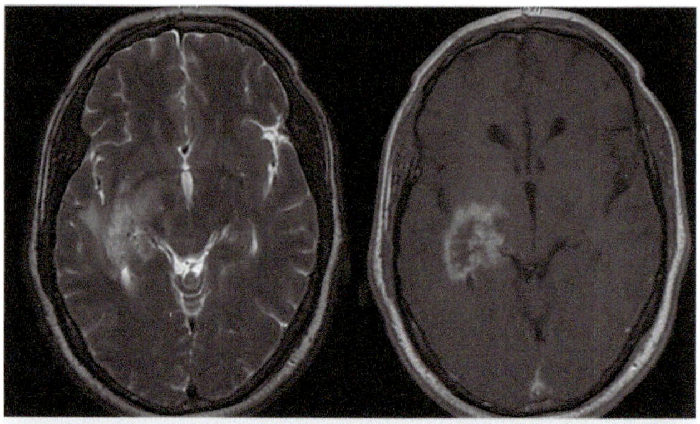

Fig. 3.28 Images from a glioma located within the deep portion of the supramarginal gyrus.

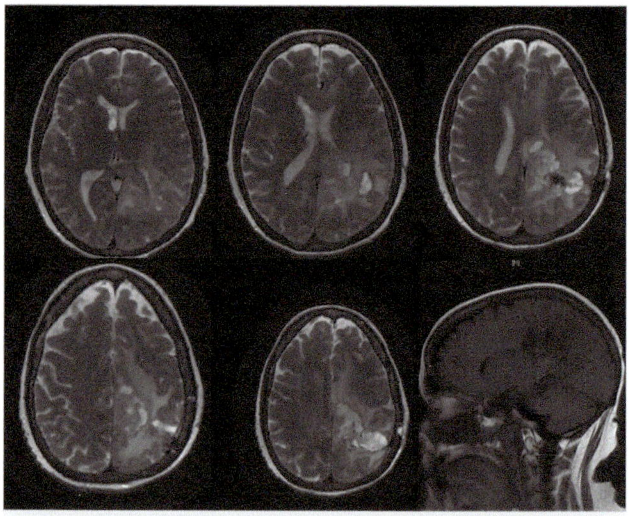

Fig. 3.30 Images from a glioma located within the posterior cingulate gyrus. Similar to the anterior cingulate, these tumors are most obvious on the coronal and sagittal images.

3.9.2 Important Distinctions in Occipital Lobe Glioma Surgery

Due to the relative lack of reliable sulcal landmarks, I limit classification of occipital lobe tumors to their involved surface. A lateral occipital tumor is demonstrated in ▶ Fig. 3.33.

3.10 Deep Cerebral Anatomy

As stated above, the relationships between basal ganglia, thalamus, internal capsule and other deep structures have been demonstrated in detail more beautifully by others than I can do myself. In many ways, the exact relationships are largely unimportant to glioma surgery; it is almost always a good idea to not be in the basal ganglia or thalamus without a good reason. Thankfully, these tumors are uncommon; for some reason gliomas tend to stay out of the basal ganglia most of the time, I have noticed. Chapter 14 discusses some advice for those few times when it is necessary to enter the deep structures.

What follows are a few observations about this anatomy, which are relevant to the other parts of the book, and which are not generally noted in basic anatomy text books.

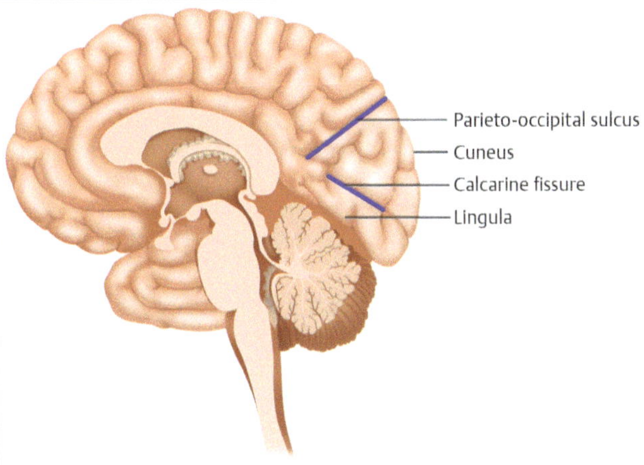

Fig. 3.31 Schematic demonstrating cortical anatomy of the occipital lobe.

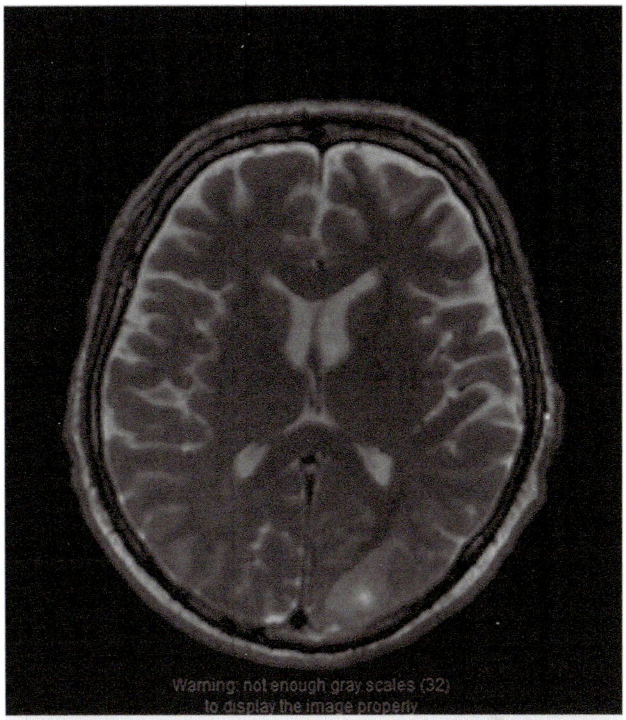

Fig. 3.32 Images from a glioma located within the lateral occipital lobe.

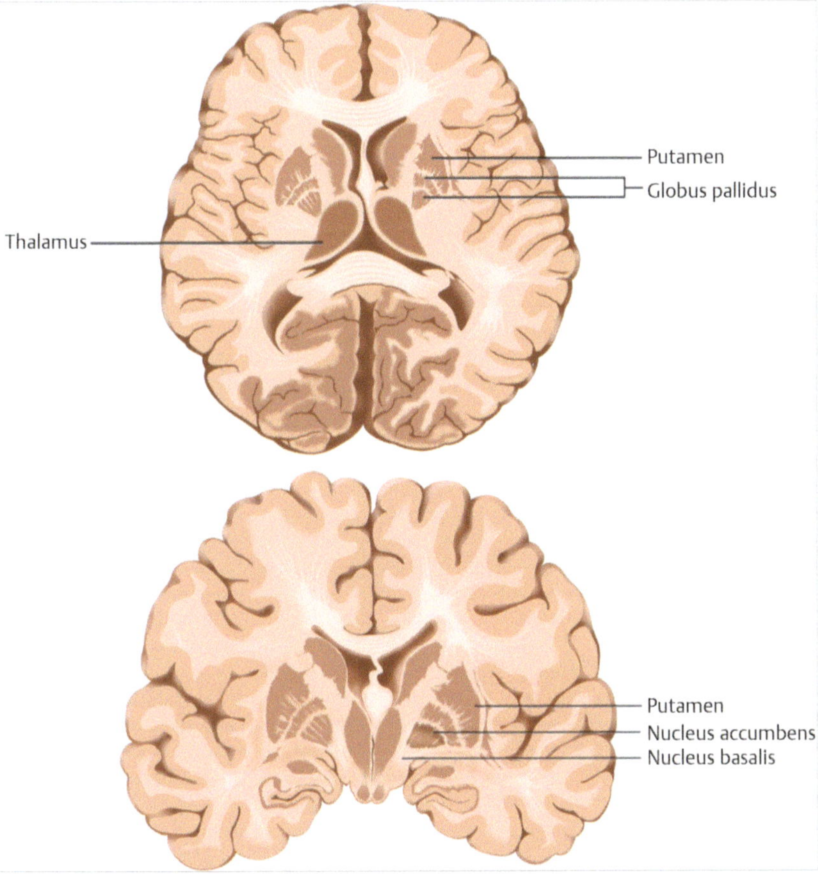

Fig. 3.33 Schematic demonstrating relationships between the basal ganglia and deep structures with the rest of the cerebrum.

1. The putamen lies directly above the temporal horn.
2. The insula is lateral to the putamen across its entire lateral surface.
3. The posterior limb of the internal capsule is deep to the putamen and lateral to the thalamus.
4. The posterior limb of the internal capsule starts medially in its anterior aspect, but by the time it reaches its posterior aspect, it is relatively laterally, and the back of the internal capsule nearly abuts in the insula near the atrium.
5. The lateral wall of the lateral ventricle is indented by the caudate nucleus and the thalamus.
6. The caudate nucleus directly overlies the anterior perforated substance. This means that as long as you are working anterior to the caudate head, you are not encountering them and the arteries you see are local ACA branches.
7. The basal forebrain structures (such as the nucleus basalis and the nucleus accumbens) are lateral and inferior to the caudate head.
8. The septal nuclei lie in the medial frontal lobe just below the rostrum of the corpus callosum.
9. The thalamus directly overlies the midbrain tegmentum, stressing the need to remain above this during thalamic surgery.
10. If you draw a six-sided cube as follows you will completely enclose the deep structures, (a) the bottom of the cube is the axial plane running through the roof of the temporal horn, (b) the top of the cube is the axial plane extending through the superior insular boundary (i.e., the top of the circular sulcus) to the body of the corpus callosum, (c) the anterior face is a coronal plane which extends from the limen insula in front of the caudate head, (d) the posterior face is a coronal plane through the atrium of the lateral ventricle, (e) the lateral face is a sagittal plane which follows the surface of the insular cortex, and (f) the lateral face is a sagittal plane which parallels the lateral wall of the lateral and third ventricles. This "cube of safety" should mentally guide you in what you should think twice about before entering. This is not to say you cannot cause problems outside of the cube, but at minimum, you are avoiding disconnecting these structures from each other or cutting across their key peduncles (▶ Fig. 3.34).

3.10.1 Functional Considerations of the Deep Structures

Basically, almost all higher brain functions require signaling through the basal ganglia and thalamus. Thus, any surgery inside of them must be undertaken with extreme caution.

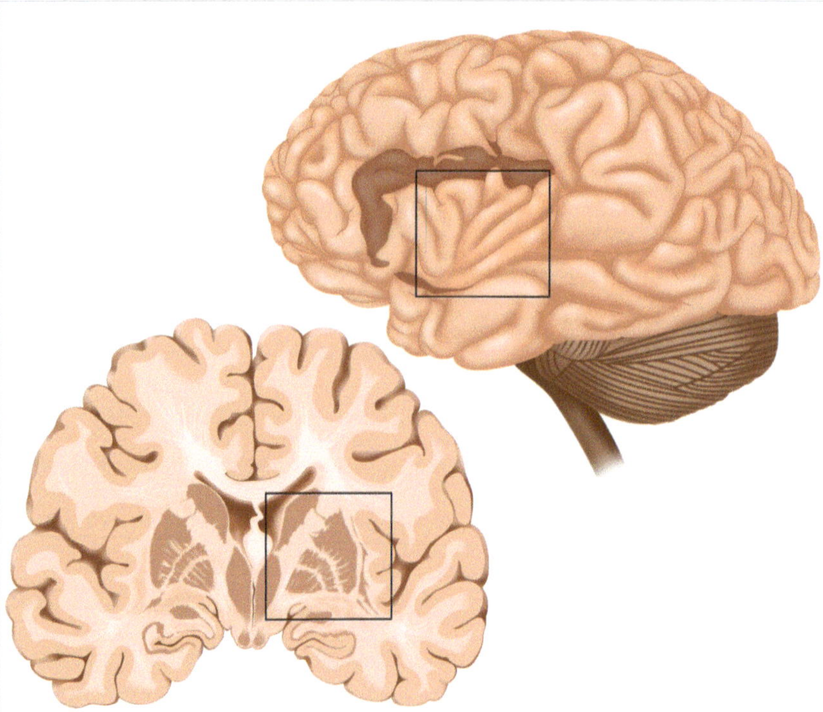

Fig. 3.34 Schematic demonstrating the "cube of safety." This "cube" demonstrates the boundaries of the portions of the cerebrum containing the deep structures such as the basal ganglia and thalamus. This is not to say that working outside the "cube" guarantees safety, or that being in it is always bad, just that visualizing this central core is helpful for thinking about how to avoid inadvertently entering these areas without knowing it.

3.10.2 Important Distinctions in Deep Glioma Surgery

As stated earlier, not all tumors in the deep areas involve the brain structures you think they do and you should examine the T2 image closely. ▸ Fig. 3.35 demonstrates an example of a tumor which legitimately lies within the putamen, which should be contrasted with other junctional temporal or SMG tumors which do not actually involve the basal ganglia.

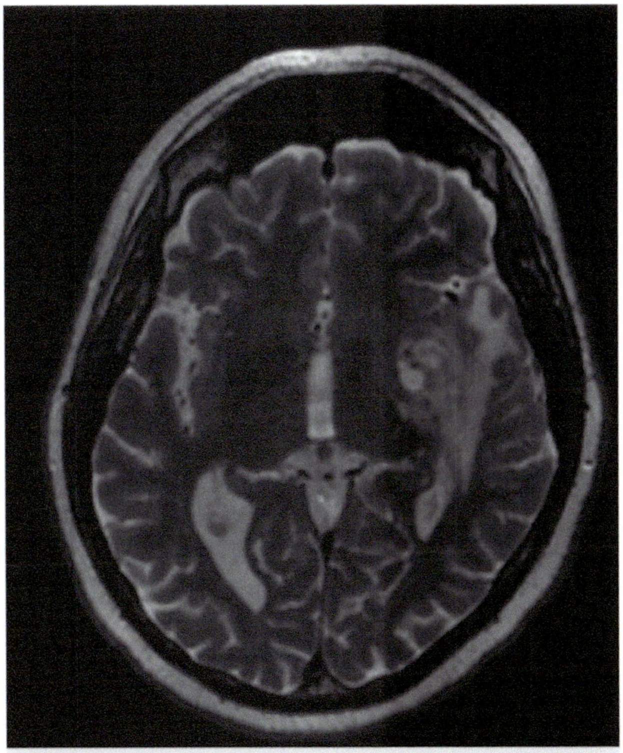

Fig. 3.35 Images from a glioma located within the basal ganglia. We have shown many examples of tumors which appear to be in the deep brain, but are not, and it is notable that gliomas often avoid entering the basal ganglia. This tumor provides an example of the exception to this rule.

4 An Introduction to Macroconnectomic Networks in Cerebral Surgery

4.1 Introduction

Macroconnectomics and functional network based thinking are the foundation of rational decision making in glioma surgery and this book and philosophy are based on them. So it is probably worth defining the terms early.

The term connectomics refers to efforts to create a connectional map of the human cerebrum. Such efforts are ambitious and likely will yield key insights into how human cognition works. However, they are of limited clinical utility at present. Beyond just the fact that they are not done, they provide a level of detail and complexity that we cannot really harness with our hands or our minds to drive surgical efforts. Until we have better lasers or better brains, we cannot use this much information to make the kind of decisions we need to make in a pinch.

Macroconnectomics is a term we coined at our center to describe the kind of connectomics we were studying in our efforts to do better brain surgery, which is connectional anatomy involving bulk information flow though large connections. In other words, we were not aiming to know every single neuronal connection, but rather the big connections and the important ones. The rationale for the macroconnectomic approach is threefold. First, the practical ability to utilize a brain map with billions of mapped connections is limited without technological advances in other areas to work at that scale. Second, it will likely be some time before a map of that complexity will be complete and annotated, and in the meantime we have a very poor understanding of even major brain connections underlying elemental brain functions such as speech, vision, and attention, so it is probably best to first work on the lower parts of Maslow's hierarchy of needs and fix the massive knowledge gaps necessary for daily practice of brain surgery prior to aiming for perfect models. Finally, it seems unlikely to me that there is a single neuron in any place in the brain that can be cut to cause a deficit, especially one that cannot recover. In other words, clinically relevant deficits generally require a significant number of neurons to be taken offline in a network before they become evident.

In short, during a macroconnectomic glioma surgery, our goal is to understand a functional network and its major connections, and to perform resections in a way that the network maintains its function.

Thinking in terms of functional networks in brain surgery means planning and executing brain surgery with the idea that higher cognitive functions require the coordination of several brain structures, each of which contribute a subprocessing component to the overall successful end output, and that functional preservation requires anatomic preservation of these structures and their interconnections.

The idea that certain complex brain functions are located in a single place or two places, is contradicted by functional imaging data which shows multiple co-activated areas during most higher tasks, by neuro-psychological data showing complex and subtle variations of neuropsychological syndromes (i.e., aphasia, apraxia, etc.) with varying injuries of often distant parts of the brain, and by the experience of most of us who have noted neuro-psychologic consequences of our surgery that "don't make sense." I would suggest that when a patient has a neuro-psychologic deficit that "doesn't make sense," that often an explanation can be found by thinking of the function in terms of a network, as opposed to thinking of brain functions being localized to a single part of the brain, or a specific gyrus.

4.2 An Introduction to Complexity and Cerebral Networks

For over a century, neurosurgery has been working in the cerebrum with a model of the brain that not only is incorrect, but I would argue cannot possibly be a basically correct view of the brain. Localizationism, the idea that certain functions are performed by specific parts of the brain, like many outdated models, does lead to some often good predictions, for example primary motor functions are usually found in the precentral gyrus in most people. However, such a model will fail one if followed blindly off the cliff, especially in patients who reorganize, and it has minimal ability to work towards a world where we do not unintentionally damage higher cognitive functions, which do not fit the ideas put forward by this model. I put forward the idea that for neurosurgery to improve our outcomes, we need to embrace "complexity" and begin to restructure our ideas around the idea that we are cutting around functional networks.

The term "complex" does not merely signify that a system has a lot of parts, that it is difficult to study, or that it is poorly understood. A cell phone is complicated; it is not "complex." Formally defined, the term "complex systems" refers to large networks of diverse, interconnected, interdependent and adaptive parts. In other words, to be "complex" a system needs to have a network of interconnected entities which react to each other's activity, usually in nonlinear ways. Most of the persistent problems we face as a society: the behavior of the stock market; economics; global terrorism; neuroscience; the proteomics of cancer; and so on, have complexity as a predominant issue. In other words, we will have trouble improving our nonlinear complex problems with linear thinking. Of note, many of the earliest seminal papers in studying complexity are less than 20 years old, and presently the mathematics are in evolution.

"Complex" systems display some unique properties not seen in linear, randomly connected, or regularly interconnected systems. Most notable, complex systems demonstrate a property called emergence, which is when a "complex" network and its nonlinear dynamics, demonstrate behavior on the macro scale which cannot possibly be predicted a priori by the simple sum of the parts and their individual interactions. Higher cognitive functions, even consciousness itself, are emergent phenomenon which cannot be predicted simply by looking at the binary fire/don't fire nature of individual neuron action potentials.

Another feature of complex networks is the presence of power law mathematical distributions within their static and dynamic structures. While most variables which are influenced by multiple independent variables vary in normal or near normal distribution (i.e., a bell curve), complex systems often vary in a power law fashion, meaning that the distribution curve has a very long broad tail. Height is a variable influenced by numerous mostly independent influences, and it is roughly normally distributed. This means that as we move several standard deviations away from mean height, that the probability of finding extreme outliers approaches zero. For example, there has never been a 10-foot-tall person in recorded history, and a 20-foot or 100-foot-tall person would be unthinkable. If height were distributed as a power law, then 100-foot-tall people would be uncommon, but occasionally we would see one. This means that very extreme outliers are uncommon but possible.

The degree of connectedness of brain nodes (i.e., the number of other areas an area is connected to), doesn't perfectly conform to a power law distribution, but it is closer to a broad tailed distribution than a normal distribution. This means that while most areas of the brain are mainly connected to immediate neighbors, a few areas (so called hubs) are extremely interconnected to a large number of areas.

Final observations about complex networks are that they are robust. Deletion studies of brain networks, where nodes are removed from a network to determine the effect on the network, have shown that power law distributed networks are highly resilient to random deletions, meaning that the path length is relatively unchanged due to the loss of individual nodes. However, targeted attack on the most highly connected nodes cause the network to fragment at relatively low numbers of nodes deleted. The parallels between the eloquence versus non-eloquence binary which has long dominated our thinking is striking, and it provides a better model I think for thinking through the problem.

Robustness may also explain the early recovery of some neurologic problems (in addition to brains swelling resolution), as the network might figure a way to perform a cognitive task without the injured area. It might also be a key way gliomas cause the brain to reorganize.

4.3 Small World Networks

One of the seminal papers of the past 20 years in science was published by Watts and Strogatz in 1998 in a paper cited over 32,000 times at the time of this book's writing. In this simple, elegant study, they studied completely regular, lattice graphs (graphs where every node was initially only connected to its neighbors), and used computer simulation to randomly rewire one connection at a time. They found that the path length (meaning the mean number of connections distance between any two nodes in the graph) decreased in a steep nonlinear fashion dropping substantially when only a small fraction of the connections were rewired. They termed this the small world phenomenon, and it has been shown to be a common organization in diverse complex networks including the internet, social networks, and the brain. In other words, complexity is governed by common mathematical principles regardless of the area of study, and that mathematics is heavily driven by small world topology.

There is abundant evidence that brain networks follow small world patterns of organization. This means that the dominant mode of connectivity is modular, meaning most areas are most connected to their neighbors, with interconnections between modules principally linked through the highly connected nodes, occasionally with linker nodes whose main function is to ensure no lag synchronization between two distant areas which need to synchronize their activity.

Complex networks have been frequently shown to be self-organizing, meaning that they usually do not have a dominant area which drives the activity or static organization of the network. For example, who really can control the global activity of the stock market. The small world organization is a logical effect of the need for the brain to achieve its static and dynamic goals with a minimal consumption of energy. Statically, it is most efficient for areas to make the shortest axons possible, and most areas should thus be mainly connected to their neighbors. However, as Watts and Strogatz demonstrated, path length drops substantially with making a few long range connections. Path length in the brain equals the number of synapses, and the increasing synapse number needed for two distant areas to communicate, slows long range conduction, increases noise, and increases energy costs. Small world networks are the result of self-organization driven around these competing demands.

There are many ways to describe brain networks; however, the one presently most accessible to us for surgery, is to focus on major white matter pathways, as they are demonstrable and disproportionately central to the proper functioning of wide-scale brain networks. Given that these tracts are the principal method by which two modules of nodes talk to each other, it is reasonable to conclude that they play a disproportionate role per mL of tissue in cognitive function.

4.4 Static versus Dynamic Connectivity

It is tempting to look at brain networks and their architecture and try to deduce a direction of information flow, and to determine that this is showing us the master blueprint of how the brain works. The reality, as usual, is far more complex. Structural connections are meaningless without understanding function, and studies of functional connectivity has taught us that the functional connections of the brain are changing constantly. For example, standard resting state fMRI provides statistical evidence that two areas coactivate with each other more than chance, and this is the basis of determining the location of functional networks. However, more nuanced analyses of so-called dynamic functional connectivity, have shown that this approach is akin to opening the camera shutter at an auto race for a few minutes and then pointing to the strongest blurs. The brain is constantly altering its activity pattern depending on context and cognitive tasks, and while areas A and B may coactivate for some tasks, areas A, C, and D may need to co-activate for others.

Obviously, sorting out an already complex static network is hard enough without accounting for the thousands of possible metastable states for all situations. This is a work for supercomputers, and the mathematical tools for working this out are in evolution. It is critical to note that the dynamic configuration of brain activities is constrained by the possibilities of the static brain network. In other words, areas A, B, and C cannot talk to each other if they are not connected in some way, either directly, or indirectly. Until dynamic connectivity is better understood, it is at least a good idea not to disconnect key parts of the network from itself. However, we should always look towards the future that to truly understand how to improve our outcomes, we need to continuously improve our models of the brain. Further, it highlights the drastic need to abandon our old models.

4.5 Nodes, Edges, Hubs and Rich Clubs

Graph theoretical metrics are not presently clinically accessible to brain surgeons; however, I have long believed that eventually they will be as they have the promise to answer questions. Thus, a short digression to define terms is worth a few paragraphs of space.

A brain graph analysis reduces the connections of the brain to a ball and stick type graphical format comprised of nodes, which signify specific brain regions, and edges, which are the lines signifying the connections between them. It does not take a high level of exposure to the area to recognize that nodes are grey matter structures and edges are axons/white matter. The concept of how to define the best way to split the brain into nodes exactly is a contentious one, but in almost all systems, most of the nodes are parts of the cerebral cortex, with nodes in thalamic and other subcortical nuclei included in some graphs. Either way, while a graph does not necessarily reflect the nature of the transformations enacted by various nodes, it does allow some basic hypothesis testing on the overall organization of the connectome.

A key question in graph theory is the definition of a hub, in other words a node which is extensively connected to many other areas, and thus assumed to be the pathway involved in numerous systems. There are several ways to define such a hub. Degree centrality refers to the number of other nodes which connect to a node. This is simple, but ignores the fact that a connection to a highly connected node should count more than a connection to a peripheral low degree node. This is corrected by measures such as eigenvector centrality and page rank centrality which take connectivity of neighbors into account. Closeness and betweenness centrality consider the number of shortest paths through the graph which traverse a node. Further, highly connected nodes which are highly connected to each other comprise a so called "rich club."

Does "hubness" indicate parts of the brain we should avoid destroying and if so what measure is best? These are unknown and in need of study. Of note some of the more well known primary cortices, such as the primary motor cortex and primary visual area, are neither hubs nor in rich clubs. Others, like area 44, known for its role in language, definitely are. Based on mathematical measurements of random versus targeted attacks on broad scale networks (such as the brain) it is likely that preserving hubs are critical in preventing cognitive networks from collapsing; however, it is unclear which hubs, and what happens if you don't achieve this.

4.6 What Parts of the Brain are Truly Eloquent

For decades, neurosurgeons have divided the cerebral world into "eloquent" brain and "non-eloquent brain" with the dividing line being whether the brain was felt to do something clinically evident when you cut into, removed or damaged it. In this conceptual model of how cerebral functions are organized in the brain, areas such as the motor strip, where an injury would cause a motor deficit, are "eloquent" and thus best avoided, while other areas of the brain, such as the anterior right frontal lobe were more "silent" and safe to cut into.

This is a system for organizing brain function which is simple, easy to teach residents, and completely inconsistent with common sense and scientific studies. I would argue that there are probably no legitimately "silent" areas of the brain. All parts of the brain probably did not evolve as a decoration, a CSF sponge, or a shock absorber, but rather evolved to perform some neurologic function. Thus, all parts of the brain are eloquent in some way and are doing something. If you are skeptical of this, spend some time talking to a family member of someone who has had a large amount of right frontal lobe damage, and you will probably become convinced that there are consequences to losing this part of your brain, they just are not glaringly obvious immediately after surgery in the recovering room.

This is not to argue that brain function is randomly distributed, or that some parts of the cortex are not more tolerant of injury than others. No inaccurate scientific model persists for years without at least some explanatory power. It's just that the model we work under presently fails to prevent neurologic problems, often especially with higher brain functions, and often with systems like motor and language.

A better explanation, again comes from network and complexity science. Studies of small world networks suggest that the problem is just more complex than that will break under our efforts to think through the problem, but rather requires the work of computers to deal with the massive parallel nature and complexity of the brain. Likely different nodes need to coordinate with different networks under different contexts in order to achieve specific goals.

4.7 How Is Brain Surgery Possible if That's True?

Of course, we know from years of experience that not all cuts in the brain lead to clinically apparent problems. Further, I am not trying to argue that we should leave glioblastoma in the brain for fear that the whole brain is eloquent. Instead I am arguing that we should make these kind of decisions based on the idea that all brain removal involves a tradeoff between tumor removal and potential functional consequences. Additionally, given the potential that a brain area could be involved in function of a network centered in a distant part of the brain, this trade off should be based on a more nuanced appraisal of the exact organization of the functional network than what the "eloquent" vs "noneloquent" model can yield. In other words, we have to remove part of the brain to remove a glioma; we should just base the decision about what part to remove based on a realistic assessment of risks to the neighboring brain networks, versus the relative benefit of cytoreduction in a specific brain area.

This tradeoff has been termed the "onco-functional balance" by Hughes Duffau, and I would argue that this is the single most important aspect of glioma surgery if it is applied rationally. Brain mapping, white matter tractography, and macroconnectomic knowledge used rationally, are all tools for balancing the anatomic and functional considerations of a specific case, and ultimately for making informed choices how far to go, where to cut, and when to stop.

It is important to note that as our understanding of cerebral functional anatomy, network organization, and macroconnectomics becomes more sophisticated, that the idea that some parts of the brain are completely without consequence or functional risk to operate in becomes problematic and should be replaced with a view that we are trying to minimize the functional consequences of surgery, and to leave functional networks as able to produce their end product as possible given the functional and oncologic starting points of a specific patient.

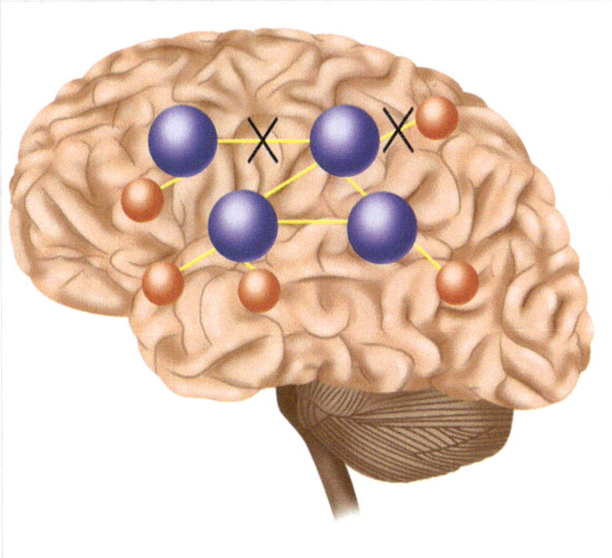

Fig. 4.1 A schematic demonstrating the concept of hodotopy in the organization of functional networks. In this conceptual framework, a functional network is made of essential hubs of the network (in blue), the associated (but ultimately not essential) nodes (in red), and their interconnections. While removal or disconnection of any part of the network can cause neurologic deficits in the short term, loss of the associated nodes (red) can ultimately be compensated for if the essential hubs (blue) are preserved. Thus, glioma surgery aims not to avoid neurologic deficits, but to leave the patient with a network which can recover ultimately.

4.7.1 Hodotopy

Hodotopy refers to the idea that a functional network may contain multiple parallel interconnected sites, but that some parts of the network may be more critical than others. ▶ Fig. 4.1 demonstrates a schematic of an idealized hodotopic functional network, comprised of central in expendable hubs, peripheral, possibly expendable, nodes and white matter interconnections. This is not to say there is absolutely no consequence to removing a peripheral node. I would argue that there is often great short term consequence to doing so, and would propose that in some cases, the temporary deficits that we have often chalked up to "brain swelling," may in fact be the effect of removing a node on overall network functioning, and that resolution of deficits, which in cases takes weeks and can extend beyond the typical time course of resolution of brain swelling, is in fact the network learning to compensate for the loss of a node. The possibility of mixed effects of this phenomenon and brain swelling is likely, and this is obviously a difficult concept to study and answer with confidence with current technology.

Thus, when trying to preserve a hodotopic network, we must understand which brain structures represent the hubs, in other words that which is essential and cannot be compensated for, and which are not. Similarly, networks often have multiple interconnections, which may or may not all be essential, and thus preserving the network our goal may not be avoidance of any white matter sectioning, but rather informed sectioning which avoids cutting essential connections in the network. In this way of thinking, brain mapping can be rethought as a systematic approach of studying the essentiality of different cortical and subcortical structures for the proper functioning of a network and for the production of its end output. In other words, brain mapping is a method for pruning a network while leaving the essential hubs and connections.

One flaw in ▶ Fig. 4.1 is that it suggests that if two connections exist between two hubs, that one of them may be redundant. This is incorrect in many cases because it is not always the case that both connections are carrying the same information. Parallel processing of different aspects of the same genre of information (for example visual information, language related information) is well described, and the role of certain brain structures in comparing information from two or more sources to modulate other outputs is also well known in neuroscience. Dual pathways

Finally, it is important to get our minds around what kind of structures can constitute a hub, and what a hub actually contributes to a network. The most obvious hubs are end effectors and primary cortices. For example, the primary motor cortex for hand is a hub in a number of systems, notably motor control and praxis, as the ability to control fine movements is essential to both functions. Similarly, injury to the primary somatosensory cortex, eliminates the contribution of this hub to the motor control system, the spatiotemporal system, and even to systems such as sematic speech as it can eliminate the ability to recognize objects by tactile cues. Thus, while these systems may be able to function to a degree without some of this input, they may not function normally.

Another type of hub is association type cortices. The contribution of association cortices to a network can be less obvious than primary cortices, as not all things termed "association cortex" in the textbooks are inviolable hubs and the deficits caused by these are not always obvious, especially without advanced neuropsychological testing. This is probably why our conceptions of brain organization have viewed these areas as "noneloquent," because they are not as obvious when there is a problem, and they can be compensated for in many instances. But association cortices are clearly hubs in many neurofunctional systems, and taking them offline in a network can cause complex problems that can be hard to figure out. Every time a family member describes strange behavior, bad judgment, or other things that in traditional neurosurgical outcome accounting would be called "following commands and moving all four," I assume there must have been some association type structure necessary for that function to occur. For example, the posterior temporal lobe (especially on the left in most patients) contains a collection of semantic knowledge about the meaning of words. This semantic area is called Wernicke's area historically, but it is a far more extensive and multifaceted area than this historical explanation gives it credit for. Its proximity to primary auditory cortex suggests a role as a cache of verbal memory and verbal processing, but its participation as a hub in numerous functional systems related to aspects of language is beyond question. Thus, while it is not a primary effector or primary sensory cortex and thus does not directly move the mouth, larynx, or hand, it still is a key hub in speaking and writing.

One final overlooked type of hubs consists of the subcortical structures, such as the thalamus, basal ganglia, and basal forebrain, among others. Corticocortical connections and long tracts are typically accounted for in most accounts of white matter connectivity, but neurosurgical teaching has traditionally neglected the fact that many parts of the brain communicate with one another through cortico-thalamo-cortical connections or through a basal ganglia circuit, a fact that is rarely included in teaching about how to safely navigate the cerebrum, and I hypothesize that our lack of attention to this likely explains some deficits that are not immediately explainable in a purely cortical world view. The fact that thalamic tumors and injuries can cause neglect syndromes similar to right parietal injuries suggest that parts of the thalamus likely are hubs in this circuit.

4.8 Redundancy

The connections of the human cerebrum are seemingly limitless. Nearly every part of the cerebrum sends at least few neurons to some part of the thalamus, and most parts of the cerebrum are interconnected in some way with most other parts. Yet, despite this fact, neurologic functions are reasonably predictable based on what part of the brain we are in. For example, despite interconnections between the frontal and occipital lobe, I have yet to see a hemianopsia from operating in the inferior frontal lobe. Besides the fact that fronto-occipital fasciculi are certainly not carrying identical information as the optic radiations, it also implies that the frontal connections to the occipital lobe are redundant with regard to elementary networks involved in visual processing.

Thus, while the number of interconnections of the brain is massively complex beyond the processing ability of the human brain, it is likely that a large fraction of these interconnections are not essential for the brain to function normally or at least acceptably. While it is probably best to maintain the entire connection one was born with, in the setting of cancer, many connections can be sacrificed without changing the overall endpoint. In some cases, losing these axonal connections might eliminate a pathway which is processed in parallel with a different connection. In other cases, cutting a part of the cerebrum might reduce the number of neurons performing a similar function, but not below the compensable reserve capacity. The latter observation is supported by clinical observations of variability of grades of weakness, or extent of visual impairment with increasing extent of damage to the motor or visual system. The fact that these injuries are not always all or none, strongly argues that it is unlikely that there is any single axon which can be cut to cause a dense neurologic deficit of any type. Thus, my approach emphasizes the maintenance of gross connection and tract integrity (much more clinically possible than accounting for every microscopic connection) under the idea that much of any of anatomy is redundant, and that our main goal is preserving major connections, and especially avoiding cutting bystander connections which are headed to different parts of the brain from what is being removed.

The bi-hemispheric nature of the brain provides the other main source of brain redundancy. While certain high brain functions, famously language, show a hemispheric preference, most are probably processed bi-hemispherically, and can compensate to some extent for the loss of the contralateral side in many cases. The fact that many patients with large territory left MCA strokes still maintain some verbal abilities, however modest, strongly argues that contralateral compensation occurs to some extent even in a highly lateralized brain function.

Despite this ability for bilateral compensation, it is important to think carefully about the contralateral side, its ability to compensate, and the potential risk of its failure to compensate, when thinking through a neurologic function and its associated network. First, I teach my residents that "bi-anything" is bad. For example:

- Bifrontal= Akinetic mutism
- Bitemporal= No short term memory
- Biparietal= Profound spatiotemporal dysfunction
- Bioccipital=Blind

The observation that a bilateral injury can bring out a profound deficit not usually seen with a unilateral deficit strongly supports the idea that the contralateral side can compensate for numerous critical brain functions, especially some higher processing functions. However, we know that at the same time, this is not always reliably true. We know from patients undergoing temporal lobectomy, the most reliably compensable lobectomy that many patients cannot carry the memory load from the other side, and they can get less dramatic, but still measurable memory problems. Alternately, the other frontal lobe cannot always carry the cognitive load, behavioral, or motivational load of the other side. The fact that the contralateral lobe cannot always carry the full load when one side is removed should cause pause in some cases when thinking through some operations, but at the same time, gliomas are a different disease with a different mandate and natural history.

Finally, going hand in hand with a view looking towards rehabilitation and recovery, it is essential to think about contralateral compensation and how this will happen, especially when working around the corpus callosum. A notable example is the supplementary motor area (SMA). Removal of the SMA causes a severe neurologic disorder which generally recovers in most patients in a few weeks. However, removal of the SMA and a corresponding portion of corpus callosum prevents this recovery from happening (I know this from experience, unfortunately), probably by preventing the contralateral SMA from compensating and taking over. Thus, if one doesn't think

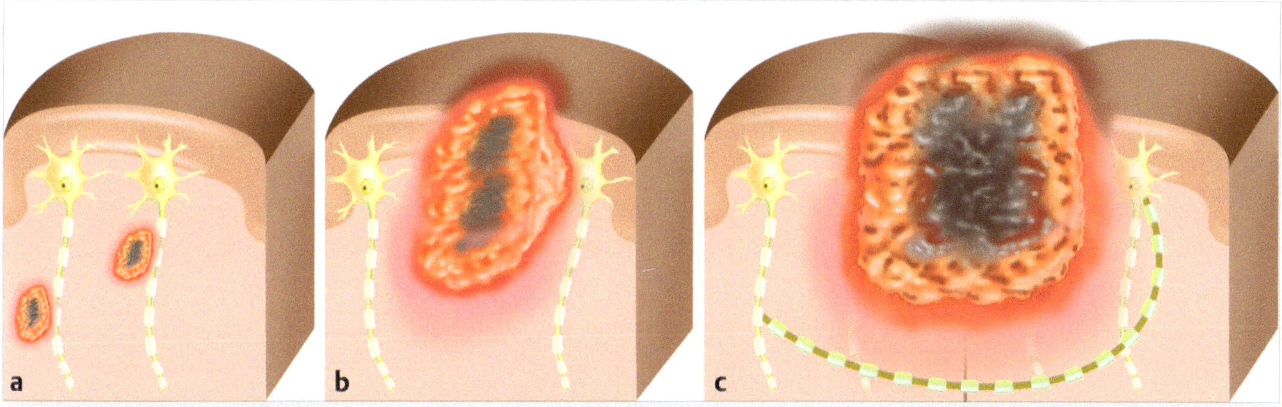

Fig. 4.2 These drawings demonstrate few ideas about how it is possible that seemingly important part of the brain can be removed without destroying a network and eliminating brain functions. Thinking about the tumor as a discrete mass, ignores the fact that a glioma filled gyrus looks like distorted brain and not as much like a clear tumor. Thus, it is essential to consider the ways how a gyrus (or other brain region) which usually is important can sometimes become unimportant. (**a**) A schematic of tumor involved cortex with two representative normal neurons with tumor cells intermixed. In this situation, the tumor has infiltrated normal brain and cannot be removed without eliminating the brain function of that area. This is the likely initial state of gliomas in their early stages, and is typical of the leading infiltrated edges of all gliomas later on. (**b**) An example of densely packed tumor cells which have displaced the normal neurons outward. Careful technique can remove the bulk of this kind of tumor situation without causing neurologic loss as in the center of this kind of tumor tissue is mostly wall to wall tumor cells without brain cells running through the middle. It is flawed to think of the borders of these tumors are being like this, as they typically are not. For example, there is no brain running through the necrotic center of a GBM, but it is foolish to assume that it may not be running through the border tissue of these tumors, and this is the enhancing part of the tumor, which is the most important part to aggressively remove. (**c**) A different example demonstrates two neurons of an area engulfed by tumor cells. Reorganization and sprouting causes an adjacent neuron to form connections which allow it to take over the function previously provided by these now tumor involved brain areas.

about the cerebrum in terms of network anatomy, compensation, and recovery, severe and permanent results can follow.

4.9 Reorganization

Reorganization is the glioma surgeon's best friend, but without awake brain mapping it can the surgeon's worst enemy. It is unquestionable that some gliomas cause often dramatic cerebral reorganization, often in the patient's favor. Any glioma patient theoretically could have reorganization, but this is more the norm in the case of low grade gliomas, and especially oligodendrogliomas. My hunch is that higher grade gliomas grow and progress faster than the brains ability to move function out of the area, though many have organized prior to the transformation event.

The bottom line is that you really cannot look at a scan of a glioma patient and predict how they are wired up, and how much of the tumor you will be able to get out as reorganization is the rule. The typical trend in reorganization is for function to move out of the tumor, or the tumor to have expanded and displaced functional tissue, but all bets are off until you test the patient.

Any idea of exactly how a part of the brain which is usually critical can reorganize to become nonessential is speculative, but some speculation follows to put some ideas out there. An older idea is that the highest density of glioma cells in the center crowds out the normal brain, and only the edges still have functional neurons in it (▶ Fig. 4.2**a**). This is probably part of the story; however, it doesn't explain why essential hubs of the network can be found in unexpected gyri, and why in some cases we are able to completely remove critical gyri (in many cases gyri that look grossly like the normal structure) in some patients without causing deficits.

Another possibility is axonal sprouting (▶ Fig. 4.2**b**), which is supported by my observation that the termination points of major tracts often predicts the location of brain functions in highly reorganized brains. One final possibility is dynamic functional connectivity changes which increase synaptic strength over time (▶ Fig. 4.2**c**). We know from fMRI work that functional connectivity in certain networks can change rapidly several times a minute in some instances, and it's possible that reorganization of functions may begin with a dynamic reorganization which strengthens over time.

4.10 Rehabilitation

If you are not getting some temporary functional problems, you probably aren't doing enough tumor resection. To reduce overall survival to avoid a neurologic deficit which improves with a few weeks of therapy doesn't make a lot of sense, and is not what most properly informed patients would choose if they had all the facts.

In a surgical paradigm based on hodotopy some parts of functional networks will be sacrificed in most surgeries for glioma, which involve resecting large parts of the brain, and in some cases, something functional will go with it. The principle goal is not to have a perfect patient the day after surgery, it is to leave the patient with something that will ultimately recover to normal or near normal with rehab. This involves leaving the hubs and key connections essential to the network, such that reorganization, compensation, and other restorative mechanisms can restore the network's function in the end. The first and second law (Chapter 2) are structured around avoiding problems which I think common leave the patient with a non-recoverable network, and thus long term disability.

We counsel patients that short term problems are likely, and that our plan is generally aimed at the long term. Rehabilitation is expected, and in the ideally we start planning rehabilitation in the preoperative period.

4.11 Escaping from Mythology

For purposes of this section, I define mythological glioma thinking as interpretations about safe, unsafe and unwise maneuvers and decisions in glioma surgery that arise from common teachings or instincts which are incomplete or inconsistent with the present neuroscientific understanding of how the cerebrum is organized and works, and/or contradict the experience of people who have actually tried those maneuvers. Like all mythology, there is some truth at the core, and it can explain some observations about the world in the absence of better models; however, like the belief that Poseidon controls the tides, mythology should eventually be replaced with better models, like the orbit of the moon controlling them.

Few people have ever put what I would call mythological glioma thinking into print a peer reviewed article or text book with their name on it; however, search your thoughts and you will recognize people in your past passing on some of the following ideas though word, attitude, or deed. This section highlights some of these ideas, which I would argue are not rare, as I see surgeries weekly come for second opinions that were likely performed under the influence of such mythological ideas. In what follows, I provide an alternate view addressing these myths with a model grounded in macroconnectomic networks, and contemporary neuroscience.

4.11.1 Myth 1: Stay Out of the Motor, Speech, and Visual, etc. Cortex and You Will be Fine

As with most commonly held, yet inaccurate, views, there is some truth in this. It is good to not transgress the motor strip during cerebral surgery, and failure to heed this will likely lead to immediate negative feedback for the surgeon confirming that this is a bad idea.

The problem with simple explanations is that while they are easy to follow and to teach, they also ignore a lot of equally important facts about how these systems work, and ultimately set some cases up for failure. For example, avoidance of the motor cortex, but yet getting your angles off and drifting into the descending motor fibers, undercutting the gyrus is certain to end in problems, often worse than transgressing the motor strip (▶ Fig. 4.3**a**). Additionally, removing the brain on both sides of the motor strip, but leaving the motor strip and descending motor fibers will similarly leave the patient hemiplegic as no motor planning systems exist to drive and control the strip (▶ Fig. 4.3**b**). Finally, the absence of inputs from the cerebellum, sensory cortex, basal ganglia (among other inputs) might leave a limb which moves but is functionally unusable. We often pat ourselves on the back when a patient is "moving

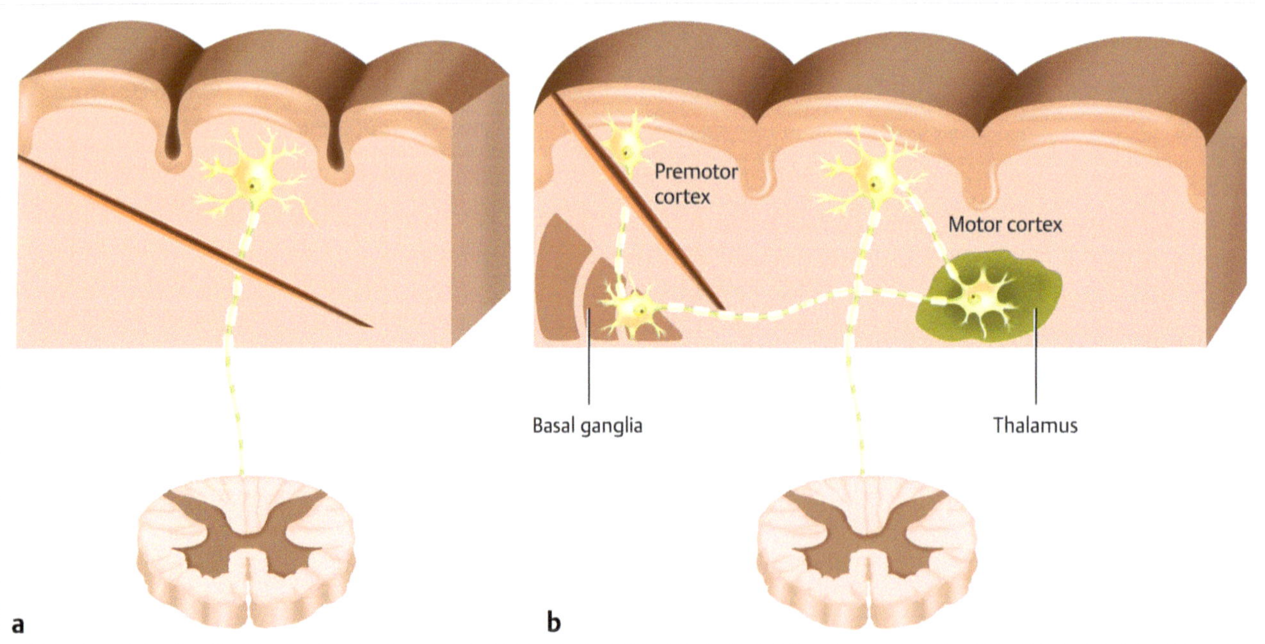

Fig. 4.3 We are typically taught that the secret to preserving motor function is to locate the motor cortex and not transgress it. This schematic depicts two ways in which only paying attention to the motor cortex can fail you, which should serve as an example from other networks. **(a)** This diagram depicts a motor neuron descending in the white matter towards the spinal cord below. A misaimed transcerebral trajectory (shown in this diagram) entering anterior to the motor cortex, but veering posteriorly into the descending motor fibers has the effect of removing a larger area of the motor cortex. **(b)** This more detailed diagram demonstrates a motor planning neuron (SMA or premotor) signaling down to the basal ganglia, which in turn signals to the thalamus, which ultimately signals to the motor cortex. This schematic demonstrates the effect of disconnecting motor planning areas from the basal ganglia, namely that it can disrupt this motor network significantly.

all four extremities," but then shrug shoulders when family ask why the patient can't ambulate or transfer without major assistance, and chalk it up to steroids, brain swelling, age, "poor protoplasm," radiotherapy, etc. The difference between that outcome, and the ideal one is the difference between preserving the motor cortex, and preserving the hubs of the relevant sensorimotor network.

The truth is complex cerebral functions require the communication of several key brain areas, including often the basal ganglia, thalamus, or other subcortical structures. Merely staying out of the most "eloquent" part is not enough to keep something working well. It may not be possible in all cases to save the network in its platonic ideal form, and "moving all four" may be the best we can do; however, we will come a lot closer to the goal if we acknowledge that this is how the brain actually works.

4.11.2 Myth 2: If the Tumor Is in an Eloquent Brain Region, It Is Inoperable

This is rarely true, and there are very few cases where a thoughtful surgery cannot make the situation better. In most cases, in cases where surgery has little to offer, the tumors are small and following a key white matter tract, such as the SLF, making the return on investment for surgery minimal compared to the consequences.

Additionally, it is important to stay oriented to the natural history of the disease, and specifically with reference to the function surgery would risk. I frequently tell my residents that the only thing worse than being hemiplegic from a glioblastoma in the motor strip, is being hemiplegic from a glioblastoma in the motor strip that is still there. Common sense argues that a patient's long term chances of walking are not improved by leaving a glioblastoma growing in the leg motor cortex, and certainly their overall survival is not helped. Thus, the decision to leave tumor in a brain area should result from a conscious thought that that function could be saved by leaving that piece of tumor behind, and that the tradeoff is in the patient's best interest. Thus, leaving part of a low grade tumor in a speech area to only achieve a 97% resection instead of 100% makes sense, while doing an open biopsy on a hemiplegic patient with a motor strip glioblastoma because it is "in the motor strip," does not. Similarly, leaving most of a grade 2 glioma to avoid subtle memory problems or trouble remember the names of colors, probably isn't an optimal trade, as malignant transformation to glioblastoma ensures those same problems eventually.

As should be obvious, making decisions about what is an appropriate trade-off can be quite complex and personal. For example, most people would trade color naming for a longer life, memory is a function with an unclear network anatomy, and it is unclear that you can sacrifice that function only without damaging a more substantial network. Additionally, the duration of functional preservation achieved leaving behind a part of a grade 2 glioma is less predictable than high grade tumors, and thus leaving some tumor can achieve functional sparing that can last years in some cases, compared to an uncontrolled glioblastoma which can wipe out the function you aimed to save in a few weeks or months.

Thus, the optimal onco-functional balance does not merely aims to spare function by leaving tumor, but rather aims to spare critical functions which can actually be spared over some reasonable time period. We should accept a reduced degree of tumor resection only if doing so will actually achieve the aim of a meaningful protection or a meaningful function. There is no reason to leave tumor to save function that is going to be gone in a week or two no matter what we do, and certainly no reason to leave tumor to save function that is lost.

4.11.3 Myth 3: To Protect Higher Brain Functions, We Just Need to Map the Brain for that Function and Not Remove that Part

This is more of a boutique myth among some glioma surgeons. Many people have an interest in protecting functions more sophisticated than just moving the contralateral side and speaking. To that end, a number of tests have been created, tested in surgery, and related to neuropsychological function.

Unlike the previous myths, this one is mostly true, and one I currently involve myself with. I do agree that we should save higher functions as much as possible, and that mapping is the way to start working towards that.

However, the myth is that we can just stimulate the brain in an undirected fashion and find what part does that function. An alternate version is that we should always test all functions and put boundaries on our resection to spare whatever we find. In reality, not all findings in tests like this are real, many are related to the testing conditions, or result from interruption of a different related functional system. For example, causing a speech arrest will similarly interfere with most other tests, making it hard to do certain types of mapping in certain brain areas.

Presently, we cannot reliably go about trying to save many complex brain functions in a reliable, focused way, and I would suggest that while this is ultimately our goal, that the following guidelines provide some framework for how we should go about introducing new ideas and tests in a way that will ultimately lead to an onco-functionally valid way to assess these functions and balance our desire to resect more tumor, against our desire to preserve brain function.

Sughrue's Guidelines for Attempting to Find and Save Higher Brain Function

For a function to be amenable to a focused effort to find it and save it, a higher brain function should:

1. Be worth saving such that it is better to reduce your extent of resection to achieve it.
2. Have a reasonably well understood functional network, with some idea of what structures are essential for performing that function and their essential interconnections.
3. Have a test of function which can be reasonably performed in the operating room by at least some patients.
4. Have a test which clearly becomes abnormal in a reliable and easily observable way when the system is disturbed.

These guidelines are discussed in more detail in the chapter on functional testing. Sufficed to say these are not the end verdict on functional testing, but it serves to temper the enthusiasm of introducing new techniques and ideas, with the reality that you cannot save a function if you lack an anatomic framework to understand this function, any more than you can avoid double vision in a central skull base meningioma surgery if you do not understand what the third nerve does and where it is. Further, it stresses the importance of practical tests with unambiguous and rapidly obtained results. Finally, it emphasizes that we are always making an onco-functional exchange throughout the surgery, and that we should not back-off our tumor resection for minor, theoretical, or unrealistic functional goals. By working in this framework, we can continually refine our technique and save more brain networks as our understanding improves, but at the same time, do not allow flawed ideas about functional preservation which reduce our effectiveness to distract from our goals.

5 White Matter Anatomy of the Cerebrum

5.1 Introduction

White matter anatomy is not a new hobby for neurosurgeons, but at the same time it is in a period of great change as new techniques and technologies allow us ask and answer questions which were not realistically possible to answer previously. Notably, with improvements in technology such as DTI and DSI, we can now ask what parts of the brain are connected by various tracts, and the relationship of different tracts to each other in 3-dimensional space. Thus, this raises the possibility of a gross anatomic understanding of functional brain networks on a macroscale, with the obviously profound implications for cerebral surgery.

This chapter is a repository of cerebral white matter anatomy. Some of the information in this chapter is described in other work, while much of this is from my own studies of smaller local white matter connections. Functional implications of these connections are discussed in other chapters, especially as it relates to tumor surgery.

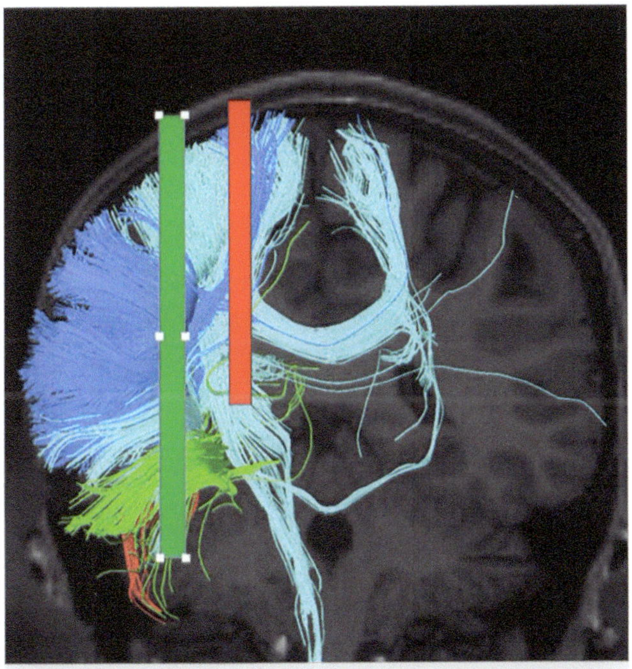

Fig. 5.1 A basic schematic overview of the white matter systems of the brain seen in coronal section. The red lines depict a set of arbitrary boundaries between the lateral, middle, medial fiber systems. The lateral systems include the SLF, the IFOF, the ILF, the optic radiations, and the uncinate fasciculus. These fibers are principally running along the anterior-to-posterior axis. The medial system includes the cingulum, fornix, and corpus callosum and run either anterior-to-posterior or commissural (i.e., the corpus callosum). The middle system includes the corticospinal tract, the thalamic peduncles and their connections with the cortex, and the cortical communications with the basal ganglia, all of which make up the coronal radiata. These fibers run along a rostral-caudal axis. There are tracts which cross these systems, namely the FAT, the MdLF, the lateral thalamic peduncle, and the crossed semantic loop; however, most tracts obey this scheme.

5.2 Major Cortico-cortical Tracts

We start with a description of the major cortico-cortical tracts both because of their major importance to functional outcome, but also because a deep understanding of these tracts provides a reference point for smaller tracts, and local subgyral white matter anatomy, which often either joins these tracts, or at least can be explained in reference to them.

A helpful way others have classified the major tracts is in reference to the corona radiata (▶ Fig. 5.1), and basal ganglia which divides the major tracts into lateral tracts, which generally run anterior to posterior, and medial tracts, which are similarly oriented in the anterior-posterior plane, but also include the callosum fibers which run bi-hemispherically. The central core fibers of the corona radiata run mainly rostral-caudal and include the corticospinal tracts, the fibers of the thalamic peduncle, among others.

Beyond just providing a classification system, this way of mentally classifying the tracts forces us to think differently about the transgressing the cerebrum as it shows us that the lateral tracts form a wall which generally blocks direct lateral approaches to deep targets such as the ventricle. This forces us to take what are counter-intuitive and longer approaches to the lateral ventricle (▶ Fig. 5.2), which avoid these large association tracts. Alternately, ▶ Fig. 5.3 demonstrates a case which shows that in an emergency, taking the easiest route to a clot is often the wrong answer for long term functional recovery, as in this case when a transinsular approach avoided the tracts in the absence of image guidance and saved the patients function in the long term.

5.2.1 Lateral Tracts

Superior Longitudinal Fasciculus (SLF)

We start with the SLF as it is the dominant lateral tract, and it dominates our thinking about functional networks and glioma surgery. It is a massive tract, which covers a great deal of ground, and its preservation is integral to leaving the patient as a functional person. There are a large number of networks whose primary hubs require communication via the SLF, including the speech, neglect, praxis, and attention networks, and this means that there are few better ways to hurt someone than cutting through the core of the SLF complex.

The SLF has been described as being comprised of 4 layers with the arcuate fasciculus being the lateral part of this tract, the arcuate fasciculus, and the SLF I, SLF II, and SLF III. In the description of functional networks, it is quite helpful to know these distinctions, as they help to reduce the mental complexity of this extensive tract to usable subunits. In surgery, these distances between systems are generally not observable or actionable, and thus distinctions are academic, and you should view the SLF as a single large tract.

It is easy to mistakenly view this as a c-shaped tract, as the bulk of it mirrors the c-shape of the hemisphere; however, by viewing it as a modified-Y shape, you remind yourself of the parietal

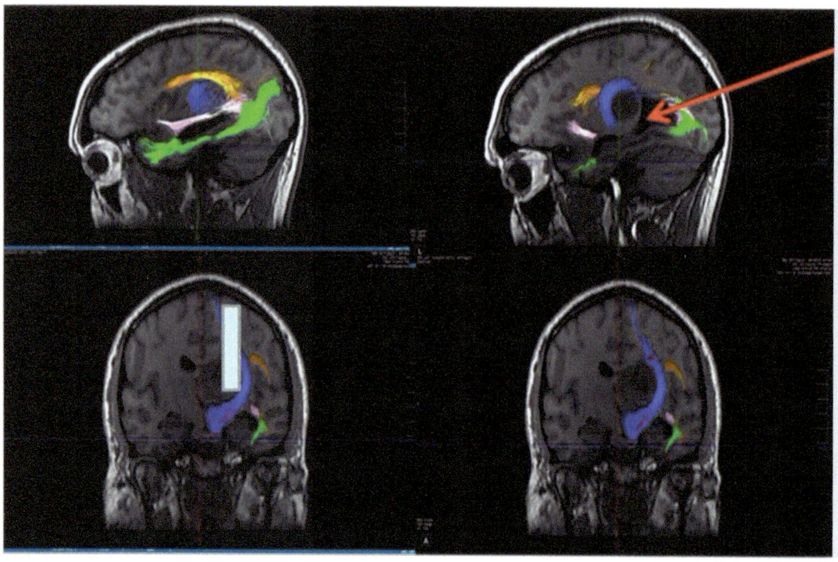

Fig. 5.2 In many cases, the teaching that the shortest path to the target is the best can be demonstrated to be incorrect with a careful review of white matter anatomy. These images demonstrate that the best approach to the atrium is not the direct lateral approach (which takes you through the SLF and optic radiations), but instead the more posterior, medial and longer approach indicated by the arrow. This approach parallels the lateral fibers and works between the medial and lateral systems, though a section of the white matter which is largely local fibers and less dominated by large range white matter connections.

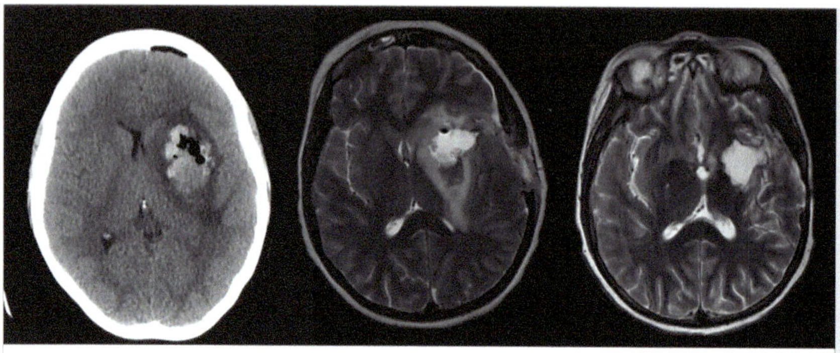

Fig. 5.3 These images demonstrate pre- and postoperative images from a remarkable case of a patient who suffered a significant hemorrhage from a left basal ganglia lymphoma. She was taken back to the operating room from the recovery room after the hemorrhage was recognized from signs of herniation. We did not have DTI images available, so we selected to take the difficult angle of working through the insular window. The clot and much of the tumor were evacuated. She made a complete recovery of motor and speech and has no clinically detectable deficits at long term follow-up. This highlights the value of remaining out of large white matter tracts even during emergency neurosurgery. It also demonstrates the anatomy of the insular window, i.e., the gap between the SLF and IFOF provided by the insula.

ramus, which is sizeable and essential for networks which engage the inferior parietal lobule, such as praxis. This ramus is the lateral margin of most medial parietal cuts, so it's critical to know it.

The most obvious enpoints of the SLF complex are the supramarginal gyrus, the inferior parietal lobule, and the middle frontal and triangularis/orbitalis parts of the inferior frontal gyri. The fact that this tract links the major language centers of the left hemisphere should be obvious to most neurosurgeons, and this is how I view the left SLF, as a highway for phonemic and syntactic aspects of speech. It is critical to note that the SLF is fundamentally more complex that this, and its carrying a great deal more information than this.

We have long ignored the SLF at our own peril. During evacuations of basal ganglia hemorrhages, it was not at all rare to see someone pick the shortest path (usually through part of the SLF) and transgress that to evacuate the clot. We then would chalk up a bad outcome to the initial bleed. Careful review of white matter anatomy makes the foolishness of this approach obvious. We now think a better approach is through a more anteromedial corridor.

The SLF creates a virtual wall over the lateral hemisphere, and often makes the direct lateral approach to deep targets challenging or impossible.

Anatomy of the SLF in Normal Patients

It is critical to note that all of the following descriptions of normal tract position and positions come from anatomic studies of patients without gliomas, and that we have seen a wide variation from this in our glioma patients with tracts in unusual places, and often with major rami not present from either destruction or re-organization. Thus, the images in ▶ Fig. 5.4 provide a basic understanding of what the SLF typically looks like, with the caveat that it is probably not exactly what your patient's SLF (or any other tract) is going to look like.

The SLF generally has an anterior-posterior core running under the sensory and motor cortices paralleling the lateral ventricle, and a genu which bends just deep to the supramarginal gyrus. There are three principle rami which contain the main termination of the tract: The temporal ramus, which terminates in the

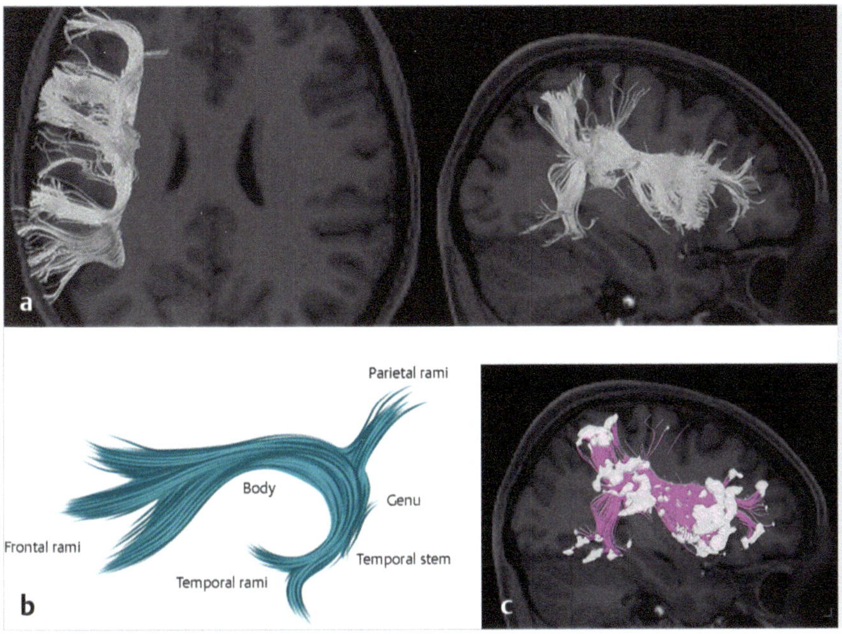

Fig. 5.4 (**a**) Anatomy of the SLF, including tractographic images and a (**b**) schematic demonstrating a simplified version of the anatomy of the SLF including its three primary rami. The image in (**b**) demonstrates white balloons on all of the termini of the tract, demonstrating its targets.

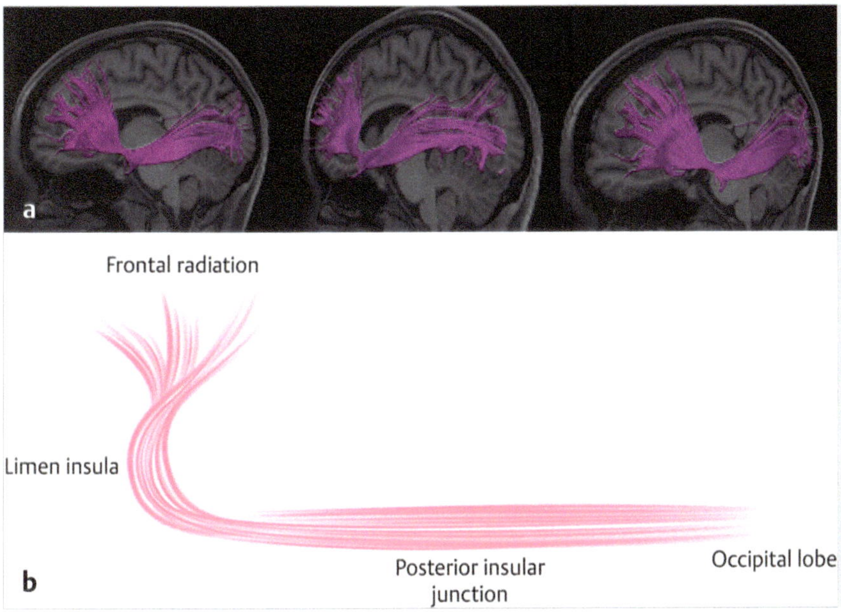

Fig. 5.5 (**a**) Anatomy of the IFOF, (**b**) including a tractographic schematic demonstrating a simplified version of the anatomy of the IFOF.

supramarginal, middle temporal, and superior temporal gyri, the frontal ramus which terminates mostly in the middle and inferior frontal gyrus, and the parietal ramus which largely ends in the inferior parietal lobule and the banks of the intraparietal sulcus.

The SLF (and most other tracts for that matter) are best viewed as a bus route rather than an airplane flight. Our methods, be they physical dissection of imaging based methods, are limited in their ability to reliably define small contributions from overlying gyri. Thus, it is likely that small contributions from many of the overlying gyri also enter the SLF at several points along its course, so it's to consider the SLF as a bus route more than an airplane flight, as there are probably multiple points of entry and exit.

One thing worth noting is that the majority of the SLF runs in the white matter core which lies deep to the depths of the overlying sulci. Only at its rami, when fibers turn towards the cortical surface does it present itself superficially. Thus, I generally do not start to look for the tract until I have reached the bottom of the relevant sulci.

Additionally, the SLF and several other tracts cross just lateral to the posterior most point of the internal capsule just posterior to the insula, and deep to the temporo-parieto-occipital junction, making this area one of the most functionally treacherous parts of the cerebrum.

Inferior Fronto-occipital Fasciculus

This tract is quite long (▶ Fig. 5.5). It runs from anterior to posterior connecting the inferior occipital and frontal lobes. Again, it's best to think of this tract like a bus route than a single connection. Its most notable feature is that it runs at the base of the insula, just above the temporal stem, and hooks anterior at the limen insula before fanning out to the frontal lobe. This fact dominates insular glioma surgery.

The occipital origins of this tract are principally in the lingula and cuneus and after hooking superiorly around the pre-occipital notch before diverging from the ILF and crossing at the TPO junction as a largely compact bundle. After bending anterosuperiorly at the limen insula, the fibers fan out. The bulk of these fibers are connected to the SFG where they interact with a large length of the gyrus. There are also communications with the IFG, and a lesser communication with the MFG.

The IFOF is similarly located at the crossing fibers of TPO junction and runs just deep to the genu and temporal ramus of the SLF and superficial to the optic radiations. Together with the SLF it frames the insula, anterior and inferior (IFOF) versus posterior and superior (SLF) and working in the insula safely working within that "frame" (▶ Fig. 5.6).

Superior Frontal Occipital Fasciculus

This fiber bundle, which was claimed to run just lateral to the cingulum was described in fiber dissections long ago and has had numerous names. Yasargil first questioned its existence stating that it was an artefact of dissection techniques. Our work with fiber tracking supports this, as we have found no evidence that there is a tract running in this region connecting the frontal and occipital lobes. Most of the communications between the processed outputs of the visual system and frontal planning areas run via the SLF, which highlights the parietal lobe's important role of translating visual information into a form useable by the motor systems.

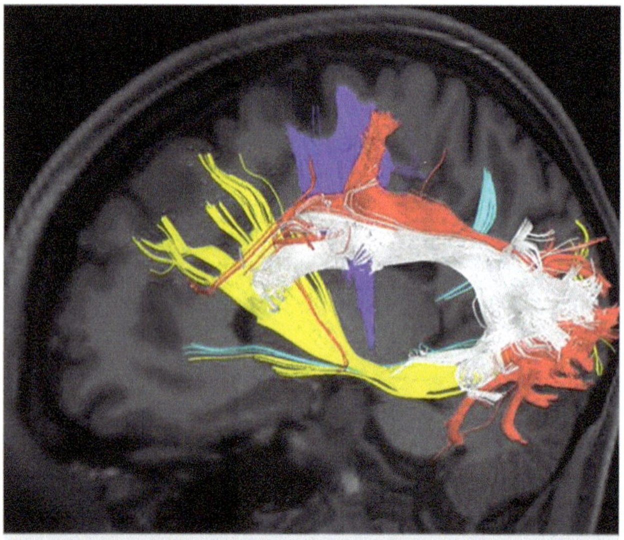

Fig. 5.6 Images demonstrating the insular window created by the SLF and IFOF, which form a frame around the insula.

Optic Radiations

These are probably one of the better known white matter tracts to neurosurgeons so I will not belabor the point (▶ Fig. 5.7). Probably the most surgically important aspect of this anatomy is that the optic radiations comprise form the majority of the lateral wall of the atrium of the lateral ventricle, a fact which radically alters the ideal approach to the atrium and similarly positioned structures.

It is also of relevance to note that the visual system probably works in large part by communications with the pulvinar which are critical in serial visual processing. These fibers generally run in the same bundle as the optic radiations. There are numerous examples of this fact worth noting demonstrated in this chapter.

Inferior Longitudinal Fasciculus (ILF)

The ILF is an anterior to posterior tract running from the occipital pole to the temporal pole running just deep to the fusiform gyrus on the inferior temporal/occipital surface (▶ Fig. 5.8). This tract does not typically block a lateral approach to a deeper target in the way other lateral tracts do; however, it is a common path for spread of gliomas.

It primarily connects the inferior temporal gyrus to the lingula, though some fibers extend superiorly into the temporal pole.

Uncinate Fasciculus

Most of us are aware that this tract is running in the limen insula and connects the frontal and occipital lobes. Specifically, it connects the inferior frontal gyrus, pars triangularis to the anterior temporal lobe (▶ Fig. 5.9).

It is laterally positioned relative to a similar bend in the IFOF, and this has caused the functions of these two tracts to become confused. Its most clinically relevant attribute is as a pathway of spread of gliomas from the temporal to the frontal lobes through the insula.

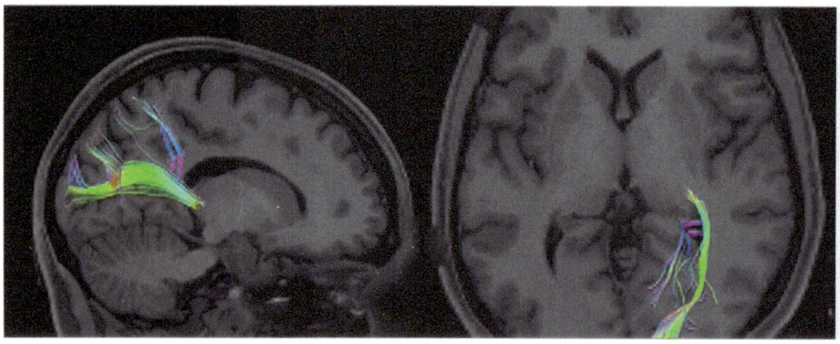

Fig. 5.7 Tractographic anatomy of the optic radiations.

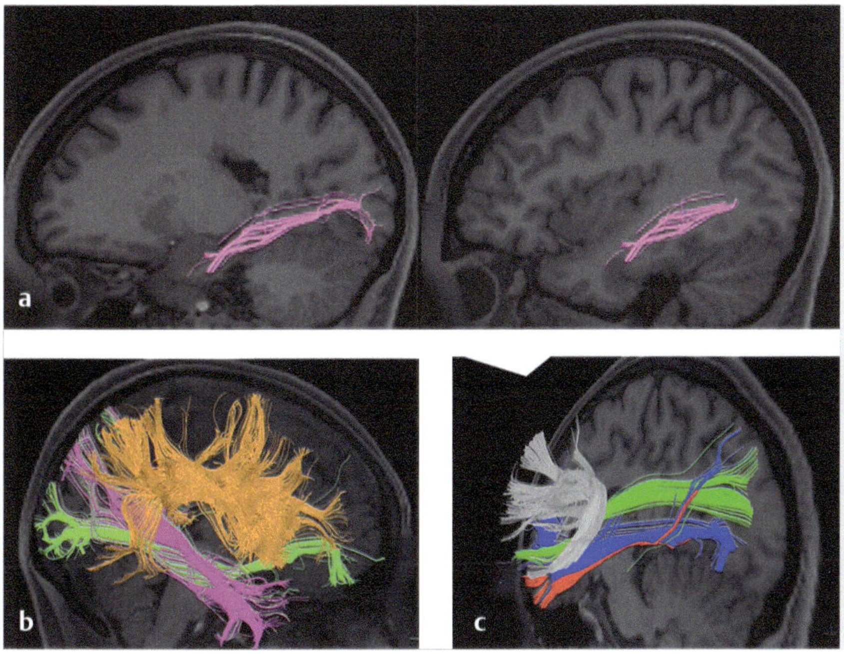

Fig. 5.8 (**a-c**) Tractographic anatomy of the Inferior longitudinal fasciculus.

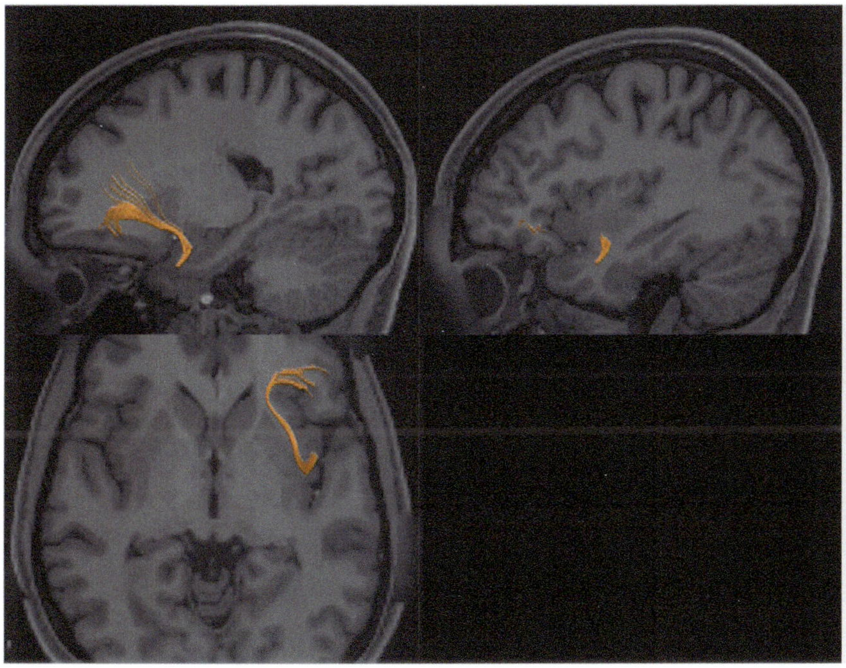

Fig. 5.9 Tractographic anatomy of the uncinate fasciculus.

About the Superior Fronto-occipital Fasciculus (SFOF)

The IFOF was so named because early fiber tract dissections suggested a small tract running from occipital to frontal lobes. Subsequent dissections raised questions about its existence, and our own work has failed to demonstrate any evidence that such a long tract exists. We believe that what was previously called "SFOF" is in reality parts of the medial SLF components, or an artefact of the U-fiber anatomy. It is important to note that there is not a great deal of information directly carrying early visual processing information to the motor planning areas (as an SFOF would be expected to do).

Because of its familiarity to us, we call the more definitively present IFOF by its historic name.

5.2.2 Medial Tracts

Cingulum

This tract is best known for its inclusion in the Papez circuit, completing the loop by connecting the cingulate cortex to the parahippocampal gyrus. While this is certainly one of the functions of the cingulum, I would argue that its role in attention networks, such as the default mode network, is of equal or greater importance when operating near the midline.

The cingulum is a c-shaped tract which runs in the center of the cingulate gyrus, the isthmus, and the parahippocampal gyrus (▶ Fig. 5.10). Its primary branches are to the superior frontal and subparietal gyri (probably part of the default mode network).

Corpus Callosum

This well-known tract is really a collection of numerous of c-shaped bihemispheric connections (▶ Fig. 5.11). The basic parts (from anterior to posterior) are the rostrum, genu, body, and splenium. The majority of the callosal fibers connect homologous contralateral brain regions. For example, large connections exist between homologous parts of the superior frontal gyrus, the superior parietal lobule, the medial occipital lobe, etc. There are homologous connections between more lateral cortices (middle frontal and inferior frontal gyri for example), and there are some connections between nonhomologous brain regions (as with what I term here the crossed FAT tract below which connects the middle frontal and inferior frontal gyri with the contralateral superior frontal gyrus).

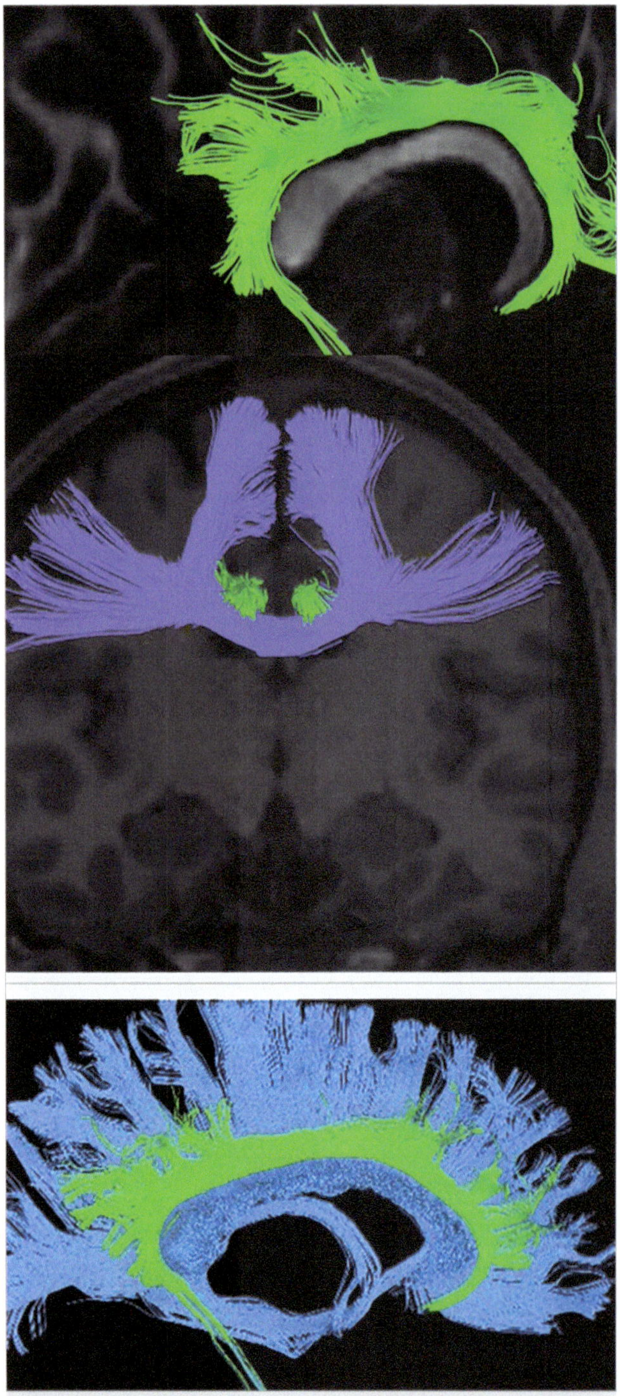

Fig. 5.10 Tractographic anatomy of the cingulum.

The connections of the callosum are easily remembered by dividing the supra-rostral parts of the callosum into fifths. The genu and anterior fifth connects medial prefrontal cortices, the second fifth connects motor and pre-motor cortices, the third fifth connect parietal cortices, and the posterior two-fifths connects occipital cortices (▶ Fig. 5.11). Equally important is the relationship between the corpus callosal fibers and the cingulate gyrus and cingulum. The corpus callosum wraps inferiorly, then laterally, then superiorly around the cingulate gyrus and cingulum towards its target (▶ Fig. 5.11). Because the cingulum and corpus callosum run roughly perpendicular to each other, they do not cross, there is only occasional cross talk between their relevant gyri (they are also different types of cortex), and they can be dissected free from each other without too much difficulty in cadaveric fiber dissections. This relationship is critical for understanding how to safely remove butterfly gliomas.

5.2.3 The "Aslant" Tracts

These tracts defy the simple grouping of tracts into medial, lateral, or vertical (i.e., corona radiate/thalamic peduncle), because they cross all of them. They are a major way medial brain structures, talk to lateral ones, and have long been ignored because they were hard to find before fiber tracking technology came into being as they don't survive fiber dissection as well.

Frontal Aslant Tract (FAT)

This tract (▶ Fig. 5.12) has been recently described, but it is clear that it is quite important, as it connects the supplementary motor area to the premotor cortices, and the expressive speech areas. It is a large tract which crosses the center of the corona radiate and connects the posterior superior frontal gyrus (especially the supplementary motor area region) with the middle and inferior frontal gyri (especially the triangularis and opercularis). It crosses diagonally across the deep white matter including the SLF, and it probably plays a role in the transition between volition and actions, including the initiation of speech. We also have recently noted a crossed FAT tract which runs in the corpus callosum and connects one SFG with the other sided premotor MFG and IFG. I hypothesize that this tract is critical for recovery of the SMA syndrome.

Middle Longitudinal Fasciculus (MdLF)

This is a misnamed tract as it is not a longitudinal tract (▶ Fig. 5.13) in the way the SLF or ILF are. It would be better termed the occipital aslant tract (the OAT), as it runs from the medial to the lateral systems similar to the FAT.

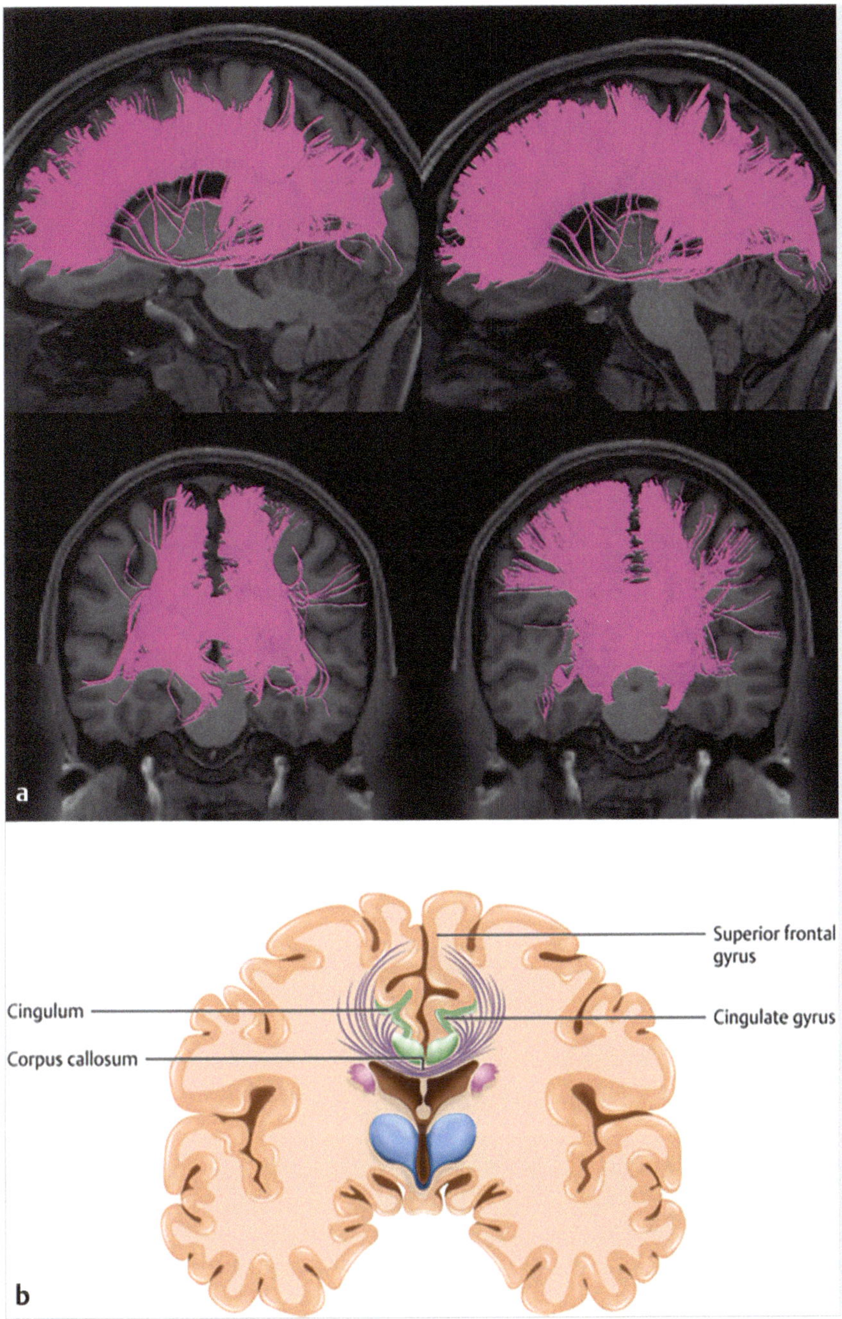

Fig. 5.11 (**a**) Tractographic anatomy of the corpus callosum. (**b**) Schematic demonstrating the organization of the corpus callosum and its relationship to the cingulum.

It principally connects the upper cuneus to the superior temporal gyrus. The most logical explanation is this is a mechanism of linking the dorsal visual pathway (which has later level processing cortices in these regions) with the semantic areas.

The Semantic Crossing Loop

This tract is one we have recently discovered in our mapping work, which is small but of clear clinical significance. It is a bilateral communication between the two semantic areas in the posterior temporal lobes, which crosses in the posterior corpus callosum just in front of the splenium, its absence probably explains the alexia without agraphia syndrome, and we presently look for it and try to preserve it during relevant subcortical mapping cases. This is better described in Chapter 6 with the section on the "two pathway" type networks.

5.3 Gyral Level Anatomic Connectivity Maps

One key to success in glioma surgery is to avoid injury to the large white matter tracts, as the amount of disconnection which occurs is generally extensive and the deficits profound. However, as I have probed deeper into white matter anatomy, I have devoted intense study towards the connection patterns of individual gyri and the often lesser tracts which link them to the main tracts and to each other. One reason for this is the idea

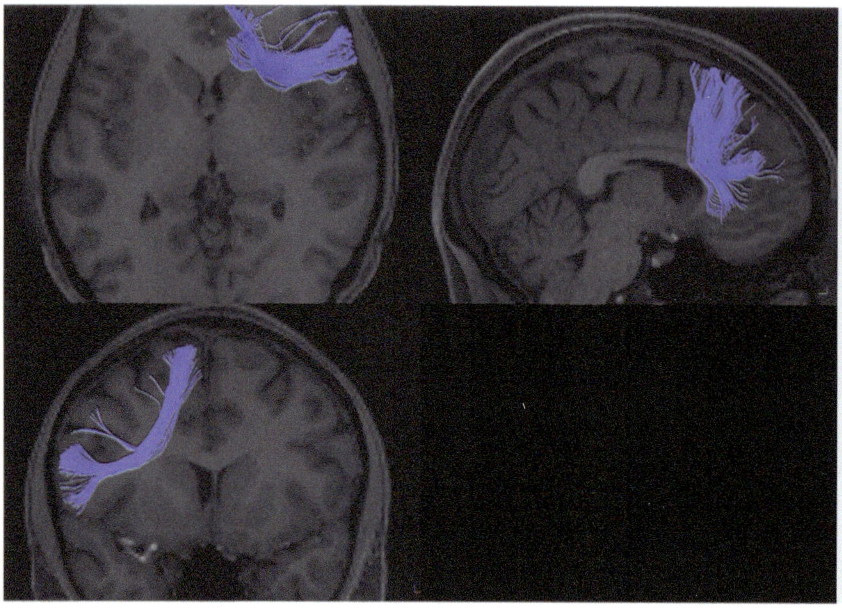

Fig. 5.12 Tractographic anatomy of the frontal aslant tract.

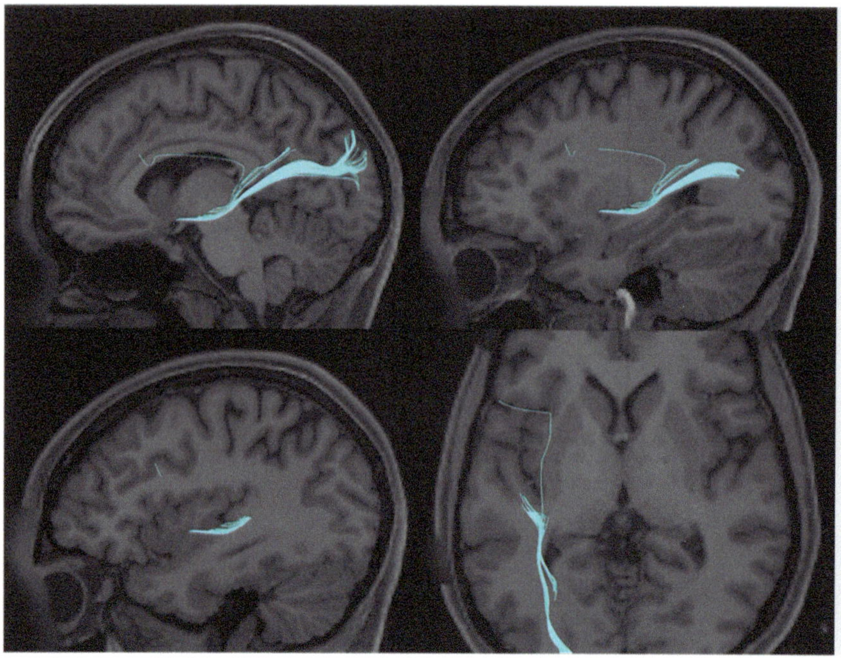

Fig. 5.13 Tractographic anatomy of the Middle longitudinal fasciculus (also known as the occipital aslant tract).

that there is no point of preserving eloquent cortex and the associated large tract if you disconnect the two just below the sulcus. Further, many brain networks probably require connections with the basal ganglia, thalamus, or other subcortical structures to work properly, and these communications are not from the large cortico-cortical tracts described above, but more through smaller thalamo-cortical and cortico-basal connections which can only been seen clearly on gyrus level maps. In addition, looking at which gyri significantly talk to each other, can lead to insights that are not obtainable through any other means. Finally, not all connections within a given network are made by long range large tracts, but many systems are quite dependent on local connections. For example, detailed understanding of how to operate in the motor system requires a good understanding of how the motor strip communicates with other nearby members of the network.

The maps provided in this section were made by our group using data from diffusion spectrum imaging data as part of the human connectome data base. This is based upon the macroconnectomic principles described in previous chapters, and thus it is certain that not all connections between brain regions are demonstrated on these maps. Many of these connections are smaller, and I am skeptical that any single neuron or small group of neurons can be cut to cause a clinically observable deficit, and for this reason I have focused my discussion of white matter anatomy on reasonably discernable brain connections. To my knowledge, no previous source of similarly detailed maps has been published accessibly.

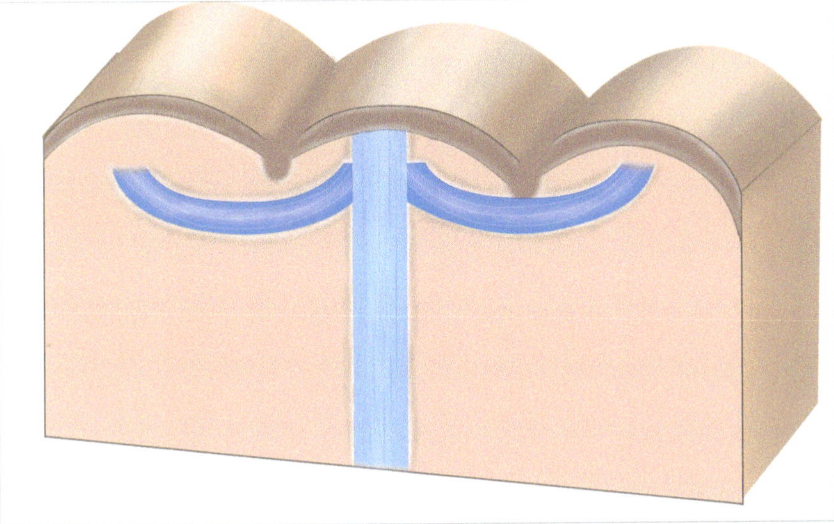

Fig. 5.14 Schematic demonstrating the basic schema of how white matter tracts leave a gyrus.

5.4 Generic Pattern of Gyral Connections

The basic intragyral white matter of individual gyri can be schematically viewed as a trident pointed at the center of the cortex (▶ Fig. 5.14). The small white matter fibers from the cortex combine in the gyrus center and this forms the center point of the trident, which then communicates with the adjacent gyrus across the sulcus through the small U-fibers. The staff of the trident represents the longer range communicating fibers, which at least initially point in the direction of the ventricle, and which are headed to other parts of the cerebrum. Moving beyond this schematic, note that the small U-fibers are not always perfectly symmetric, they do not always leave the formal gyrus they originate in; note that a gyrus is a concept, and thus a gyrus often is discontinuous and interrupted by sulci, with their own short U-fibers which never leave the formal gyrus as we define it. Further, the staff is not always straight or singular, and may branch and/or bend often significantly to join longer range tracts. Regardless, conceptual diagrams are a helpful starting point for reducing complexity, and ultimately this reminds us of the general initial orientation of tracts leaving a gyrus.

The long distance fibers are highly complex but generally can be thought of in three types, as follows:

Cortico-cortical: These include the commonly described tracts listed above as well as many smaller regional connections.

Corticobasal: Smaller tracts connecting cortex to basal ganglia structures. Usually these tracts are afferent from the cortex to the basal ganglia.

Thalamo-cortical: These can be afferent or efferent and can serve as primary relay of sensory input to primary cortices, or often are cortico-thalamo-cortical loops indirectly facilitating signaling between two cortical areas.

The latter two fibers types are rarely large fiber bundles in their own right, at least peripherally in the immediate subgyral white matter. Often they follow other corticocortical pathways within the same system. As these tracts approach their targets, they are often running in the middle of a large connection of crossing tracts, often lack clear landmarks to locate them, and often can blend into other larger tracts headed to a similar area and running in the same direction, making them harder to describe and classify. However, it is unquestionable that many cortices talk to each other through basal ganglia and/or thalamic circuits, or at least some networks need these circuits to work properly. Thus, these maps make a specific point to identify the location of significant cortical communications with deeper structures whenever we can.

5.5 Specific Gyrus Anatomy

5.5.1 Frontal Lobe

Superior Frontal Gyrus

For clarity, our maps divide this huge gyrus into 4 parts along its anterior to posterior axis. We also include parts of the posterior medial part of this gyrus which contains the supplementary motor area, in discussions motor region anatomy which is its more obvious home.

The medial frontal pole region (▶ Fig. 5.15**a**) is predominantly oriented anterior-posterior and mostly consists of local interconnections and connections with superior frontal gyri. Its principle long connections are through the genu of the corpus callosum to its homologous gyrus.

Moving slightly posterior in the SFG (▶ Fig. 5.15**b**), we find that the tracts run more rostral-caudal and communicates with the lingula of the occipital lobe via the IFOF. These fibers exit posterolaterally to join the orbitofrontal fibers entering the IFOF. There is a medial set of fibers which cross just superior to the genu in the corpus callosum and connect to the homologous parts of the contralateral SFG. There are also small fibers which communicate with the caudate head and ventral putamen mainly heading to the anterior limb of the internal capsule. It has numerous internal u-fiber connections as well as some local connections to the adjacent parts of middle frontal gyrus.

The third portion has its apex pointing rostral-caudal (▶ Fig. 5.15**c**). The FAT is its main output and this makes a lateral bend to connection to MFG and IFG laterally. There are also connections to the contralateral SFG through the anterior body of the callosum. In addition to the internal interconnections, there are connections to the anterior cingulate, which probably

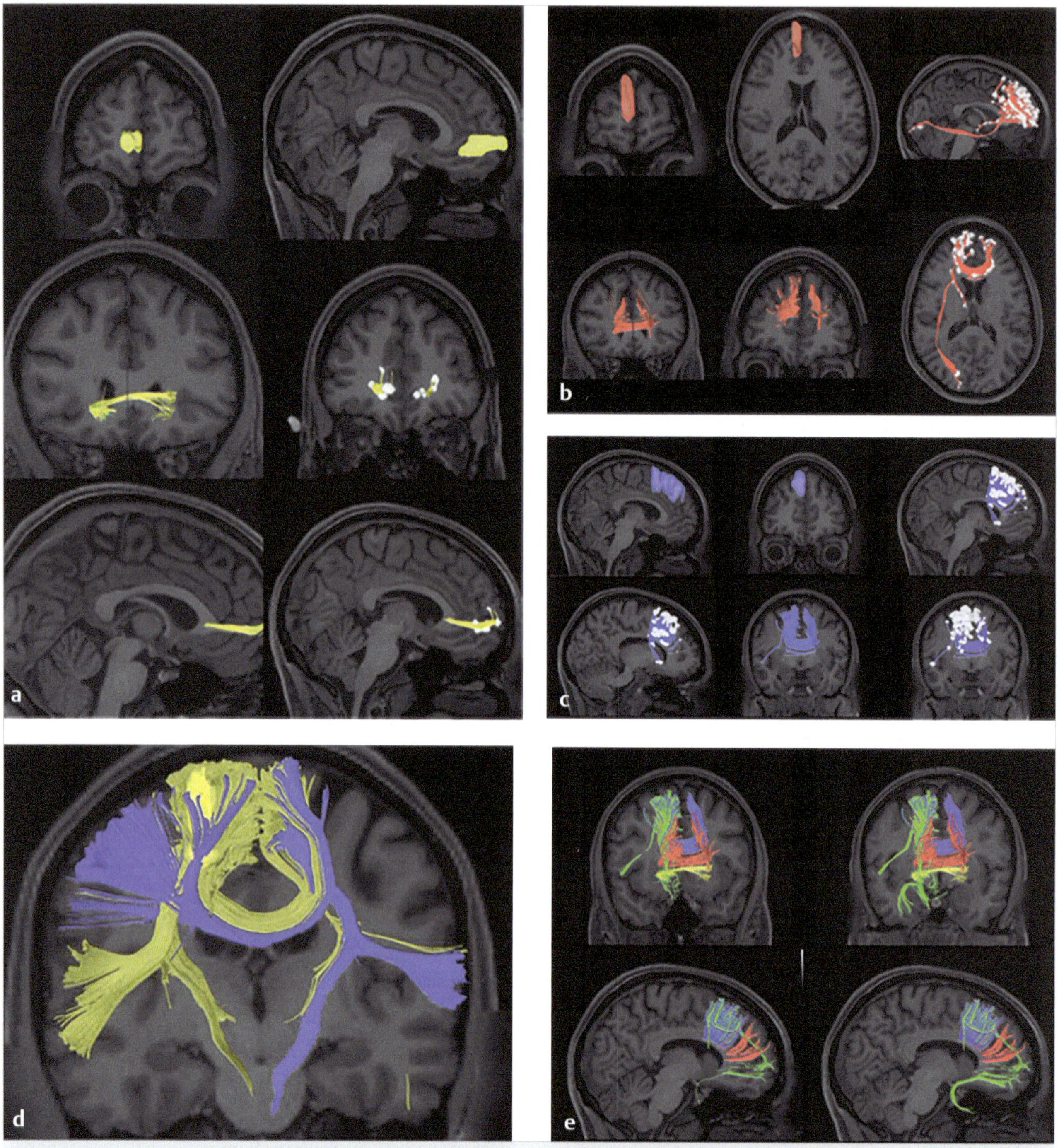

Fig. 5.15 Tractographic anatomy of the SFG. The images are divided into quarters for simplification. (**a**) ROI of the anterior quarter. (**b**) ROI of the next quarter. (**c**) ROI of the third quarter. (**d**) ROI of the posterior quarter (the SMA). (**e**) Combination of all four ROIs.

are part of the default mode network. The communication with the basal ganglia and thalamus is not major.

The posterior SFG (▶ Fig. 5.15**d**) has a much larger contribution to the FAT which leave this part of the gyrus heading gently anterior and inferior to the MFG and IFG. The corpus callosum fibers communicate with the contralateral SFG as well as the contralateral MFG and IFG in a tract we call the crossed FAT. I personally think this tract is essential for recovery from the SMA syndrome, but of course this is hard to test. It also has small communications with the cingulate gyrus and MFG.

Middle Frontal Gyrus

Our maps similarly divide the MFG into four parts. The anterior portion (▶ Fig. 5.16**a**) is mostly a set of local connections with the anterior SFG and pars triangularis of the IFG. There is a minor contribution to the SLF.

Moving posteriorly (▶ Fig. 5.16**b**) the connections are mostly with the caudate head and thalamus which exists the gyrus inferoposteriorly en route to the caudate head. The contribution to large cortico-cortical tracts is less prominent, and most of the other connections are local.

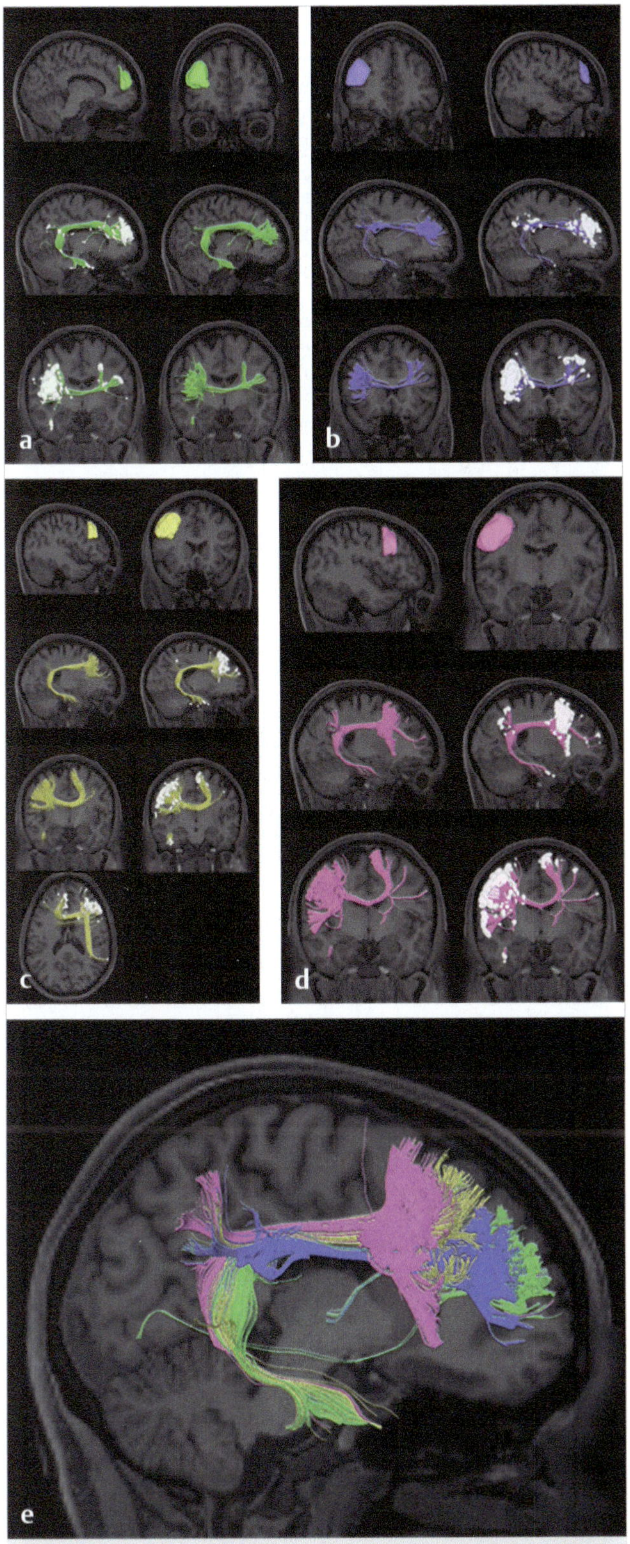

Fig. 5.16 Tractographic anatomy of the MFG. The images are divided into quarters for simplification. (**a**) ROI of the anterior quarter. (**b**) ROI of the next quarter. (**c**) ROI of the third quarter. (**d**) ROI of the posterior quarter. (**e**) Combination of all four ROIs.

The next section of the MFG (▶ Fig. 5.16**c**) comprises a major contribution to the SLF and has connections to its parietal and temporal termini. This ramus exits the gyrus posteriorly and medially and curves to join main tract. This exact frontal bend is a key anatomic point for saving the SLF in posterolateral frontal lobe resections. The callosal connections are mostly to the contralateral SFG with some fibers to the contralateral MFG and anterior insula. There are also connections to the ipsilateral SFG via the FAT. A small portion of these fibers bend towards the thalamus just before entering the callosum. There are numerous local connections with the other parts of the MFG and IFG pars triangularis, as well as a small connection with the insula.

The posterior MFG (▶ Fig. 5.16**d**) also makes a significant contribution to the SLF and these fibers run superior and later posterior to the fibers from part 3 as they move posteriorly. Similarly, its callosal fibers connect to the contralateral SFG and MFG. Unique to this part is a large descending ramus to the inferior frontal gyrus.

Inferior Frontal Gyrus

The anterior portion (▶ Fig. 5.17**a**) is an anterior-posterior oriented set of fibers. A large superior contribution of this gyrus to the SLF connects to the supramarginal gyrus, fusiform gyrus, and the inferior temporal gyrus. There are also connections to the lingula via the IFOF and connections to the contralateral SFG/MFG through the callosal genu.

Moving posteriorly into central par orbitalis (▶ Fig. 5.17**b**) the connections are mostly follow the IFOF which exit the gyrus straight posteriorly en route to the lingula and inferior insula. There are communications with the orbitofrontal gyri, but minimal communication via the callosum.

The pars triangularis portion of IFG (▶ Fig. 5.17**c**) sends out a posteromedial branch to the SLF and has connections to its parietal and temporal termini. There are also connections to the ipsilateral SFG via the FAT which is its major output. It has extensive connections with the local MFG and orbitofrontal cortex. In most cases, it connects to the contralateral SFG.

The pars opercularis (▶ Fig. 5.17**d**) anatomy was surprising to us. We had expected this to connect principally to the SLF and other speech sites given this area's reputation as Broca's area, but it really doesn't appear to be the case. The majority of large cortico-cortical connections of this area connect to the SFG via the FAT. There are some local connections to the MFG and the insula, as well as intragyrus connections. The challenges of resolving this crossing has likely led the FAT vs SLF crossing at this area to be difficult to separate out, but DSI tractography makes a distinction like this possible.

Gyrus Rectus

The majority of this gyrus (▶ Fig. 5.18) connects to the superior temporal gyrus via the uncinate fasciculus which exits the gyrus posterolaterally. There are minimal callosal or local connections, and we could not find large connections with the basal forebrain, caudate, or thalamus.

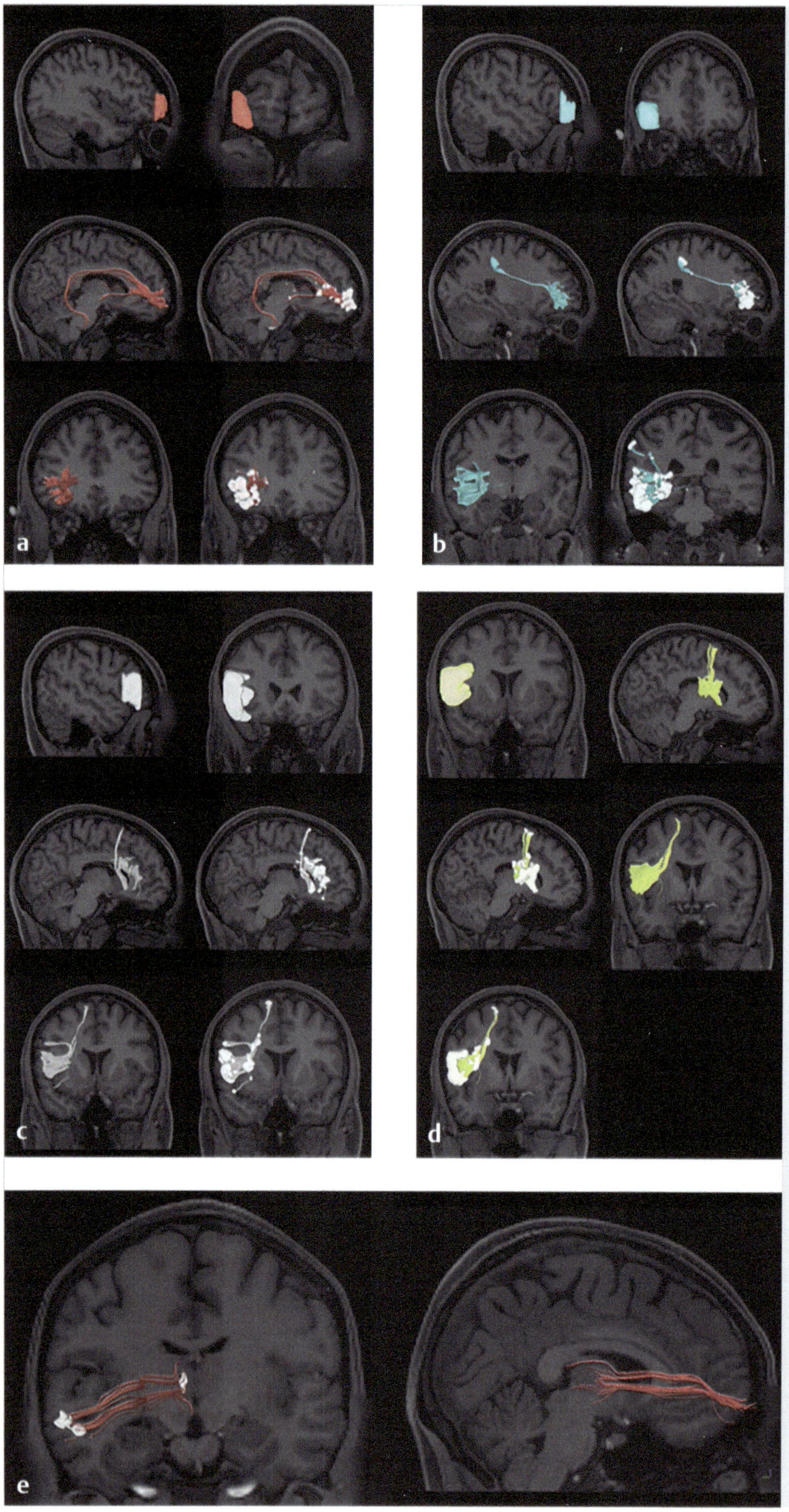

Fig. 5.17 Tractographic anatomy of the IFG. The images are divided into quarters for simplification. (**a**) ROI of the anterior quarter. (**b**) ROI of the next quarter. (**c**) ROI of the third quarter. (**d**) ROI of the posterior quarter. (**e**) Combination of all four ROIs.

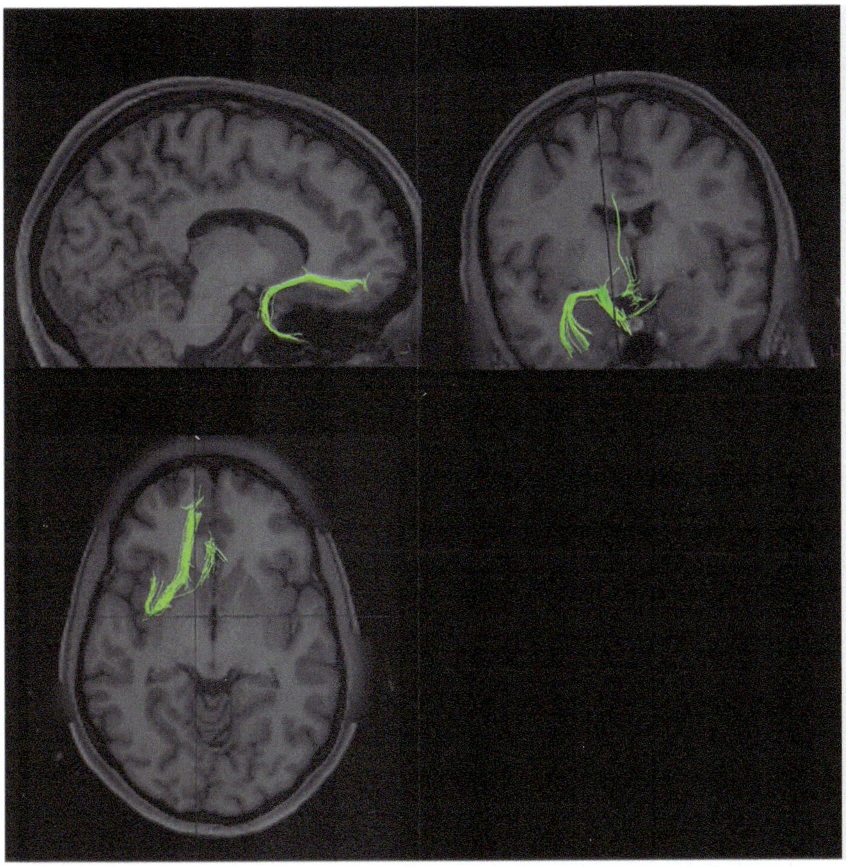

Fig. 5.18 Tractographic anatomy of the gyrus rectus.

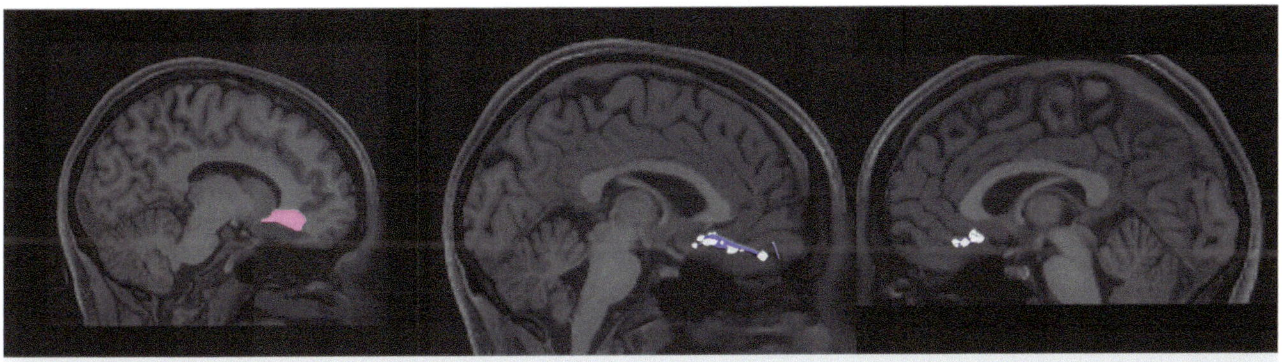

Fig. 5.19 Tractographic anatomy of the subcallosal gyri.

Subcallosal Gyrus

This small gyrus (▶ Fig. 5.19) has some small internal connections as well as some small fibers to the subcallosal cingulate gyrus. It lacks clear evidence of large size fibers with the basal ganglia.

Orbitofrontal Cortex

These gyri are described as a unit divided into thirds from anterior to posterior. The majority of output in all of these gyri leaves the area via the IFOF. The anterior third sends most of its fibers to the MTG in IFOF with some of these fibers bending laterally to this gyrus (▶ Fig. 5.20**a**). It has a reciprocal u-fiber connection with the middle third of the orbitofrontal cortex.

In addition to local connections, the middle third (▶ Fig. 5.20**b**) sends fibers just lateral to the anterior third in the IFOF which also terminate in the MTG.

The posterior third of the orbitofrontal cortex (▶ Fig. 5.20**c**) also exits via the IFOF, but these fibers reach the lingula and STG more prominently than the MTG.

None of these cortices have large fibers to the basal ganglia or thalamus.

5.5.2 Temporal Lobe

Superior Temporal Gyrus

The STG primarily sends its output in a large ramus which courses superomedial over the superior optic radiations to

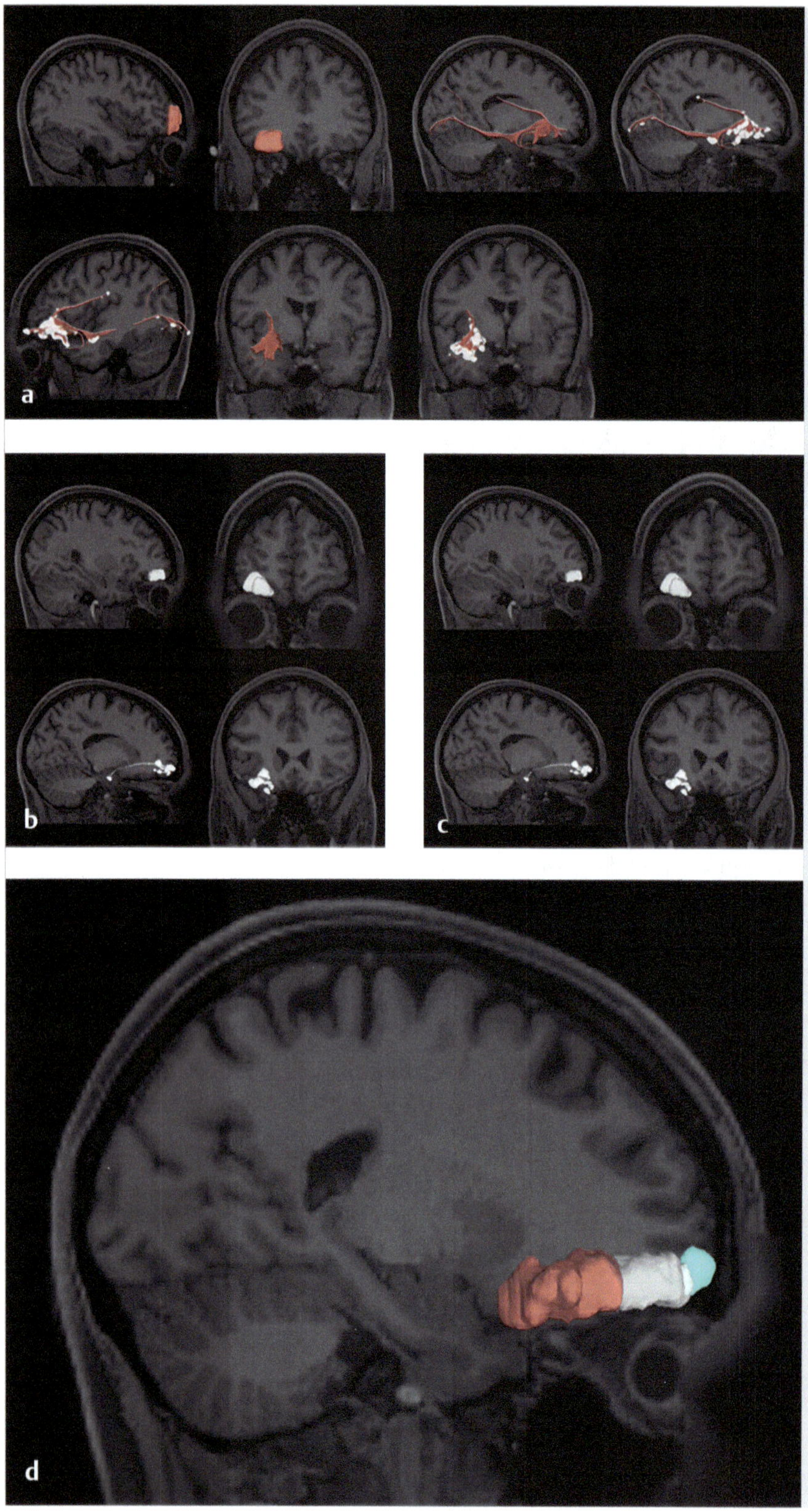

Fig. 5.20 Tractographic anatomy of the orbitofrontal cortex. The images are divided into thirds for simplification. (**a**) ROI of the posterior third. (**b**) ROI of the middle third. (**c**) ROI of the anterior third. (**d**) Image demonstrating the ROIs used.

connect to the superior parietal lobule, cuneus, and precuneus (▶ Fig. 5.21). It has smaller connections to parallel parts of the MTG and ITG. We did not find many connections with the angular gyrus. Though it does connect to the SLG and supramarginal gyrus.

Middle Temporal Gyrus

The anterior half of the MTG (▶ Fig. 5.22) has a similar large posteromedial ramus which ends in the lingula after passing over the optic radiations. It similarly has connections to the orbitofrontal cortices via IFOF, in addition to other local connections.

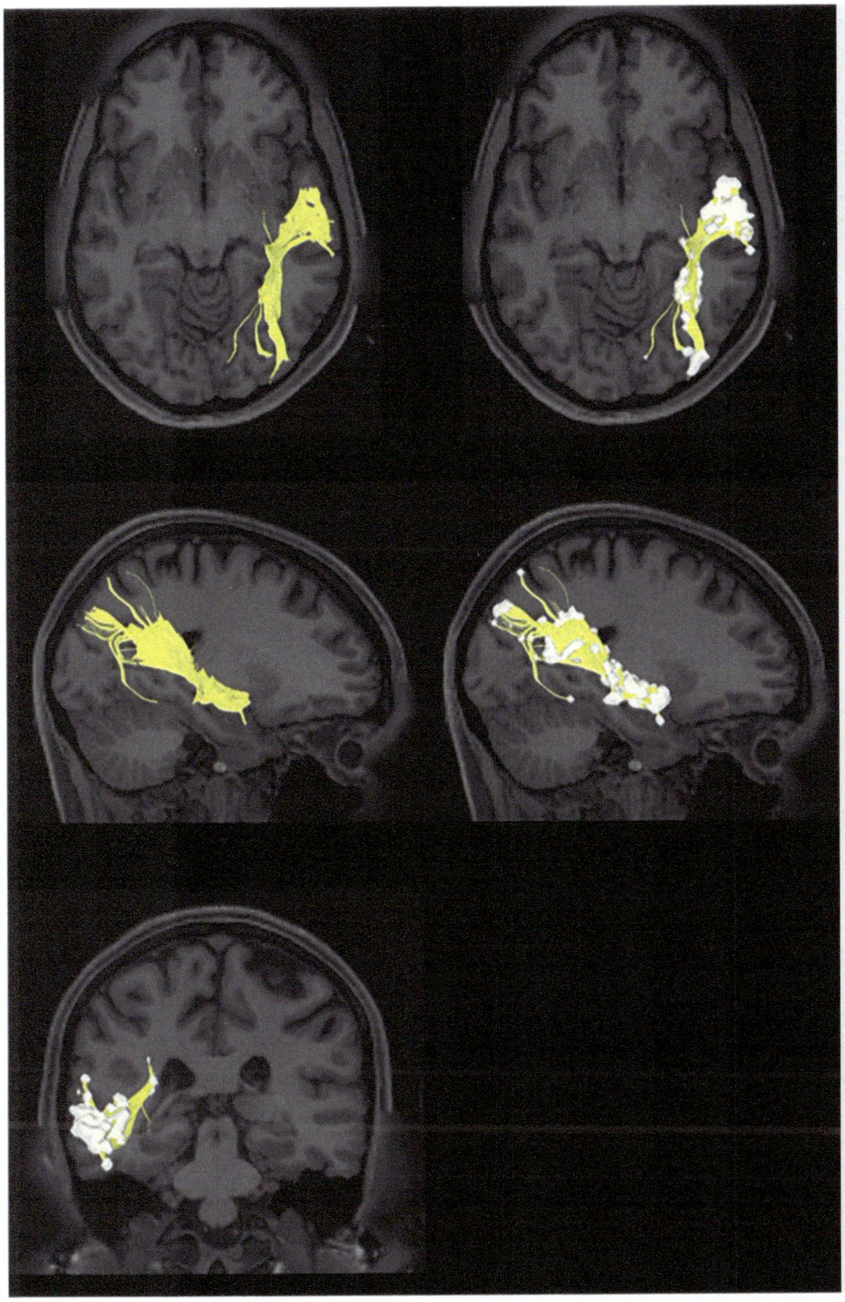

Fig. 5.21 Tractographic anatomy of the STG.

The posterior half (▶ Fig. 5.22) has the same large ramus, which in this gyrus connects to the cuneus and superior parietal lobule via the MdLF.

Inferior Temporal Gyrus

This gyrus has connections entering the SLF (▶ Fig. 5.23), which connect it to the IFG and MFG. As well, it has local connections to the angular gyrus as well as STG and MTG.

Fusiform Gyrus

The fusiform is a difficult gyrus to track fibers in and at present we are still working out the anatomy of this gyrus.

Angular Gyrus

Despite the general belief that the angular gyrus plays a role in speech networks, we did not find much evidence that this gyrus has significant connections to either the SLF or IFOF (▶ Fig. 5.24). Its major connection projects down and medially hooking toward the posterior MTG in a large bundle running lateral to SLF. This of course doesn't eliminate its possible link to speech, as it could be part of a greater semantic network, but it does suggest that it does not have a direct connection to these networks.

It has some connections with the superior parietal lobule.

Supramarginal Gyrus

This gyrus (▶ Fig. 5.25) principally contributes its fibers to the SLF connecting it to the IFG and STG principally. These fibers

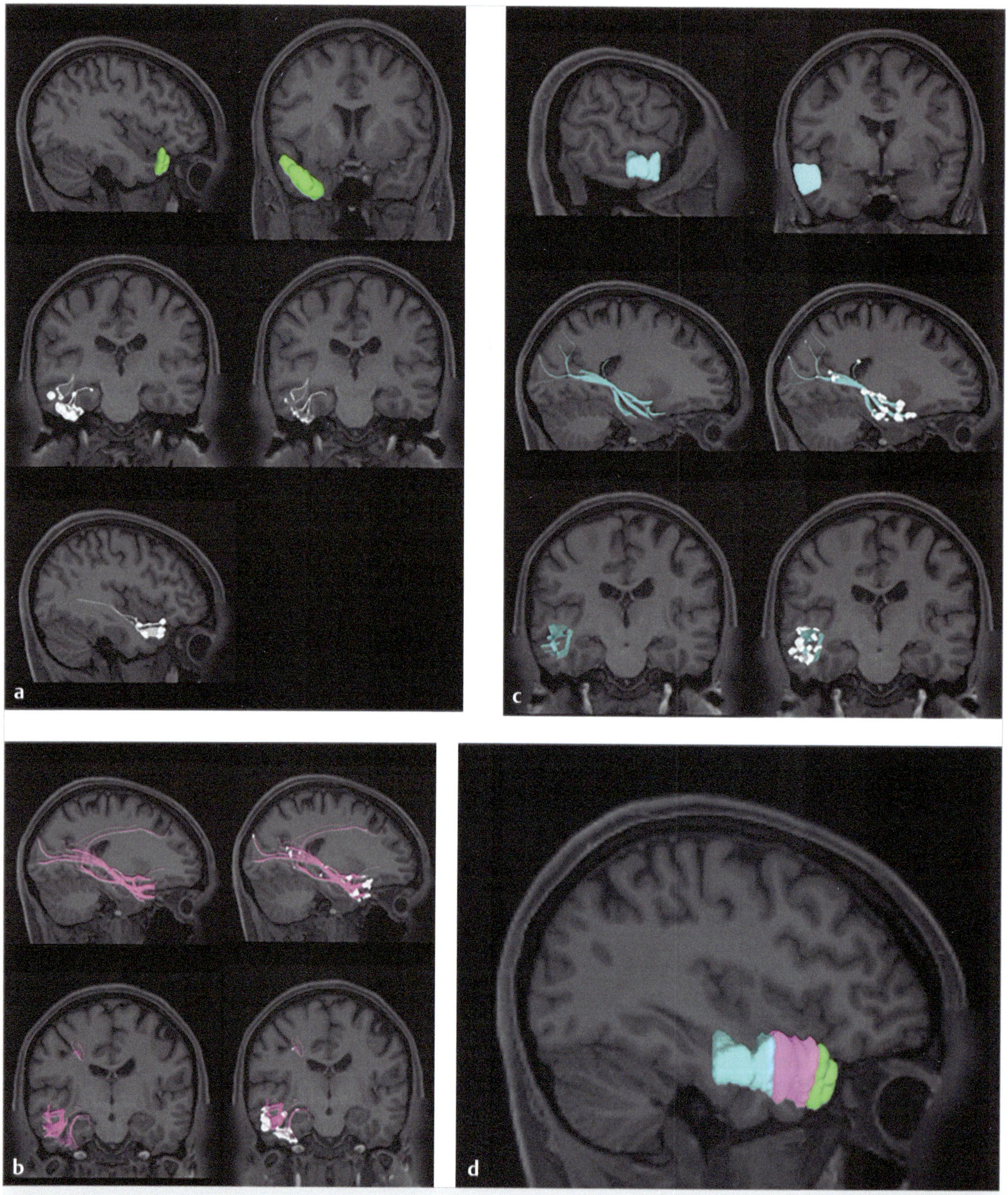

Fig. 5.22 Tractographic anatomy of the MTG. The images are divided into thirds for simplification. (**a**) ROI of the anterior third. (**b**) ROI of the middle third. (**c**) ROI of the posterior third. (**d**) Image demonstrating the ROIs used.

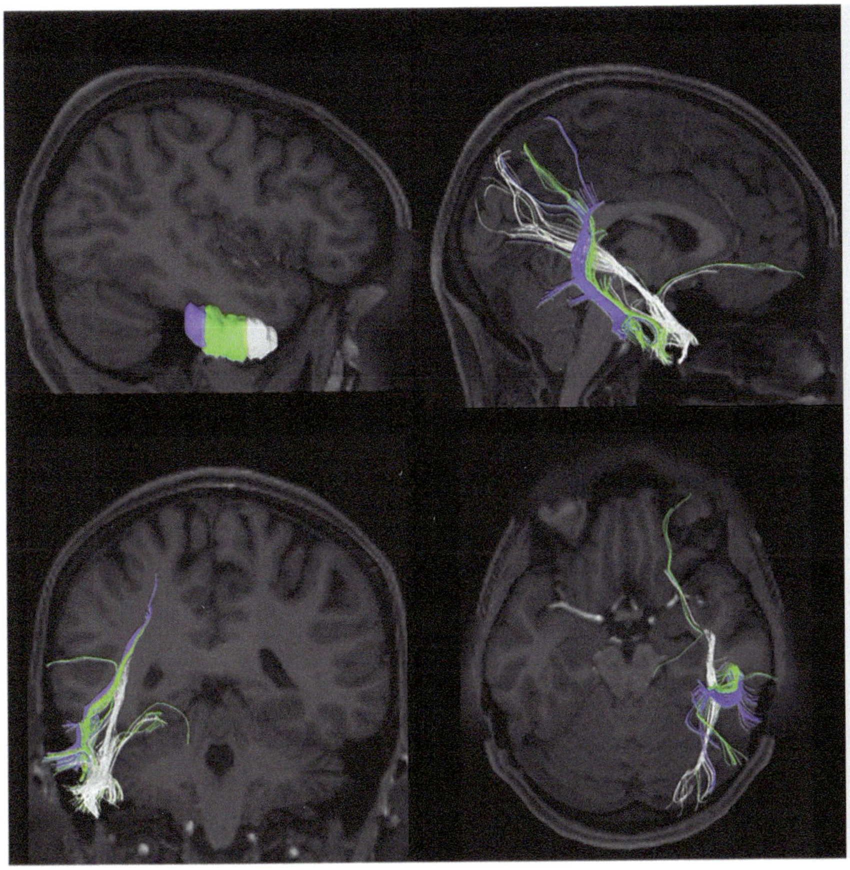

Fig. 5.23 Tractographic anatomy of ITG with all three ROIs demonstrated on the same image set.

are principally located in the inferior part of the arcuate/SLF. This gyrus also has local connections to the parietal lobe, especially the intrapartetal sulcus.

As ▶ Fig. 5.25 also demonstrates, the SMG and angular gyrus have a unique, hydra shaped orientation of their fibers as they exit the gyri to join the subcortical white matter.

5.5.3 Occipital Lobe

Cuneus

We study the cuneus in two parts, one which involves the primary visual cortex, and the other part superior to this. This is because the optic radiations dominate the latter when they are combined making it hard to study where things are going.

The superior cuneus (▶ Fig. 5.26**a**) has a large ramus which first hooks laterally from the gyrus before hooking anterior into the deep white matter. In a pattern repeated throughout the medial occipital lobe, the medial section of these fibers hook medially to cross in the splenium and connect to the homologous part of the contralateral cuneus, while the medial fibers head anterior into the posterior thalamic peduncle to enter the pulvinar and LGN. There are numerous local connections with the lingula and the lower cuneus.

The lower cuneus (▶ Fig. 5.26**b**) not surprisingly receives the optic radiations. It also has a similar medial, then anterior projecting ramus which splits into splenium crossing fibers to the contralateral cuneus and lingula, and lateral fibers which continue to the pulvinar. It also is richly interconnected to the lingula and neighboring cuneus.

Lingula

This unique gyrus has surprisingly more connections than the lower cuneus other side of the calcarine sulcus (▶ Fig. 5.27). In addition to the optic radiations, the fibers into the splenium, and the anterior ramus to the thalamus and pulvinar, the IFOF connects the lingula to a number of brain structures including the orbitofrontal cortex, the MTG and STG, the MFG (i.e., the frontal eye fields), and possible the caudate head. This extensive connection puts the lingula into a number of different neurofunctional systems.

Lateral Occipital Cortex

The lateral occipital lobe generally lacks a stereotypic pattern of gyral/sulcal organization and for this reason, the anatomy is described as a single unit (▶ Fig. 5.28).

The lateral occipital lobe is densely interconnected with itself via u-fibers. Its output/inflow forms a semicoherent bundle at the anteroinferior boundary, which can be identified as leaving in two major directions. Some fibers head to the TPO junction, joining the IFOF. A larger number of fibers bend inferiorly to the inferior temporo-occipital junction. These are likely the fibers of the ventral "what" visual pathway (see Chapter 6).

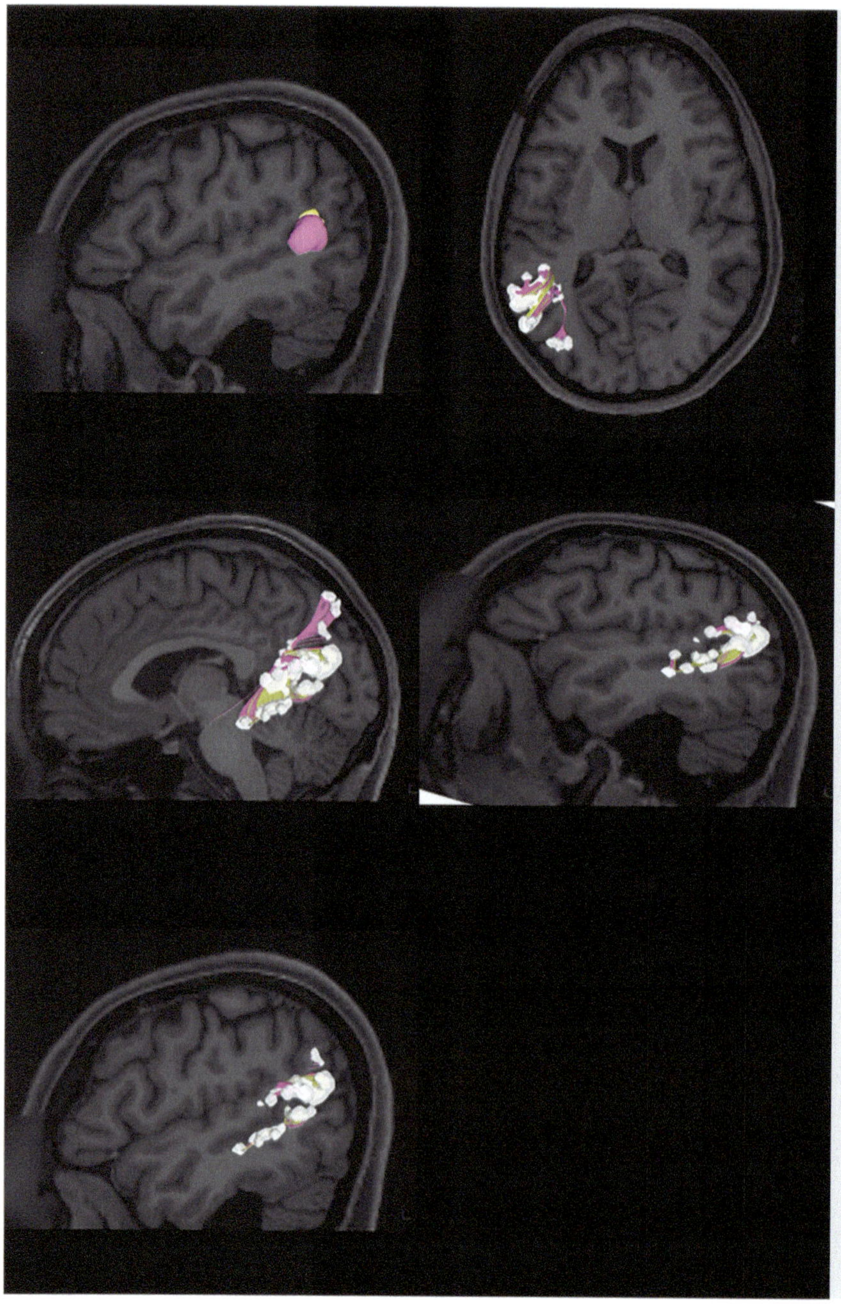

Fig. 5.24 Tractographic anatomy of the angular gyrus with two ROIs demonstrated on the same image set.

5.5.4 Parietal Lobe

Superior Parietal Lobule

The superior parietal lobe has a complex and diverse set of interconnections, which is not surprising given its role in multimodal sensory integration (▶ Fig. 5.29). In addition to internal interconnections, the SPL interconnects with the superior precuneus, likely receiving information from the dorsal "where" pathway, which is a series of serial interprocessing gyral sites on the superior paramedian occipital cortex.

Its most obvious interconnection is its anterior ramus, which connects to the sensory strip, and the posterior MFG (likely premotor areas for the hand) via the medial SLF. Direct connections with the motor strip are usually minimal. In all likelihood, that this communicates processed locational visual information with motor planning areas, which is modified by somatosensory and proprioceptive input from the somatosensory areas, in this bidirectional pathway.

There is also a large inferiorly directed ramus which communicates with the thalamus and head of the caudate.

Finally, there is a large lateral ramus, by which the SPL, communicates with the posterior angular gyrus.

Precuneus

The precuneus maps (▶ Fig. 5.30) were somewhat surprising to us. The majority of the connections of the precuneus were with the thalamus, basal ganglia, and brainstem, with only local connections with neighboring gyri. There are contributions to the

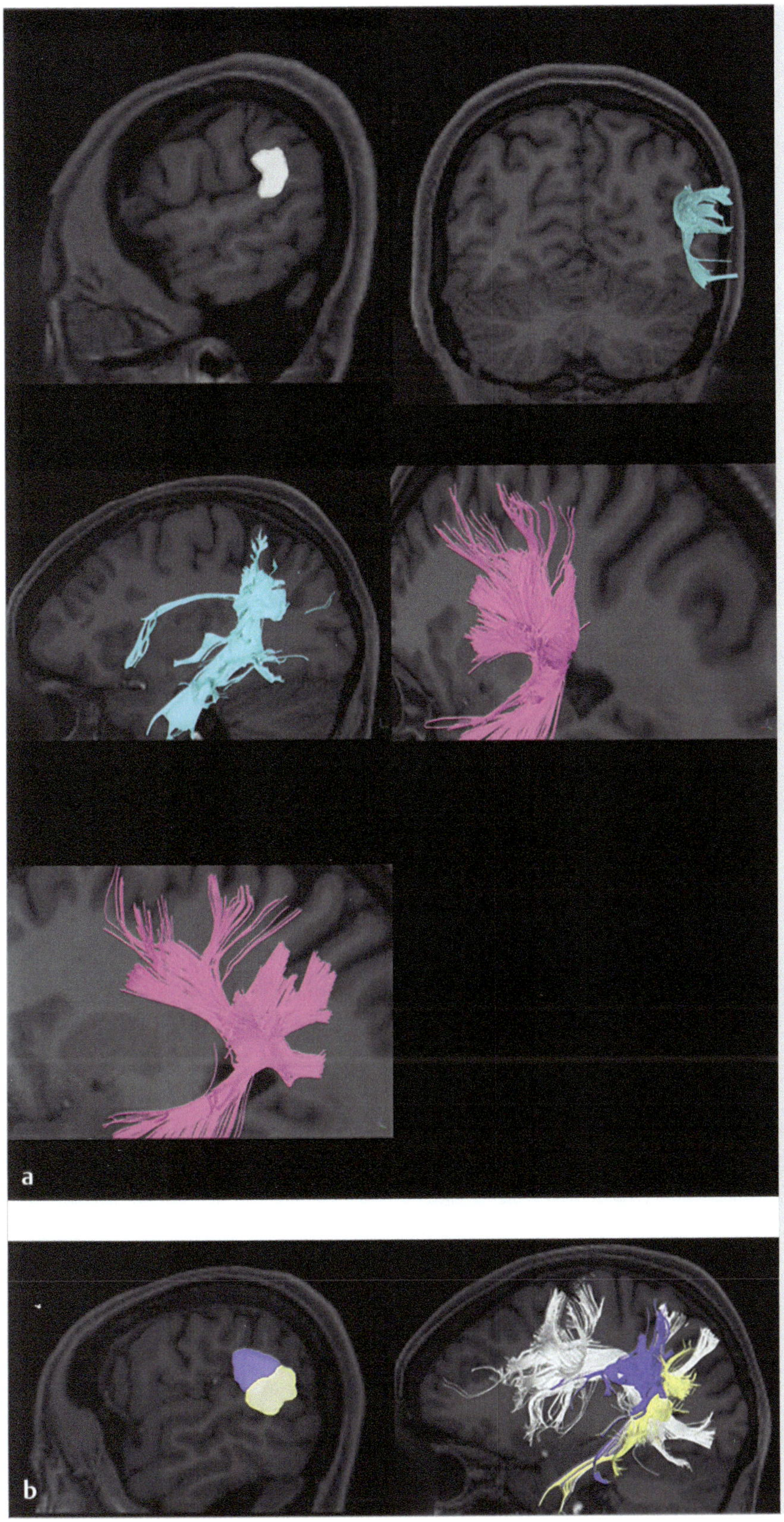

Fig. 5.25 Tractographic anatomy of SMG.
(**a**) Demonstrates the anatomy of the SMG in two ROIs the lower panels in pink demonstrate the a zoomed in view of the fibers leaving the gyrus.
(**b**) A comparison of the white matter anatomy of the SMG (blue), and the angular gyrus (yellow). The SLF proper is displayed in white to demonstrate what part of the tract these gyral connections form.

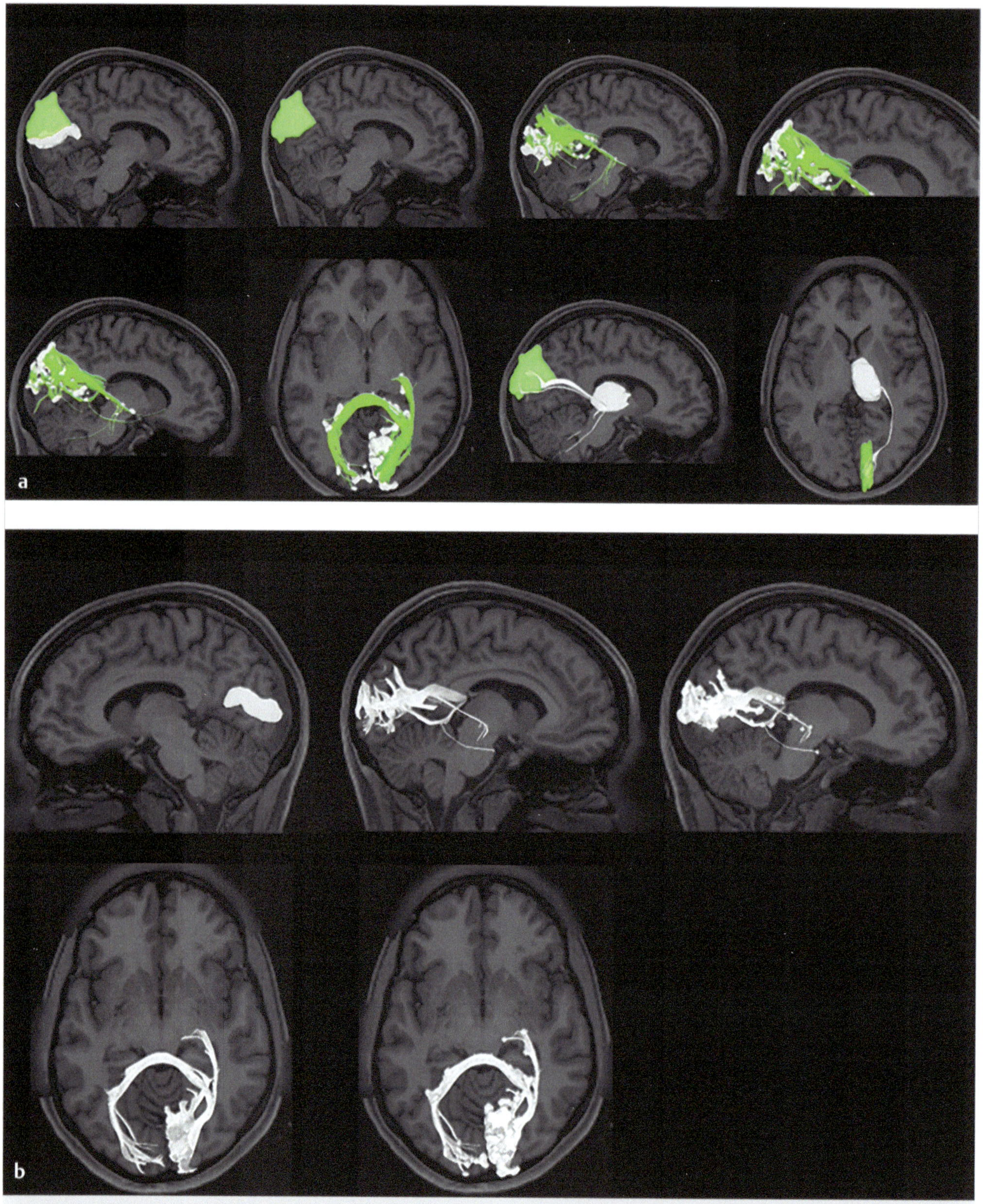

Fig. 5.26 Tractographic anatomy of the cuneus. (**a**) Demonstrates the anatomy of the upper cuneus (i.e., that which is not part of the primary visual cortex), a connection with the thalamus is demonstrated. (**b**) The anatomy of the lower cuneus which straddles the calcarine sulcus.

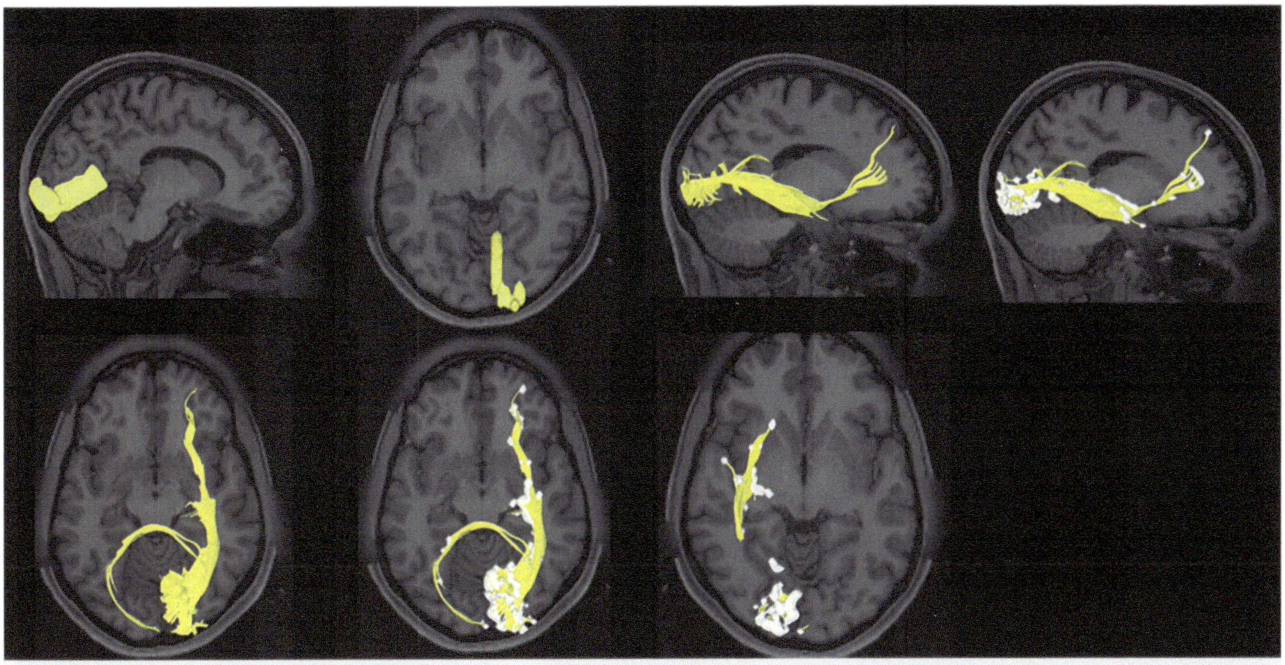

Fig. 5.27 Tractographic anatomy of the lingual.

dorsal visual processing stream on its superior border, but its connections are mostly with the lower structures, and less with long range cortico-cortical connections, at least based on our early work. The significance of this is unclear.

Subparietal Gyrus

Despite its close proximity to the SPL and precuneus, the subparietal gyrus (▶ Fig. 5.31) has an entirely different pattern of connections. The majority of its connections are with the anterior medial superior frontal gyrus, through the cingulum. This is quite likely a part of the default mode network, which is discussed in more detail in Chapter 6.

Sensorimotor Areas

Sensory Strip

I have divided the maps of sensory strip macroconnectivity into two parts (▶ Fig. 5.32), which demonstrate different connection patterns. The upper two-thirds has a "bouquet" type appearance, with a stem exiting the thalamus and widening into the entire strip. The sensory strip has communication with the motor strip and the SPL, as well as connections with the contralateral brain.

The lower third (the facial portion) receives its thalamic input in a smaller, laterally curving ramus. It has extensive local connections with the supramarginal gyrus, the motor cortex, and the IFG (premotor areas) via the lateral parts of the SLF. The relevance of this input for the speech network is obvious.

Motor Strip

▶ Fig. 5.33 demonstrates the motor cortex connections divided into three parts. The upper portions are extensively interconnected with the basal ganglia, the thalamus, the contralateral motor cortex, as well as the sensory cortex, the SMA and premotor areas, in addition to its contribution to the corticospinal tract.

Moving slightly inferior, we note that the principle communications are local U-fibers with the sensory cortex, and the premotor areas, including some communication with the pars triangularis. The contribution to the corticospinal tracts are less well visualized with our methods.

Finally, the lower motor cortex principally communicates with the middle motor cortex, as well as premotor, and sensory cortices. The premotor cortex in this region is largely the "Broca's area."

Supplementary Motor Area

This complex area has been described above (▶ Fig. 5.15**d**) but is repeated for emphasis. The SMA is the medial SFG. Fibers leaving/joining the SMA leave in three bundles: The medial bundle, which crosses in the corpus callosum to connect to the contralateral SMA and premotor areas (the crossed FAT), the middle bundle which communicates with the basal ganglia and contributes to the corticospinal tract, and the lateral bundle which forms the Ipsilateral FAT. Its long range fibers mostly run in the coronal plane, and it has only smaller U-fiber connections with adjacent cortices anterior and posterior to it.

Cingulate Gyrus

The cingulate gyrus is a seemingly simple gyrus with seemingly simple connectivity (▶ Fig. 5.34): it is a C-shaped gyrus, and the majority of its connections run in the cingulum with minimal interconnections with the surrounding gyri. The major exceptions to this are the frontal rami, where fibers exit the bundle to connect with the medial SFG, and the parietal rami which ascend to join the subparietal gyrus among others.

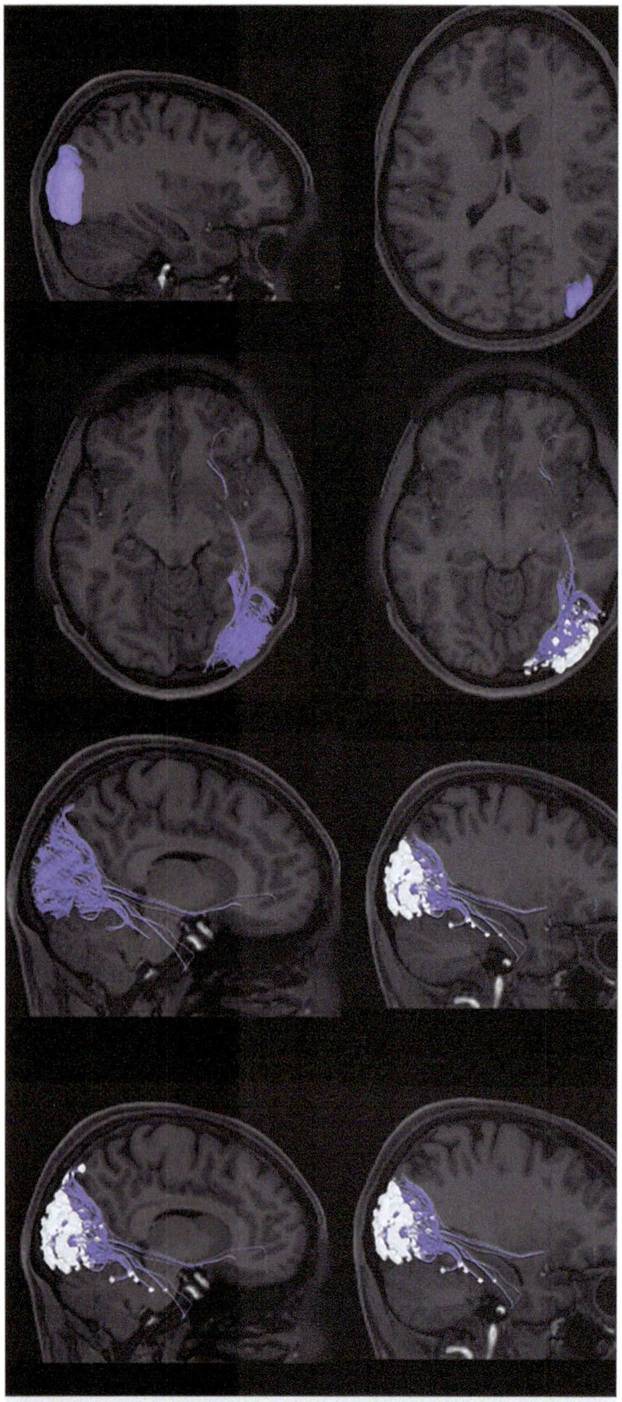

Fig. 5.28 Tractographic anatomy of the lateral occipital cortex.

With these exceptions in mind, the cingulum otherwise is a long connection interconnecting the basal forebrain and septal structures with the cingulate gyrus cortex, eventually terminating in the parahippocampal gyrus.

Connections to the Deep Structures

Caudate Nucleus

The majority of the bulk of the caudate nucleus is located in the head. The head predominantly projects anteriorly in a series of rami predominantly aimed at the anterior part of middle frontal gyrus (▶ Fig. 5.35). There are some connections with the SPL as also.

Putamen

Not surprisingly, the putamen receives widespread communication from a large variety of cortical sites (▶ Fig. 5.36). Interestingly, the majority of these seem to come from relatively paramedian cortices, including dense connections with the SMA and SFG areas as well as commication with the superior parietal lobule and apparently the contralateral SMA. Other maps of networks (Chapter 6) demonstrate some connection with the premotor IFG, but these are seemingly smaller than those from the SMA.

Thalamus

Fibers enter/exit the thalamus in five major bundles; the thalamic peduncles (▶ Fig. 5.37). The anterior peduncle passes through the anterior limb of the internal capsule and heads to the anterior frontal lobe. The superior peduncle is broad and remains medial to the corticospinal tract and lateral to the cingulum as it heads upward to connect with the cingulate gyrus, the SFG, motor and sensory cortices, and paramedian parietal lobe. The posterior peduncle begins just anterior to the atrium and hooks around it on its way to the occipital lobe. It is carrying the optic radiations, as well as bidirectional communications between the visual system and the thalamus. The inferior peduncle is somewhat shorter, and is headed to the orbitofrontal cortices, the amygdala and insula. Finally, the lateral peduncle passes laterally to communicate with the lateral temporal lobe, including the STG and SMG.

5.6 Crossing Points

Moving back to the macro scale, it is important to make a few overall observations about global tract patterns which are critical to understanding cerebral anatomy and how to plan safe surgeries. In that regard, ▶ Fig. 5.38 highlights some of the key conflict zones in the cerebrum, where large tracts or key connections cross in close proximity to each other. In other words, at crossing points it is possible to disconnect several brain areas by removing a small volume of brain.

The most notorious crossing point is at the temporo-parieto-occipital (TPO) junction which lies at the back of the insula just deep to the posterior most parts of MTG and STG. Here, in a small area one has the opportunity to cut (from superficial to deep) across the connection between angular gyrus and MTG, the SLF, IFOF, the optic radiations, the posterior thalamic peduncle, and parts of the posterior limb of the internal capsule. This should give pause to anyone venturing into this area.

Another crossing point occurs deep to the posterior parts of inferior and middle frontal gyrus, particularly near the plane of the anterior insula. In addition to the Frontal rami of the SLF, there are branches of the IFOF, and the bulk of the FAT and crossed FAT all in a small area.

A final major crossing point of note involves the midline posterior frontal lobe. Here, as we descend inferiorly from the superior surface, we can cut across the FAT, parts of the corpus

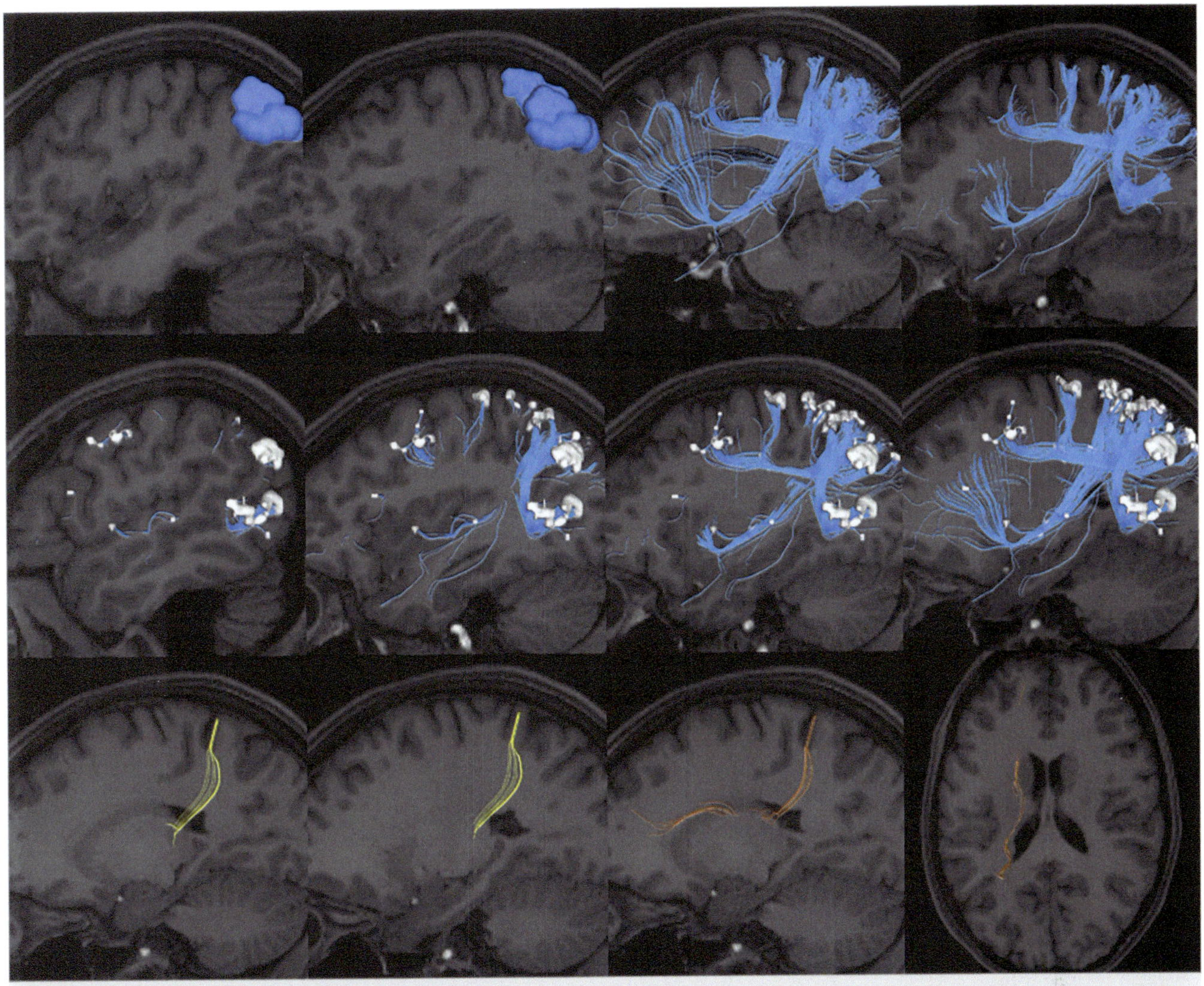

Fig. 5.29 Tractographic anatomy of the superior parietal lobule.

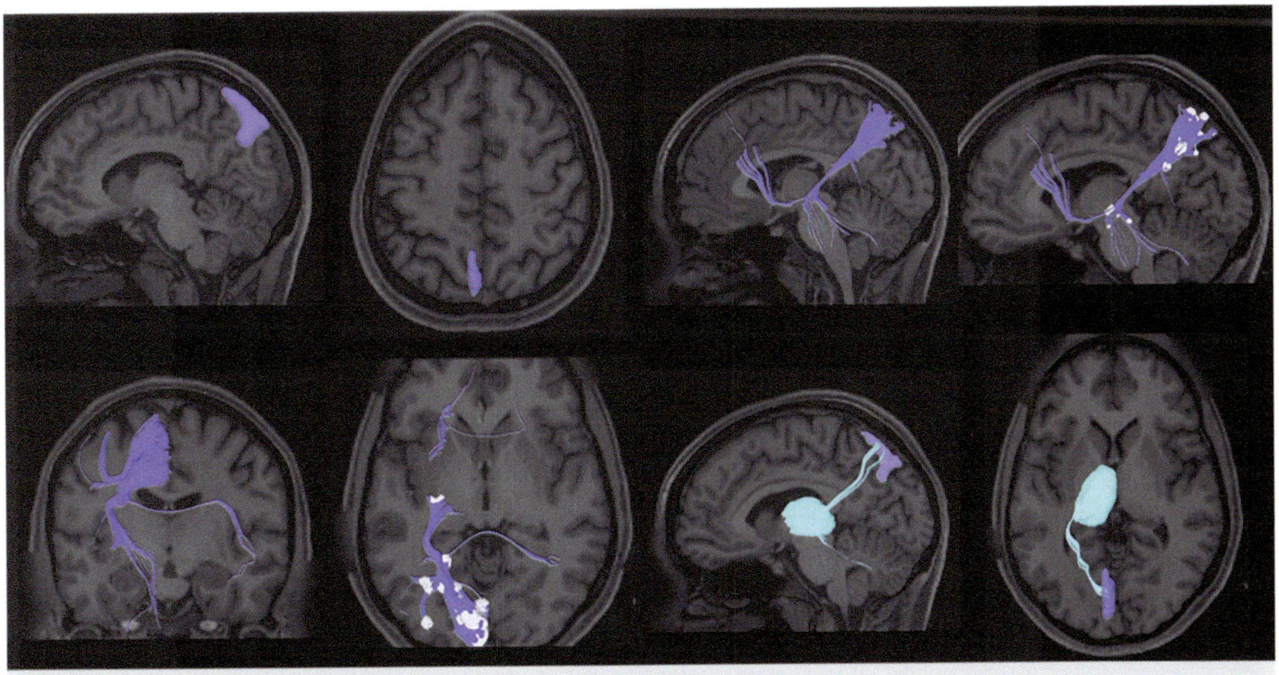

Fig. 5.30 Tractographic anatomy of the precuneus.

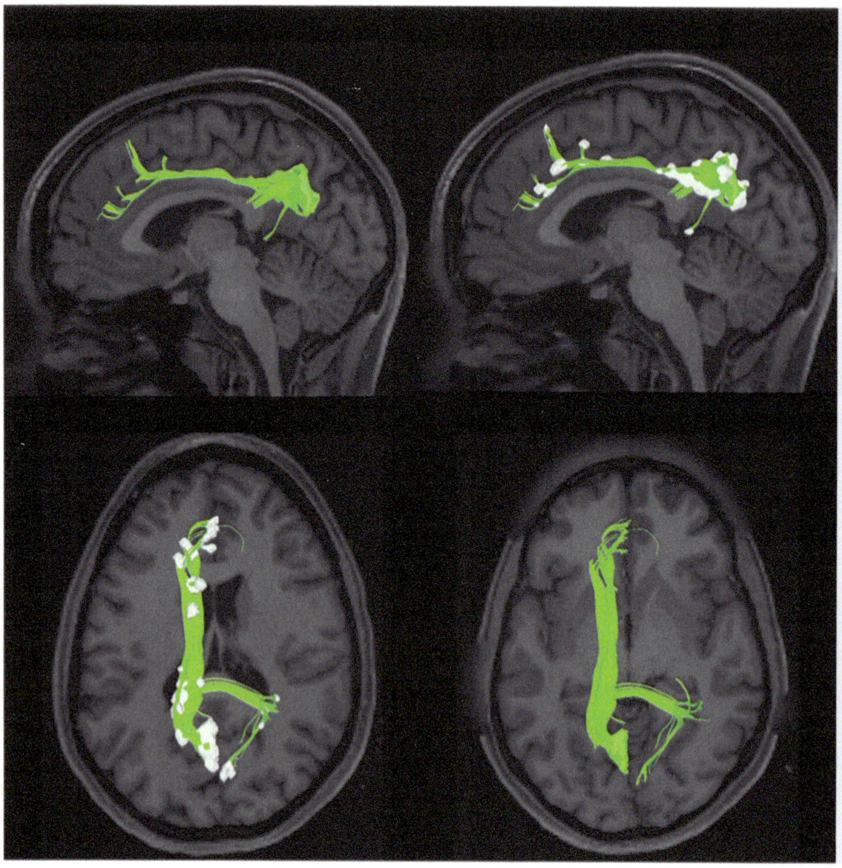

Fig. 5.31 Tractographic anatomy of the subparietal gyrus.

callosum connecting the SMA regions, the cingulum, and parts of the thalamic peduncle.

I'll end this chapter by pointing out that the crossing points underlie areas typically associated with eloquence, such as the so-called Broca's and Wernicke's areas, and the SMA. This in my opinion is one of the great cofounding problems with using lesion data to ascribe function to specific cortical areas, as lesions at crossing points have the ability to cause widespread network damage with small lesions.

5.7 Final Points

This is the most detailed analysis of specific white matter anatomy that I am aware of to date. It is not an all-encompassing atlas of all white matter anatomy of the cerebrum, and is tailored to the specific needs of this book. For example, I did not spend time describing the fornix or the corticospinal tract, which I assume more readers of this book are familiar with. Additionally, I did not include anatomy of the insula, the fusiform, or parahippocampal gyri for technical reasons: they are challenging to map with tractography, and we are still working out the details, and I didn't elect to put speculative details into this book, especially when the areas involved are generally not critical brain regions with lower margins of error. This is just a detailed set of images not available anywhere else at present, which begin the discussions which follow.

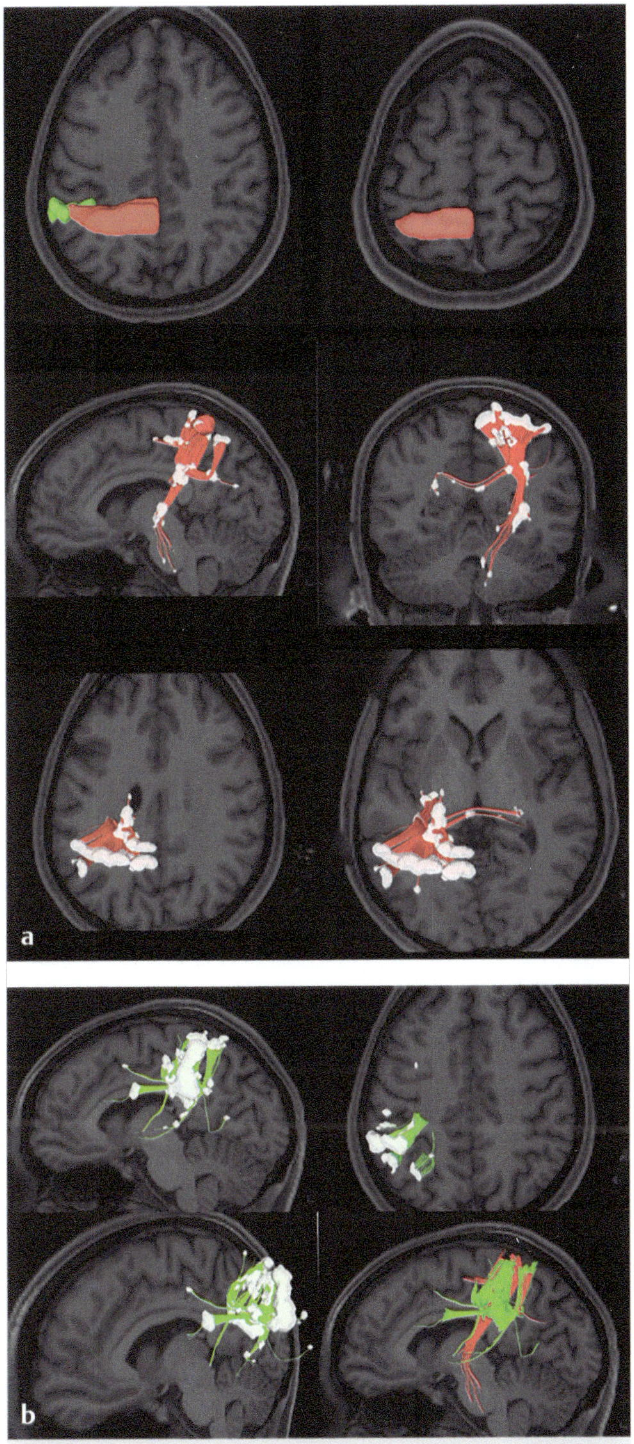

Fig. 5.32 Tractographic anatomy of the sensory cortex. The images are divided into halves for simplification. (**a**) ROI of the medial half. (**b**) ROI of the lateral half.

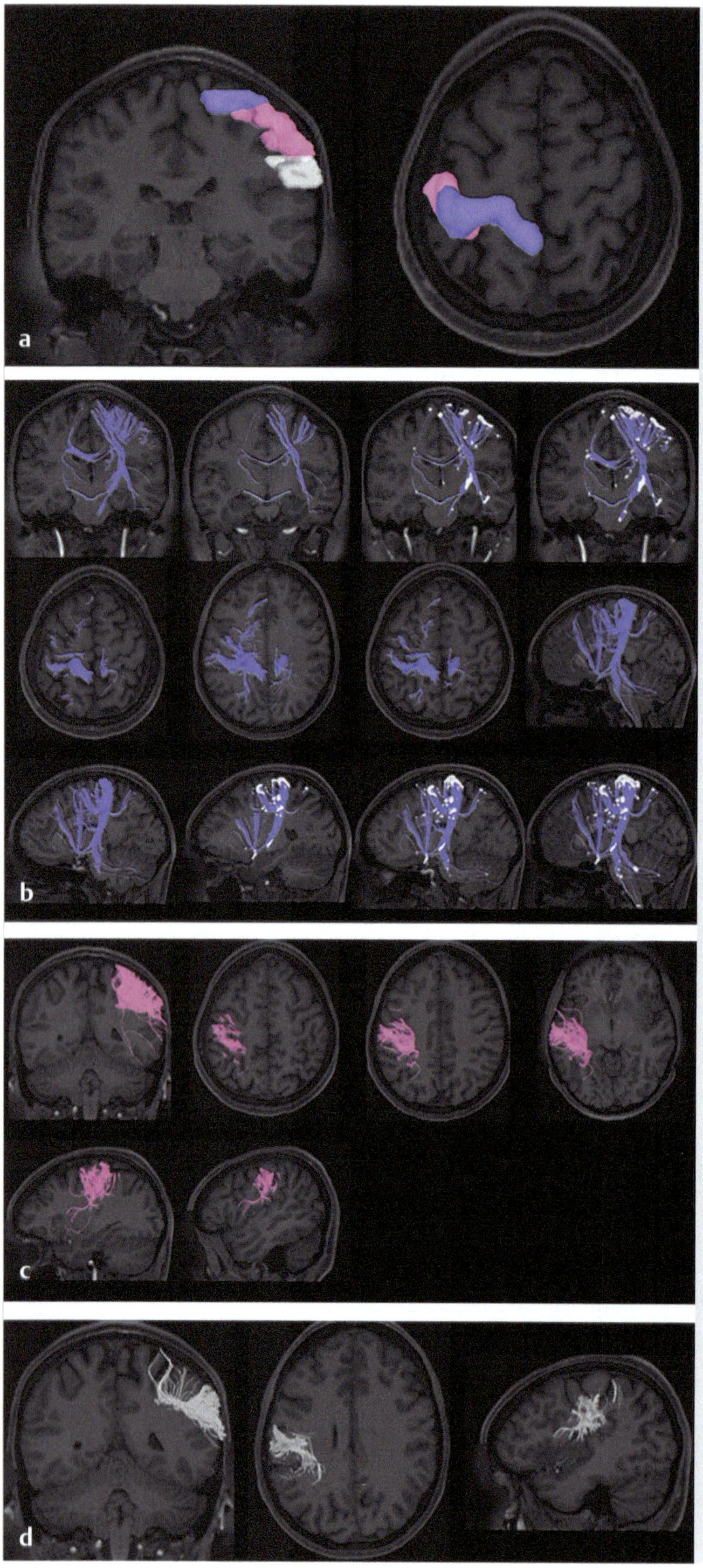

Fig. 5.33 Tractographic anatomy of the motor cortex. The images are divided into thirds for simplification. (**a**) Image demonstrating the ROIs used. (**b**) ROI of the medial third. (**c**) ROI of the middle third. (**d**) ROI of the lateral third.

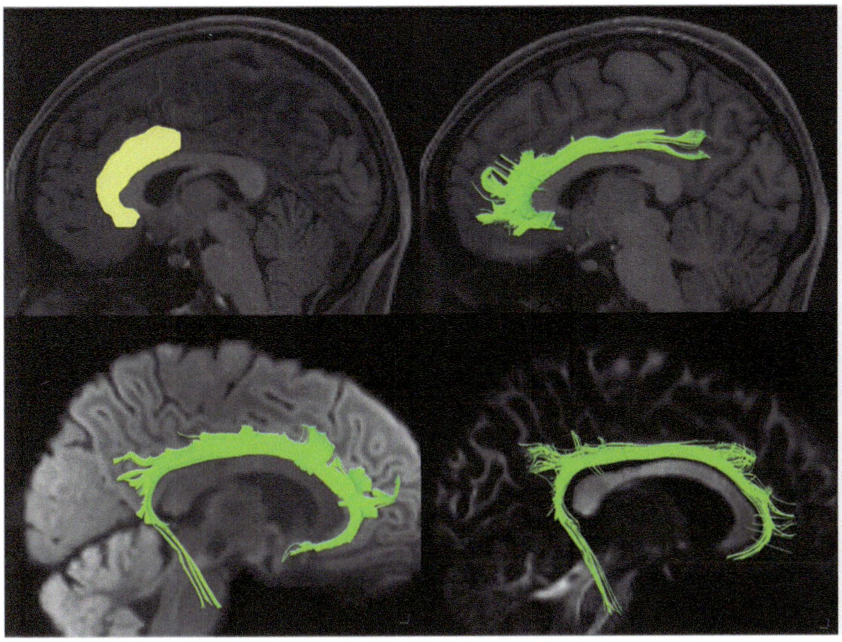

Fig. 5.34 Tractographic anatomy of the cingulate gyrus.

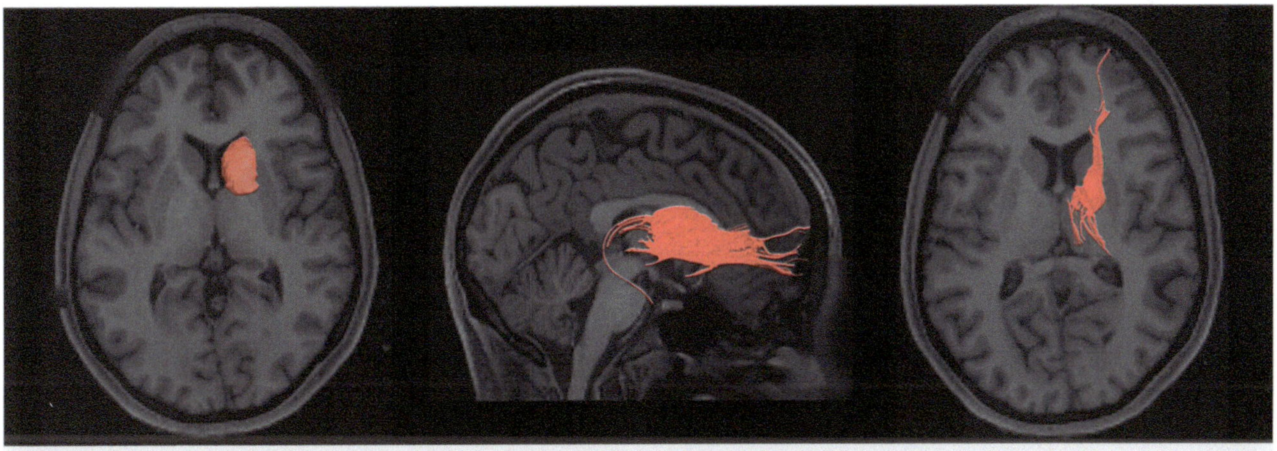

Fig. 5.35 Tractographic anatomy of the head of the caudate nucleus.

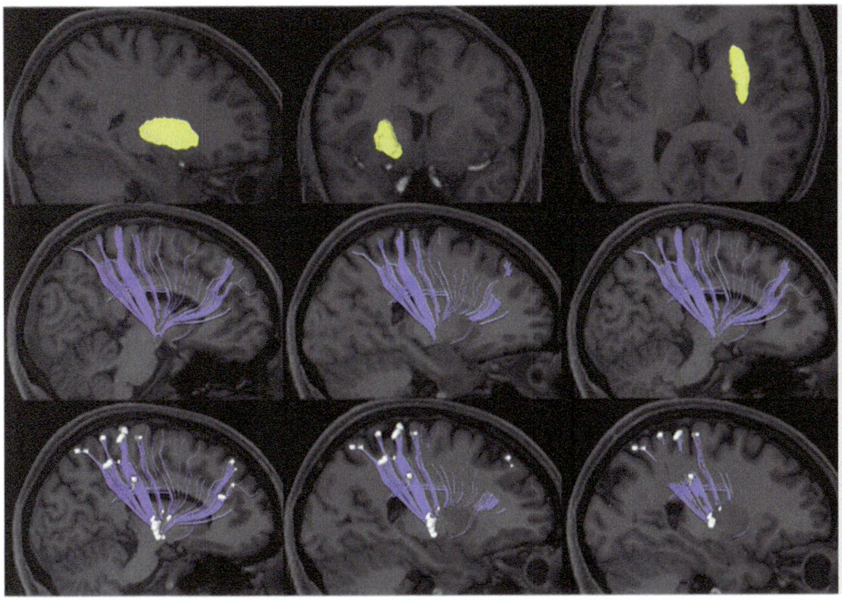

Fig. 5.36 Tractographic anatomy of the putamen.

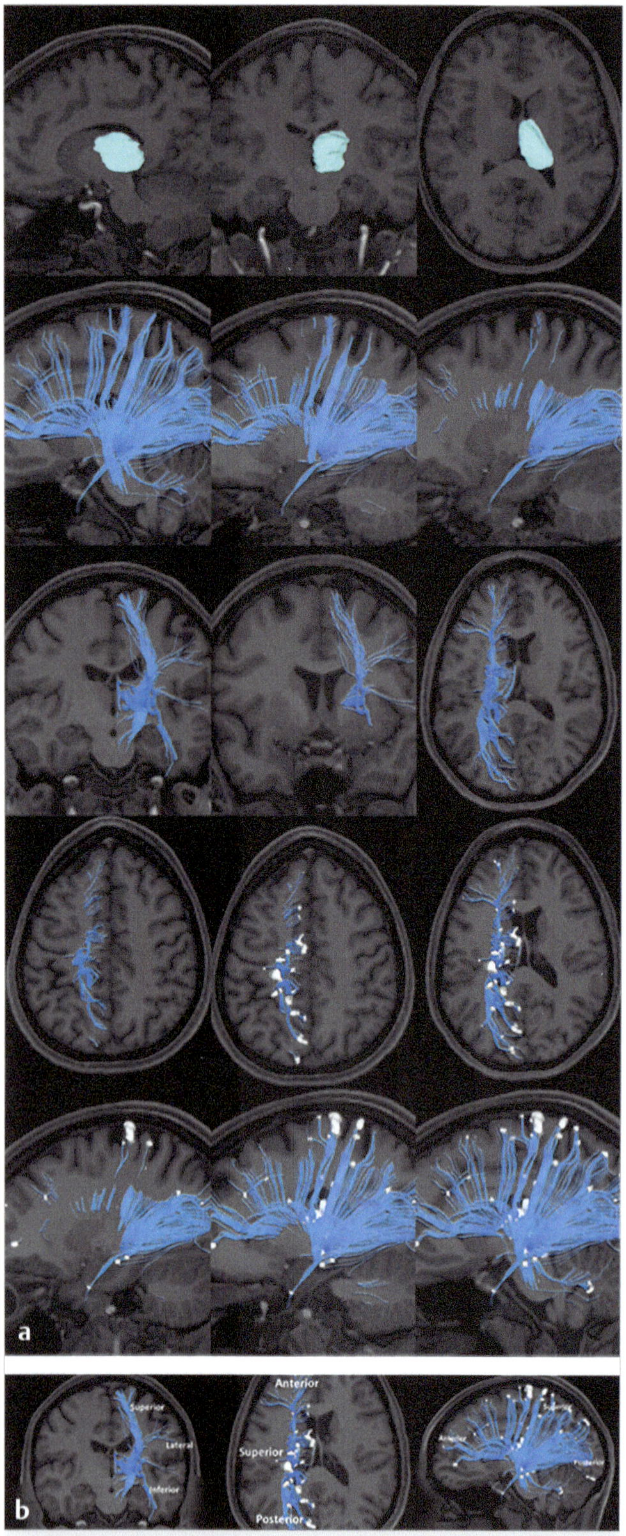

Fig. 5.37 (**a**) Tractographic anatomy of the thalamus. (**b**) Labeled diagram demonstrating the 5 thalamic penduncles.

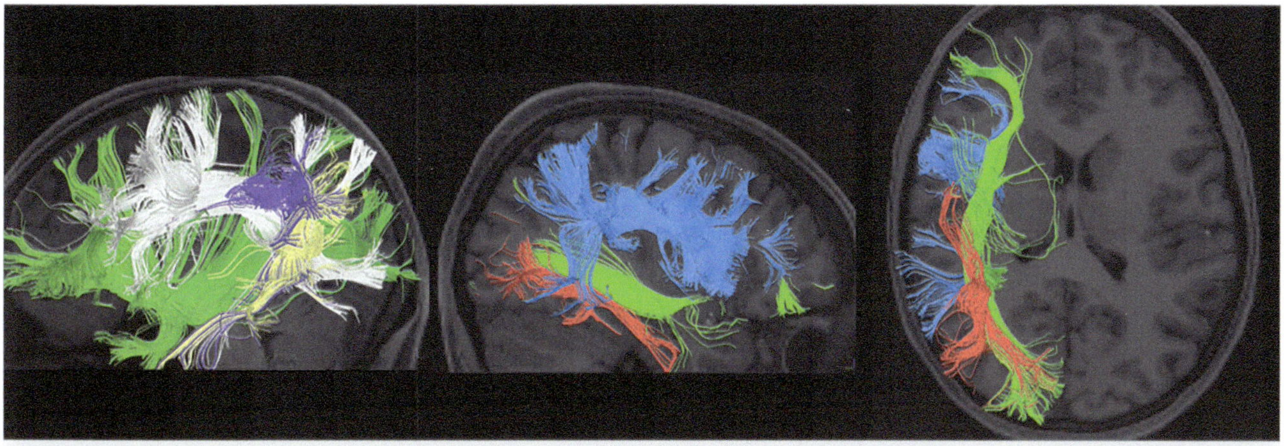

Fig. 5.38 Tractographic anatomy demonstrating multiple lateral tracts on the same images. Note the significant number of tract crossings deep to the SMG and the inferior frontal gyri.

6 Functional Networks of the Human Cerebrum

6.1 Introduction

In this chapter, I take the ambitious step of trying to cobble connectomic data into a coherent model of human brain networks. It should be acknowledged that by doing so, I am putting out some data which may need to be revised in the future. Quite simply, we are still working a lot of these data out.

Despite the challenges of working with incomplete data to try to create a world view of how higher brain functions, there are some major potential rewards.[1,2] Presently, we do surgery on the brain without more than cursory models of how the brain works, many of which date from decades ago which predate MRI let along functional imaging. It is almost certain that an incomplete anatomic model is better than no real model. Further, while functional MRI and other types of brain mapping have provided some insight into how some of these functions are organized, often the exact anatomy is imprecisely defined and the exact connectivity is poorly understood. Knowing that the function is grossly located in the lateral frontal lobe may work in research, but millimeters count in surgery.

The goal of this chapter is to provide an advanced anatomic framework of the gross cerebral anatomy underlying specific higher brain functions from which to base any further discussion on how to preserve cerebral functions in surgery. You can't validate or invalidate an idea with no clear hypothesis, and you can't build a model without attempting to synthesize existing data into coherent frameworks. This chapter is the first that I know of to try to demonstrate the anatomy of higher brain functions in a surgically and anatomically useful framework, and hopefully, it will be the beginning of a long future of critically revising and refining these models.

6.2 Methods and Assumptions

If you look at maps which attempt to summarize every single connection in a network, such as the motor network, the complexity is stunning, and it strikes you that we will never be able to meaningfully use something so complex in daily practice.[1,2] Further, it is likely that almost every part of the cerebrum has at least some connections at a microscopic level with almost every other one. Despite this, we as neurosurgeons know from experience, that you can make a significant transgression without destroying observable brain functions in any tragic manner, so it is certain that many of these connections are redundant, or at least compensable. It is likely that there are no individual neuron or small collections of neurons anywhere in the brain that cannot be cut without causing a deficit, assuming that other similar neurons remain to compensate for its loss.

These networks do not strive to account for every possible connection in the human cerebrum between sites of relevance, nor do they attempt to include every area of the brain which has been noted to be activated in one study or another. It is probable that the basal ganglia, basal forebrain, the ascending seratoneric system, and or the cerebellum could probably be put somehow by someone into every single one these circuits based on some study, again, we have to cut somewhere, and we want to focus on what is necessary or central to maintaining the brain function of interest. There are no bonus points for adhering to strict interpretations of connectionism, and what matters is whether the patient can do the function you aim to preserve after the surgery or not.

We have grounded all of our work with connectomics in the Human Connectome Parcellation scheme. It is not the only way to divide up the human cortex into segments; however, it is based on extremely high-quality data, and it is a sensible, data-driven scheme which correlates many previous schemes in addition to identifying new regions. Examples of the parcellations can be seen in the figures in Chapter 3; however, thoroughly describing these areas is beyond the scope of this book and would require a book of its own.

With the idea that these models are aimed at clinically useable as opposed to comprehensive maps of brain function, I went about making these maps in the following manner:

1. We utilized neuropsychologic and functional imaging literature paired with my own experiences with awake brain surgery to create a basic idea about what the networks should roughly entail.
2. We performed coordinate meta-analysis to determine statistical locations of activation in a standardized coordinate space. This techniques allows one to combine the published coordinates from the fMRI and lesion literature to make a statistical map of significant sites of brain actuation.
3. We converted the Human Connectome project parcellation scheme to create ROIs of the parcellations in this coordinate space. We then matched these ROIs to the activation estimates yielded by coordinate based meta-analysis to figure out which areas were being activated according to these studies.
4. We then utilized tractography to identify which fibers, if any, joined these areas. This creates a backbone for the network. It is important to note that the term backbone does not imply that we have identified all possible sites involved in the network. It is certain that the creation of higher human abilities involve interactions between networks. For example, interactions between visual, semantic, and face motor systems are necessary to name objects.

6.2.1 The Motor Network (▶ Fig. 6.1, ▶ Fig. 6.2, ▶ Fig. 6.3)

This system is the most familiar to neurosurgeons, as we have been making sure patients were "moving all four" for our entire careers. Thinking in terms of basic motor cortex issues is not foreign or novel to us; however, I would argue that most of us have a relatively overly simplistic view of the motor system, which overestimates how great a patient who is "moving all four" is really doing from a motor standpoint, and in some cases, puts our goal to use all four extremities at serious risk. In short, you cannot leave motor strip, disconnected from the rest of the network, floating in the air, and expect it to move the

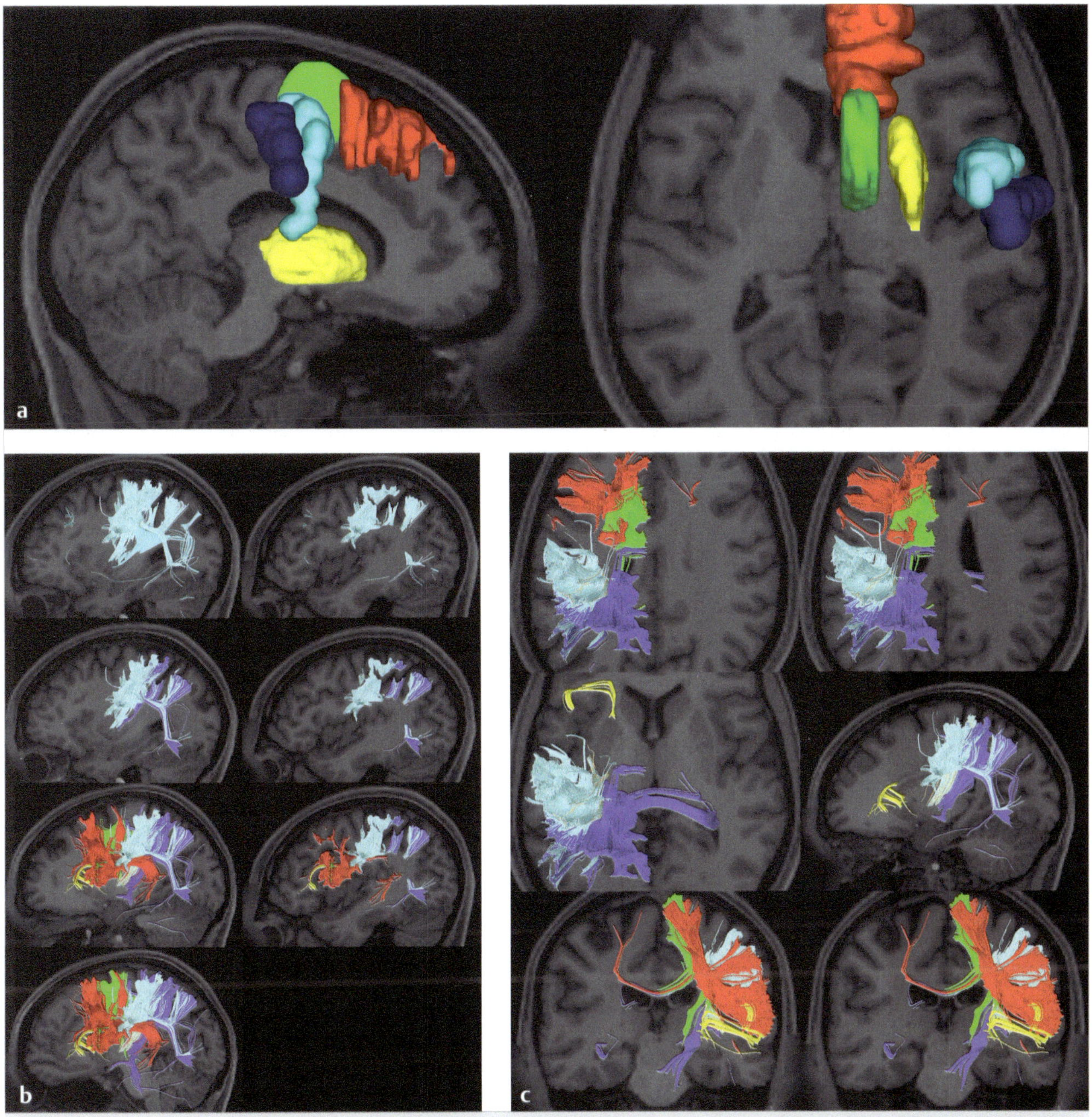

Fig. 6.1 Gross anatomy of the motor system. The model is gradually built in these sequential images in a sequential manner so that the relative contributions of each component can be distinguished. Face motor areas (**a**) demonstrates the ROIs used to build this model which include the face motor cortex (in light blue), the face sensory cortex (in dark blue), the premotor cortices (in red) and the SMA (in green). These colors are used for the corresponding tract throughout the map. (**b**) Sequential building of the network: 1) the upper panels demonstrate the face motor cortex fibers in light blue. The curved medial bend of the fibers into the descending motor fibers can be visualized bending into the page to run around the insula, 2) the second set of panels demonstrate the addition of the sensory cortex communications in dark blue. The bidirectional communication between these two cortices is striking, 3) in the third set of panels, we add the premotor cortex in red. Note that in addition with communication with the SMA via the FAT, and with the motor cortex, there is a communication via the lateral SLF with the SMG running over the top of the insula. The yellow fibers highlighted demonstrate communication between the premotor cortices and the basal ganglia. This would represent a communication between the so called "Broca's area" and the basal ganglia on the left side, 4) the bottom panels demonstrate the addition of the SMA in green. The FAT communication with this network running perpendicular to this network and the fibers are headed into the page. (**c**) Different views of the final network and of the communication with the basal ganglia. (*Continued*)

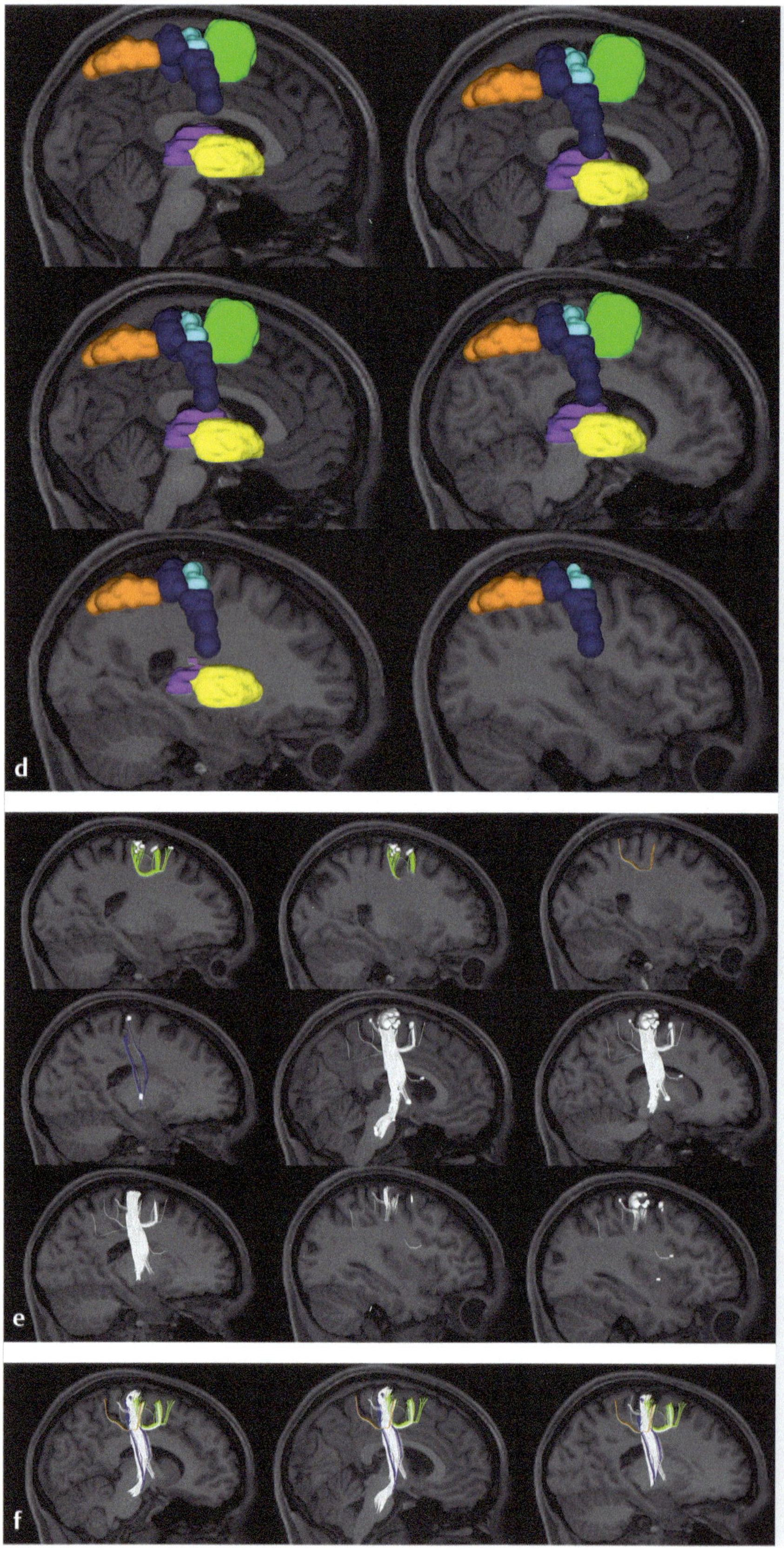

Fig 6.1 (*Continued*) Hand/arm motor system. The model is gradually built in these sequential images in a sequential manner so that the relative contributions of each component can be distinguished. (**d**) Demonstrates the ROIs used to build this model which include the handmotor cortex (in light blue), the face sensory cortex (in dark blue), the premotor cortices (in red) and the SMA (in green). These colors are used for the corresponding tract throughout the map. (**e**) Sequential building of the network: 1) the upper panels demonstrates the face motor cortex fibers in light blue. The curved medial bend of the fibers into the descending motor fibers can be visualized bending into the page to run around the insula, 2) the second set of panels demonstrate the addition of the sensory cortex communications in dark blue. The bilateral communication between these two cortices is striking, 3) in the third set of panels, we add the premotor cortex in red. Note that in addition with communication with the SMA via the FAT, and with the motor cortex, there is a communication via the lateral SLF with the SMG running over the top of the insula. The FAT communication with this network running perpendicular to this network and the fibers are headed into the page. (**f**) Different views of the final views of the network and of the communication with the basal ganglia.

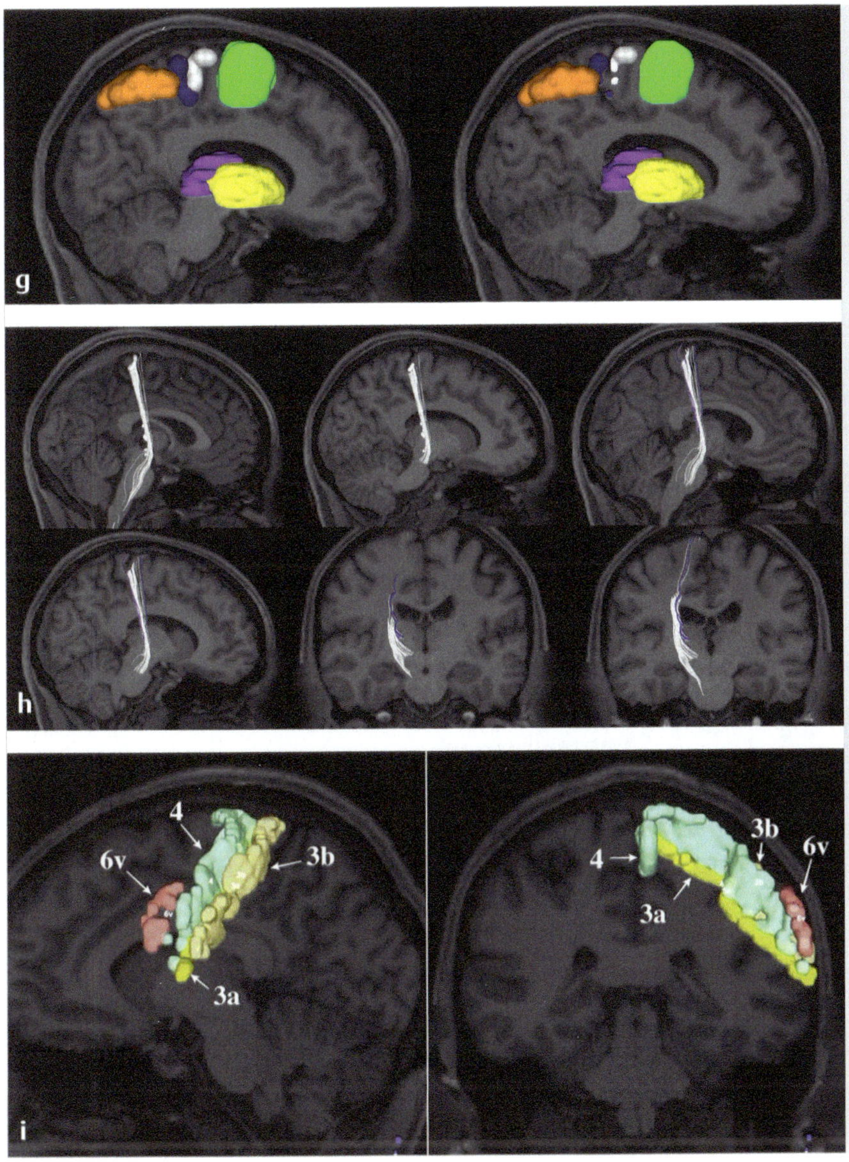

Fig 6.1 Leg motor system. The model is gradually built in these sequential images in a sequential manner so that the relative contributions of each component can be distinguished.
(**g**) Demonstrates the ROIs used to build this model which include the handmotor cortex (in light blue), the leg sensory cortex (in dark blue), the premotor cortices (in red) and the SMA (in green). These colors are used for the corresponding tract throughout the map. (**h**) Sequential building of the network: 1) the upper panels demonstrates the leg motor cortex fibers in light blue. The curved medial bend of the fibers into the descending motor fibers can be visualized bending into the page to run around the insula, 2) the second set of panels demonstrate the addition of the sensory cortex communications in dark blue. The bilateral communication between these two cortices is striking, 3) in the third set of panels, we add the premotor cortex in red. Note that in addition with communication with the SMA via the FAT, and with the motor cortex, there is a communication via the lateral SLF with the SMG running over the top of the insula. The yellow fibers highlighted demonstrate communication between the premotor cortices and the basal ganglia. This would represent a communication between the so-called "Broca's area" and the basal ganglia on the left side, 4) the bottom panels demonstrate the addition of the SMA in green. The FAT communication with this network running perpendicular to this network and the fibers are headed into the page. (**i**) Different views of the final views of the network and of the communication with the basal ganglia.

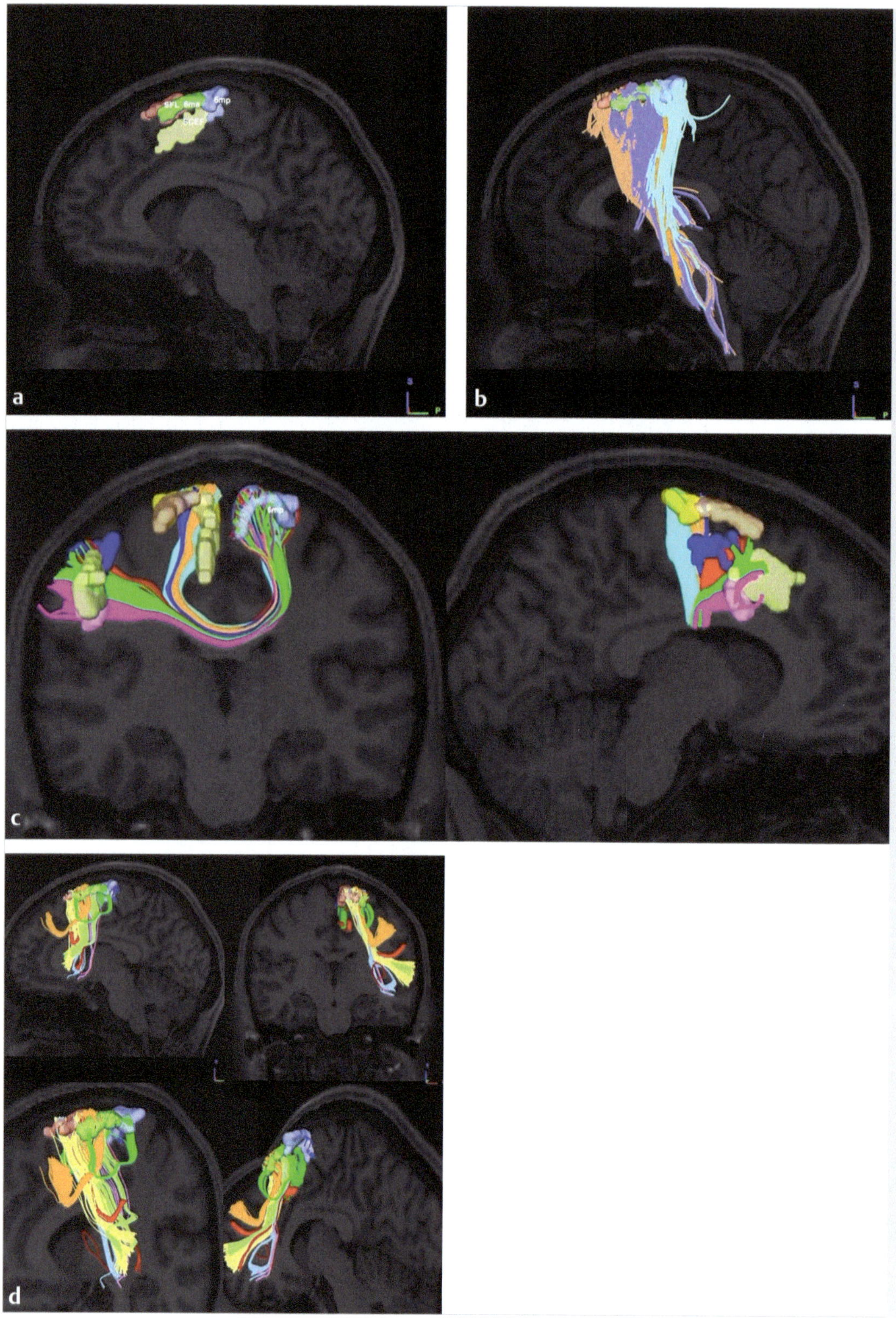

Fig. 6.2 Network map of the supplementary motor area. (**a**) The SMA contains 4 principle subunits: Supplementary and cingulate eye field (SCEF), superior frontal language area (SFL), 6ma, and 6mp. (**b**) Demonstrates the connections of these areas to the descending corticospinal fibers. (**c**) Demonstrates the connections with the contralateral SMA regions as well as the contralateral premotor areas. (**d**) Demonstrates the connections of these areas to the FAT system.

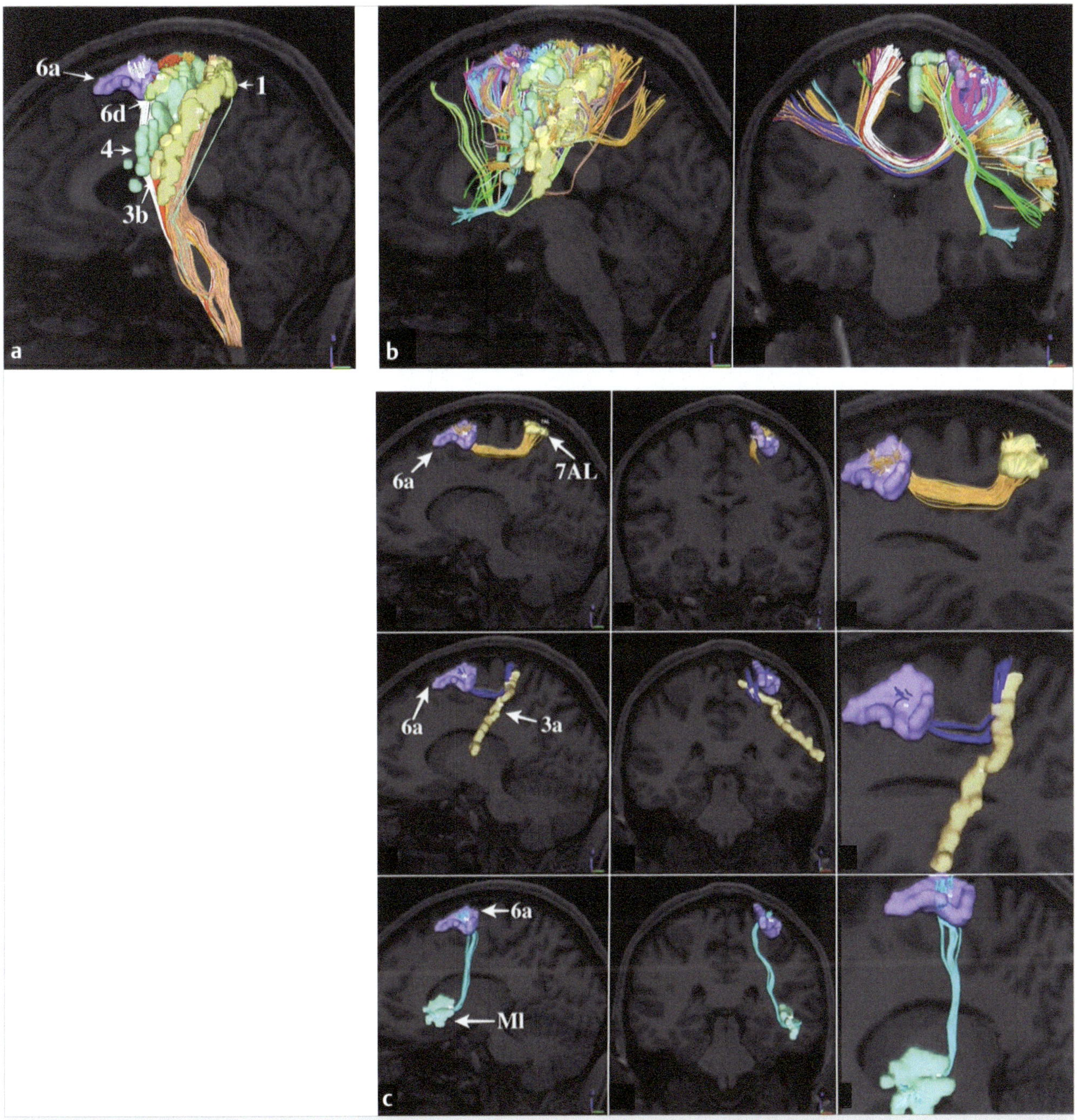

Fig. 6.3 Network map of the dorsal and ventral premotor areas. (**a**) The dorsal premotor network lies in areas 6a, and 6d and in their connections with areas 1-4 in the sensorimotor cortices. All areas contribute substantially to the corticospinal tract. (**b**) Demonstrates the mechanism of connections between these areas and their communications across the callosum. (**c**) Demonstrate the distant external connections of 6a via the FAT, corpus callosum, and crossed FAT. (*Continued*)

hand. The failure to apply these facts has been at the root of many episodes where the arm doesn't work and no one can quite figure out why.

We discuss the motor system first because it is the center piece of many of the other networks, as motor output is essential for many of these networks to manifest that they are working. It is probable that most core neurofunctional units of the cerebrum must access the motor system at some point to make a clinically observable output, however indirect that may be. For most systems below the sublime intellectual and the limbic, this is a short and direct path, so it's valuable to know this system in detail before moving on.

The Major Players

The Primary Motor Cortex (M1)

For most neurosurgeons, the motor system is synonymous with M1, the corticospinal tract, and probably if asked, we would

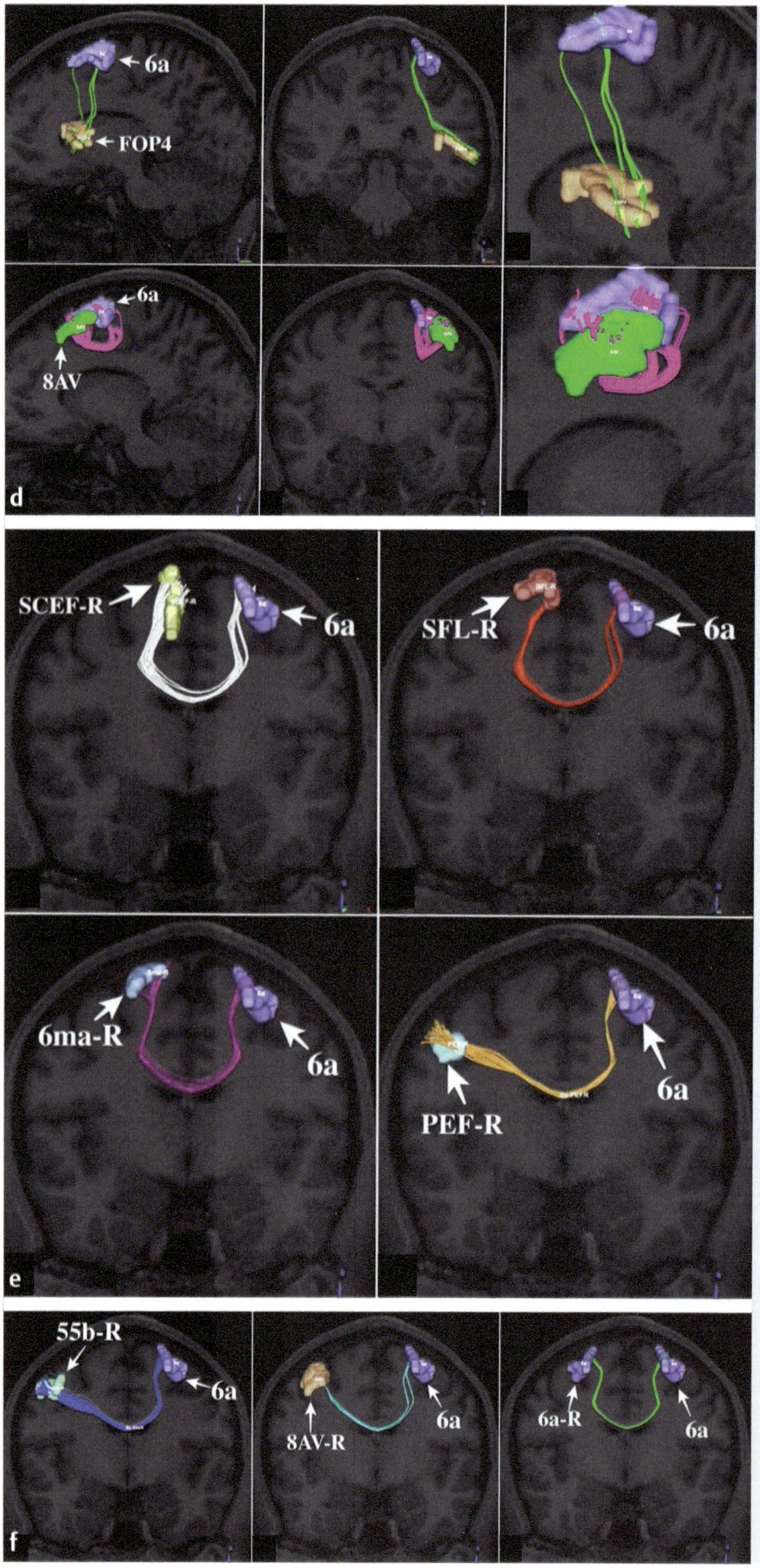

Fig 6.3 (*Continued*) (**d-f**) Demonstrate the distant external connections of 6a via the FAT, corpus callosum, and crossed FAT.

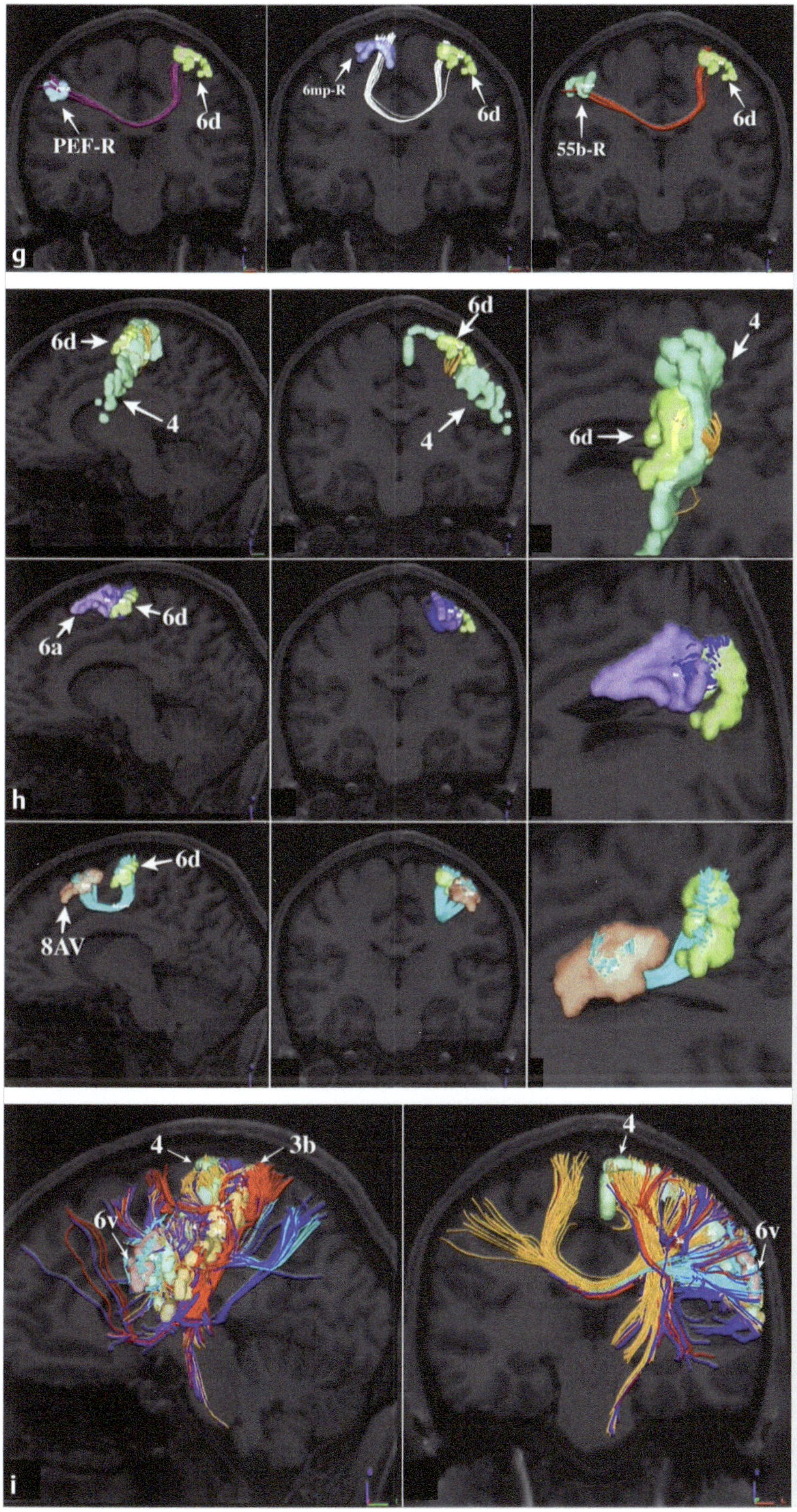

Fig 6.3 (**g,h**) Demonstrates the external communications of area 6d. (**i**) Demonstrates the interconnections of the ventral premotor network.

throw in the basal ganglia, and the cerebellum. It does not need to be restated here that this gyrus is a critical end effector of motor function as it provides the lion share of corticospinal axons, and its injury is clinically obvious.

What is interesting is that there is evidence that it is not the original motor site during evolution as it comes from a phylogenetically younger lineage than the supplementary motor area (SMA), which also contributes to the corticospinal tract. This is logical given its key role in coordinating complex coordinate movements such as alternating finger movements, which would not be needed in lower animals which hemibody movements may suffice. It also, in my opinion, argues why SMA syndrome in its early stages appears so much worse of a motor problem than motor cortex transgression.

The somatotopic organization of the motor cortex should be quite familiar to anyone planning on doing complex glioma surgery, and I will not belabor this point.

The Supplementary Motor Area (SMA)

This is located in the medial bank of the posterior SFG just anterior to the motor cortex. This area has been known to play a role in motor planning for decades, and although its exact role in this is still being elaborated, I think it's safe to say it is an important player in motor initiation given how bad SMA syndrome looks at least initially: usually some combination of dense hemiplegia and mutism.

The literature tells us that SMA syndrome improves around 90% of the time in long term follow-up, and in my experience it often does improve, but I think some observations should give us great pause prior to charging in there to get a little bit more tumor out of the SMA areas. First, it has been my experience that recovery is not always complete, i.e., these patients often do not reach a normal baseline either from a motor, speech, or volitional standpoint, and I suspect that in many studies, these patients were counted in the 90% "recovery." Second, even with that liberal definition, 10% of patients are left hemiplegic and/or mute permanently. Third, recovery probably involves the contralateral motor system taking over, and cutting the corpus callosum fibers can prevent recovery from happening (see Chapter 17). Fourth, and most salient, the idea that the SMA was a part of the brain you could sacrifice and then just ride it out until they recover, comes from the epilepsy world, where resections are usually cortical, and there is no need to do any other treatments on a time schedule. Gliomas are not purely cortical, and the patients need to get to adjuvant treatment in most cases in a time frame much faster than SMA syndrome usually recovers.

In most cases, I would argue that its best to leave it in the network, the amount of increased resection obtain by taking it out is usually very small and doesn't justify the problems it causes.

The area traditionally viewed as SMA is really four areas: 6 medial anterior (6ma), 6 medial posterior (6mp), superior frontal language area (SFL), and supplementary and cingulate eye field (SCEF).

Premotor Areas (PMA)

These portions of the inferior and middle frontal gyri just anterior to the motor cortex, are the point of access to the motor system for numerous neurofunctional systems, including the speech, praxis, and spatiotemporal systems.

In addition to its well-known role in organizing motor signals to be sent to downstream effectors such as the motor cortex, a common way it interacts with other systems is as a judge which compares and assesses information deciding the relative importance of various streams of information.

The Human Connectome Data suggests that original Brodmanns area 6 on the lateral convexity can really be viewed as 3 clusters:

- Dorsal premotor area: 6 anterior (6a) and 6 dorsal (6d) which lie on the posterior SFG near its junction with the motor cortex.
- The MFG cluster: these lie in the precentral sulcus near its junction with the MFG and includes the frontal eye field (FEF) and premotor eye fields (PEF) that surround area 55b, which is clearly a new language area.
- Ventral premotor area: these include areas 6 rostral (6r), and 6 ventral (6v) which lie in the opercularis portion of the IFG.

Basal Ganglia

The putamen, globus pallidus, subthalamic nucleus and substantia nigra are well known to all as key parts of the motor system. This is not a book about movement disorders, so we will not belabor the details of the direct and indirect pathways of circuitry and their roles in the regulation of smooth movement and movement initiation. Sufficed to say that in general you should not be working between parts of the basal ganglia if your goal is preserve good motor function, though this can be done in specific circumstances which are described in Chapter 14.

More important to the practice of glioma surgery is the observation that the basal ganglia receive input from the motor planning areas, among other areas, and if you undercut the motor planning areas such that you disconnect them from the basal ganglia, it is probable that the motor circuit is significantly disturbed.

Cerebellum, VA/VL Nuclei of the Thalamus

The need for cerebellar input to achieve coordinated and smooth movement is well known, and needs no introduction. Most relevant to the supratentorial brain is the descending corticocerebellar tract, which parallels the corticospinal/corticobulbar fibers, and the ascending inputs which enter the motor unit via the VA/VL thalamic nuclei, which send fibers in the motor system via the thalamic peduncle.

Somatosensory Cortices

For years, I was under the impression that the goal of brain mapping and finding the sensory strip, was to have a clear idea where the motor strip was. It was best, obviously, to avoid the sensory cortex, but at worse the issue would be a numb leg and/or hand. I suspect many still think in these terms today, though if asked on the boards no one would suggest this is a good idea out loud.

The problem with this idea is that the central sulcus is not the Sylvian fissure, a deep aneural cleft, but rather there are dense, bidirectional communications between the motor and sensory cortices. It should not surprise anyone that proprioception and touch are key to useful control of movements, especially for the hand. It makes no sense to preserve movement in a hand which one has no control over and then applaud yourself because they are "moving all four." Neurosurgery is difficult, and we shouldn't and can't dwell on all problems we cause, but at the same time we shouldn't ignore that they are there and refuse to strive for better results.

This fact highlights a key flaw in our thinking that can only be exposed by careful thought given to the study of brain connectivity. For years, we have strived to be less damaging to the brain, and have devised many techniques to cut less brain to get to a lesion. Exploitation of subarachnoid spaces is one such approach. Using a trans-sulcal approach to minimize brain trajectory length is another. In many cases trans-sulcal approaches make a great deal of sense, but like all dictums, they should not be applied blindly. Remember that the bottom of a sulcus is not like the floor of the third ventricle, it is not aneural but rather it is cortex and transiting U-fibers, and that a trans-sulcal approach down the central sulcus in some cases, may be more damaging than a slightly longer brain path which does not disconnect the sensory and motor cortices from each other. The shortest path is not always the best.

Superior Parietal Lobule and Banks of the Intraparietal Sulcus

As described below, higher level visual processing has generally been described as flowing out from the occipital lobe in two basic streams: The Ventral "what" pathway and the Dorsal "where" pathway. The dorsal stream ("where") is progressively processed in the precuneus and neighboring occipital lobe before sending its output to the superior and inferior parietal lobules. While these two lobules are both known for spatiotemporal processing, they are quite different functionally, as the inferior parietal lobule is phylogenetically much newer (these cytoarchitectural areas probably do not exist in macaques and lower monkeys), and its damage causes a very different syndrome that superior parietal lobule damage. For this reason, the inferior parietal lobule is included with other networks.

Because the direct input from the visual system to the motor system is at best limited, the superior parietal lobule probably is involved in integrating visual, proprioceptive, and somatosensory inputs and feeding this information forward to the motor system where it helps shape movements. Numerous studies have especially linked the intraparietal sulcus and its banks to maps of personal and extrapersonal space, and their roles in visual guidance shaping of hand movements to conform to targets during reaching, grasping and manipulation.

It seems likely that the superior parietal lobules functions are densely bilaterally connected as its transgression is generally well tolerated, though the phenomenon of optic ataxia, meaning difficulty and inaccuracy moving the hand to visually directed targets should point out the possibility that parts of this gyrus may be important for use of the hand, and we have encountered poor coordination when working in this area before.

The role of the intraparietal sulcus and its banks, which in likelihood is where our spatiotemporal maps of the world are stored, should give us pause before choosing this sulcus as a route to the atrium of the lateral ventricle. This is in addition to the frequent location of the medial parts of the SLF deep to this sulcus in some patients.

6.2.2 The Anatomy of the Network (▶ Fig. 6.1, ▶ Fig. 6.2, ▶ Fig. 6.3)

Using the SMA as a starting point, the SMA fibers exit the gyrus in three primary bundles. The lateral bundle is the FAT which connects the SMA to the Premotor areas in the posterior portions of the MFG and IFG. The middle bundle descends vertically to contribute to the corticospinal tract, and to communicate with the basal ganglia. The medial bundle enters the corpus callosum, wrapping around the cingulate gyrus and cingulum en route.

The callosal fibers are interesting as they have a mix of homotypic fibers which interconnect the bilateral SMAs, and heterotypic fibers which connect the SMA with the contralateral MFG and IFG (which we call the crossed FAT pathway). I suspect this pathway is necessary for the SMA syndrome to recover (it allows the other side to take over). This is also the principle reason why I think mid-callosal butterfly gliomas are probably still largely inoperable, or at least you can't get much of them out safely.

The FAT is one of the principle components of the motor planning system as it is the principle way the SMA and PMA communicate, and I suspect it is one way to cause hemiplegia without entering the motor strip, though I have had great respect for it ever since I learned about it.

The motor planning sites communicate through vertical, apically directed small tracts aimed at the basal ganglia. Thus, the descending fibers of the motor system generally begin anterior to the motor cortex. They also have U-fiber connections directly linking the motor planning areas to the motor cortex. The thalamic peduncle carries this information back up to the motor strip.

Sensory information probably enters the motor network through two routes. First, the central sulcus contains U-fiber communications between the primary sensory and motor cortices. In addition, the Superior parietal lobule and banks of the intraparietal sulcus send processed information to the middle frontal gyrus via the medial parts of the SLF.

Ramifications of this Anatomy for Surgery Near the Motor Network

1. The motor network is more extensive than just the motor strip and its fibers, and thus motor mapping should start well anterior or posterior to the motor strip, and the end point we are looking for ideally should integrate numerous aspects of movement, more than just moving "yes/no." decisions. We cannot always save proprioceptive function in some cases, but we should base these decisions on facts on the ground, and should think about motor mapping as a study of the overall integration of all aspects of motor function.
2. The cuts around the motor system are largely coronal and straight cuts which parallel the descending and ascending pathways between the motor cortices and their basal ganglia, thalamic, and cerebellar sources.
3. Cutting through the medial SLF can have motor ramifications.

4. If you find that you have entered the body of the lateral ventricle through a lateral approach, you probably have screwed up. There are too many tracts blocking that route. At minimum, you have transgressed the superior thalamic peduncle.

The Two Pathway Networks: Language, Praxis, and Neglect

Conceptual Framework

I have grouped these three networks together as they share remarkable parallels in anatomic organization, the involved cortices, and more interestingly, in the way they process information. Thus, understanding one system provides major insights on how the other ones work.

I have speculated that this similarity comes from the evolution of the semantic areas of the cerebrum namely the posterior temporal lobe and inferior parietal lobule. In short, animal psychology has long postulated that the idea that animal intelligence can be accurately depicted as a fraction of the global human intelligence is inaccurate. In many cognitive domains, animals perform quite close to humans, while others they lack entirely. This suggests that increasing intelligence with evolution was achieved not merely in the increase in cerebral volume, but also by the creation of new brain areas and networks.

While monkeys such as macaques have an inferior parietal lobule and intraparietal sulcus, cytoarchitecturally these structures are better characterized as analogs of Brodmann's area 7, and thus the supramarginal and angular gyri and posterior temporal lobes are substantially bigger in humans than monkeys.[3] In fact, in addition to the fold increase in the relative size of the prefrontal cortices, this is one of the most conspicuous area of difference with the monkey to human leap. Thus, it is not surprising that a large number of human like brain functions localize strongly to this part of the brain. Interestingly, while it will not surprise you that experimental brain lesioning in macaques has failed to provide an acceptable model for aphasia or apraxia for tool use, it is of interest that the cortical lesioning in macaques is also unable to recreate human hemineglect, as lesioning the parietal lobe merely leads to an optic ataxia like syndrome similar to that seen with lesioning of the superior parietal lobule.

6.3 Speech Network

We have been taught for decades to view speech in terms of two cortical areas, Broca's and Wernicke's, connected by the arcuate fasciculus which has something to do with repetition. Like any persistent but incorrect model, there is some predictive power in the model, as the most prominent parts of the speech network in normal people cluster in these two regions, so it will often lead to correct predictions, and this leads us to reaffirm our belief. However, the model fails miserably when put to critical scrutiny, especially when used for glioma surgery where functions move and cortical anatomy is a poor predictor of functional anatomy. I can think of nothing else in neurosurgery other than bone wax which comes from the 1800s which is still being used in daily neurosurgical practice, and it's time we put this model into the dustbin of history as it is dangerous.

It is clear from decades of study of aphasias that speech disturbances are far more complex than these simple models predict, notably that semantic speech problems (dysnomias or problems naming objects) often dissociate from phonemic speech problems (problems with paraphasias, agramatism, perserveration), and that they tend to degrade in comparable ways within their own domains. This is especially true with dementia related aphasias, where primary nonfluent aphasias are prototypical with Alzheimer's disease, and semantic dementia (general anomia and loss of semantic knowledge with preserved fluency) is a known subtype of frontotemporal dementias.

Careful quantitative research has shown that speech tends to degrade in phoenemic versus semantic networks in a neighborhood reduction pattern. This means that speech is often clustered in closely related neighborhoods of phonemes and/or semantic concepts and that progressive non- catastrophic damage typically manifests by a cluster becoming richer and more narrow. In semantic loss, this manifests as hammer being described as a "tool" or a "thing," suggesting that these ideas are clustered in a group, and that the patient has lost their ability to subdivide concepts within that neighborhood, or that they are pulling ideas from other intact neighborhoods. In phoenemic problems, this involves paraphasias, where the loss of one phoneme leads to its replacement by a closely related one (such as calling a ball a "pall") suggesting that paraphasias are not random.

6.3.1 Speech versus Language versus Semantics

One notable point of confusion which has made discussion about language anatomy impossible to make sense of is worth a section of discussion. It is beyond doubt that the final product of human communication requires the interaction of numerous systems, including the motor systems of the human face, tongue, palate, and larynx, the visual and auditory systems, systems of meaning and semantic functions, and higher cognitive systems of executive control and verbal memory. It is likely that many of these systems depend on somatosensory and proprioceptive input as well as that which involves parietal areas. Thus, any discussion of the topic needs to begin with the idea that the term "speech" refers to the motoric interaction between face, tongue, palate, and larynx muscles to produce language, likely guided by somatosensory, proprioceptive, and auditory input, and that the term "language" refers to the interaction between cognitive and semantic systems to determine the content of speech. Semantic function, the ability to classify words based on meaning, is obviously a key aspect of the language system but also is critical in understanding, and comprehension and language are tightly linked, but clearly can be decoupled by some injuries.

It is clear that intraoperative mapping is excellent for identifying and preserving speech areas. Speech arrest caused by direct electical stimulation is likely disturbing the motor-production of language. Studying naming and anomic arrests is closer to what we would term language, but clearly this is not syntactic nor is it really drilling down on the cognitive aspects of speech. It is also possible that language is more redundant and adaptable than speech. Either way, it is critical that we begin calling speech and language different things.

6.3.2 The Major Players (▶ Fig. 6.3)

The Semantic Areas

In a theme that will be repeated over and over in this chapter and elsewhere, these areas comprise a densely interconnected local network which lies at the hub of numerous networks. Their function is probably as a storehouse of concepts that the brain has acquired over time, which it can draw from to perform higher abilities like talk, figure out a tool, or figure out the shape of things around you. Cognitive neuroscience terms this semantic memory, which is probably useful given its proximity to the temporal lobe, and its role in storing information based on experience, but this can be confusing because they are not explicit memories such as who your kindergarten teacher was, but instead what the word bird means, the phonemes that create that word, what a bird looks like, and facts about birds (or at least connections to the place where those ideas are stored).

It's critical to note that the neuropsychologic observation about neighborhood density, highlights the idea that there are multiple sites which can be involved in semantic storage. Indeed, this is often the case in speech mapping, where multiple naming sites are often found and can span a significant area of the posterior temporal lobe. It should also alert you to the idea that you need to test suspected sites more than once before concluding they are negative: just because the work "ball" isn't stored there, doesn't mean other words aren't.

The semantic parts of the brain are located in the posterior STS and MTG in HCP areas STSdp, TE1p, and PHT. It is important to note that these are not located within the semantic stream.

Premotor Areas

If you stimulate the left ventral premotor area with enough current, you will cause a speech arrest. Typically, this site is found in the back of the inferior frontal gyrus in most people, but it is important to not assume where it is based on gyral anatomy alone, especially with glioma patients.

This area obviously gives commands to the motor cortex telling it which face, mouth, tongue, pharynx, and larynx muscles to fire to make the sounds which comprise speech. However, the presence of the dual pathways suggests that it may play a corrective or comparative function in linking these two streams into coherent speech.

Basal Ganglia

Anyone who has caused an artery of Heubner infarction, with injury to the caudate head, has some idea, whether or not they fully acknowledged it, that the basal ganglia play a role in speech. While the frequent improvement of caudate mutism suggests that this can be compensated for, this suggests that we should consider the basal ganglia in our network.

SMA

Mutism is a striking component of the SMA syndrome, and the complete or near complete failure to produce speech (as opposed to aphasias where speech is usually present but bad) strongly implicates the SMA in the production of volitional speech. While the frequent improvement of caudate mutism suggests that this can be compensated for, this suggests that we should consider the basal ganglia in our network.

Motor and Sensory Cortex

Beyond the obvious need to move the mouth and tongue in order to talk, recent work has linked these cortices to some cognitive aspects speech production. The motor strip is especially linked to action verb production, which is surprising but logical as it is the site of action. Note that the SLF runs directly underneath both of these cortices.

Area 55b

This area located in the precentral sulcus just behind the MFG was primarily highlighted in the HCP parcellation effort, and is clearly a language-related site. We presently believe it is a laryngeal motor cortex.

It's notable that the visual network is highly bilateral, the posterior 2/5 of the corpus callosum is dedicated to ensuring this. This is important towards understanding the essential parts of IFOF I believe.

Auditory Network

This system in STG and greater Heschl's gyrus is connected both to the semantic areas and to area 44 directly. It obviously has a role in comprehension; however, its direct connections to area 44 suggest a more complex role in regulating the tone and pitch of speech, or a more interesting role.

Areas 8C and IFJa

These areas in the posterior MFG and IFS is likely an executive control type area, and shows connections to other language areas, raising some interesting questions about its role in language production.

The Parietal Lobe

Since Geschwind first suggested this area in his maps of human language, its role in language is unclear, and it is even possible his stroke data resulted from injury to the SLF arcuate system. Our data suggest that several parietal areas, including angular area PFm (which doubles in the DMN), intraparietal sulcus area AIP, and SMG area Perisylvian language area (PSL) all play a part in language production. Whether this is necessary for providing sensory integration for speech production or a more complex function is presently unclear.

6.4 The Anatomy of the Network (▶ Fig. 6.4)

6.4.1 The Two-stream Model and Limits

The observation that patients with frontotemporal dementia often develop a fluent language disturbance with a general loss of meaning which localizes to the left temporal pole began a series of efforts to define a "two stream" model of language, modeled after the dual stream model of visual processing from the macaque (never mind the fact that such a model does not very well explain features of human visual processing, such as a

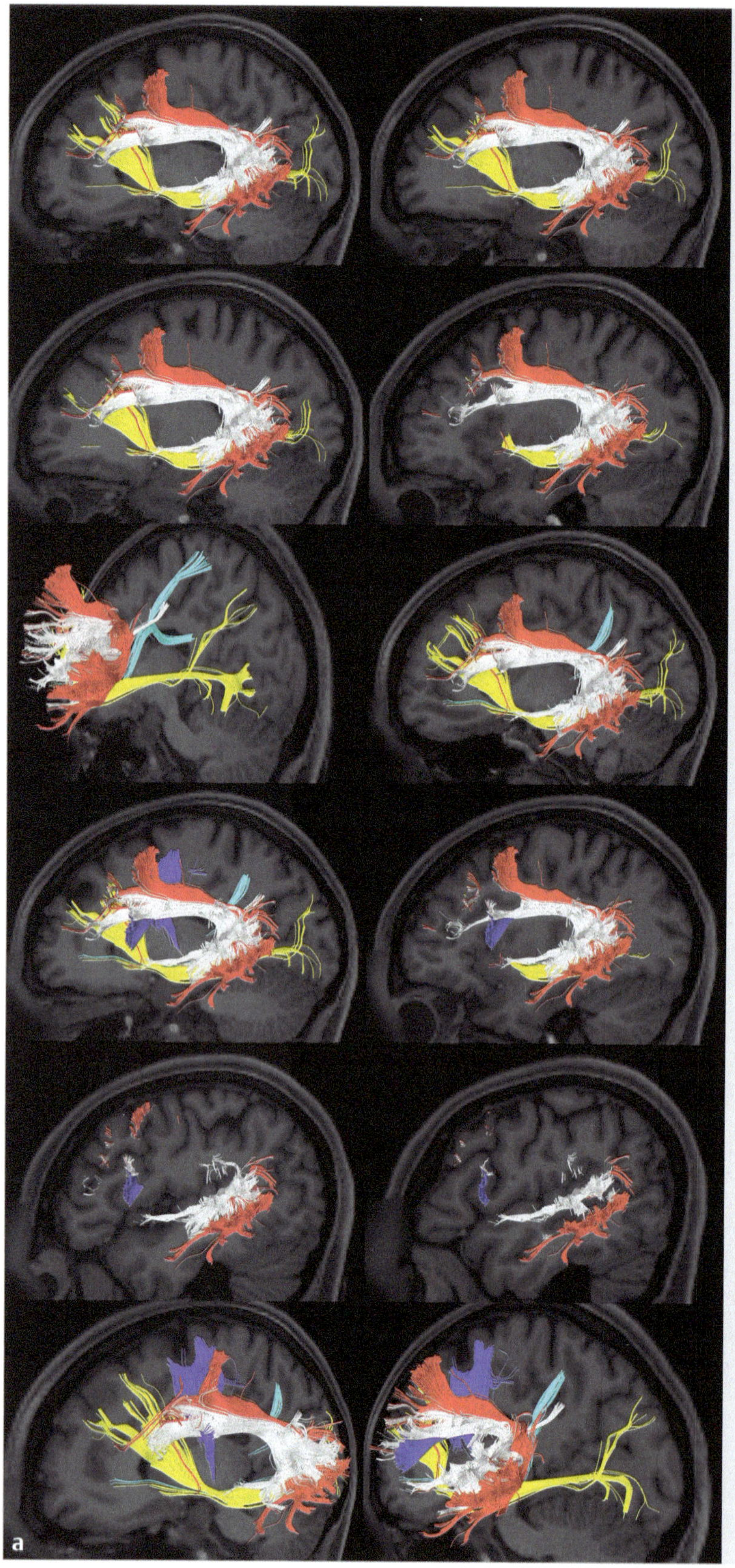

Fig. 6.4 Network map of the language network. The first three images demonstrate proposed models for a two stream model of language; note all models agree about the role of the SLF/arcuate system in phonemic and syntactic aspect of language and differ only in their proposed mechanism of semantic transfer. (**a**) The Duffau model posits the semantic pathway to be carried by IFOF.

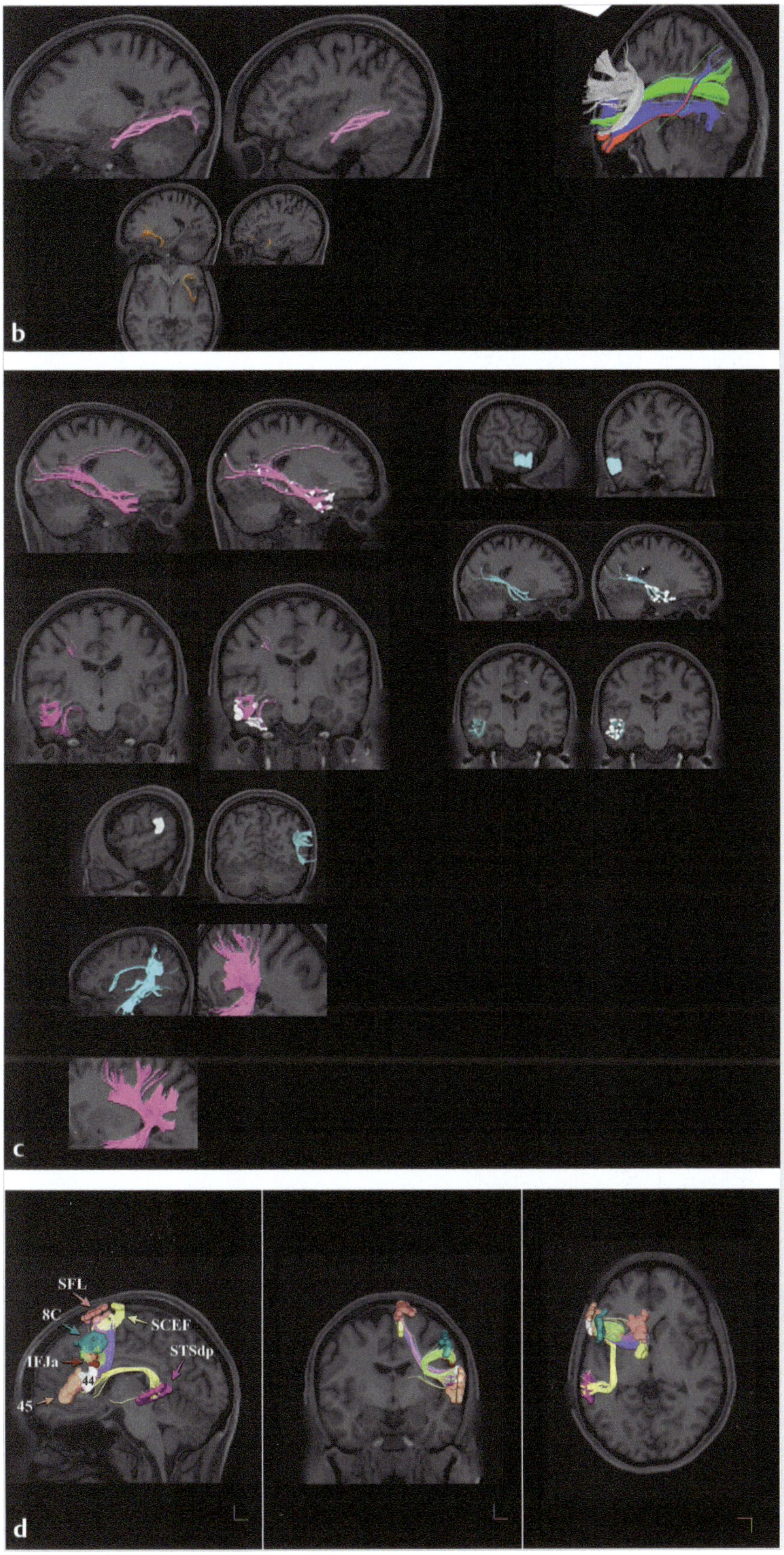

Fig 6.4 (**b**) The Mesulam model posits this stream to first involve visual transfer to the temporal pole via ILF and then transfer to area 45 via the uncinate. (**c**) The Catani model suggests that semantic information flows anteriorly to the pole via small fasciculi in the middle temporal gyrus to the temporal pole which then communicates to area 45 via the uncinate. (**d,e**) Our model based on metaanalysis suggests a different mechanism. The semantic areas seem to be in the posterior temporal sulcus (STSdp), and posterior MTG (TE1p, PHT), and these communicate with area 44 and 55b respectively, via the arcuate (44) and SLF part 2 (55b). Note the connections of areas 8C and the S. We can find no evidence of any direct communication of these areas with the temporal pole or with fibers of the IFOF, suggesting that the primary semantic pathway is connected to the SLF system. (*Continued*)

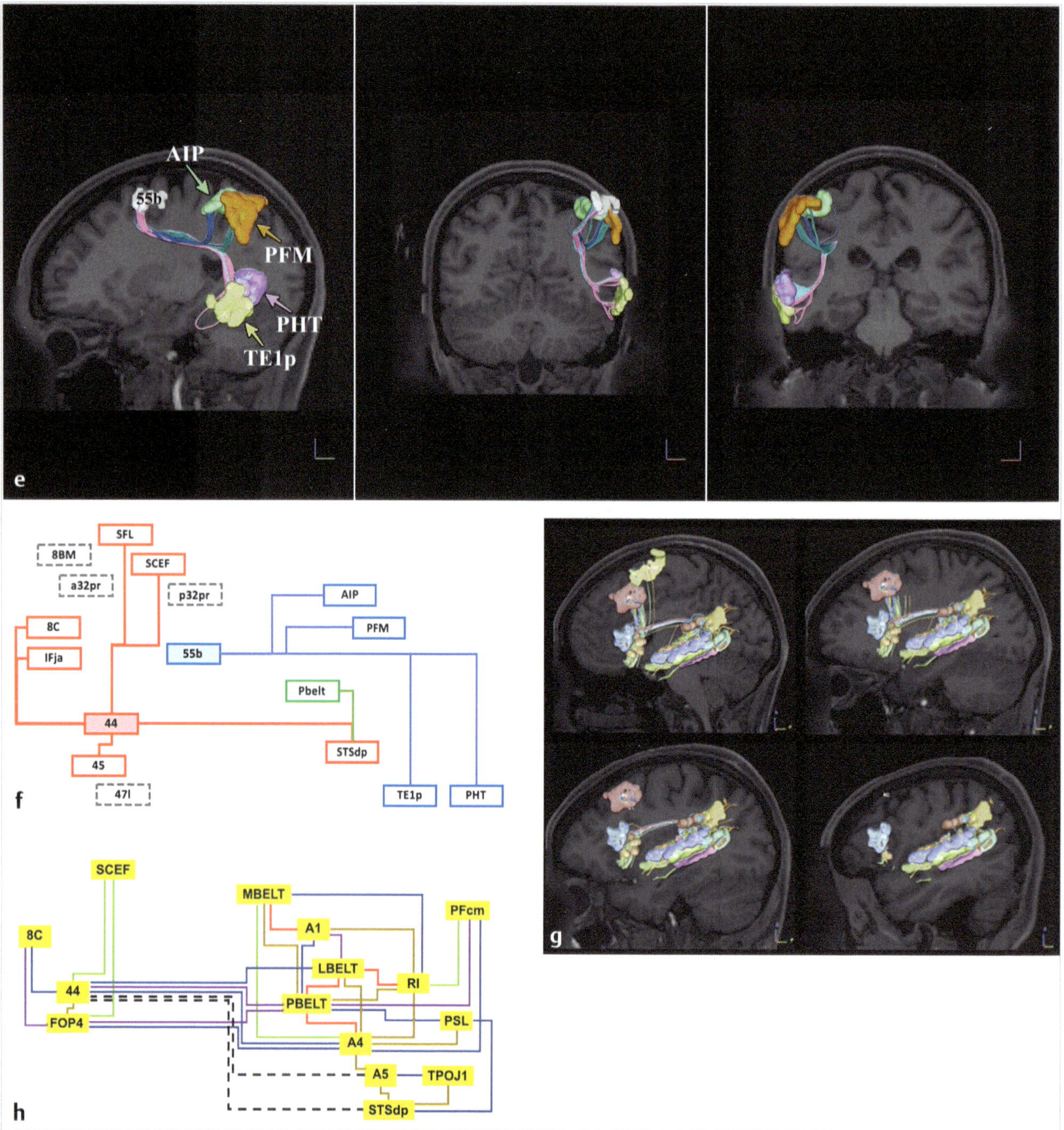

Fig 6.4 (*Continued*) (**d,e**) Our model based on metaanalysis suggests a different mechanism. The semantic areas seem to be in the posterior temporal sulcus (STSdp), and posterior MTG (TE1p, PHT), and these communicate with area 44 and 55b respectively, via the arcuate (44) and SLF part 2 (55b). Note the connections of areas 8C and the S. We can find no evidence of any direct communication of these areas with the temporal pole or with fibers of the IFOF, suggesting that the primary semantic pathway is connected to the SLF system. (**f**) A map of these connections shows the main connections of the semantic areas. (**g**) The auditory network also has a parallel set of connections to the language area. (**h**) A map of the auditory network.

prominent lateral occipital system in parallel with both streams, and the fact that both dorsal and ventral streams are densely interconnected to each other via the VOF). Coupled with the verbal deficits seen with temporal lobectomy, initially blamed on the hippocampus which, after not being seen with laser ablation of this structure, must now be attributed to something sectioned at surgery, and with awake brain mapping with direct electrical stimulation demonstrating anomic events in the sub-insular areas, it is clear that our models need revision to account for some structure in this area.

No one doubts the role of the arcuate/SLF complex and its components in the left posterior IFG and left posterior temporal lobe, where the models differ is in their hypothesized nature of the ventral stream, frequently termed the semantic stream. A variety of dual stream models have been proposed, at least in talks I have attended, and can be summarized as follows.

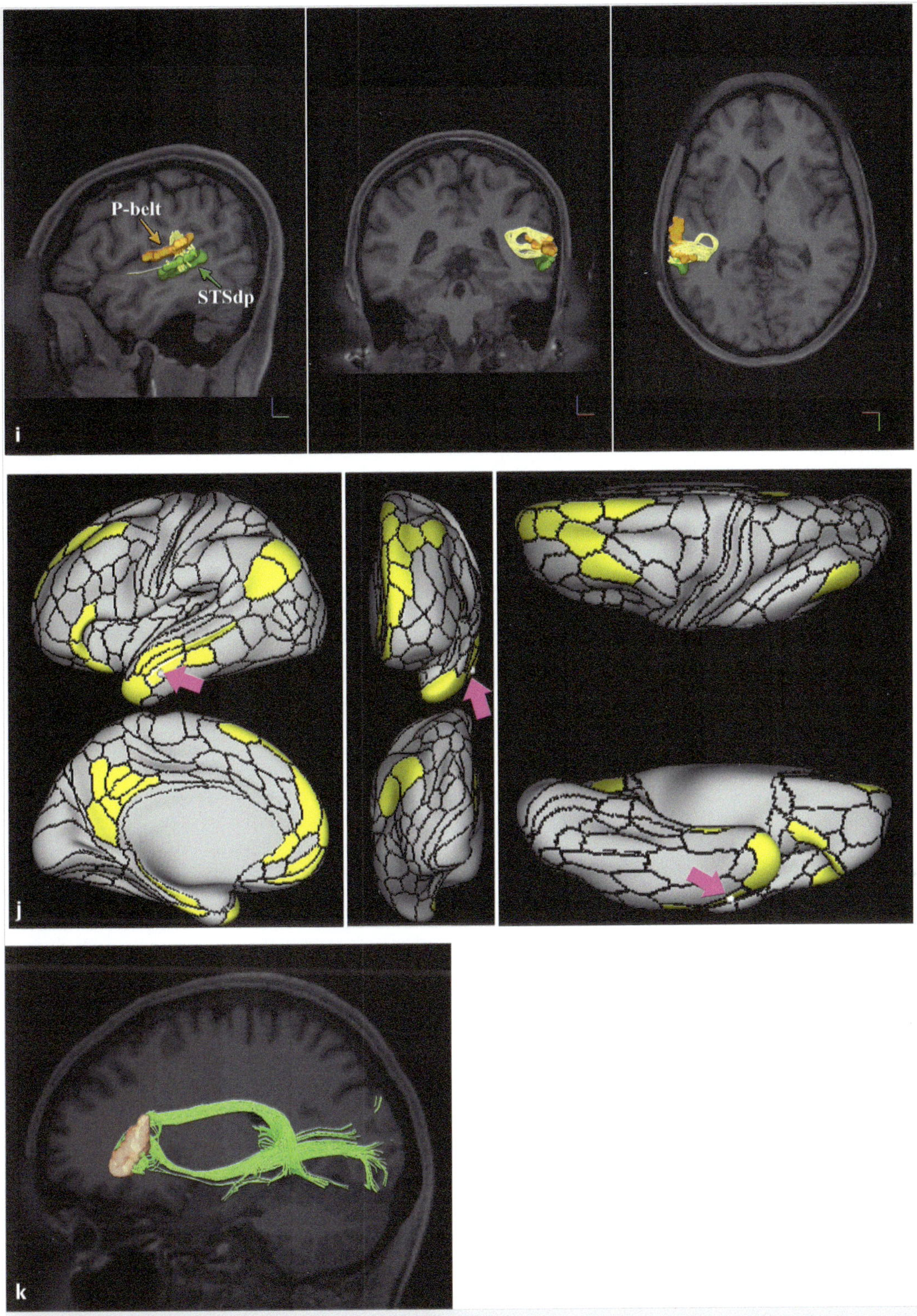

Fig 6.4 (**i**) This image demonstrates that the subinsular area contains a communication between PBelt in the Heschl's gyrus and the STSdp, a semantic area in the STS. (**j**) Resting state functional connectivity map showing areas which coactivate with area TE1a in the anterior middle temporal gyrus. This map suggests that the temporal pole and anterior MTG co-activates with the semantic area STSdp, and area 45, which would support the Catani model, but also it is strongly linked to areas of the DMN. Taken together with the observation that these areas do not activate during semantic tasks, but rather with verbal memory-related tasks, we would suggest that the role of the anterior temporal area is more complex than merely a second stream, and may be part of the default mode system. (**k**) Tractography from temporal polar area TGd, and area 45. These maps demonstrate that these areas connect via the uncinate and connect to the occipital pole via ILF (TGd) and IFOF (45). While this would seemingly support the Duffau or Mesulam model, it is important to note that these connections are almost entirely to areas V1-4, which are very early visual areas, suggesting that the relationship is a bit more complex than merely visual to semantic transfer.

6.4.2 The Duffau Model (▶ Fig. 6.4)

The ventral stream is carried by IFOF which carries semantic information to the IFG with minimal contribution from the temporal pole.

6.4.3 The Mesulam Model (▶ Fig. 6.4)

The ventral stream involves a communication between the visual system and the temporal pole via the ILF. This communicates to the IFG via the uncinate.

6.4.4 The Catani Model (▶ Fig. 6.4)

The semantic areas of the posterior temporal lobe communicate to the temporal pole via a series of local fibers in the MTG. The temporal pole communicates with the IFG via the uncinate.

6.4.5 Our Own Models

Meta-analysis of activation sites during semantic tasks (ones which require sorting objects based on meaning), activate the expected areas in the left STS (STSdp) and posterior MTG (TE1p, PHT), as well as area 44, 8C, 55b, the parietal lobe areas PFm and AIP, and the SMA areas. These can easily be shown to be directly connected via the arcuate and SLF systems (▶ Fig. 6.4; ▶ Fig. 6.4; ▶ Fig. 6.4). We found no reports of activation of the temporal pole in semantic functioning.

The auditory system involves the greater Heschl's gyrus area and the STG (▶ Fig. 6.4; ▶ Fig. 6.4) and this are direct connections to area 44 and other language areas in parallel to the semantic system. It also directly connects to STSdp via a large bundle of U-fibers (▶ Fig. 6.4).

We have found no direct connections between any semantic area and the temporal pole. We have also not found any connections between IFOF and the semantic areas. It is possible these are too small to be detected by tractography, but it is hard to hypothesize this is really the semantic pathway so important that its loss causes a deficit, when so many large fiber connections can be detected using the high-quality HCP DSI data we are using. It is also hard to hypothesize that a multiconnection pathway runs in parallel with a single connection pathway to achieve the same basic output (language), as the timing is likely off with such a dual pathway. While neither contention is impossible, it seems to me to be unlikely as these explanations are inelegant in comparison to connectional observations which have proven to be robust.

What is the Temporal Pole Doing in Language, Then?

▶ Fig. 6.4 demonstrates a resting state functional connectivity map for area TE1a in the anterior MTG which demonstrates that there is a small strip of the MTG and temporal pole which seems to functionally connect with both the STSdp semantic area and the temporal pole. These areas, interestingly, also seem to fire on the same wavelength of the DMN. We have studied these areas and they seem to play a role in verbal working memory and memory retrieval. The DMN is increasingly thought to play a role in some cognitive aspects of language and so may explain this. It also argues that while these areas may play a role in the cognitive aspects of language processing, they are not a stream, in that there is no flow of information in the same sense of serial visual processing.

What about the ILF and IFOF? Clearly these connect to interesting areas like TGd in the temporal pole (ILF) (figure 6-4k) and area 45 (IFOF) (figure 6-4L). While these are interesting ideas in the stream idea, the devil is in the details as these connections are almost entirely connecting these areas to areas V1-4, which are early visual processing areas. It seems unlikely to me that a higher function such as language can utilize visual information such as the direction of lines (the level of resolution of V1-4), to name objects and assign meaning. The better explanation is that these areas are playing a top down role in visual processing. At least it seriously problematizes the idea of a stream.

Mechanisms for Applied Language Function (Naming, Reading, Writing)

Naming involves visual to semantic to language transfer. The most likely points of communication involve communication between visual hubs FST and PH (see ▶ Fig. 6.8), and their neighbors PHT and TE1b, as well as FST's and PH's connections to the SLF system.

Reading (▶ Fig. 6.5) utilizes similar visual to verbal links as naming, but pure lexical processing sites I have found are often rather more posterior and more inferior in the temporal lobe than semantic sites. The Occipital temporal system and the ventral visual stream seem to be strongly associated with this, in a way naming is less associated with it.

Writing obviously is a different task involving a verbal to grapheme transformation which does not require visual input. It probably arises from the semantic system a similar fashion to spontaneous speech, and cross talks with the praxis system discussed below.

Ramifications for Surgery Near Speech Network

1. It should be apparent by this point that the speech network is extensive, as numerous parts of the brain need to inter-

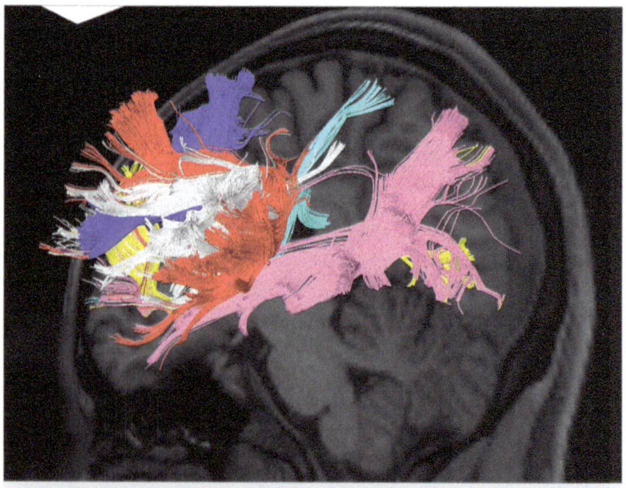

Fig. 6.5 Possible model of the mechanism of reading. Note the contribution of the ventral visual stream via the occipitotemporal system. Note this model is based on the Duffau model.

communicate to perform all of the potential actions of the language network. This is one reason why speech tasks are worth testing in most parts of the brain.
2. The speech network dominates the surgery for left insular glioma as both networks run in close proximity to the borders of the insula.
3. The syndrome of alexia without agraphia, where occipital injury combined with splenial injury causes the inability to read without affecting writing, is generally accompanied by an anomia without agraphia as the visual disconnection mechanism is the same. I have found that this seems to be due to involvement of the crossed semantic loop.
4. While speech is typically a left-sided function in most people, the network is bilateral with interconnections of both the motor and visual systems at minimum (even if speech comes from the left, the left tongue and mouth, etc. need to move as well as the right to talk normally). Thus, while this is more pressing in right speech patients, the network should be studied on both sides.

6.5 Praxis System

Apraxia is a left-sided problem in most people and it clusters with the aphasias to a substantial degree. So, it doesn't take a logical leap to suggest that praxis might occur with similar circuitry, and work on an analogous network.[5]

Since its early descriptions, apraxias have generally been classified in the following manner:

1. Ideational: The inability to plan, and sequence multistep tasks, which has been classically linked to diffuse brain diseases, such as neurodegenerative disorders.
2. Ideomotor: The inability to plan and execute single step motor tasks that is not due to visual disturbance, motor weakness, or other confounding deficits. An example would be the inability to use a hammer.
3. Limb kinetic: Traditionally, the inability to accurately perform overlearned fine motor tasks accurately.

Ideational apraxia is not well understood and likely irrelevant to all but the most aggressive glioma, so I will not try to account for this in our models.[5]

Otherwise, I will scrap this classification as it is generally confusing for most people, and what most of us think of as apraxia, is basically ideomotor apraxia. Within ideomotor apraxia, there are a variety of types, which are probably more informative towards mechanism. These include apraxias which involve failure to imitate other actions, apraxias which prevent pantomiming the use of a hypothetical tool without the device present, apraxias which involve failure to use an actual tool, and global apraxias which involve impairment of all of these.

Interestingly, recent work has separated out how praxis occurs in the first place into two interconnected mechanisms[5]:

1. Mechanical knowledge: This is a collection of observations about shapes of objects, physical properties of objects, and mechanical angles. For example, experience teaches one that a flat bladed firm device can fit into a screw head, and turn the screw. This is how we can figure out that a substitute device of similar properties might work for the issue, and how we discard using a piece of paper or a toothbrush for the same task, as they lack the right shape, and strength to do the job. Mechanical knowledge is a collection of facts we use to figure things out.
2. Functional knowledge: This is a collection of facts about tools and actions and how they work. For example, most of us can verbalize that a screwdriver is used to drive a screw, or how to perform a military salute, even if we are not in the presence of this device. In other words, this is semantic knowledge about tools and actions.

Interestingly, problems with mechanical knowledge and functional knowledge can double dissociate. One example are patients who cannot describe what a tool does, or pantomime its use, but who are able to use the tool when it is actually there (because they have mechanical knowledge to navigate the task). Conversely, there are people who can name a tool and describe a tool's use, but not successfully use it.

6.5.1 Anatomy of the Network (► Fig. 6.6)

The final common pathway for praxis related activity is the motor network, especially the hand motor areas. The key hub of this network seems to be the intraparietal sulcus and it communicates to the rest of the system via the SLF. Interestingly, the frontal targets are areas 44 and 8C, making it quite similar to speech; however, its SMA component is 6ma and not SFL.

Ramifications for Operating Near the Praxis Network

1. In most cases, saving speech means saving praxis as the networks are so tightly linked. Note that poor cooperation with mapping tasks can be due to aphasia or apraxia, and this should be considered during surgery.
2. Praxis is more prominently parietal, and should be tested in these regions even if speech mapping is negative, as the cortical sites may not entirely overlap, and the findings can be subtle.

6.6 The Neglect Network

Neglect is like pornography, we all know what it is but it's hard to nail down a definition which fits all of its traits. In fact, when thinking what to name this network, I decided to keep it just neglect, as it is not purely a spatiotemporal problem, though those issues are certainly involved, and it is not purely an attentional problem, though obviously attention is involved with the problem. It's best, I think, to not try to oversimply what the missing function is doing in normal people.

First, it's essential to get up to speed with recent advances in our understanding of neglect, and namely what it is not. First, it is not extinction, meaning an inattention to contralateral stimuli when presented with an ipsilesional stimulus. Extinction runs with neglect in big lesions, but the two have been found to double dissociate, as extinction is a superior parietal lobule problem. It also probably is not synonymous with deviation on line bisection tests, which also double dissociates with neglect, and localizes more posteriorly into visual processing areas and the

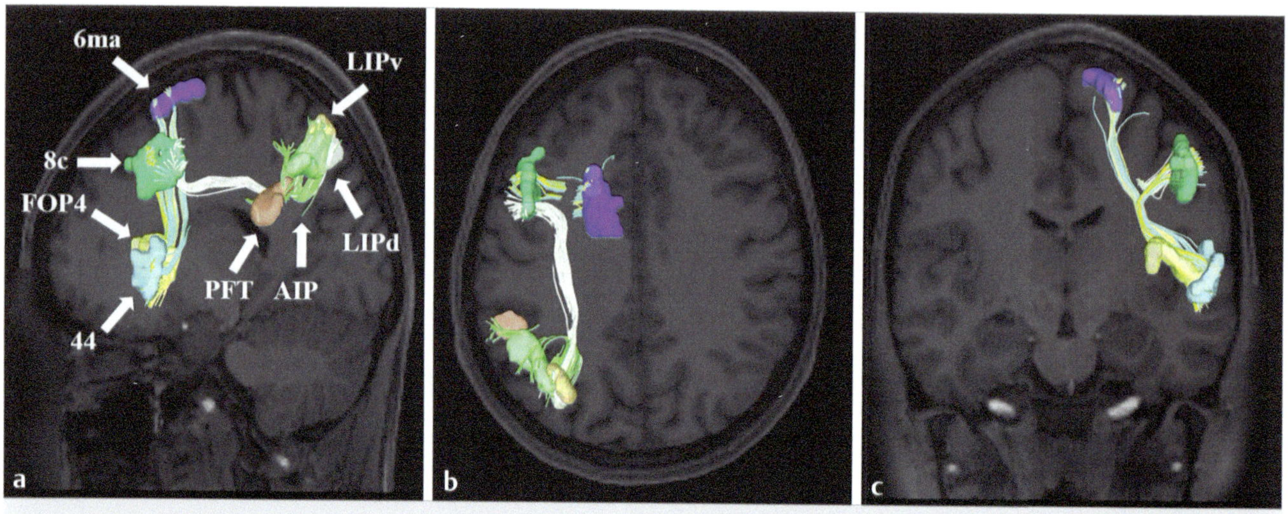

Fig. 6.6 (a-c) Network map of the praxis network. It is a left-sided network based on the SLF, essentially involving the intraparietal sulcus, and many semantic/language type areas such as 6ma, 44, and 8C.

angular gyrus, probably causing people to see the left side of the line as shorter than the right. The frequent co-existence of these syndromes with neglect is likely due to the physical proximity of these areas which often lie within the same vascular territory.

True neglect is a hemispatial inattention syndrome manifested in motor and/or sensory forms. The sensory inattention forms have several subtypes. One form is termed egocentric neglect (alternately called spatial centered neglect), which is the form we typically associate with neglect. These patients ignore objects in their left hemispace, fail to read words on the left side of a page etc. The other form is allocentric neglect (also called object centered neglect). This subtype of patient does not neglect the entire left side in pure form, but rather neglects the left side of objects. Interestingly, these patients will neglect the left side of an object even if it is placed within the right visual field, strongly suggesting that there is a dual pathway which processes spatiotemporal awareness both from an egocentric perspective on a coordinate system relative to the individual, and an allocentric perspective where individual objects are analyzed as whole entities and the coordinate system is relative to the object. Importantly, a very recent article (released a week before the day I wrote this) has linked egocentric neglect to the SLF/arcuate complex, and allocentric neglect to the IFOF. Further, previous articles on neglect have demonstrated that recovery from stroke induced neglect depends on the degree of white matter injury of the periventricular white matter, strongly tying neglect into a white matter network disease.[3]

6.6.1 About the Sidedness of Neglect[3,6,8,9]

Although left-sided injury can cause neglect, especially to the thalamus, neglect is overwhelmingly a right-sided problem, especially with regards to cortical injury of the parietal lobe. The easiest first thought is that this is a right-sided network, and this is why right injury causes the problem and that's the end of it. The problem with viewing this as such is that unlike language, which is substantially lateralized such that a unilateral injury involving both sides (aphasics cannot talk using the left side of their mouth), unilateral injury to the right side only causes left neglect as opposed to neglecting both sides. This strongly argues that the network is bilateral to some extent, but that the right side is dominant and that the left cannot compensate for it if it goes down.

The interesting hypothesis that I will put forward is that the neglect system was the original use for the SLF and IFOF in lower animals, and that as speech and praxis began to evolve, they began to crowd out the neglect system from these tracts, eventually leaving a left side which was unable to compensate for the right should it go down. Obviously, this is hard to prove, but it's an interesting idea.

What Is Neglect Actually?

Clearly the easiest thing is to term this network as the spatiotemporal network, as it is likely results in part from the failure to transmit information about coordinates about 3D space on an egocentric and/or allocentric grid. But the presence of neglect in some patients with thalamic or medial frontal injuries calls into question that there is not an attentional component. Further, the superior parietal lobule similarly processes the dorsal visual stream, and not only is it in parallel with the 2-pathway model of the inferior parietal lobule/STG/MTG/Angular system, but it (the SPL) is also is generally tolerant to some damage without as drastic a clinical syndrome as with the more lateral system, which calls into question the idea that this is a purely spatiotemporal system.

I think in the absence of more information about the exact anatomy of this problem, our best way to view this is that this part of the parietotemporal junction involves a transformation from the complex multimodal and comparative signal of association cortices, which provide various types of processing of visual input (including directionality, motion, rotation specific neurons among others), auditory input, somatosensory, cerebellar, proprioceptive (eye, head, neck and arm position data needed to create a grid), converting this information to simpler outputs needed to interact effectively with the motor system.

The Key Players

The Supramarginal Gyrus

This is not consistent; however, it is likely part of the network, especially of egocentric representations of 3D space.

Superior Temporal/Middle Temporal Gyrus

These gyri are classically part of the semantic network, which probably performs an analogous transformation to the left side, only with object recognition being transformed into coordinates centered on that object, instead of creating a name as with the left side.

Premotor Areas

These are the principle connection partners of the SLF network and I have found neglect sites in these cortices with target cancelation tasks.

Thalamus

Thalamic injuries and lesions can cause neglect syndromes. This strongly suggests a role for the thalamus in allocating attention resources towards different sensory aspects, and that thalamic deprivation can lead to misallocation of resources.

The Network (▶ Fig. 6.7)

Our meta-analysis of injury patterns of published studies of neglect demonstrated statistical linkage to areas in both the grey and white matter of the right hemisphere. Tracing the white matter regions, demonstrated that they were all in the SLF/arcuate system and all of them could be traced to the same grey matter areas seen in the grey matter regions of interest.

The final network is quite interesting. First, we compared it to the VAN and DAN described below, and found that while there is some overlap at points, they are not the same areas, and neglect is its own network. That network contains components of the semantic system seen in the language system (STSdp, AIP), the auditory network (A4), the central executive (aka control) network (PF, 46, p9-46v), the sensorimotor network, and the piriform cortex. This strongly suggests that neglect results from damage to a network of the SLF/arcuate system which binds sensory functions into a coherent reality for executive systems to utilize.

6.7 Visual System (▶ Fig. 6.8)[10]

The overall organization of the visual system can be described as four basic clusters in the occipital lobe: early, dorsal stream, ventral stream, and lateral system; and their connections with the rest of the brain. It has been known for some time that visual information in higher mammals leaves the visual cortices and feeds into other networks in two streams. The ventral stream or "what" pathway, processes information related to object recognition. The dorsal stream or "where" pathway processes information relation to object position.

It is likely that this basic two stream model needs some modification for humans. First, the lateral occipital system is only partially associated with either stream, and contains well known areas such as MT and MST, as well as highly connected hubs such as FST and PH. Second, the two streams are highly interconnected via the vertical occipital fasciculus or VOF. Thus, we utilize convention, with the understanding that the reality is a bit more complex.

From a pure anatomic standpoint, the internal connections and functional connectivity map of the visual system is rather boring. It is a series of areas connected to their neighbors by U-fibers, located in the same lobe, all of which fires on a similar timescale. In other words, the entire occipital lobe fires together. Its topology is quite interesting: it is a collection of four small world type modules. Basically, these areas are mainly connected to each other, with a few hub areas which are highly interconnected to the rest of the brain. We focus on the external connections and the hubs in the rest of this discussion.

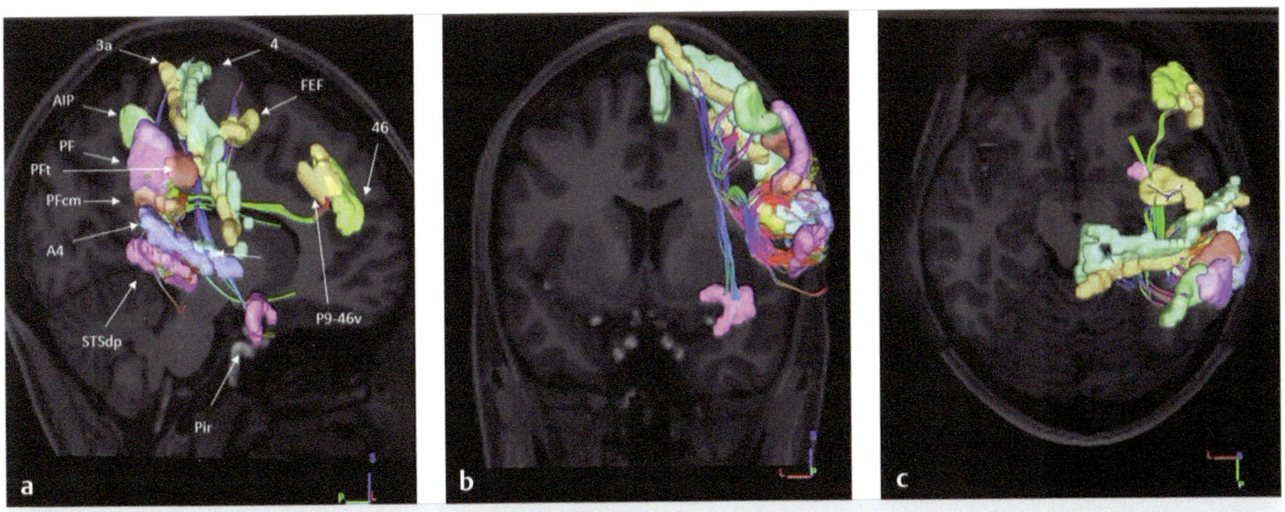

Fig. 6.7 Network map of the neglect network. (a-c) These areas demonstrate the results of a meta-analysis of areas commonly reported in studies of patients with neglect. This network is a unique combination of components of other diverse networks such as the central executive network (PF, PFt), the sensorimotor networks (3a, 4), the auditory system (A4), the semantic system (STSdp), the Frontal eye fields (FEF), executive areas (46, p9-46v), and the piriform cortex (Pir). Its relative lack of substantial overlap with the attention networks is interesting, and suggests that its role is cross modal binding more than attention.

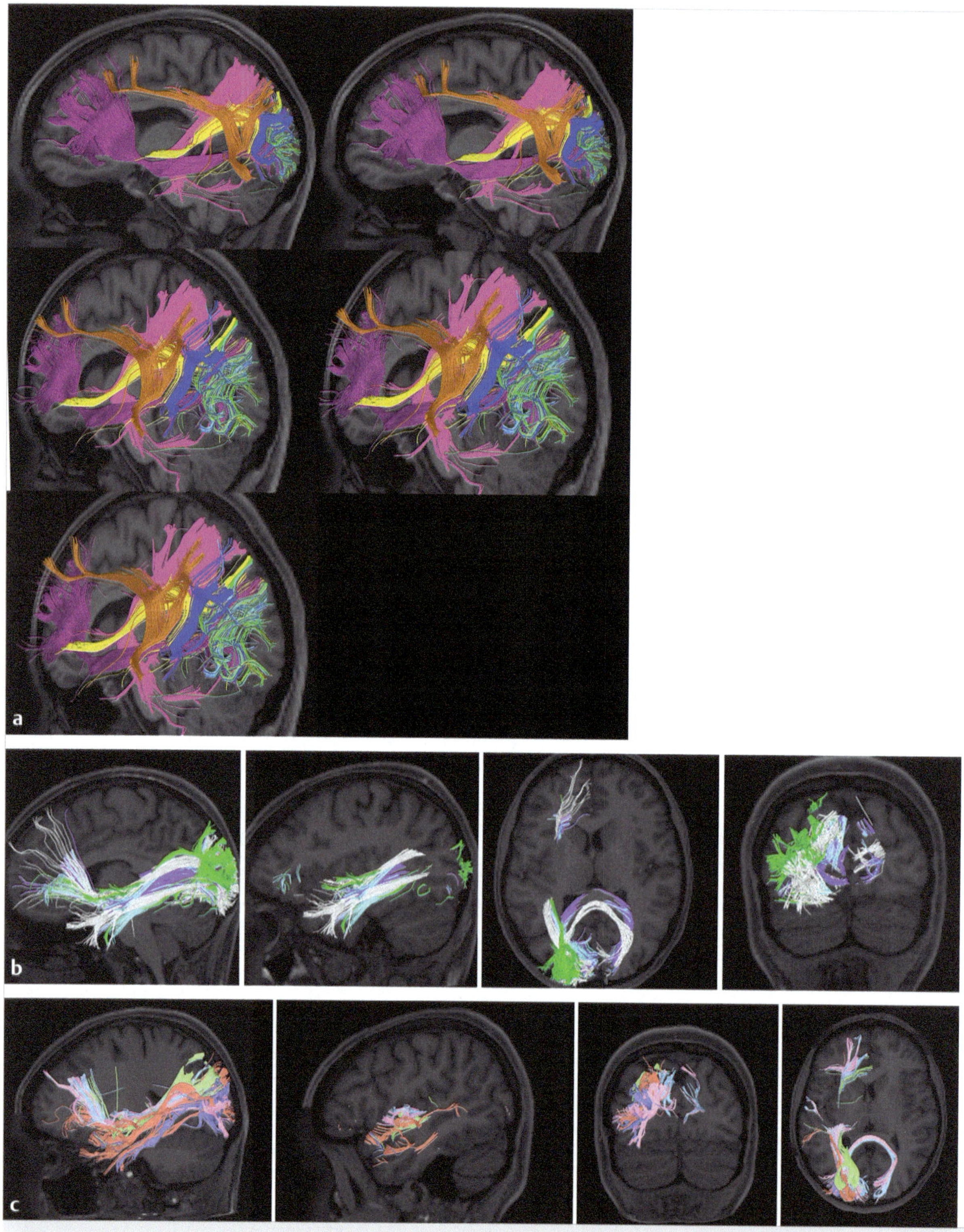

Fig. 6.8 Network maps of the visual system. (**a**) The tractography of the overall system. You can see the extensive network local interconnections between areas typical of a small world network topology. Note the vertical occipital fasciculus (VOF) connects the ventral and dorsal streams. Also note the outflow pathways: the MdLF, the IFOF, and the ILF, as well as some areas which communicate with the SLF. The occipitotemporal system (OTS) is a collection of serial connections of large U-Fibers which connect the ventral stream to the posterior temporal lobe. (**b**) It is most interesting to study the pathways and visual areas which interface the visual system with the rest of the brain. This tractography image demonstrates the connections with V1-4 which include IFOF and ILF. It is stunning that such a large part of the brain interfaces with the earliest steps of the visual pathway. (**c**) The dorsal stream sits at the junction of the medial and lateral faces of the superior occipital lobe.

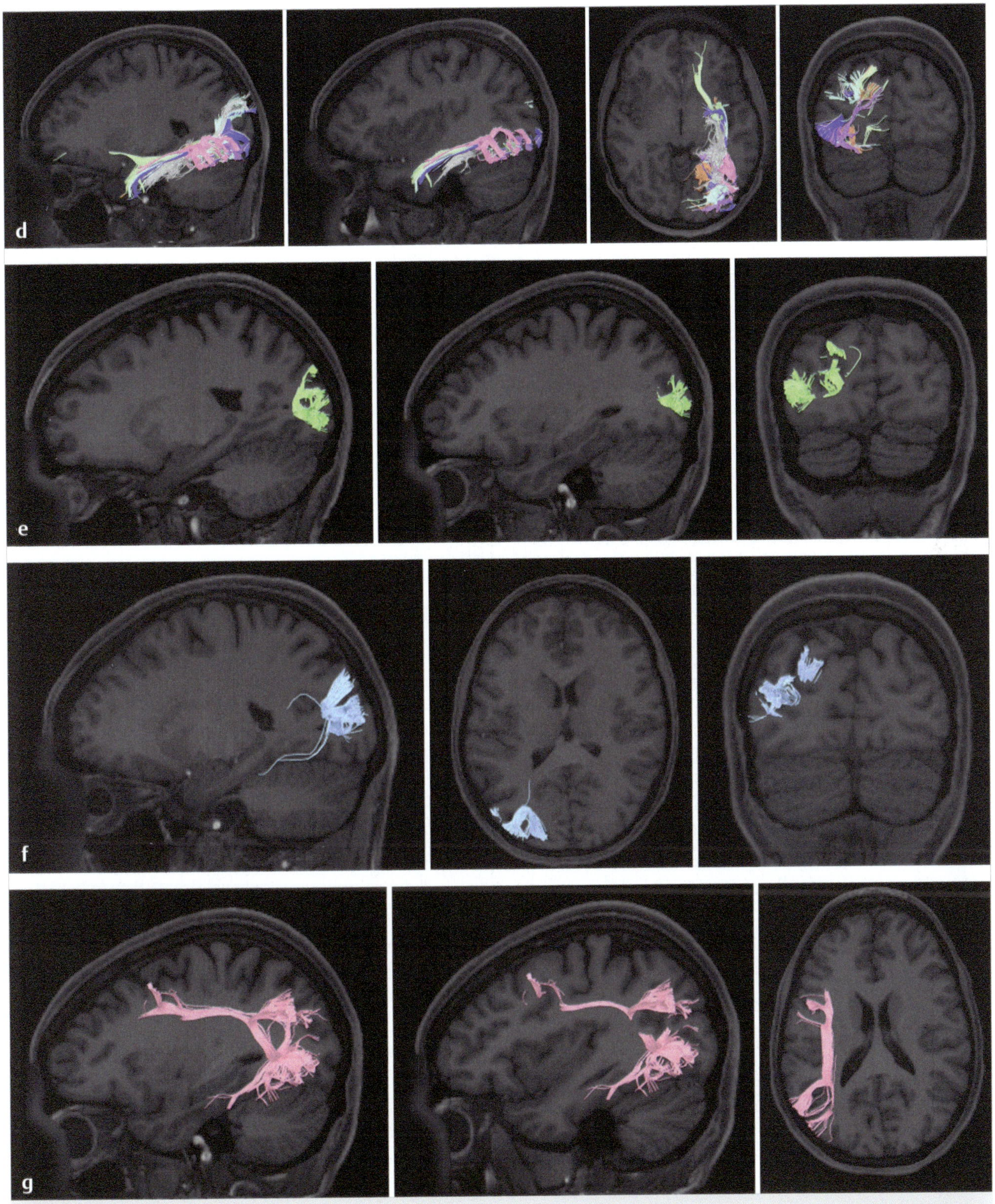

Fig 6.8 (*Continued*) The outflow is highly complex, including MdLF and IFOF outflow, and communication to the ventral stream via the VOF. (**d**) The ventral stream areas of the basal occipital lobe communicates mainly through the OTS but also the ILF and to a limited extent the IFOF. (**e**) The lateral occipital lobe is the prototypical small world network, these tractography images from lateral occipital area V3 cd, and (**f**) LO3 demonstrate that most areas communicate primarily with their neighbors. In contrast hub areas like (**g**) FST (*Continued*)

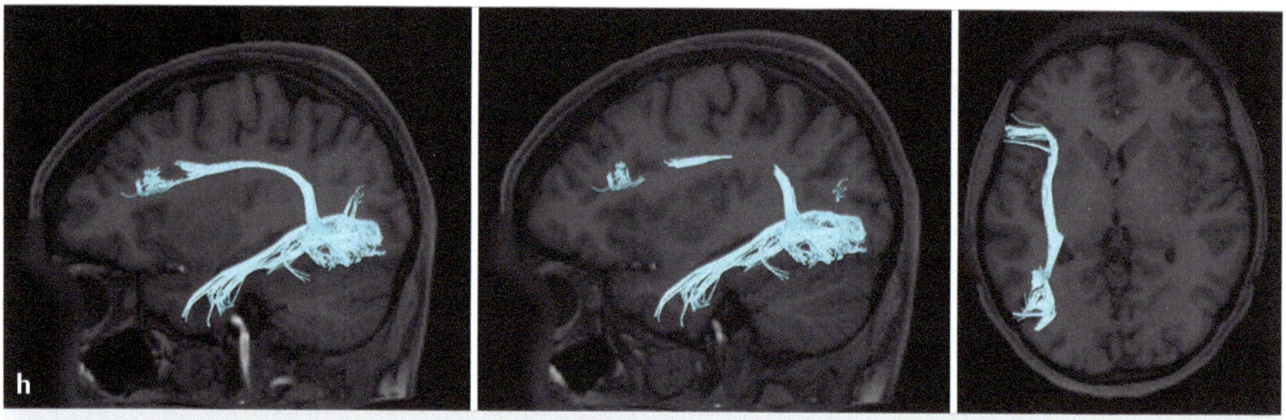

Fig 6.8 (*Continued*) and (**h**) PH demonstrate widespread connections.

6.7.1 The Early Visual Areas

V1-4 cover the medial face of the occipital lobe. They principally receive input from the LGN via the optic radiations, and have extensive interconnections with the pulvinar via the same basic pathway into the posterior thalamic peduncle.

What is most interesting is a substantial fraction of the communication the occipital lobe has with higher cognitive areas in the frontal and temporal lobe via the IFOF and ILF is to areas V1-4. The most plausible explanation is that this is somehow related to top down control of visual processing, but it is nevertheless a fascinating point of neuroscience that areas which look at visual input in terms of very crude levels of resolution have direct communication with some of the most abstract areas of human cognition.

The Dorsal Stream

The "where" pathway contains areas V3a, V3b, V6, V6a, V7, and IFS and straddles the interhemispheric cleft between the medial and lateral occipital faces at their superior angle. The external communications with these areas are highly complex, and involve parts of the IFOF, and the MdLF which joins these areas to the early auditory areas. It also communicates with the ventral stream via the vertical occipital facisculus (VOF) which again is quite an interesting observations as it largely bypasses the lateral occipital lobe.

The final termini of the dorsal pathway are the precuneus and superior parietal lobule. The connections of the SPL to the motor networks are described earlier. The exact reason why the precuneus, which has a large number of connections with deeper structures and fewer with the rest other cerebral areas, intervenes between the V7 and the SPL (the latter which is the likely end user of these data), is unclear but I speculate that this has something to do with modifying visual locational information to account for head and eye position information to make a stable visual image.

The Ventral Stream

The ventral stream proper lies on the basal surface of the occipital lobe, primarily involving the posterior fusiform cortex, the occipitotemporal sulcus, and parts of the collateral sulcus and PHG. It includes areas posterior inferior temporal (PIT), V8, fusiform face complex (FFC), ventromedial visual complex (VVC), and the three ventromedial visual areas (VMV1, VMV2, and VMV3). It principally talks anteriorly to the inferoposterior temporal lobe via the occipitotemporal system (OTS) and to the temporal pole via the ILF.

The Lateral Occipital System

This area of visual areas includes the well known MT and MST areas which play a key role in visual processing in macaques. It is relatively modular as most areas only communicate with their immediate neighbors. MT and MST have some external connections; however, the obvious hubs are FST and PH in the anterior aspect which are widely functionally connected and have extensive communications via the SLF system.

6.8 Ramifications of the Visual Network Anatomy for Surgery

The complexity of these systems requires a great deal of thought about how to deal with them in a way that makes rational tradeoffs of function vs resection.

The question of how visual information makes it to relevant effector systems such as the semantic networks and the spatiotemporal system which informs the motor networks, is only partially addressed by these maps. What is not entirely clear to me is how the brain compensates for various insults, especially to later cortices in the pathways, without losing function. We know that while damage to the primary visual areas, or the optic radiation, causes a field cut, otherwise unilateral injuries, up to a point, do not impair the patient's ability to access visual information without a second injury. The exact way visual information can reach the relevant areas which need them in the setting of an occipital lobectomy or similarly large damage to the visual system, is of critical importance to surgery in the parieto-occipital region. Some information flow lost by damage to the ventral stream can clearly be compensated for by contralateral semantic flow from the cross semantic loop, but the existence of alexia with left-sided ventral stream lesions argues that this is not always enough. Further, dorsal stream compensation in the setting of superior parietal lobule or precuneus insult is not immediately obvious to me and deserves more thought.

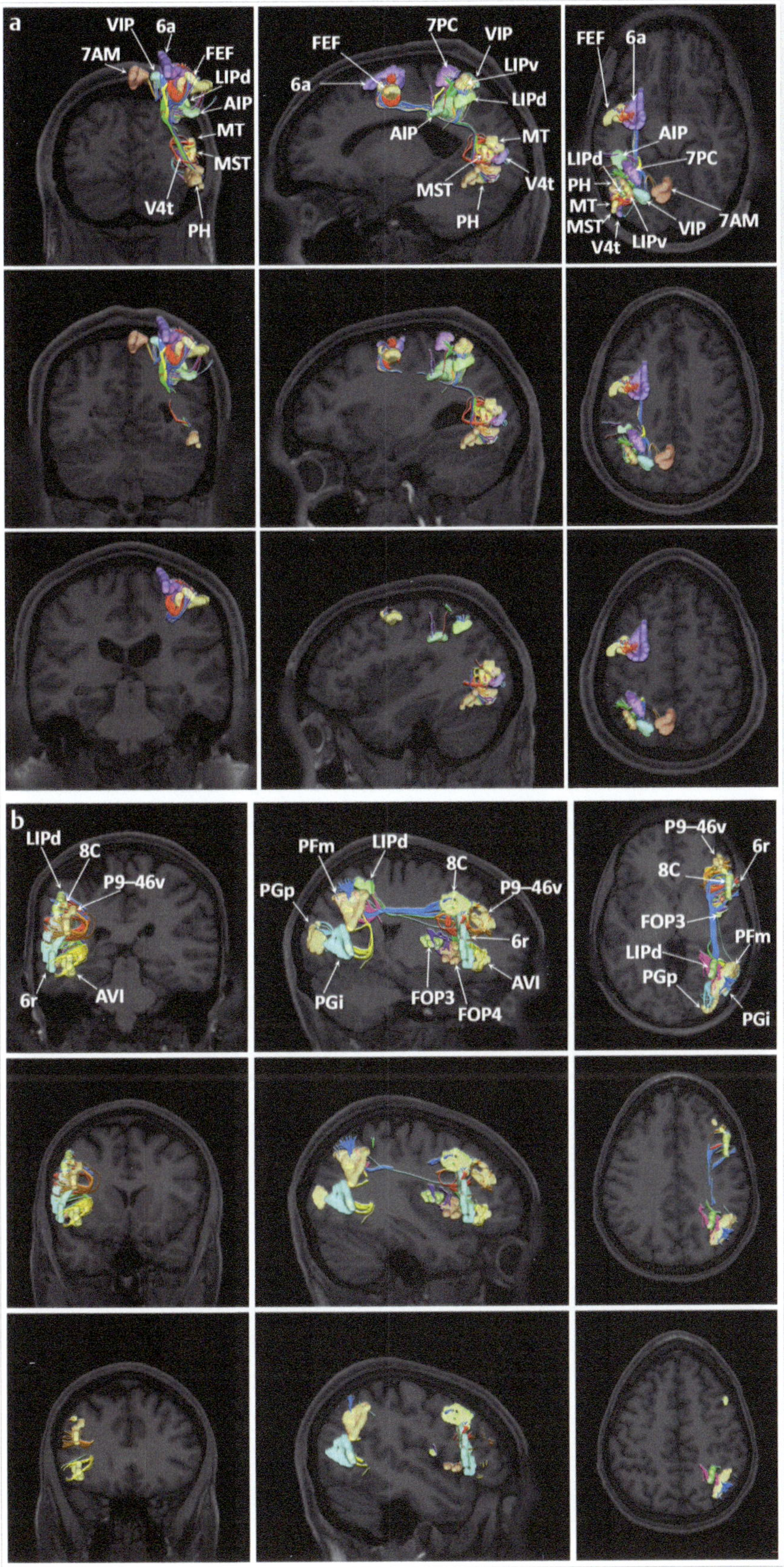

Fig. 6.9 These images show the network map of the DAN and the VAN. (**a**) The DAN is a bilateral network involving connections of the frontal eye field (FEF) and premotor area 6a connected to the intraparietal sulcus and postcentral sulcus area 7PC, and to the lateral occipital areas such as MT, MST, and PH. (**b**) The VAN is a right-sided network which links posterior frontal and opercular areas including ventral premotor area 6 R to the parietal parts of the DMN which include PFm and PGI as well as parts of the inferior parietal lobule and intraparietal sulcus.

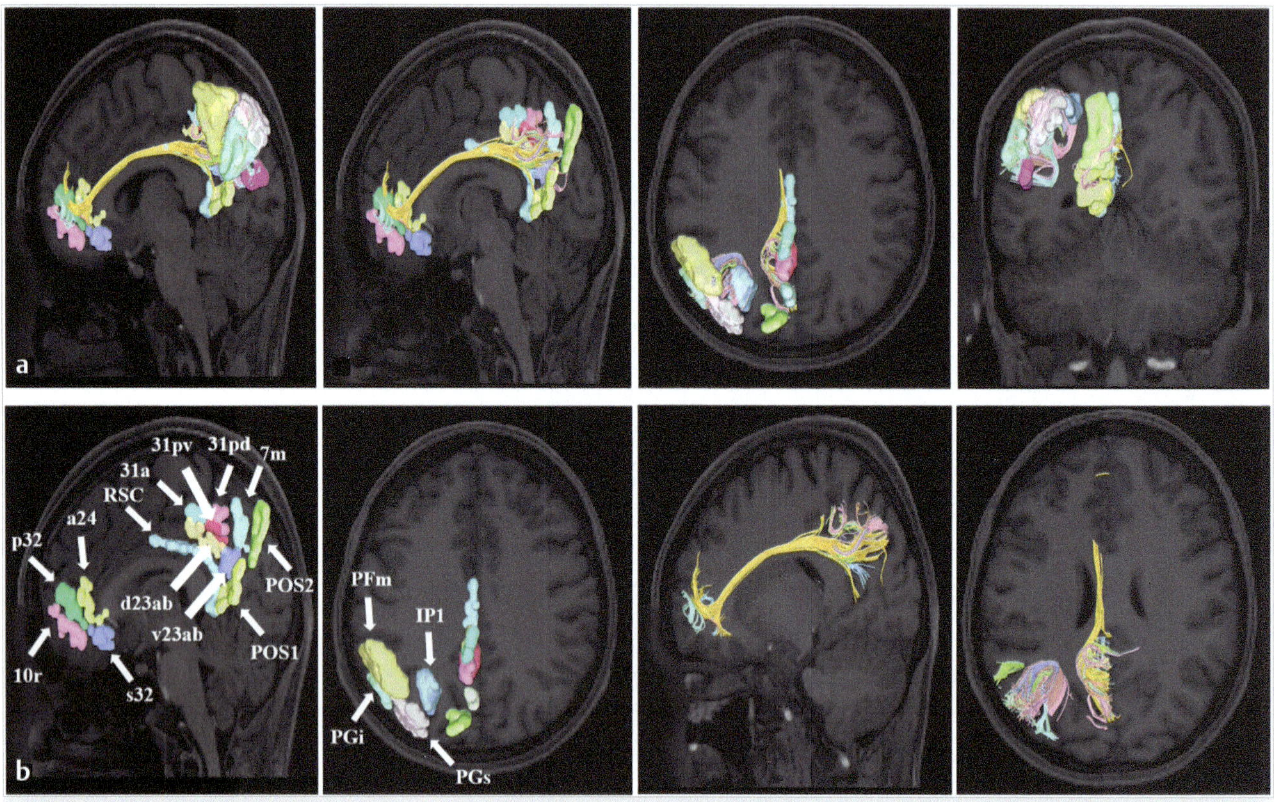

Fig. 6.10 The network anatomy of the default mode network. (**a**) ROIs demonstrating the key hubs of the DMN. (**b**) Connections of the DMN.

6.9 Attention Networks

To paraphrase Yoda from Star Wars, attention is like the force, it flows through everything and influences everything. It is important, therefore to define and understand what it is exactly.

This digression is to point out that almost all parts of the cerebrum depend on attention type mechanisms to work properly, and all parts of the cerebrum can contribute to directing attention in some way or another.[3,6,8,9] The reason for this is simple: pyramidal processing is the only way the cortex can realistically process all the information it receives.[1] There aren't enough neurons to do this otherwise. Pyramidal processing is well described for the visual system where each stage of neuron processes a combined aspect of previous neurons. For example, while an earlier stage of neurons may process point information, a later stage may combine those points into an individual neuron which only fires when a line is oriented a specific direction, and so on as neurons in later stages develop quite complex reactive fields. There are also a great deal of feedforward and feedback mechanisms which focus and enhance certain inputs, and suppress other ones.

Computational neuroscience informs us that one of the features of a pyramidal system like this is information loss on the periphery at each step.[1] This is compensated for by serial redirections of attention to salient features on the periphery to eventually fill in gaps left after a single observation. In the visual system, this redirection is known as a saccade. In other systems, such redirection also likely occurs but is less well understood with the visual system where it is easy to study such things.

Thus, attention is a mechanism for dealing with information limitations of a pyramidally processed system.[11] But parts of the brain must be dedicated to determining how to redirect attention. Some of these parts include lower structures, notably the thalamus, which gate out certain information based on information and goals fed to it from other brain areas. These lower structures can also modulate cortical functions in certain areas to change their gain and receptive fields. There are also within system cortical areas which feedback to earlier parts of the network to emphasize certain features and de-emphasize others depending on salience or other features. Other longer range cortical areas can change the gain of a certain cortical area for various reasons. All of these mechanisms are necessary to ensure the proper functioning of a brain region.

Despite all of these mechanisms which change the gain of output from a particular brain area, we still need to formally adjust our global direction of attention. Using the example of vision, our eyes are typically drawn to the most salient feature, often by precortical information from structures such as the superior colliculus. They then scan based on a hierarchy of salience to fill in the gaps provided by the first eye position. A part of the brain must keep track of where the attention has been directed, and where it should go next, or otherwise attention would unproductively be repeatedly redirected to the most salient feature. This information is termed a salience map, and part of the brain which keep these maps and thus guide attentional direction as their specific functions are part of formal attention networks.

There are two well described networks dedicated to attention: the dorsal attention network (DAN) and the ventral

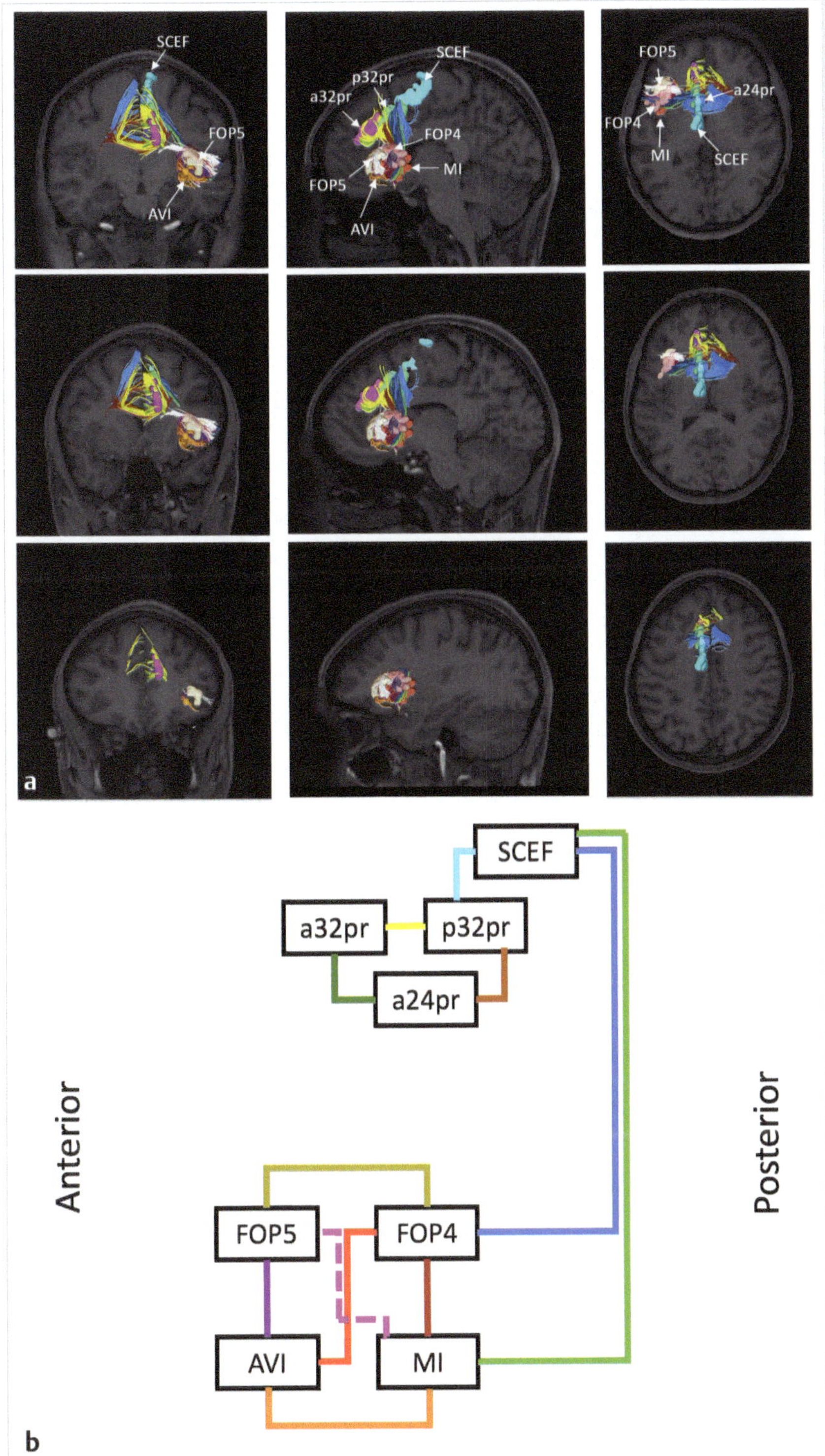

Fig. 6.11 The anatomy of the salience network. (**a**) ROIs demonstrating the key hubs of the salience network. (**b**) Connections of the salience network.

attention network (VAN) (▶ Fig. 6.9). The DAN is a bilateral network, and the VAN is a right-sided frontoparietal network.

6.9.1 Dorsal Attention Network

This network is the best-known attention network, and is made up of areas in the intraparietal sulcus 7PC, AIP, VIP, LIPv, LIPd), and the frontal eye fields (FEF and its neighbor 6a), which lie at the back of the middle frontal gyrus just in front of the motor strip, and lateral occipital areas (PH, MT, MST, V4t) These are easily shown to be linked by the SLF.

The striking overlap between areas active during attentional redirection, and areas involved with moving the eyes, argue strongly that the frontal and parietal eye fields' primary roles are as salience maps and to redirect attention, part of which

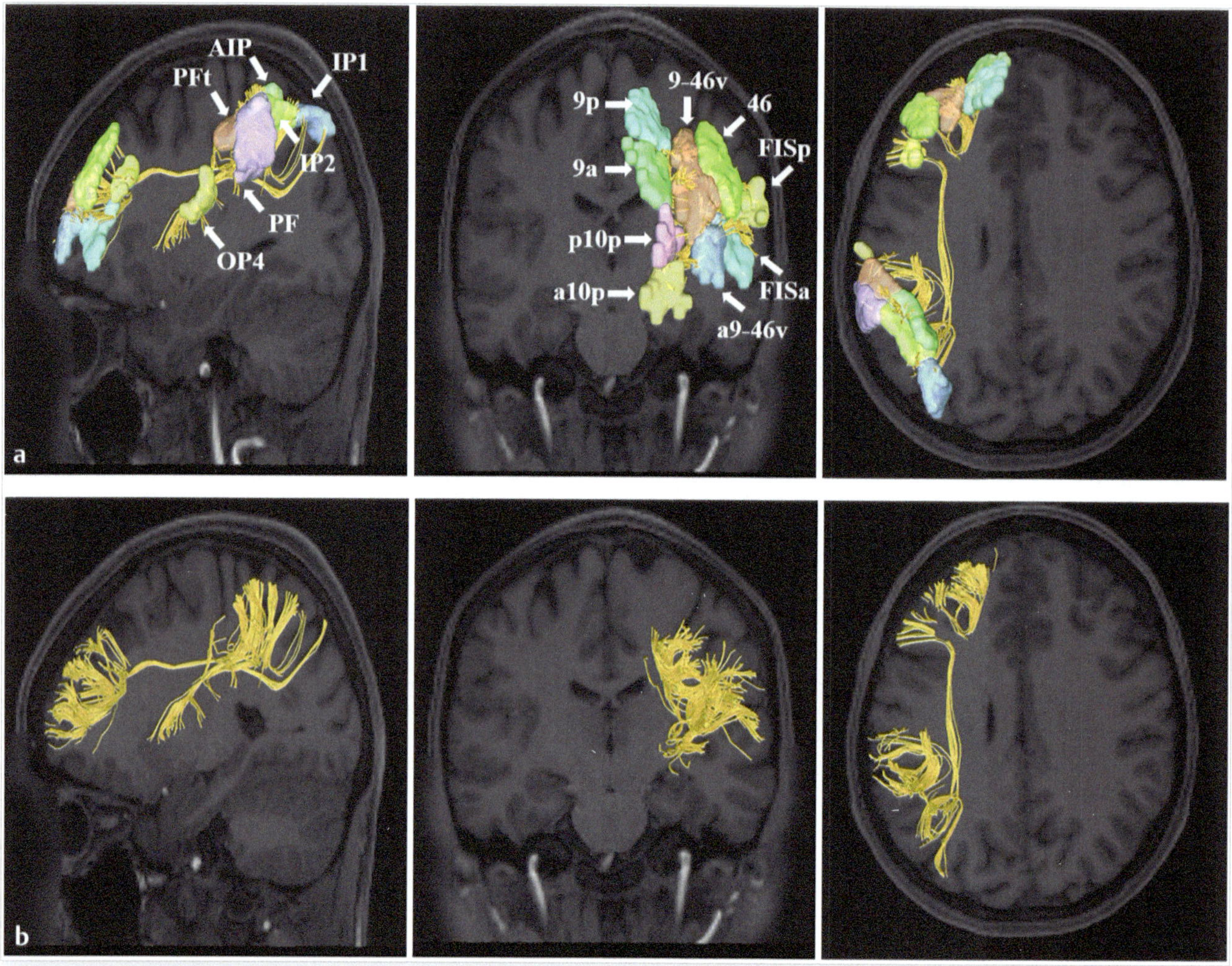

Fig. 6.12 The network anatomy of the central executive network (aka control network). (a) ROIs demonstrating the parcellations of the CEN. (b) Connections of the CEN.

involves moving the eyes, as opposed to a primary site for eye movement alone.

6.9.2 Ventral Attention Network

The VAN is a right-sided frontoparietal network consisting of frontal executive areas such as 8C, p4-46v, ventral premotor area 6r, insula opercular areas FOP3, FOP4, and AVI, which communicate via the SLF with parietal areas PFm, PGi, PGp, and LIPd. PFm and PGI are components of the lateral parietal component of the DMN.

The VAN is thought to be involved in redirection of attention away from irrelevant stimuli. At first glance, it would seem that the overlap of the VAN with the areas involved with neglect is striking, and of course raises the issue that this is in fact the neglect network. The data does not bear this out, as the networks only overlap in places and neglect seems to be its own network.

6.10 The Large-scale Executive Networks

Three networks which have emerged from resting state functional connectivity data, the default mode network, the salience network, and the central executive network, clearly play some role in the transition from nondirected to goal directed behavior.[12] In the traditional model, the default mode network (DMN) functions when there is no goal directed behavior taking place, the salience network is activated when something demands goal directed attention, and the central executive network (CEN) is then activated (and the DMN inactivated) by this process. A brief description of these networks follows. Studies have demonstrated that these networks lie at the top of a hierarchy of networks which define an axis of human cerebral function, with other networks functions heavily defined as lining up with the control (CEN) axis or the DMN axis. It should not be surprising then that the components of these networks show up in other networks.

6.10.1 Default Mode Network

The DMN is the most consistently identified network on fMRI and contains three core components: the posterior inferior parietal lobule, the ventromedial frontal lobe, and posterior cingulate cortex (PCC). The network map shows that the lateral parietal part involves areas PFm, PGs, and PGi. The medial frontal component contains posterior 32 (p32), subcallosal 32 (s32), anterior 24 (a24), and 10 rostral (10r). The PCC component is large and contains area 7 medial (7m), parietooccipital sulcus areas 1 and 2 (POS 1/2), the retrosplenial cortex (RSC), and all of areas 31 (31a, 31pv, 31pd), and 23 (v23ab, d23ab, 23c, 23d). The PCC is one of the most widely functionally connected parts of the human hemisphere. The frontal and PCC components are linked through the cingulum. We cannot identify any direct connections with the lateral parietal components, and speculate that the control and salience network connections may play a role in shaping this component. (▶ Fig. 6.10).

The DMN is involved in numerous aspects of high brain function and parts of the MTG; the hippocampus and the PHG can often be part of this network. I first became interested in it when it became clear to me that preserving the anterior cingulate was essential to obtaining good outcomes with butterfly and other medial frontal tumors. Interestingly, my recent work has led me to think that the junction of this network in the anterior cingulate with the salience and executive network may be the key point of problems with these patients if injured.

6.10.2 Salience Network

This is a relatively poorly understood network, but its components seem to involve the posteromedial frontal lobe notably its hub is area SCEF, and the middle cingulate, and the insula, namely parcellation MI. The FAT is the best candidate for the connection linking these modules.

The DMN is connected to the salience components via the cingulum, and the CEN may also have components in the anterior cingulate. My current thinking is that this junctional area is the key switch point where these networks talk to each other, and its preservation is paramount (▶ Fig. 6.11).

6.10.3 Central Executive Network

The CEN is best defined as the network most highly anti-correlated with the DMN (meaning when the CEN is on, the DMN is off and vice versa). It essentially involves the polar frontal lobe, including areas 9 anterior (9a), 9 posterior (9p), anterior 10 polar (a10p), posterior 10 polar (p10p), inferior frontal sulcus anterior and posterior (IFSa, IFSp), area 46, 9-46 dorsal (9-46d), and anterior 9-46 ventral (a9-46v); which is connected to the inferior parietal lobule and intraparietal sulcus, including areas PF, PFt, AIP, IP2, IP1 (the latter two are located on the inferior bank of the sulcus), and parietal opercular area 4 (OP4), which are linked via the SLF (▶ Fig. 6.12).

6.11 Final Observations

1. It should be obvious by now that the SLF is involved in a large number of networks (speech, praxis, neglect, CEN, DAN, VAN, and the motor network). Cutting across it during glioma surgery should be as undesirable to us as cutting across the optic nerve during meningioma surgery. I would argue that it is as bad as it can be to rob the patient of much of their higher brain function in a way that blinding one eye never can.
2. The overlap of networks like the DAN and CEN or the neglect and VAN is striking and raises some questions of what these functions really are.
3. These networks are constructed using data from people with normal brains. It is almost certain that your glioma patient will have a network that differs from these maps in some way, tracts will have moved, cortical sites can change, but without a framework, it is impossible to work through what the network is doing in an individual case. If they are able to talk, move the arm, etc, then the brain has some network organized to do the basic aspects of the task, either ispilaterally or from the other side.
4. There are numerous other brain functions which we did not try to map. Some of this is due to the complex number of ways a function is defined (like memory, which memory do you map?), others due to the poor understanding we have of the ability (what part of the brain is involved with judgment, other than a generic statement that it is in the frontal lobe somehow), or the extreme complexity of the problem. A first start, and where I decided to dedicate my time, is toward understanding the backbone of key networks, or elementary functions, which can both be used to build more complex models of brain function, and to determine what is left that isn't in these models, which may be the modules of human cognitions.

References

[1] Mangun GR. The Neuroscience of Attention: Attentional Control and Selection. Oxford University Press; 2012

[2] Bressler SL, Menon V. Large-scale brain networks in cognition: emerging methods and principles. Trends Cogn Sci. 2010; 14(6):277–290

[3] Farah MJea. Parietal Lobe Contributions to Orientation in 3D Space. Berlin: Springer-Verolag; 1997

[4] Chang EF, Raygor KP, Berger MS. Contemporary model of language organization: an overview for neurosurgeons. J Neurosurg. 2015; 122(2):250–261

[5] Goldenberg G. Apraxia: The Cognitive Side of Control. New York: Oxford University Press; 2013

[6] Pouget Aea. Parietal Lobe Contributions to Orientation in 3D Space. Berlin: Springer-Verolag; 1997

[7] Vaessen MJ, Saj A, Lovblad KO, Gschwind M, Vuilleumier P. Structural white-matter connections mediating distinct behavioral components of spatial neglect in right brain-damaged patients. Cortex. 2016; 77:54–68

[8] al Be. Parietal Lobe Contributions to Orientation in 3D Space. Berlin: Springer-Verolag; 1997

[9] Gentrilucci Mea. Parietal Lobe Contributions to Orientation in 3D Space. Berlin: Springer-Verolag; 1997

[10] Goodale MA, Milner AD. Separate visual pathways for perception and action. Trends Neurosci. 1992; 15(1):20–25

[11] Sestieri Cea. The Neuroscience of Attention: Attentional Control and Selection. Oxford University Press; 2012

[12] Sridharan D, Levitin DJ, Menon V. A critical role for the right fronto-insular cortex in switching between central-executive and default-mode networks. Proc Natl Acad Sci U S A. 2008; 105(34):12569–12574

7 Awake Brain Mapping: Goals, Methods, and Logistics

7.1 Introduction

It is likely that most neurosurgeons (even some who have never done awake-surgery) could briefly describe the basic steps of awake brain surgery and summarize what it is trying to accomplish. In short, you are trying to stimulate the brain with an electrode during testing (classically speech and motor) to locate eloquent brain regions and prevent yourself from injuring them, while removing a tumor or other lesion.

What is less clear to people who don't do this kind of surgery often or at all is how to actually go about doing this. The challenge comes from how to go about finding critical areas, how to know what you are seeing is reality (and how to decide to ignore something), and what to do with the information once you have a map. Pushing an electrode into the brain is not a physically challenging maneuver on par with placing a clip on an aneurysm or removing tumor off the brainstem, but brain mapping is far more than just stimulating the brain with an electrode randomly, but instead is an intellectual challenge of figuring out what is real, and how to incorporate this into a mental map which summarizes what you are actually seeing.

This chapter (and the next) provides practical information about how to get the information and how to determine if it is real. The rest of the book is about what to do with the information.

7.2 What Are Your Goals with Brain Mapping?

Brain mapping is performed to determine if a cut into a cerebral structure (cortical or subcortical) should or should not be made before it happens. Note that the term cut has both global and local meanings that are both valid in this context, as the global cut of a glioma surgery (termed disconnection in Chapter 9) is in fact made up of a series of smaller cuts being made, ideally based on hundreds of decisions based on what should be or should not done next. Thus, performing a disconnection with brain mapping involves as large number of mini-mapping events to decide whether each individual part of the cut is ok or should be moved.

Over my career, I have seen numerous presented examples of different cases that various surgeons have "mapped," I think it's worth pointing out what brain mapping isn't good for. Note it seldom makes surgery worse to test the brain; it's just that it doesn't add much. By understanding cases where mapping is largely useless, you have a better understanding of what it actually is useful for.

1. Mapping a meningioma invading eloquent brain: I am not saying this is commonly done but I have seen it and it's worth discussing why this is not helpful. First, meningiomas obviously are not infiltrating tumors, so there is no chance functional brain is running through the tumor. In addition, even if the tumor is invading the motor strip, and you stimulate the surrounding the brain and prove that it is the motor strip, knowing this fact does not mean that tell you that remaining on the tumor border will or will not be a safe method of removing the tumor or not (it may be possible to separate them without damaging the brain and it may not possible.), nor does it provide additional information of how to find the plane. In order words, it's not to say that it's not reasonable to leave meningioma tissue behind in the motor cortex if you believe it is invaded and is in the patient's best interest; it's just that mapping doesn't help you accurately make that decision about how to manage the borders. Just because it stimulates doesn't mean that it is not safe to carefully separate it out.
2. Mapping a non-infiltrating tumor which presents to the cortical surface: Many series on brain mapping contain a number of metastatic tumors (or other non-infiltrating tumors) mixed in with gliomas. This is not to say that mapping is never indicated for these tumors, in many cases it is. However, it is important to recognize that these are non-infiltrating tumors, and the role of mapping is to find a safe cut into the tumor when it is deep to the surface and the best way into the tumor is not immediately obvious. Once you are inside the tumor, good microsurgical technique and staying within the lesion boundaries is usually more than enough to avoid injury to the surrounding brain. Again, it is unclear how the information from stimulation mapping makes that part of the resection safer, the boundary is the boundary and is visible most of the time.
   When a tumor like a metastasis is on the surface, not only does mapping not help you with the tumor boundary definition, but you do not need it to find a path into the tumor. Thus, any information you get does not necessarily change your strategy, but may inappropriately scare you off prior to doing what needs to get done.
3. Mapping something you cannot sub totally resect: Here arises the thorny issue of arterial-venous malformations (AVMs) in eloquent brain. These lesions can have functioning brain in the center of the nidus, which makes them different than non-infiltrating masses like metastases. However, AVM resections ideally are en bloc removals around the margins, as cutting across the nidus is generally unwise, and there is no evidence supporting a benefit for subtotal resections of AVMs. This fact makes the surgery into an all or none event: you either take it all out, or you probably should consider not operating at all. It's unclear in most cases how brain mapping would change this much.

Of course, there are exceptions. Mapping can help find a plane into a deep nidus, or allow removal of certain cortices which could help with resection. But in general, brain mapping is a tool for intelligent subtotal resection and AVMs aren't very good candidates for subtotal resection.

Thus, brain mapping is most obviously helpful for gliomas, which are always infiltrative to some extent, are always subtotally resected to one degree or another, and lack clear boundaries which you need functional techniques to define. The vast majority of my brain-mapping cases are for infiltrating gliomas as mapping guides your decisions in featureless and potentially treacherous brain regions.

7.3 Which Gliomas Should be Done Awake?

Awake glioma surgery has traditionally been undertaken when the tumor is so close to the speech areas that there is significant risk to being asleep. In other words, awake surgery is something best avoided unless forced.

I am of the alternate view that almost all glioma patients should undergo surgery while awake, with the only exceptions being patients who cannot handle being awake, and patients undergoing repeat surgery for a small recurrence where it is very unlikely function will be meaningfully risked.

A rationale to keep essentially all patients awake:

1. If you only do awake brain surgery when absolutely forced to (i.e., back of left temporal or left inferior frontal lobe), you will be bad at it and your staff and anesthesiologist will be bad at it. When someone really needs it, you will be less effective at it. When you do awake surgery all the time, everyone is better at it.
2. It is quite easy to cause a lot of havoc in parts of the cerebrum besides the speech and motor areas. If the patient is asleep, you are not monitoring any of this, as you cut into deep brain areas with complex anatomy (if you doubt the complexity of an area like the occipital lobe, glance at Chapters 5 and 6 again).
3. There is almost no such thing as a glioma which can be done better asleep than awake. There is more to life than moving your arm and following commands. Being awake creates the possibility of protecting other functions, or taking a margin around the tumor. Being asleep just saves the patient two hours of work, and risks their higher functions to improve comfort slightly. No rational person would rather have a neurologic deficit in higher brain function or an inferior resection, than work for 1–2 hours awake.
4. No anesthesia=no anesthesia related problems=quicker recovery.
5. No anesthesia=no chance that anesthesia interferes with your mapping.
6. Patients with poor preoperative function (who many people don't map because they are hard to map) are the patients who need what little function they have the most, and the ones who have their tumor closest to bad brain areas.

In short, I map all possible patients undergoing glioma surgery because I do not see any way in which asleep surgery for gliomas improves the quality of surgery done, and I do not agree with the idea that somehow that awake surgery done by an experienced team with a good field block is somehow so bad for the patients that we should risk neurologic function to try to avoid it.

Finally, here is a brief word about asleep motor mapping. I would argue that the terms "asleep" and "motor mapping" are mutually exclusive terms; meaning that either the patients are asleep or you can map motor function. The techniques termed "asleep motor mapping" are too fraught with issues to be compared to the quality of motor system preservation that one can obtain with awake techniques. For example, the technique of motor mapping using "phase reversal," where a strip electrode is placed on cortex and studied by an electrophysiologist who determines the location of the motor cortex by EEG phase reversal, may locate the primary motor cortex, but provides little information about where the descending corticospinal tracts are running, and it is unlikely even with the addition of motor evoked potentials that you will get as reliable an early warning as one gets with the double task performed in an awake patient. Further, direct stimulation mapping asleep fails to provide insight into the rest of the motor system, including premotor areas, the SMA, and the cumulative effect of the impact of a planned cut on inputs from the sensory system, the basal ganglia, the cerebellum, etc. As I noted in Chapter 4, a disconnected motor strip connected only to the spinal cord does not drive the anterior horn cells, and a moving but functionally useless hand is only slightly better than a plegic one. In an awake patient, all of these systems can be studied using ground truth, i.e., the patient doing a task, as opposed to a surrogate measure, or partial testing of a system. Finally, asleep motor mapping can be completely thwarted by too much anesthesia, low body temperature, as well as other physiologic problems, which is not a problem in fully awake patients.

In short, I do all patients awake because I almost always can do a more complete, and/or safer surgery awake than is possible asleep.

7.4 Set Up

As with all neurosurgical procedures, positioning is a critical detail. In brain mapping, bad positioning makes the case impossible, as it can prevent the patient from participating in testing. I also teach my residents that uncomfortable patients don't map well. As will soon become obvious, extensive subcortical mapping requires a cooperative patient for hours sometimes, and an uncooperative patient provides only slightly more information than an asleep one.

I position all patients on their side with the lower arm off the bed slightly and placed on an arm board which is slightly below the level of the bed to prevent the lower shoulder from being kinked (▸ Fig. 7.1). The Mayfield bed attachment hooks under the arm board to fixate the head.

One key point in glioma surgery is that most head positions used in other neurosurgical approaches are basically unwise in awake brain surgery. Extreme head rotation, flexion, or extension, not only is uncomfortable, but it makes it hard to see the testing examiners. Also one of the key things to avoid in glioma surgery is not accounting for head rotation in your assessment of proper trajectory during the disconnection phase of the mapping (see Chapter 9) which can lead to disastrous cuts made based on a flawed understanding of the anatomy. Almost all neurosurgeons (whether or not they are conscious of it) think of the cerebrum from the classic side view, and it is best to put the head as neutral and close to that as possible to eliminate or at least minimize the need to rotate the images in your head during the surgery.

This leaves us with basically four awake head positions: (▸ Fig. 7.2)

1. Head neutral: This is the default approach for opercular tumors or tumors in neighboring gyri.
2. Apex tipped upward: By tipping the apex of the head upward with the head otherwise neutral (no rotation or flexion/extension), you place the SFG, MFG, top of motor/sensory strips, and superior parietal lobe into easy view. It is also

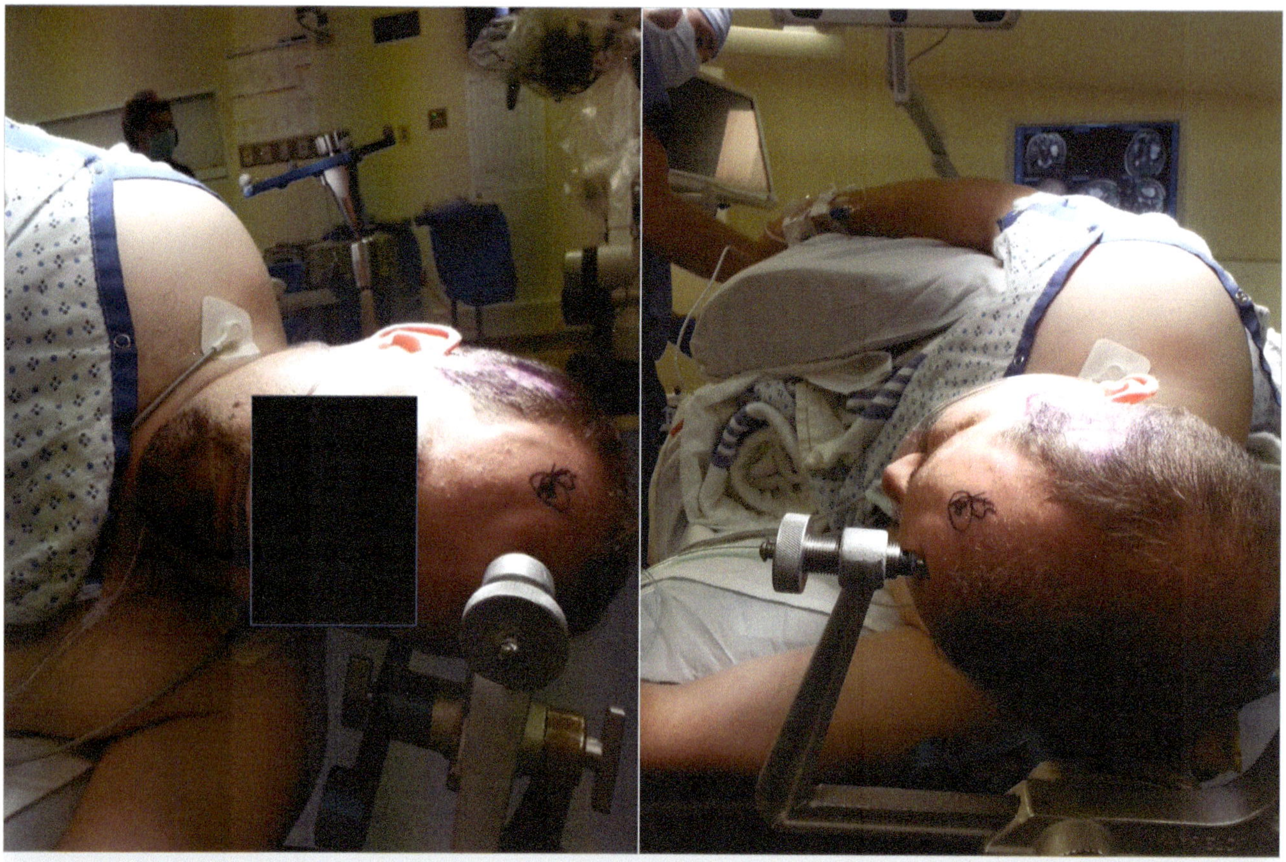

Fig. 7.1 These two pictures depict the typical patient position we utilize for awake brain surgery. The head is in the head holder and placed in a neutral position (meaning not rotated in most cases). The patient is in the full lateral position with an arm board placed below the level of the table (so that they are not laying uncomfortably on their shoulder), and bolsters used on the back and abdomen so that they patient does not need to support their own body weight. The contralateral leg and arm are available for testing. There is a viewing screen used to hold the drape out of the patient's face. Similarly, the image guidance is placed so it is not in the patient's line of sight.

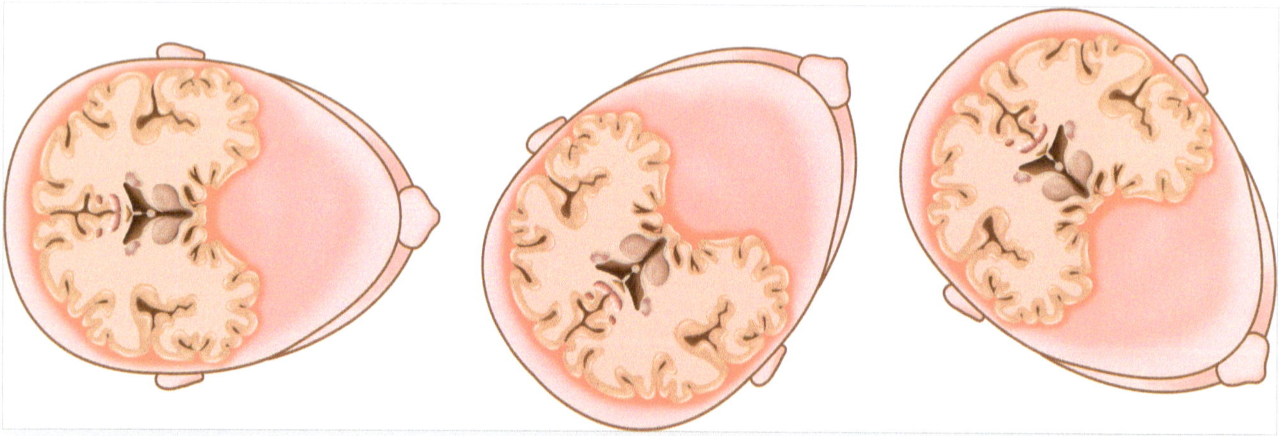

Fig. 7.2 These schematics demonstrate the three basic head positions for brain mapping cases. The most common position is the neutral position, with the head neither tipped up nor down. This is useful for maintaining orientation and is the default position. The tipped down position (center) is useful for looking up underneath the temporal lobe, especially in insular and hippocampal cases. The tipped up position is useful for frontal and midline parietal tumors, as well as sensorimotor and some insular tumors.

helpful for accessing the insula from the superior transopecular approach when that is the appropriate angle.

3. Apex tipped downward: Tipping the apex slightly downward in the neutral position is key for lower temporal and occipital tumors, especially when access to the hippocampus, fornix, atrium, and parahippocampal gyrus is desired. A transopercular approach to the insula from the temporal side should also be positioned this way. If the head was positioned apex

up, the shoulder would block working at this inferior to superomedial angle, making life miserable.

4. Slight contralateral rotation: This is the position of last resort as it makes mapping harder. However, when the angle of approach comes from the posteromedial parietal lobe or the upper occipital lobe, as with superior parietal lobule approaches to thalamic tumors, or approaches to splenium tumors, a neutral position causes the brain to fall across the field tying up a hand retracting the cut edge of the brain. If this position is needed, you should account for this constantly to remain oriented, and try to keep the rotation to a minimum.

We have a custom-made square-shaped bar to hold the drape off the patient's face and we tightly attach the drape to the bar so we can use this as an attachment point for hooks. It is also important that the image guidance attachment to the Mayfield not cross the patient's line of sight.

Finally, whenever possible, anesthesia should avoid placing lines in the contralateral arm or foot as this can severely hamper arm use and make higher level testing difficult.

7.5 Local Field Anesthesia

A pain in pain maps badly or not at all, and the lack of accurate mapping invalidates many of the fundamental assumptions of this book, vis-à-vis what is safe to do. Learning to achieve good local pain relief is the key to success.

I utilize a mix of Marcaine (long term), lidocaine with epinephrine (quick acting), and bicarbonate (less sting) for local blocks, and always have some extra medicine on the field for additional blocks of the muscle and dura as needed. The Mayfield pin sites also need to be blocked prior to pinning.

A generous field block 360 degrees around the planned incision is usually more than enough to achieve comfort, given that it is reasonably wide of the incision. I have once injected low enough to get a transient facial weakness from injecting below a temporal limb of an incision. It is usually best to start by blocking the roots of the main scalp nerves (▶ Fig. 7.3) going to the area and then generously connecting them into a circle around the incision, followed by injecting the incision.

Turning the bone flap is usually going to hurt on a first time craniotomy, so it's best to go fast until the dura can be exposed and numbed. Besides this, the only other common source of pain is making contact with the dura of the orbital roof, middle fossa floor, or falx, which in some procedures is unavoidable. Fortunately, it is uncommon that more than a short amount of critical mapping work is needed in these areas, and I save those parts for last, or after the patient can go to sleep. The only time dural pain is unavoidable, is in some cases of surgery for recurrent tumor. I have seen the brain scarred to the dura in many places making touching anything painful. In those cases, making a disconnecting cut which quickly prevents what you are working on from pulling on the dura somewhere else can help.

7.6 How to Map the Cortex

The exact testing paradigms are described in Chapter 8 and this section instead discusses concepts of electrical stimulation common to mapping any neurofunction system.

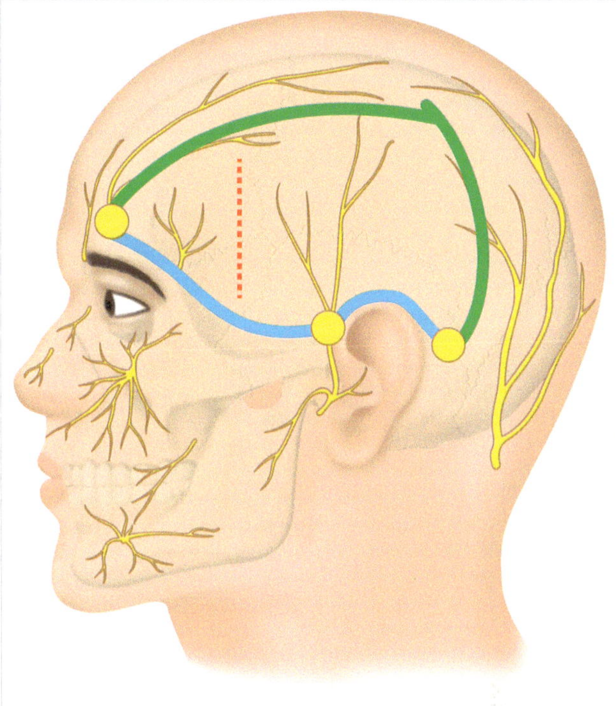

Fig. 7.3 This schematic demonstrates the field block for an awake surgery. This is the generic block for most frontal, temporal, and insular tumors. It is best to start by placing large wheals of local anesthetic at the supraorbital, auriculotemporal branch of the trigeminal nerve, and the posterior auricular nerves (shown in red circles), as this reduces the pain at the rest of the injection sites. I then connect these sites with multiple injections across the bottom of the head (blue). Finally, I inject around the incision (green) to complete a 360 degree block, before injecting the incision. This can obviously be modified based on incision location, notably, occipitoparietal blocks should include the occipital nerve and exclude the supraorbital.

Stimulation of the cortex is usually performed with a bipolar electrode, though under the right conditions, monopolar stimulation can be effective with a lower risk of seizures but it's easiest to start with a well-established method early on. Bipolar stimulation to the primary motor cortex can cause some involuntary movements of the contralateral side, stimulation of the sensory strip can cause a shocking sensation in the contralateral side, and stimulation of the optic radiations can cause visual phenomena. With these notable exceptions, bipolar stimulation typically deactivates the area being stimulated.

Thus, I think of stimulation as a way to turning off an area I wish to cut, and seeing if the patient can function without that area. In this line of thought, stimulation helps determine if a cut is safe to make before you make it. This is the main reason awake surgery is superior to most existing extraoperative functional testing, like task based functional MRI, as most other methods tell you what brain areas are active during as task, but cannot tell you accurately how a system would work without the part in question. This may surprise the reader to hear given that I am writing this sitting in a conference about fMRI brain mapping, as this is a key interest of mine. I think the potential of functional neuroimaging, especially multinetwork studies such as resting state fMRI, to radically change what we do is real; however, I think we need to be realistic that there is a big difference between knowing a few areas which light up on an fMRI task study for speech, and really knowing what has to stay and what does not in an infinitely complex set of networks. This difference between "active" and "essential" is often the difference between "inoperable" and "operable."

7.6.1 How High Do You Set the Current?

The current setting is a balance between the desire to make sure negative sites are truly shut off during the testing, which in turn means making sure the area being stimulated is inactivated by the current, which can be assured by turning the stimulation current high; against the risk of causing an intraoperative seizure, which increases with increasing current. The best rule of thumb is to start low and escalate early in the mapping process. Based on experiences of people who do largely positive mapping with large craniotomies, in general it is uncommon to not find a positive site in a fully awake patient when stimulating with 3 mA current. Because I do negative mapping, I generally go a bit higher to ensure the map is truly negative, but have never found a benefit for going over 4.5 mA, but have seen more seizures at higher currents. I start at 2 mA and increase until I find a site or reach 4.5 mA.

7.6.2 Big Craniotomy (Positive Mapping) vs Smaller Craniotomy (Negative Mapping)?

The long standing argument has its proponents on both sides. I do negative mapping because I want glioma surgery to be as minor of a deal a possible, because I don't wish to see or scar brain areas for future operations which I don't plan on operating on, and because I have yet to encounter a case where it was clear that fully awake negative mapped patient suffered an adverse outcome due to not having a complete map of a large area of the cortex. As negative mapping techniques have been repeatedly refined and validated, it is unclear why having a positive site is essential for success in mapping given our improved understanding of anatomy.

I was trained to use electrocorticography and did so for years to make sure the current was high enough, but have recently stopped as it makes the case unnecessarily complex (try getting someone to read ECOG on Friday at 4pm) for a for only minimal gain in technique. If the current is at 4.5 mA in an awake patient, it's pretty safe to assume that your negative sites are really negative in my experience. The safety of negative mapping has been validated by others also.

7.6.3 When to have the Patient Awake versus Asleep

There are a number of "asleep-awake-asleep" type protocols for managing the patient around the mapping. My protocol is better described as "kind-of sleepy, awake, awake, awake, awake, asleep." My thinking is that if mapping is important (it is), then it should be done well, and having a patient be mostly asleep under general anesthesia prior to trying to map them, only can make good mapping less likely to happen. This is especially true for patients with marginal preoperative function, as even short runs of general anesthesia can sabotage their ability to map for hours, and these are the patients who have the most threatened systems with the highest risk of losing them.

Further, the idea that our goal is to get the patient back to sleep as fast as possible, again discounts the idea that anything in the subcortex is worth saving, and that mapping is important for saving function. Either you believe in mapping or you don't.

We give the patient only light sedation for opening and do not give any sedating medicines until the entire subcortical disconnection is done. If it's important (it is), then we shouldn't compromise it being done well.

7.7 How to Manage Stimulation Induced Seizures

If you and/or you anesthesiologist are not ready to manage a seizure in a mapping case, you are not ready to map because they can happen even in patients without a seizure history. I do not routinely place glioma patients without seizures on prophylactic anti-epileptics, but I do load patients going into a mapping case because I want to avoid seizures if possible. I also go up on the current slowly, and do not exceed 4.5 mA as I do not think the risk-benefit favors doing so.

Even then it can still happen. We always have ice cold irrigation on the table in case, as this can abort the seizure. If this doesn't work, alone, a small dose of Propofol can also help but will likely halt the mapping for a while. Intubation with an LMA airway and conversion to general anesthetic is a last resort that we have only had to do once for a few minutes to break a seizure. In a bad generalized seizure, until the seizure breaks, the surgeon needs to minimize injury to the head in pins (which may require disengaging the table attachment), to keep an eye on the brain to ensure it is not extruding outward, and ensure someone is continuously irrigating the brain with cold irrigation. After breaking the seizure, it is time to inspect the head clamp to ensure it hasn't pulled out (it will usually pull out of the skull rather than injure the neck), see if the image guidance is still accurate (we have been able to re-register with surface tracing, inspect the brain for injury, and reorganize the field. Finally, you should be aware that the hyper-metabolism caused by seizing in a tight brain can cause a delayed sudden brain swelling, and you should be aware of it.

After a seizure, get prepared to wait a while for the patient to map again, I have seen it take 2 hours once. As you can tell, avoidance of seizures is best, but you must be prepared to handle them if they occur.

7.7.1 Handling Other Intraoperative Problems

Awake brain surgery creates anesthetic issues which are beyond the skill set of most anesthesiologists who lack specific experience. Most notably, inadequate balance of anesthetic can lead to patient discomfort, or at the other extreme, loss of the airway or inability to map the over sedated patient. At our hospital, only specific anesthesiologists are allowed to staff these cases.

The anesthesiologist should examine the final head position to ensure that they can place an LMA or other airway if needed, while in pins. LMA placement can allow you to deal with respiratory depression from over sedation, seizures, intraoperative swelling, patients with extensive scarring to the dura (especially high grade recurrent temporal lobe tumors) which hurt to peel out, or patients who freak out during the case and need to covert to general anesthesia.

Brain swelling is generally worse in awake patients, especially high grade gliomas. It is rare that with a small craniotomy that external herniation of the brain will happen outside of seizures. Giving mannitol can reduce this risk. There are surgeons who advocate against this as it can cause minor changes in image guidance accuracy. I would note that a swollen brain leaving the skull also does this (so does removing the tumor), and that this level of dependency (milimetric) on image guidance is better replaced with deep anatomic understanding and a philosophy of resecting up to anatomic and/or functional boundaries (Chapter 9), which makes image guidance a helpful adjunct, but not a crutch.

Hyperventilation can also reduce brain swelling, and it's good to pause for this if the dura is tense, before proceeding to open it. In problem situations, taking some tumor out can also help, but it's not a good idea to commando out the tumor because you are afraid of brain herniation injuring the cortex as you can do a lot worse things to the arteries and deep white matter in the melee. If the brain really won't relax, placing an airway and paralyzing the patient will usually allow you to work on a relaxed brain, but generally I have not had to stop the mapping for this problem and try to get the disconnection done before resorting to an LMA.

7.8 Subcortical Mapping

I do not begin cutting into the sub cortex until the diagnosis of glioma is certain or at least non-operative diagnoses like lymphoma or metastasis can be reasonably ruled out, either from previous biopsy or from a frozen section that I try to send at the earliest reasonable moment. I do not want to find out it was a lymphoma after cutting next to the SLF.

I do all subcortical cutting under the microscope, as it provides superior perspective for keeping my subcortical cuts oriented along their intended trajectory, and for avoiding injury to an artery in the sulci that ends the mapping before it has started. Subcortical mapping requires continuous testing throughout the disconnection phase and continues until the entire cut is well clear of anything at risk in all directions. The task selection is based on the functional network or networks at risk, and is paired with one other task type (the double task in Chapter 8) and should switch as you move between relevant regions.

7.8.1 How and When to Subcortically Stimulate

This is a technical point which is not entirely obvious at first thought and deserves some discussion. I think about using the stimulator in the sub cortex to turn off the area of white matter I am about to enter to see if it is safe to proceed. If you stimulate only the visible edge, you are stimulate brain which has already been cut, so it is important to push the stimulator inward so the current stimulates and functionally disrupts the next area of deeper brain you wish to cut (▶ Fig. 7.4). The current which found a positive site at the cortex is usually enough to work in the subcortex. If an area of subcortex maps negative, then I usually assume that this clears the next layer of white matter for about the length of the stimulator probe tip. I have no data to back that up, it has worked for me. If an area of subcortex maps positive (meaning that the patient stops doing the test every time I stimulate or work there), I deflect my cut angle away from the conceptual idea of where the tracts are likely to be, which I base on DTI tractography. Image guidance linked to tractography is an extremely helpful tool for understanding these relationships in real time, but if you think you are close to a tract, it's good to stimulate frequently to clear an area before proceeding deeper. In other words, DTIs are very helpful, but don't follow them off a cliff.

7.8.2 Awake Subcortical Mapping as Monitoring

It is important to clear specific areas of white matter before proceeding deeper in the proximity of key tracts. But to stimulate every cc of white matter prior to proceeding deeper along the entire cut, needlessly adds steps which eat up a patient's mapping time, which is a scare resource as most patients will tire out eventually and stop working as hard. In less risky areas, I speed up the white matter dissection by viewing mapping in these regions as monitoring. A patient doing two tasks at once will begin to struggle with the task as soon as you get near the tract, giving you warning well before you cut the tract, assuming you are proceeding cautiously and not rushing the approach. This allows you to focus stimulation on areas which are truly close to key parts of the network, and not waste time which the patient may not give you, stimulating every step

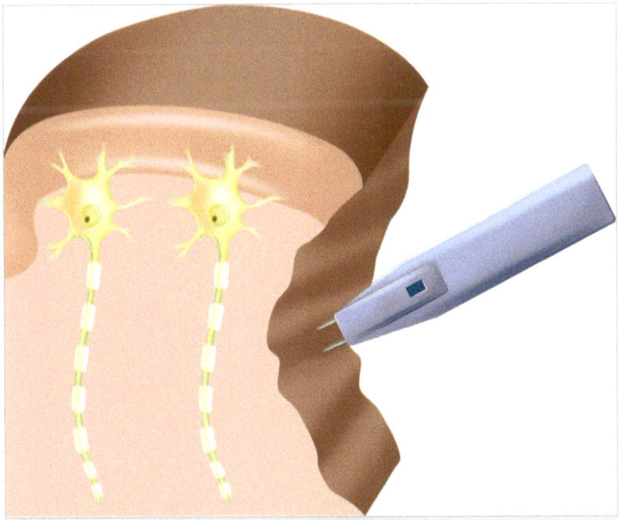

Fig. 7.4 This diagram demonstrates the goal of subcortical stimulation. When you begin doing subcortical stimulation, it is common to think the goal is to stimulate the visible cut edge of subcortical brain, but this does not make sense, as this area is already cut, and your goal is to figure out if you can proceed deeper. A more useful stimulation technique is to push the stimulator a few mm's into the subcortical tissue ahead of where you plan on stimulating, to see if it is safe to proceed.

along the way. The guide to when to start thinking about stimulation comes from DTI, understanding of anatomy, and experience.

Awake subcortical monitoring is a critical step forward in glioma surgery and has made numerous previously inoperable cases possible, as well as teaching us much more about how the brain works.

What to Do If the Patient Stops Doing the Task

The first few times this happens to you, it will be unsettling. The key is to not panic, as the majority of the time, this loss of function just means you are getting close to a connection, and the physical manipulation is interfering with an important connection (▶ Fig. 7.5).

When a patient begins to fail on a task, I react by first stopping my work in that area to allow the brain to rest. I irrigate the brain with cool irrigation, and put verapamil on the arteries in case vasospasm is ongoing. I give the patient a break, and work on some unrelated part of the case (removing tumor from brain await from the combat zone, gaining hemostasis, removing hemostatic agents, checking positioning with the image guidance, taking stock of why I think they are having this problem and what I should do, etc.). Most the time (about 90–95%), this problem resolves within a few minutes and some prompting.

If the deficit improves, but subsequently the problems keep happening when I touch a part of the brain that I think is not the area of interest, I spend a few minutes to disconnect the offending area from where I think the tracts likely are. This often stops the problem from returning and lets me continue mapping, but it's also important to figure out what structure the manipulation was probably pulling on to because the problem as this is key information (▶ Fig. 7.6).

If somehow, the patient does not return to a mapping state within a few minutes, I make a judgment call of the needs to be done, and convert the case to a conservative resection. A large percentage of the time, these problems go away over a few days and are not reflective of a long term problem if the onset of problems was sudden and not near the high risk area. What will slow this recovery is a large residual tumor, and edema, so you should try to get at least a decent resection with the mapping information you have gathered, but you are flying blind, and you cannot make cuts you would considering making with the patient awake and mapping.

7.9 The SMA Syndrome and Mapping

One problem that never dawned on me until I began to map the mid-line frontal lobe, is the possibility of SMA syndrome, and its effect on mapping. The SMA syndrome (and other similar syndromes) can come on very rapidly, and can be caused by edema that will resolve within a short time (unlike the true syndrome which takes a bit longer usually). The mutism and hemiplegia which typifies this syndrome makes mapping impossible. Similar problems are possible near the basal ganglia and occasionally the cingulate gyrus, but are worst near the SMA. Thus, I always perform this part of the mapping and disconnection last, as it can make the other mapping cuts impossible if SMA syndrome kicks in.

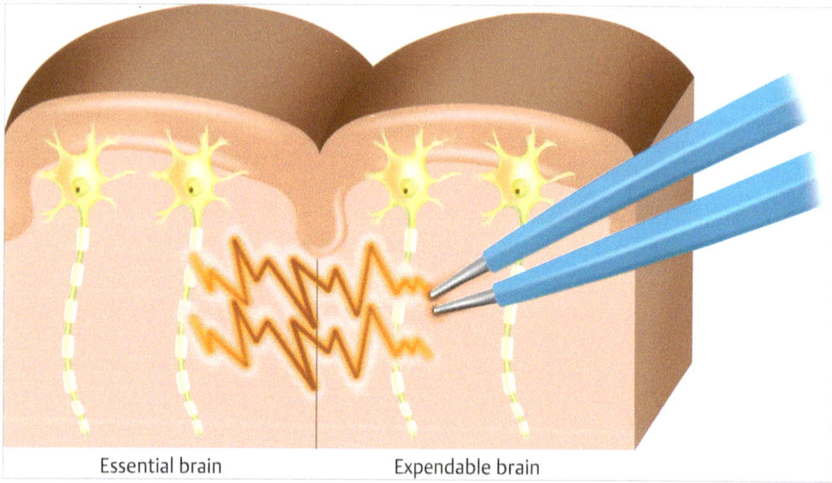

Fig. 7.5 When you are working in the subcortical brain, and you approach an essential tract for whatever function the patient is performing, they will begin to struggle well before you have actually reached the tract. This diagram aims to explain the mechanism behind that phenomenon. Note that in this figure, we are working with the bipolar in nonessential brain, but that vibration, physical deformation, and possibly heat are being transmitted to the deeper essential brain areas (cortex or tract), causing it to fail. When this happens, the majority of the time this will improve with time and some cold irrigation, but it provides a warning that you are getting close to something important for that task, or for global cognitive function (like attention).

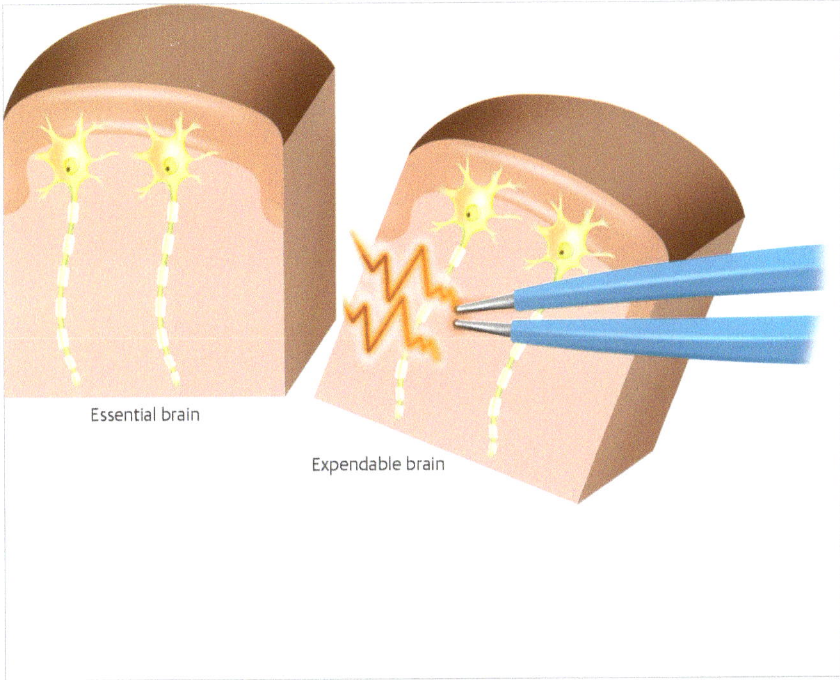

Fig. 7.6 Sometimes during subcortical work, you begin to get problems with a test in an area that you are pretty certain is not part of the network. You should always reconsider that your understanding of the network could need adjustment, but sometimes this keeps happening, and you are sure this is not due to being actually close to the tract. This is usually due to transmission of vibration or manipulation over a distance (as in ▶ Fig. 7.5), and is common in repeat cases where scar tissue can transmit forces over an undesirable distances. This can make it difficult to proceed as every move is giving you false positive feedback through an indirect mechanical effect. As this figure shows, when you are sure that an area giving you problems is not real, then making a disconnecting cut to free the area you are working on from the functional area being pulled on to cause the false positive, can allow you to proceed in peace. Note that performing such a maneuver requires a deep understanding of anatomy and network organization to know that this area is safe to attack despite what your monitoring is telling you, but also to know what area likely is the functional area.

7.9.1 Resisting Your Nature after the Mapping Is Done

It is in most neurosurgeons' nature to make decisions on the fly, and to want to try to do the best possible tumor resection. This nature can work against us in brain mapping, as it is our instinct to see the tumor, and want to remove it. This is fine when the patient is awake; however, at some point the mapping may stop, either because the patient stops cooperating, tires out, develops SMA syndrome or another problem, or develops pain or brain swelling issues which require a conversion to asleep, or when you think you are done and put the patient to sleep. All of these are reasonable reasons to stop mapping, but sometimes you will see some suspicious tissue after mapping is done, and it is very tempting to remove it.

You must resist the temptation to do something with the patient asleep that you should do awake. Thus, even if I see some tumor against the SLF area after putting the patient to sleep that I think I might be able to take out, if I think it should be mapped to be safe, I force myself to stop.

Either mapping is important for preserving function (it is) or it's not.

Part II

Applications

II

8 Functional Testing for Brain Mapping

8.1 Introduction

Many of the greatest challenges in brain mapping are epistemological. In other words, our great challenge is figuring out how to gather meaningful information, how to assess its quality, and what to do with that information. This chapter addresses the nature of our information about the brain and its function, especially with regards to functional testing, both before and inside the operating room, and when relevant provides some practical information on how we do the testing presently.

8.2 What Tasks Should You Test?

As a surgeon, you by definition won't be doing the testing during surgery, but you need to understand the task, specifically what functional systems it is (probably) testing, what task to do when, and when to ignore information versus acting on it. Also if the program is not firmly established at your hospital, you will probably have to guide the early efforts.

A common (mis)conception people have about brain mapping is that you simply have the patient do some task, stimulate the brain, and if you find something, just stay away from that part of the brain. That paradigm works reasonably well for areas with simple anatomy, such as some aspects of speech and motor function. The problem is that finding a cortical site, doesn't fully protect you if you then go on and cut that area's connection in the sub cortex, or remove another area in that network necessary for the task (for example math skills are poor in a densely aphasic patient). You will also be disappointed at times, as most higher brain functions require multiple interconnected brain areas working together in order to produce the function, so the test will often not provide you the black or white result you expect, say with something like arm movement.

Another problem with just testing a part of the brain in an undirected fashion is that you may not find a site, especially if you are looking for it in the wrong part of the brain. In addition, it may not be something so critical that it's worth leaving a great part of the tumor in the head to save the function. For example, it would be nice to name colors, but I am not certain, it is more important than treating the GBM.

Finally, not all functional tests translate well to intraoperative brain mapping. Some are too complicated or long. For example, a long figure construction based neuropsychological test would require a long period of brain stimulation before you know for sure whether that function was successfully performed or not, which of course can eat up valuable time (most patients will not do testing indefinitely) and which can increase the risk for seizures especially with longer periods of cortical stimulation. Other tests don't have a clear yes-no answer (which you need when you need to make a call of whether or not to make a cut). For example, a test which evaluated as a 1–30 score and then compared to normative data is cumbersome and cannot be continuously monitored, which limits its utility. Finally, not all tests reliably become abnormal when you approach the structure of interest.

Interestingly, we have found that most tests can be successfully performed in the operating room with the patient in the correct position with access to both arms. Obviously, you cannot test gait or balance, but most cognitive tests are possible, including some complicated tasks of real life activities. But not all that can be done in surgery is useful.

I term the process of creating an intraoperative test from an office based neuropsychologic test "miniaturization." Restating information from Chapter 4, below are a few guidelines I use for selecting, creating and integrating new tests into my mapping cases:

8.2.1 Sughrue's Guidelines for Attempting to Find and Save a Higher Brain Function

For a function to be amenable to a focused effort to find it and save it, a higher brain function should:

- Be worth saving such that it is better to reduce your extent of resection to achieve it.
- Have a reasonably well understood functional network, with some idea of what structures are essential for performing that function and their essential interconnections.
- Have a test of function which can be reasonably performed in the operating room by at least some patients.
- Have a test which clearly becomes abnormal in a reliable and easily observable way when the system is disturbed.

These aren't scientific laws, but they help us think about how to expand our mapping in a way that is logical and practically achievable.

8.3 The Testing Team

Brain mapping is often done by neuropsychologists, but I have found that physical and speech therapists are often better at these cases. First, they often have more flexible schedules than neuropsychologists, which is an important issue when you do 6 awake surgeries a week which is not uncommon for us, but is equally important as you are starting to do awake surgery, as nothing can kill interest in doing awake surgery then when logistics make the cases impossible. More importantly, therapists are great at encouraging and pushing the patient to keep going. The longer they map, the more you can do safely, so the skill of motivating patients is key to successful mapping. Plus a physical therapist has a broader experience in assessing the nature and quality of movement, which increases the sensitivity of your motor system testing. Finally, in an ideal world, they can also begin the rehab process in an integrated manner from the beginning. Every center is different ultimately and the best person to do these cases is one who is dedicated to these cases.

8.3.1 Preoperative Testing

In the preoperative evaluation, the patient meets the testing team and is familiarized with the process. Most importantly they are taught the tests, as the time to learn how to do them is not in a head holder as you are coming out of light sedation. The patient is educated about the possible problems which can be caused in the short term by brain swelling, and about the long term plan for rehabilitation.

Finally, the patient's preoperative baseline is assessed. It is important to know what tests are not available for use due to deficits, but also what parts of certain tests should be taken out of the test for that patient. For example, a non-English speaking, non-American patient unable to name an American football team is not anomic, and shouldn't be tested on this. Similarly, a patient with language problems shouldn't be tested in the operating room on naming objects that they can't name in an office.

Diffusion Tensor Imaging (DTI)

During the preoperative period, we obtain a DTI image and examine the tract anatomy which together with the tumor anatomy and the patient's preoperative function, helps us make a plan for what we are going to do (see Chapter 9).

Because DTIs (and its relative diffusion spectrum imaging (DSI)) are such a dominant feature of this book, it's worth mentioning a few details here about what these images are, as brief understanding of these modalities is helpful for understanding their limitations (I promise that I am not about to break into an engineering discussion). Both studies are MRI images which utilize a feature termed fractional anisotropy to characterize the bulk movement of water in the brain. Water moving in an organized direction is typically following a white matter tract, and this feature is exploited to describe tract anatomy.

DTI images quantify tract direction by determining the dominant eigenvector (i.e., the basic direction most of the water is moving) for each voxel. The limitation of this method is that it oversimplifies the data at crossing points by assigning one direction to the entire voxel even if there are more than one. There exists some software which compensate for this by dense data acquisition and liberally seeding the tract data so that the crossing point issue becomes less relevant (i.e., it accurately shows tracts on both sides of the crossing point) but it does limit the ability to trace a tract from origin to target.

DSI images are able to resolve tract crossings and are obviously the major image source of images for the anatomy sections of this book. The challenge with their use in routine clinical use is their long acquisition time, which can add over an hour to the end of preoperative volumetric imaging. There also are not seamless integration programs for linking this to image guidance programs presently (as there are for DTI). Also there are not studies validating their accuracy at predicting functional anatomy (there are with DTI). It is a great research tool, but we presently use DTIs for our cases.

The key point with both tests is that brain edema can wreck the regional tract quality with either test (purportedly worse for DSI, but I have never got a satisfying answer why that is), which is a major issue with high grade tumors especially. Thus, it is important to use tractography as a guide to the basic location of the tract, as opposed to a millimetric representation of the tract anatomy.

8.4 The Tests

8.4.1 Motor Testing

Testing the motor system is unique in that you can see positive and negative phenomenon relevant to the motor system. In fact, the presence of positive phenomenon is one of the greatest impediments to progress in intraoperative motor testing, in my opinion, as it is so obvious that it discouraged neurosurgeons from considering that there is anything else worth looking for besides the location of the motor cortex. I repeatedly emphasize in this book that a disconnected motor strip is synonymous with a paralyzed contralateral side.

If the motor system is in the surgical field (i.e., it is near a disconnecting cut I wish to make), I always test it first, before testing other systems. This is for two reasons. First, it is easy to find an unambiguously positive site early, and this allows us to confidently use as low a stimulation current as possible. Second, because of the role of the motor system as the final output of most other networks (for example, speech requires mouth and tongue motor function), it is important to know where the motor system is to subtract its contribution from other findings. One common example is that stimulation of the face motor cortex can make the patient unable to talk due to positive contraction of the face or mouth muscles, and knowing where this is ahead of time makes understanding the speech areas of the posterior frontal lobe easier (they usually are slightly anterior to this site).

The Basics

Positive motor mapping typically localizes to the motor cortex and manifests as involuntary face, arm, or leg movement. Smaller movements can be seen at lower currents, and in that case I turn up the current until it is obvious because I want to ensure I am disrupting sites later in the mapping. Even in patients with some invasion of the premotor or motor cortex causing hemiplegia, it is often possible to get muscles to fire that are palpable to a physical therapist, and I have restored function in some patients by preserving a compressed but not destroyed network, though obviously, this is inconsistently possible.

Negative motor mapping involves having the patient perform spontaneous contralateral movements, and stimulating to look for arrest of that movement (negative motor sites). The simplest form is simultaneous arm-leg movement, but it can be a more complex movement in higher functioning patients like playing an instrument. Some have stated that negative motor sites are expendable, but in many cases I have found them to be coterminous with the SMA or premotor areas, and while these might remap, I try to save them to avoid motor planning problems like SMA syndrome. SMA syndrome does not always improve despite the literature claim that it does, and at minimum, a hemiplegic mute patient with a GBM is probably not getting to radiotherapy as promptly as one who does not have SMA syndrome. I feel the small improvement of extent of resection by taking out the SMA is not worth the problems, and that this syndrome is usually avoidable.

A More Nuanced View

Finally, it is important to note that quality of movement is an important thing to consider in mapping the motor system as discoordinated movement it is often a sign of mild dysfunction (a sign you are getting too close), or compromise to important proprioceptive or other related planning inputs to the motor system needed to maintain meaningful use of the limb. Coordination requires various elements or muscles of the body working together to effectively complete an action, smoothly and efficiently. This likely means the networks responsible for inhibiting and the network responsible for actively contracting muscle are not acting appropriately together, therefore presenting a decrease in control. Coordination requires a balance of activity of all involved muscles.

In our motor testing paradigm, we take into the consideration the following aspects of a movement being performed, in addition to whether the arm is or is not moving.

1. Concentric control. This refers to control during shortening of a muscle. A loss of concentric control is manifested as a weakness or slowing of the movement not related to attention of neglect issues.
2. Eccentric control. This refers to control with lengthening of a muscle, measures some form of inhibitory control of a muscle. In surgery, problems with eccentric control manifest as the patient dropping the limb or hand to the initial position as opposed to lowering it in a controlled fashion.
3. Kinesthetic awareness. This refers to awareness of a limb's position as it moves in space. In surgery, this presents as the patient taking a random appearing and awkward path to the target.
4. Coordination. The presence of dyskinesia, or uncoordinated movements.
5. Attention to task. This can be affected by problems with one of any number of networks.
6. Speed of movement. Movements can become slower or less coordinated as a system begins to be affected by your presence near by the relevant network.

It is not entirely clear to me at present how any of these specific findings line up with a specific pathway or specific network. We have found problems with many of these features of movement well away from the motor strip, descending motor fibers, or the sensory strip, highlighting the extent of the cerebrum which contributes to normal motor function. It is not also clear how careful we need to be just because of an event like loss of eccentric control or lack of kinesthetic awareness, as not all patients who we continue pushing the resection after such an event lose useful limb control, though some clearly do, and likely we would find more subtle problems with limb control with more sensitive and rigorous measures.

Again the beauty of awake versus asleep motor testing is that you can meaningfully assess the end product, as opposed to just knowing that you are not cutting into the motor strip. It is critical, however, for the therapist doing the testing to push the patient to ensure these mild problems are not due to a lack of effort. Also, this is not to say that I always back off at the first sign of an issue, but I always consider this in the overall plan for the patient as I remove the tumor. In other words, if it keeps happening every time I touch a certain area, I consider the possibility that leaving that part of the tumor might be a better way to preserve function. That judgment is dependent on tumor grade, our available adjuvant treatment options, preoperative function levels, and how much tumor will be left. I do not think leaving a large amount of enhancing tumor in a motor area of a recurrent GBM case is a good strategy to avoid mild incoordination (the tumor will often go on to finish the entire motor system if we can't control it, but leaving a small amount of low grade tumor might be a good trade).

8.4.2 Speech Testing

As described in detail in Chapter 6, normal speech function involves the integration of several overlapping subnetworks, making speech production a highly complex network.

I test speech in every single glioma patient. People have asked me "Why test speech in the right hemisphere when most people are left side dominant." A few reasons follow:

1. Not everyone (including the rare right hander) have left-sided speech. It's hard to argue that it's worth leaving a patient densely aphasic because we didn't bother to look.
2. The idea that speech areas are located on only one side of the brain even in "left dominant" patients is a simplistic and outdated concept. First, a right SMA or caudate injury often causes mutism, which can be permanent in some cases. Also, brain mapping often will find speech sites on the right side (speech arrest or naming), even if the network is probably mostly left sided, which may be compensable if removed (experience with right-sided brain injury says they probably are), but which probably would worsen the overall quality of the speech network. If you are going to go for it and take these sites out, you should at least be aware of the trade you are making, instead of throwing your hands up in surprise where there is a problem. Finally, the fact that very aphasic left MCA stroke patients often gain the ability to say some words or phrases, argues that most people have at least some speech on the right. The bottom line is that excellent speech function involves coordination of several areas including some on the right side of the brain, and that our overall target of speech preservation should always be maximization of the overall end product (which reflects the integration of all relevant functional networks related to the function), not rigid adherence to individual teachings.
3. I map right-sided cases for preservation of other systems anyway (like spatiotemporal functions), and speech serves as an excellent second task for many double tasks paradigms, which allows us to strain the other system. If you test speech during the cortical mapping portion of the case, then the patient is ready when you want to add it to another test. (A similar logic applies for nontraditional areas such as the anterior frontal lobe.)
4. Speech mapping in a low risk area takes about 3–5 minutes if you are experienced and the patient is cooperative.
5. It is a warmup for more complex tests which follow.

Speech Arrest

This is the first speech test I do because it is the easiest and you need to know where this is to interpret the speech network as a speech arrest will eliminate other functions like naming and reading (it is part of the final common pathway for all of them). This test involves having the patient counting, and a speech arrest site occurs when the counting stops. This site is probably the motor planning area for the face and tongue and is just anterior to the face and tongue motor cortex in most cases. The frontal rami of the SLF and the terminus of the FAT will usually help you find this area in short order as the site is usually within about 1 cm or so of these termini.

Naming

Anomia is a disability, but in and of itself it is not a terrible one, as some patients are unaware they have it. Thus, it is good to avoid it in its own right; however, the biggest reason to find naming areas is that they show you where the rest of the speech network really is.

The naming sites are typically in parts of the posterior temporal lobe, which represents the semantic networks. As described at length in Chapter 6, the semantic areas are a library of concepts and words, and this area is capable of linking sensory input to the meaning of words, and which can be accessed by numerous neurofunctional networks for various purposes. In most normal people it is located around and just inferolateral to the primary auditory cortex in Heschl's gyrus, but in glioma patients all bets are off on exactly where the semantic network is. Tractography is extremely helpful in getting an idea of where this is, as the SLF and IFOF networks will be nearby these networks which they must access.

Naming testing requires some patience and interpretation as it is rarely as black and white as speech arrest testing (▶ Fig. 8.1). First, it is important that the patient get into a rhythm before you try to interrupt the circuit, as you need to know that negative results are really due to the stimulation and not poor effort. Second, you need to start stimulating the brain before the patient sees the object, or they will be able to name it even if you are stimulating the site, as the information has entered the network. An audible cue which precedes time that the object is shown to the patient is programmed into our naming software, and this is our cue to start stimulating. You need to continue stimulating until they name the object or it is clear they can't. The therapist needs to be trained to give loud immediate feedback to the surgeon on events like this. Third, you need to stimulate sites multiple times. Remember that the semantic areas often contains multiple sites on multiple gyri (I have seen seven sites before), and thus stimulating only once may cause you to stimulate during an object whose engram is stored at a different part of the network. A general rule is a site that causes anomia two-thirds of the time is probably real though an occasional stimulating site flanked by real sites is also probably real. Also a site that lines up perfectly with the DTIs is also worth leaving alone even if it doesn't clear the cut-off, especially if it's the only site.

Having the patient precede the naming with the phrase "This is a ..." is helpful for distinguishing between phonemic problems (more SLF) from semantic (more IFOF) problems which is especially helpful deeper in the subcortex where these pathways can cross.

Checking naming anywhere you are considering making a cut is a good idea because it tests multiple parts of the speech network and can show up in unexpected places. It double checks your work in the posterior frontal lobe near speech arrest sites, and can be affected by working near the caudate nucleus near IFOF's superior bend. It is a key part of the double task.

Reading

Reading testing (▶ Fig. 8.2) is performed almost identical to naming testing and is done with the same paradigm. It can overlap with the naming areas, as any stimulation which disrupts the speech functions will also affect reading, but more commonly, specific reading sites are found in the posterior inferior temporal lobe, near the anterior parts of the ventral stream. Some mapping studies have localized reading to the parietal lobe, but this is likely a nonspecific feature of semantic function or the SLF, as fMRI data link reading to the ventral stream.

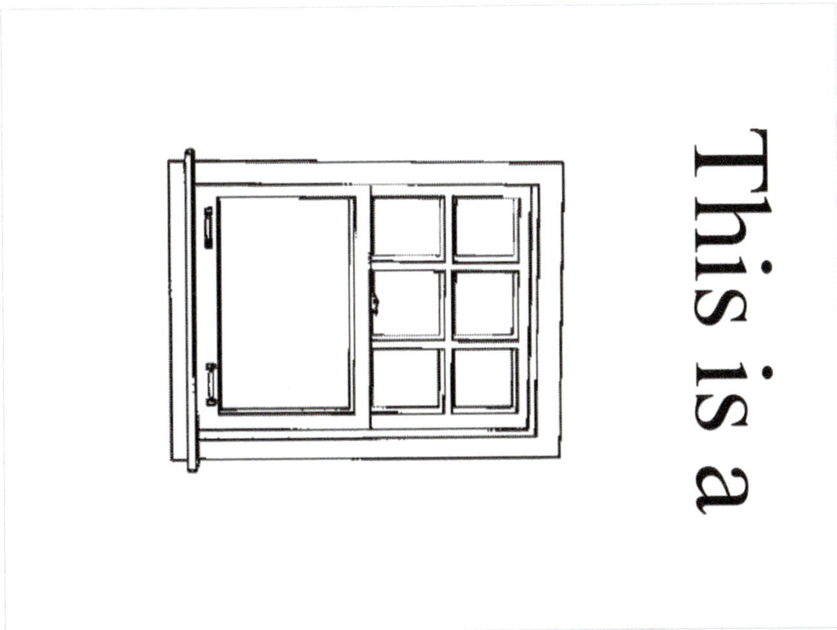

Fig. 8.1 An example of an item from the naming task. Note that it has a prompt to start with, "This is a," which helps to determine anomia from speech arrest. It is also on its side, as are all tests as this is the patient's position at surgery.

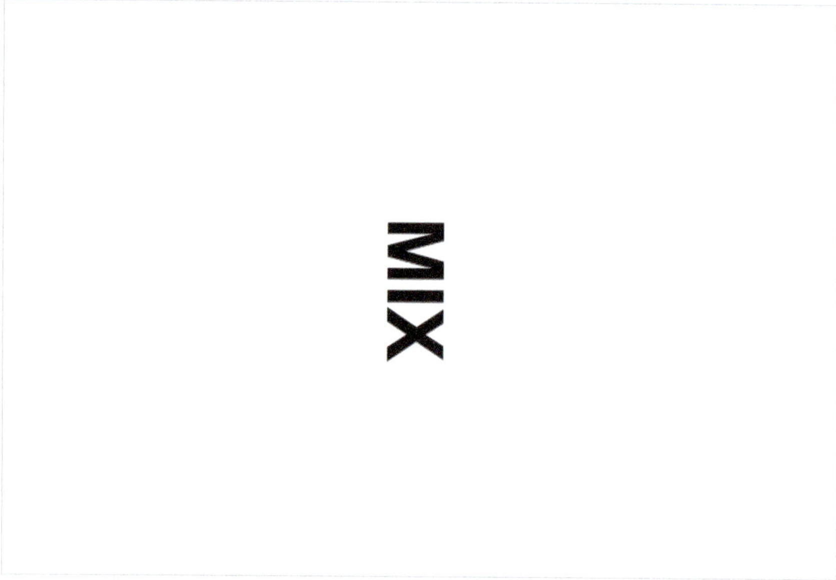

Fig. 8.2 An example of an item from the reading task. Note that it has a prompt to start with, "This is a," which helps to determine anomia from speech arrest. It is also on its side, as are all tests as this is the patient's position at surgery.

8.5 Mapping Speech in Aphasic Patients

I was taught in my training that if a patient did poorly on their preoperative testing, they were "not mapable" and it was not indicated to try to do so. Certainly, these are challenging patients to map, and this requires patience, and the acceptance that you are doing salvage surgery which may not end in a celebration of a perfect outcome as with a completely intact low grade glioma patient. But these patients can be mapped to some extent in most cases and I would argue have the most to gain from doing so, as they can make significant improvements in some cases with cytoreductive decompression, and they have the most to lose by not trying to map them and mitigate the damage, as they have tracts which are threatened or compromised, and less capacity for forgiveness if you make them worse.

Here are some strategies I use for these patients:

1. You need therapists who are experienced at pushing the patient to do whatever testing they can.
2. You need to come into the case with the right mindset and some patience.
3. They can almost always do some testing unless they are mute from a midline frontal mass. Even counting only testing can help you avoid further injury to their remaining speech network which is better than nothing.
4. If they cannot do speech testing as a double task, convert to a single speech task when anatomically relevant.
5. Minimize all anesthesia from start to finish. Even low doses can make them impossible to map for hours.

8.5.1 Neglect Testing

Spatiotemporal function problems, like motor neglect, in many ways are worse than pure motor problems. A patient who neglects the left side is functionally hemiparetic, in addition to the numerous other neuropsychological problems they suffer from related to the neglect. They are also hard to rehabilitate.

I have found that mapping aimed at preserving the right SLF system (at least that is the part which cannot be compensated for) can generally avoid this problem. The fact that this system runs deep to the parietal lobe likely explains the previous thinking that this was a purely right parietal function, but we have found neglect sites in the STG, MTG, and even the posterior frontal lobe. Neglect can also be caused in the thalamus.

8.5.2 Line Bisection

This is the easiest test to implement, and the one that has been more published as an intraoperative test, but it is the harder test to interpret, and it is likely that this is not as much a test of neglect as it is a test of visual processing. In other words, patients probably deviate because disruption of higher visual centers cause them to view the left side of the line as shorter, not as much because they are inattentive to the left side.

We use a touch screen program to have them bisect a line which is oriented along the horizontal plane of their vision (▶ Fig. 8.3) with their finger. Stimulation needs to begin before they see the line and end only when they have done the task. It is critical to get them into rhythm before testing in this task, as well as this is a difficult task to do perfectly enough in the operative conditions. Preoperative training is key to making this easier.

An abnormal test involves more than 1 cm deviation (usually leftward) at the line's midpoint. However, this test suffers from the need to place the screen in the midposition of the patient's line of sight which can be hard to judge. Visual field cuts can further confound this test. It is important to first establish a patient's baseline performance on this test and to optimize it in the operating room prior to placing too much trust in this test.

It is very difficult to subcortically map using line bisection as it does not pair with a double task well (it's hard to name and bisect at the same time), and does not rapidly provide feedback which is key to using subcortical mapping as monitoring. It is also key to mentally subtract out the role of weakness, dysphasia, poor attention, and other relevant neuropsychological problems from your interpretation of these tests.

Fig. 8.3 An example of the line bisection. This is done on a touch screen tablet so it makes a visible line.

8.5.3 Target Cancelation

We "miniaturized" this task because we wanted a way to monitor spatiotemporal function subcortically in real time, because we wanted a more unambiguous task then line bisection, and because it tests different aspects of spatiotemporal function than line bisection. Note that in cases where spatiotemporal function is most at risk, we do both.

Our touch screen program (▶ Fig. 8.4) simultaneously displays different shapes in both visual fields and requires the patient to rapidly cross out a specific shape type on both sides. Normal patients may miss one shape, especially in the contralateral superior hemifield, but true neglect involves multiple contralateral misses. Similar to line bisection, the stimulation must span the entire time they are seeing the objects or it will be invalid. Having an audible sound for when the stimulator touches the cortex is helpful for the therapist to time this well.

This test can be tested in real time to protect the subcortical parts of the network, and is easy to rapidly interpret. It must be interpreted in light of other findings, which is why I test speech and motor first.

8.5.4 Attention Testing

Specific attention testing is difficult to conceive of, attention is best noticed in its absence. Further, as outlined in Chapter 6, attention is part of the processing functions of numerous parts of the brain and its function is inseparable from its effect on other system. The visual system cannot process without it, and the neglect system involves a cross modal combination of spatiotemporal functions. Thus, while there are tasks of attention, such as digit span, this is really a test of working memory that poor attention interferes with.

Despite the difficulty we have in describing it, it is certain that we know when a patient lacks it, as their functional ability is often drastically decreased. It is well known in neuropsychology that poor attention is often best characterized as a limited ability to participate with testing of any area. This highlights the critical need for experienced and informed testers in these cases, as they need to be aware of what attentional problems look like, namely that a patient performs poorly at any task.

For some time, I did some glioma surgeries asleep, due to my own inability to understand what we could gain by being awake and testing function in some parts of the brain. For example, what can you test to save anterior medial frontal lobe function. Stimulating the brain and giving the patient a test of whether they are focusing is unlikely to yield a reliable and useful result, as most patients having a craniotomy have decreased attention compared to their baseline, and as I described above, tests which rely on comparing a quantitative score to normative data do not yield the kind of fast and decisive results needed to decide whether a system is dysfunctional when I am manipulating it.

Attention is part of most higher cerebral neurofunctional systems. We know this from akinetic mutism which causes the patient to do very little, despite having systems to speak and move which are functional. Presently, I study attention by placing a heavy demand on attention and continuously testing it when I work near these systems. Problems with attention will cause the patient to stop performing the task, or to at least put less effort towards doing it well.

The best attention task I have found involves having the patient perform a real life, complex task while I remove the tumor. Examples of what we have used include: playing an instrument, knitting, assembling auto parts, and performing accounting calculations. Initially, I thought these tasks were entertaining, but the neuropsychology underlying them was too dirty to be useful. In fact, that dirtiness of cross modal testing is the brilliance of the test. A patient able to play the guitar is not paralyzed or neglecting, does not have profound apraxia, and is not an akinetic mute. Thus, real life testing, though subtle, monitors a number of neuropsychologic systems, and especially tests attention, which is a part of all of those systems.

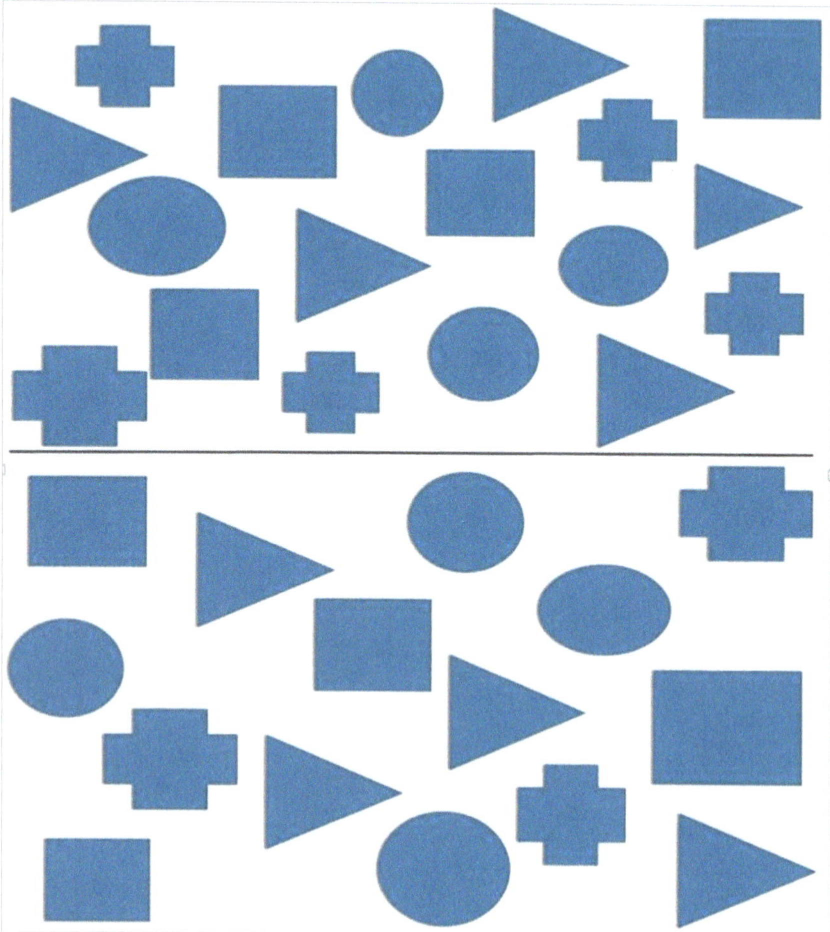

Fig. 8.4 An example of the target cancellation test which we designed for surgery. The patient is expected to mark out all of the shapes of one type on both sides of the line.

For lower functioning patients, a double task (described later) also hits on many of the same issues. If the patient struggles when you are operating in an area, it is important to deduce whether this struggle is due to problems with the primary systems (i.e., naming and arm motor or whatever you are testing), or due to lack of attention. This can be figured out often by anatomy, and by discussion with the therapists. If they know what to look for, they can give valuable insight into what is going on.

I map almost all gliomas because there is almost always something we could be saving, or taking more of a margin if we are testing.

8.6 Higher Level Functions

We have tested a number of higher functions in glioma patients. These are usually high functioning patients with low grade gliomas who have higher brain functions that they state that they would rather compromise tumor resection than lose. While when something is very important, you can monitor it throughout the resection to make sure you are not specifically eliminating that function, more often problems with the test during subcortical disconnection stem from a more elementary function, such as impairing speech while working near the SLF. In general, I try to permanently incorporate new tests based on the guidelines listed earlier, as I do not wish to compromise tumor resection based on anything less than clearly thought out functional considerations.

A list of higher functions we have tested:

1. Facial recognition: Prosopagnosia generally results from a bilateral injury; however, the possibility of not knowing family members terrifies some patients and it's easy to test if they bring in labeled pictures from home.
2. Mathematics: Classically, a left parietal function, most of the time this function gets overshadowed in these cases by the common risk to speech in these cases. But it is easy to test and preserve in high-functioning patients.
3. Judgment: This surprisingly can be tested by describing situations and gauging the patient's responses which can be assessed quickly and, though subjective, can be reasonably assessed as appropriate or not. This is obviously a test for high functioning people and the challenge is figuring out what to do with the information, as much of the right hemisphere is potentially involved with this uncertain circuit. As well, the definition of what judgment is, as opposed to emotion regulation, empathy, attention, or even some agnosia or dysphasia, is challenging to say the least.
4. Color naming: This is easy to test, but it is unclear what the circuitry really is, and also whether it is better to leave tumor then lose this function if the related systems are intact.

8.6.1 Monitoring Tasks

A monitoring task is one which can be repeatedly performed throughout the disconnection to keep an eye on a function at

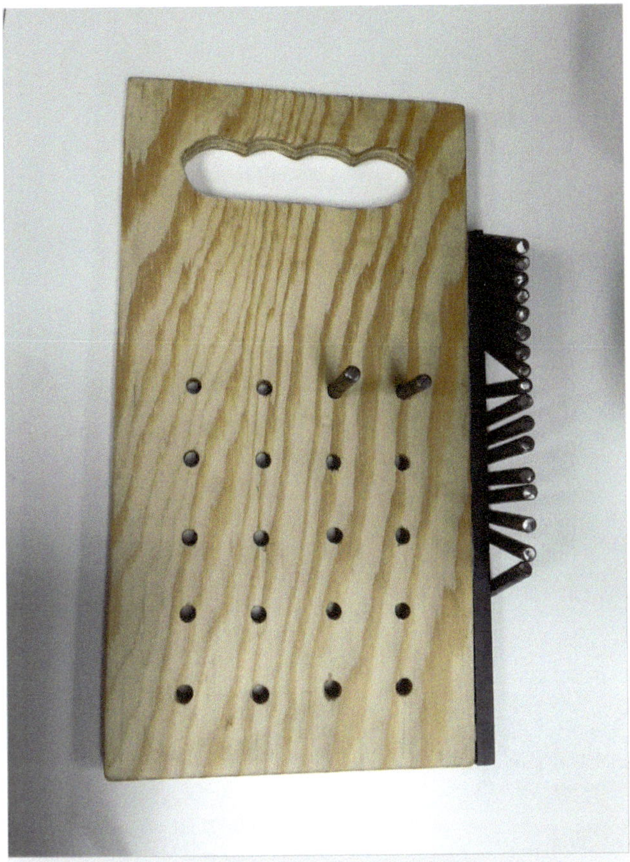

Fig. 8.5 Image demonstrating the device used for the grooved pegboard task.

risk, and ideally to note a problem before you have permanently damaged part of a neurofunctional system.

Double Task

The double task is my default monitoring task. Classically, this is a combination of moving the arm and naming objects simultaneously during the subcortical work; however, any two tasks from different neurofunctional systems can be paired. The combination stresses the two systems, by dividing attention between them, and makes each more sensitive to perturbation. Impaired patients, or ones with decreased concentration can be switched to a unimodal single task if needed.

Depending on the goals of the mapping, different tests can be paired and it is common to switch tasks during different parts of a large disconnection. For example, working near the motor strip, it is often necessary to alternate between leg and arm movement as both are at risk and we don't want to injure leg motor because we are only looking at arm.

Grooved Peg Board

This is a test of fine motor coordination of the hand, which also stresses the attention systems. It is especially helpful when motor is at particular risk, but generally a task like naming cannot be done during it (▸ Fig. 8.5).

Complex Real Life Tasks

Many real life tasks, like playing instruments, working with tools, etc. can be done in the operating room. Complex multimodal tasks test numerous simultaneous systems, including motor planning, neglect, attention, and fine motor skills and can serve as the most reassuring monitoring task.

9 Going from Scan to Plan in a Glioma Surgery

9.1 Introduction

This is the most critical chapter in the book, as it serves as the bridge between the theoretical and applied parts of this book. Most unsuccessful glioma operations fail at the stage of conceptualization of where the tumor and functional systems really are, and of formulating a plan of attack for how to safely remove as much tumor as possible.

In this chapter, I will outline the framework which will serve as the organizing principle for the rest of the book when we describe how to remove gliomas from different parts of the brain. While it's impossible to create a satisfactory universal system for glioma surgery, this chapter addresses themes common to the planning of most glioma surgery so that planning these cases can proceed in a structured and organized fashion. A plan consisting of "Get in there and take it out" is seldom a recipe for technical excellence.

9.2 The 3 "Ds" of Glioma Surgery

1. Define.
2. Divide.
3. Destroy.

9.3 How Thinking in Terms of the 3 "Ds" Aids with Glioma Surgical Planning

The 3 "Ds" represent the three phases of a glioma operation, and the transition between phases brings changes in surgical technique. More importantly, a transition in phase represents a change in the philosophy of what one is trying to accomplish. For example, dissection is usually slow and cautious during the "divide" phase, and speeds up during the destroy section, when the eloquent regions and subcortical white matter tracts are separate from the planned tumor specimen.

To define our terms (▶ Fig. 9.1):

1. **Define:** This is a non-destructive phase of the operation where the principle goals are cognitive, and which begins prior to skin incision and only ends when the brain begins to be cut. The sulcal patterns are studied closely to determine exactly what anatomy is exposed and where the tumor is. Image guidance and DTI are used to tentatively plan a cut and determine the goals of the cortical mapping. Cortical mapping is then done to determine safe entry points, and to determine the cortical termini of white matter.
2. **Divide:** This phase is the most challenging, and the most critical portion of the resection. In the division phase, the brain is divided such that the bulk of the tumor specimens is separated from the eloquent brain regions which will be left in place. This is accomplished with ongoing functional mapping of the subcortical white matter and is continued until the cut extends unequivocally past the critical regions.
3. **Destroy:** Following the division phase, the remaining tumor volume is essentially a non-eloquent brain tumor and can be removed using standard anatomic techniques, such as temporal lobectomy.

The relative length, complexity, and importance of these three phases are obviously case dependent. For example, the approach to deep tumors expose and transgress a small amount of often tolerant cortex, leaving the "define" phase far shorter than that needed for a tumor of the temporoparietal junction where this phase can be long and complex given the arterial and multimodal functional anatomy. The "division" phase usually is long, but in large insular gliomas we plan for this to last hours.

9.3.1 The "Define" Phase in More Detail

Understand the Cortex

Whether you are doing your third glioma or your five hundredth, it is imperative that you consciously stop and think exactly what gyri are involved with tumor, and where functional areas, white matter tracts and major arteries lie relative to them. Having a false concept of your location is the first step in making incorrect assumptions and, in turn, bad decisions.

Gliomas come in many forms; however, a large number of them greatly expand a portion of the anatomy relative to neighboring brain, often placing the tumor in the region of something that initial raises more concern than warranted. Examples of these distortions include an enlargement of the fornix which appears to involve the thalamus, or enlargement of a parietal gyrus which displaces the motor strip making it appear at first glance that one is dealing with a motor strip glioma when in fact it is not.

Close examination of the T2 weighted images is almost always helpful for sorting these issues out. Sulcal boundaries are more obvious, and a disciplined approach will usually reveal where the tumor really is located. In a system like the one described, which is centered around the idea that anatomic resection is generally the most complete resection, sulci can serve as critical guide posts in a world with few reliable landmarks.

Executing this plan intraoperatively requires you to take an assessment of what gyri you have exposed after you open the dura. While minimalism is fully in line with my philosophy, note that the keyhole principle predicts that you will struggle if superficial targets needed for the surgery (like cortex you plan to map) are not exposed. A small bone flap extension should not be resisted, if warranted.

Also, a mapping case can be derailed quickly into the case if an en passage artery is injured on the way into the subcortex. This is especially true near the Sylvian fissure, where arteries often interdigitate with the opercular clefts on their way to their often critical targets. Even worse are arteries contained within tumor, especially high-grade gliomas, as these are at very high risk for injury by the unaware.

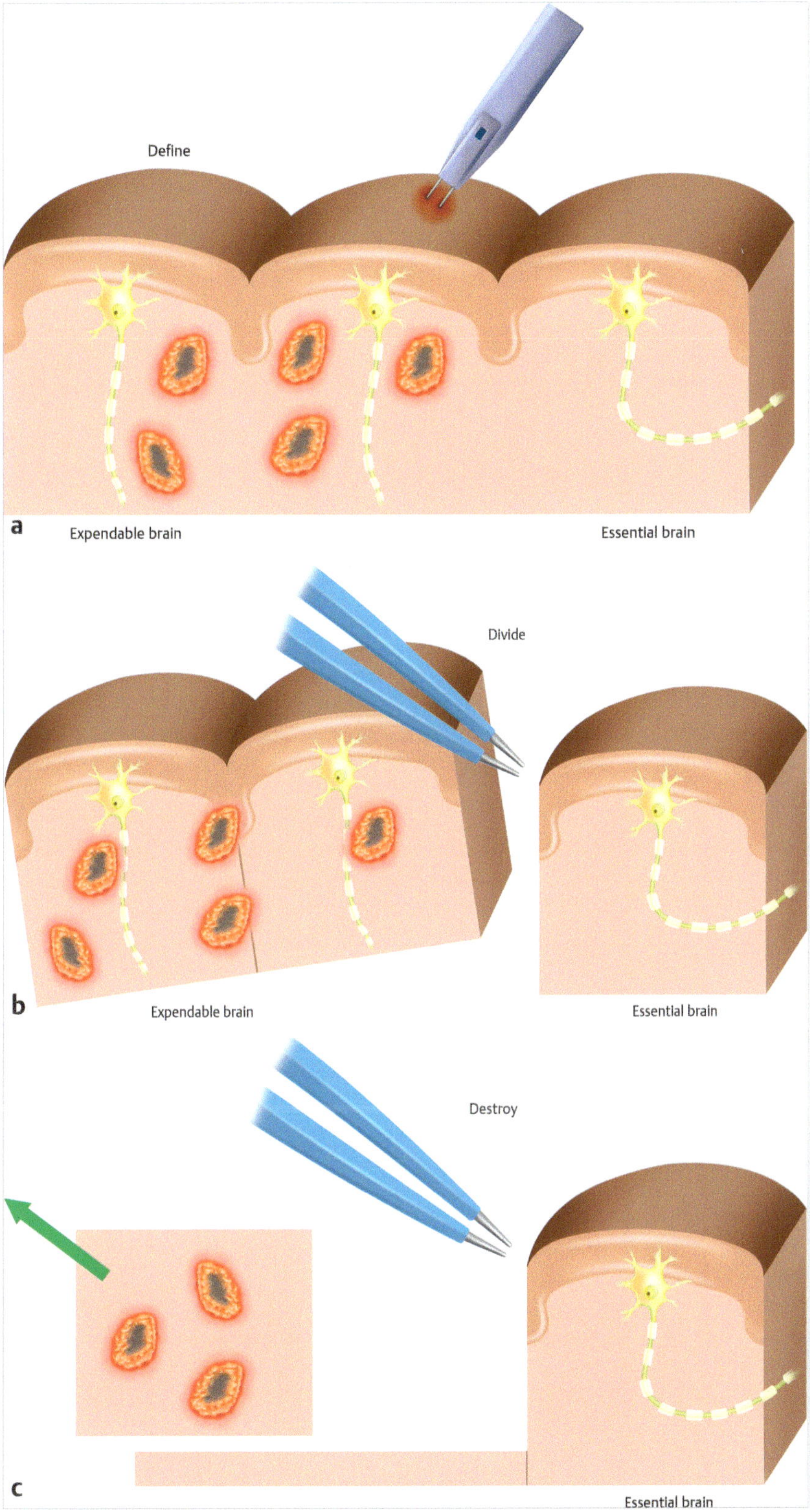

Fig. 9.1 Artistic schematic demonstrating each of the "3 Ds of glioma surgery." (**a**) In the "define" phase, we examine and map the cortex, and plan our goals, (**b**) in the "divide" phase, we perform a disconnecting cut which separates the tumor involved brain we plan to remove from the eloquent brain regions that we plan on saving, which renders the resection area essentially noneloquent, (**c**) in the "destroy" phase we perform a formulaic resection of the disconnected brain up to anatomic and/or functional boundaries.

Tumor Spread along White Matter Tracts

It is well known that glioma progression often follows white matter tracts. This is the principle reason these tumors are not surgically curable, but it also provides insight into how to best achieve anatomic resection. The very reason gliomas can be classified and described in a systematic way is that white matter spread so dominates their nature that it forces certain order and predictability on them.

By determining the pattern of spread, it is possible to make sense of the tumor anatomy and to identify a route by which an anatomic resection of these areas of higher tumor density could be removed. In other words, it is helpful to take the tumor out the way it went in, by following the involved tracts as much as possible.

Conversely, tumor spread down certain white matter tracts can often be a trap lying in wait. For example, lateral temporal tumors can often follow the SLF, which generally cannot be removed without deficit. Identifying this high risk situation is the key to avoiding it.

Mapping the Cortex

When I trained, and at many places I am aware of, "cortical mapping" and "awake brain mapping" were basically synonyms, as the patient was put back to sleep at the end of the cortical mapping in most cases. While presently my system reduces cortical mapping from its previous lofty position, it still is a critical step.

Cortical mapping obviously defines certain "no fly zones," such as speech and motor cortices. More importantly, it demonstrates the point of origin of a functional network which can then be followed inward towards the major tracts. I explain this to trainees as analogous to following a small cortical artery into the Sylvian fissure to locate the MCA trunks. The difference in this case is obviously that one cannot see these fibers, and thus function is your only true map.

As well, cortical mapping is the time to get the patient in the rhythm of doing the tests, when you are not cutting on the brain. Most patients take some time to warm up, and this is the time to get them there.

Task selection is obviously location based: we don't expect to find naming sites in the medial right frontal lobe and motor firing in the right temporal pole. With that being said; I typically test motor and speech in all cases. First, this is because even if my goal is to avoid injury to motor fibers, I would like to use speech as part of the double task to stress that system during the division phase, and cortical mapping gets the patient up to speed with the naming task.

Also, it's important to note that most higher human actions engage more than one functional system, and while the site you are operating in may not be the primary site for that function; its removal may interfere with its performance. For example, we know that semantic and lexical memory needed for naming is not primarily located in the posterior right frontal lobe; however, without motor planning ability (it might be there) it is difficult to talk. Thus, while speech mapping in the right frontal lobe is unlikely to yield a true anomia site, it helps to better elucidate the anatomy of that area in different ways. Note that higher activities of the cerebrum involve the use of multiple brain networks.

9.3.2 The "Divide" Phase in More Detail

Division is the most important part of a glioma case as this is where decisions are made regarding the boundaries of what is going to stay and what will go. Here, white matter anatomy becomes key as these tracts often define the boundaries of cuts, and conversely, provide the greatest source of risk to the patient's function.

I have found that planning the dividing cut often is what defines planning the craniotomy, planning the mapping, and ultimately planning realistic goals of the surgery. One does not need to take the craniotomy up to the temporal tip, but the cut should be front and center in your field.

Intraoperative Monitoring

We keep the patient fully awake and performing functional testing throughout the duration of the division. As described in previous chapters, the test(s) of choice are tailored to the location at risk, and the patient's functional capacity for the domain at risk. Ideally, the patient should be performing at least two simultaneous tasks using different functional systems at the same time. By splitting attention and cognitive resources between two systems, the actions are more sensitive to any interference, and thus usually providing some warning prior to performing an irreversible injury to critical portions of the white matter pathways. I think the mechanism for this involves mechanical stress on the neighboring tissue which is increasingly transmitted to the important fibers in the adjacent layer causing the test to fail prior to you actually physically coming in contact with the fibers (a diagram of how I think this happens in found in ▶ Fig. 9.2). Regardless, in my experience, performing double task type monitoring gives you the warning that we have long wished neurophysiologic monitoring like motor evoked potentials would. In other words, you get one or more warnings prior to doing something you regret.

The default task we utilize is the double task described by Hughes Duffau, which involves moving the arm and naming objects. However, we have found it necessary to tailor the task to the patient and the location at risk. For example, working near the leg motor cortex requires a double task involving leg movement and not arm. When spatiotemporal function is at risk, a neglect centered task, such as target cancelation is better, and can be combined with a different task depending on the patient. One trap I have fallen into once, has taught me to periodically alternate between arm and leg double tasks when the division takes me near the border zone between arm and leg motor cortex. It is easy to get into a sense of security when the arm is working, yet you are unknowingly drifting into leg motor fibers because you aren't actively monitoring them.

One task type which I have found is ideal for monitoring more complex cases are high level tasks such as knitting, playing an instrument, assembling a mechanical part, etc. When we first began doing it, I thought of it solely as a task of motor function, as it was unclear to me how much someone's life would really be altered by losing guitar playing abilities in the light of a glioma. However, as I began thinking about the functional anatomy of such a task, I realized that this type of task monitors a great number of functional systems simultaneously, including attention, praxis, fine motor skills, and spatial orientation, making it a superb monitoring task, whenever possible.

Making the Cut

There are many sources advocating subcortical mapping, but in my experience few sources which explain how to actually perform this and utilize this technique to improve outcomes. As a result, when I began performing this, I would typically spend far less time with this step than I do presently. To a large extent this is because a conceptual framework of what you are trying to accomplish makes it obvious how much work you really have to do to get this right, and how unclear the path really can be. I now view this as the most important step in the operation, and continue it until I have completed every conceivable millimeter of it. It is undesirable to have put the patient to sleep, only to find later in the "destroy" phase that there is still a portion of the white matter tracts still at risk.

I have found that as trainees begin to transition to my paradigm of glioma surgery (i.e., the disconnection followed by anatomic resection based paradigm), that the first disconnection performed is typically in one plane, and along too short of a front. As one gains experience with subcortical disconnection, I have found the cut becomes longer, deeper, and multiplanar, as one begins to understand how long of a segment of the critical white tracts are actually at risk in a given disconnection, and as a result how much disconnection really needs to be done.

Making the cut safely can be challenging as there are few landmarks, and few boundaries to orient the surgeon of where not to go. I compare it to trying to navigate in the center of the ocean, with the difference being that you can use functional mapping and DTI to lay ropes and buoys to guide yourself to a safe landing zone. In the same vein of this analogy is the need in the planning phase to plan for a safe landing spot, or in other words to have an idea of how you will determine that your disconnecting cut is complete (▶ Fig. 9.2). The ventricles are the most common landing spot, as it is certain that the white matter cannot run through the ventricle, and also does not run randomly to the other side of the ventricle. Thus, one can be sure that a disconnection to the ventricle has adequately separated functional tissue from the future specimen. Similarly, dividing up to non-neural anatomic landmarks, such as the temporal floor, the orbit, the falx or tentorium provides a similar assurance of completeness. Sulcal and fissural boundaries can serve as useful boundaries, as resecting opercular tumors typically involves subpially removing the opercula until you encounter the Sylvian fissure. The basal ganglia serve as the deep margins in the insula, parts of the frontal lobe and a few other cases. Finally, previous resection cavities are excellent boundaries to finish your cut in. The most challenging situation is when there are no obvious acceptable anatomic boundaries, as we often see in the motor strip when continuing the resection to the ventricle would take you across the corticospinal tract, the SLF and the thalamic peduncles. In these cases, functional feedback and DTIs are your only guide for when to stop.

Further, when landing at your boundary, it is not enough just to see the first sign that you have arrived and then stop mapping. Instead, you need to continue to utilize this safe plane until you are certain you are out of trouble and all important portions of the white matter are separated from the future specimen. For example (▶ Fig. 9.3), the disconnection of a superior medial frontal glioma from the motor and SLF systems should not stop at the first CSF flush from entering the frontal horn, but instead should continue until the L-shaped cut of this disconnection (lateral cut to separate from the SLF rami and posterior cut to separate from the motor system) extends to the ventricle along its entire length, ending at the midline and continuing anteriorly until you are well frontal to anything critical. In another example, the posterior temporal cut for an anterior temporal glioma should not just reach the temporal horn, but continue until the horn is widely opened and the cortical incision extends near the temporal floor. In both cases a complete cut ensures that the white matter tracts are separated and unquestionably out of harm's way before the patient is put to sleep and a lesionectomy is performed.

Another thing to be aware with thinking through how you are going to perform your cuts is to maintain a correct orientation of your planes (▶ Fig. 9.4). Inadequate orientation of the plane of your cut can often lead to an inadequate resection, or worse one which inadvertently transgresses a white matter tract. I often instruct my trainees to "make all circles into

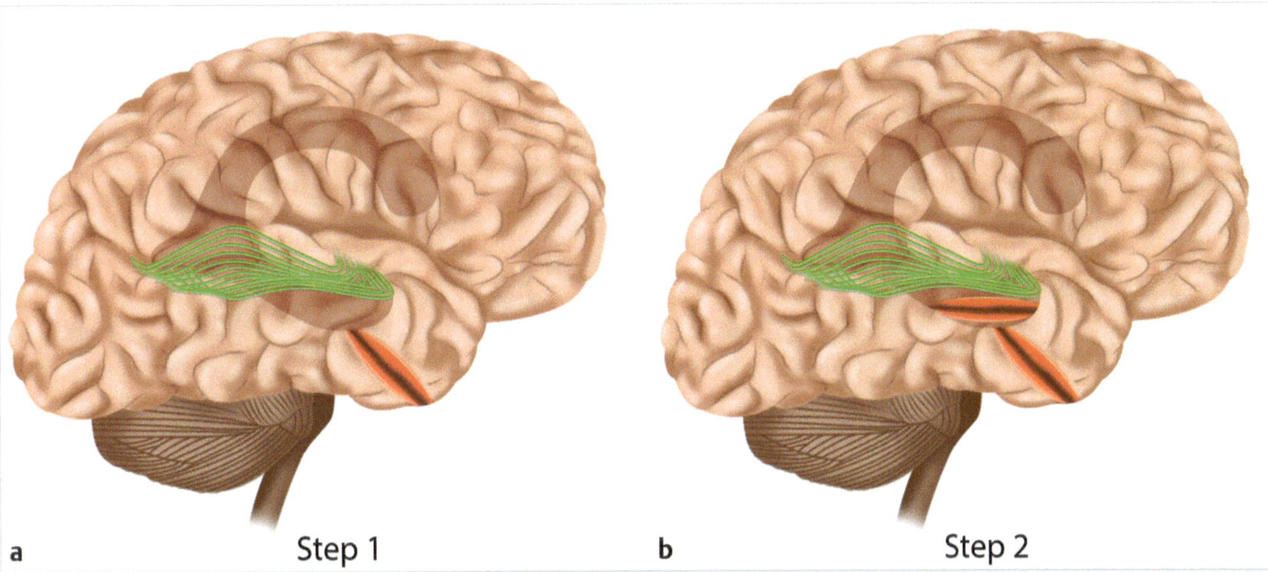

Fig. 9.2 These diagrams demonstrate the need to maximally expose your target endpoint structure (which lets you know when you are clear of the tract at risk) during a disconnecting cut. In this case, we are operating in the posterior temporal lobe and our goal is to cut anterior and near the SLF until we enter the temporal horn. Our instinct (**a**) is to breathe a sigh of relief once we see the rush of CSF as we know we are clear, and to put the patient to sleep. However, clearing the tract in one place does not mean your cut has cleared it everywhere else. The appropriate time to stop mapping (**b**) is when the cut has widely opened the ventricle until it the tract is completely free of the specimen.

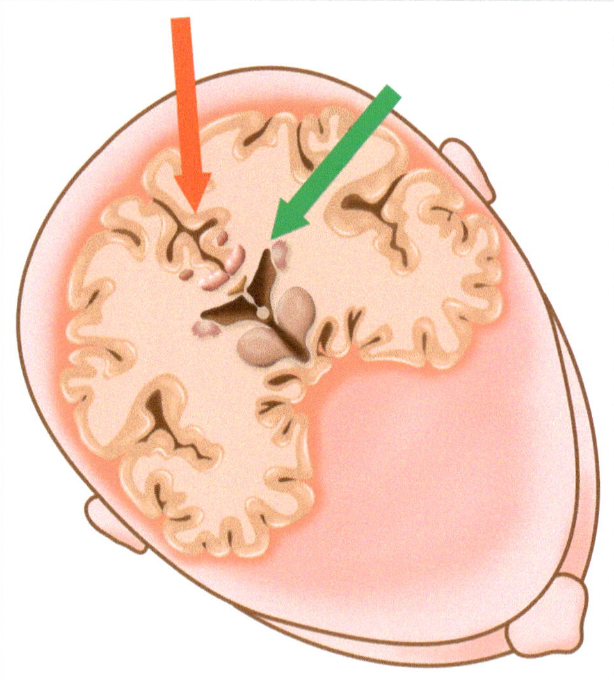

Fig. 9.3 It is critical to maintain your cuts in the proper orientation relative to the rest of the brain, so you do not veer off into critical brain structures or alternately so you do not perform an inadequately conservative cut. This is especially easy to accidentally perform in the frontal or parietal lobes for two reasons. First, they contain large amounts of white matter with few landmarks to redirect you. Second, in the lateral position, your natural angle (even with the head tipped upward) takes you downward towards the falx (*red arrow*), and not perfectly square with the true sagittal plane. I check my orientation during a cut with image guidance and using visual cues dozens of times during a disconnection to defend against this (even though often I don't need to at this point), as it usually will cause the cut to be inadequate, and thus will cause the resection to be underwhelming. The proper cut should be square with the axial, coronal, or sagittal plane as much as the functional anatomy will allow. In the frontal lobe, the proper angle for the lateral part of a medial frontal disconnection is depicted by the green arrow.

squares." By this I am pointing out that the natural tendency is to drift inward towards the middle of the cavity as we go deeper, making a resection cavity in a bowl shape. This is probably due to our discomfort as we go deeper into the brain without clear visual guidance on where we are at, the fact that a bowl shaped resection is easier, and finally the fact that minor changes in angulation at the surface lead to ever increasing misalignment of the actual plane and intended angle as you descend into the white matter. Even the most meticulous attention to head position will still lead to some minor rotation of the head position from that of the anatomic text book position our brains think in terms of. Without repeatedly checking your angles, and forcing yourself to redirect towards an ideal square plane (at least as much as the functional anatomy allows), your disconnection and ultimately your resection directed by it will fall short of the ideal.

A good plane as much as possible will try to follow the planes of the brain, and will parallel the trajectory of the sulcus into the brain. By attempting to continue the direction the sulcus would take if it continued into the brain, at minimum you are keeping the cut square and not bowl shaped. Often the first maneuver is to subpialize sulci on the margins to provide a frame of reference.

When and How to Subcortically Stimulate

This is often a confusing point for people attempting to incorporate subcortical mapping. It certainly was for me. If one subcortically stimulates every millimeter of subcortex before cutting it, there is little chance you will mistakenly come across a tract without knowing you are doing this. Like getting a daily MRI of the brain postoperatively, this is neither necessary nor practical. Remember that you will get a finite time of cooperation and quality testing out of a given patient, and you do not want to waste that time being extra-safe in low risk regions. Remember, also that maintaining a slow but steady pace using continuous double tasking or other monitoring tasks, provides you some warning that you are approaching an important

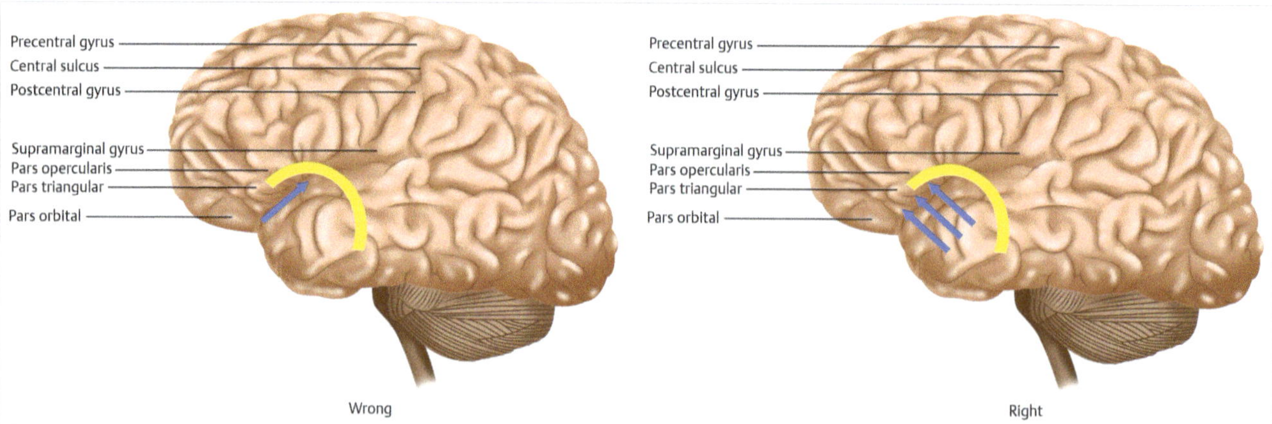

Fig. 9.4 Similar to the issue addressed in ▶ Fig. 9.2, one mistake I made when I first began mapping the subcortex was to work deeper until I found the tract, and then back off in fear. This seems like it would be a safer way to be than making a big cut and finding the tract multiple times; however, by finding a tract in a deep hole, and then trying to never come back (*left*), not only are you doing an inadequate resection, but also you can lose track of the tract and then go on to injure it somewhere else. The better way (*right*) to deal with this is to proceed along a broad front, and allow the functional feedback to guide you away from the tract along the entire three-dimensional plane.

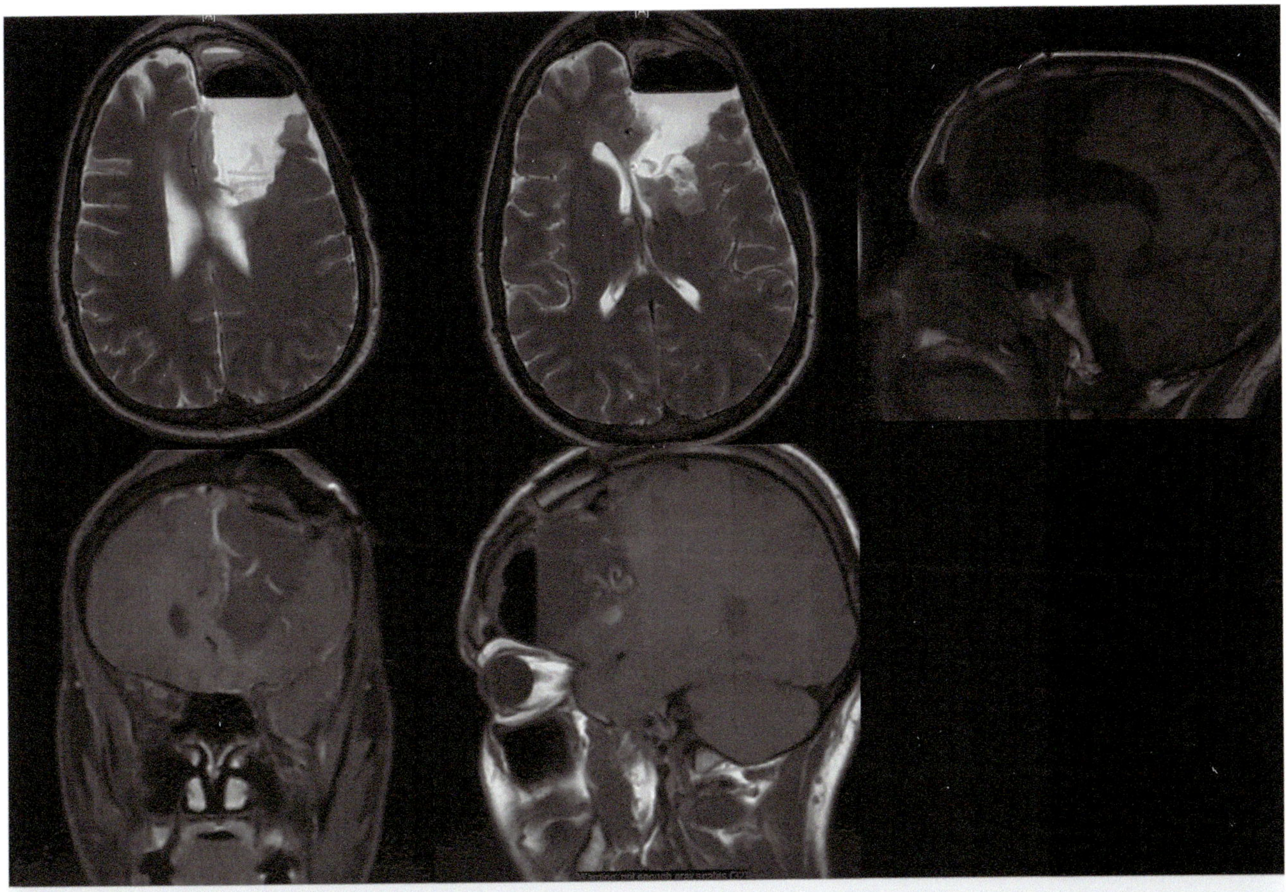

Fig. 9.5 The basic scheme of a medial frontal disconnection.

tracts. Thus, the way to stimulate is occasionally as targeted by the anatomy.

Conversely, it is unwise and inappropriate to rush up to the presumed region of the tracts, break out the stimulator a few times, find the tracts, and then move far away from them. This is paradoxically both over aggressive and under aggressive, as you would like to separate the tumor from the tracts along their entire length, not just at the bottom of hole, and dangerous, as you might hit the tract in one place, in your quest to find it somewhere else (▶ Fig. 9.5). In my experience, the biggest challenge in subcortical mapping is knowing how to interpret the results, positive or negative.

I use subcortical mapping to check the next area I am going to cut to make sure it's safe to proceed in an area where critical white matter could reasonably be. It is critical to push the probe into the brain somewhat so that the area beyond what you see is being stimulated (and thus deactivated). It is a mistake to stimulate only the white matter you see, because in essence, what you can see has already been cut. A negative test tells me I can go about as far as the probe went deep. I do not believe electrical spread is predictable in its depth, and only believe that an area has been cleared as expendable when I have stimulated it directly.

In short, I do some disconnections without very little stimulation, while others (such as the motor strip, TPO junction, and other situations of being "surrounded on all sides" by eloquence) are repeatedly stimulated.

Common Disconnections

Each chapter discusses different disconnections and their applications in more detail; however, some common ones are provided here to get you thinking about the concept.

Medial Posterior Frontal (▶ Fig. 9.6)

This is an L shaped cut which separates the specimen from the motor system posteriorly and the speech networks laterally. It needs to parallel the convexity surface as much as allowed by the subcortical functional anatomy. It is designed to land in the frontal horn with the caudate head as another important landmark. Medially, it extends to the midline and falx.

Lateral Posterior Frontal (▶ Fig. 9.7)

This is a J-shaped cut with the convex part of the J facing medially in the coronal plane. The goal is to separate the posterior margins from the speech networks posteriorly. The opercular pia and Sylvian fissure are inferior landmarks. Sometimes, the insular sulcus can orient your deep margin and occasionally the basal ganglia can as well. Often there is no deep landmark to guide you.

Posterior Temporal (▶ Fig. 9.8)

This is a workhorse disconnection which generally starts as a straight line across the lateral temporal lobe to disconnect the

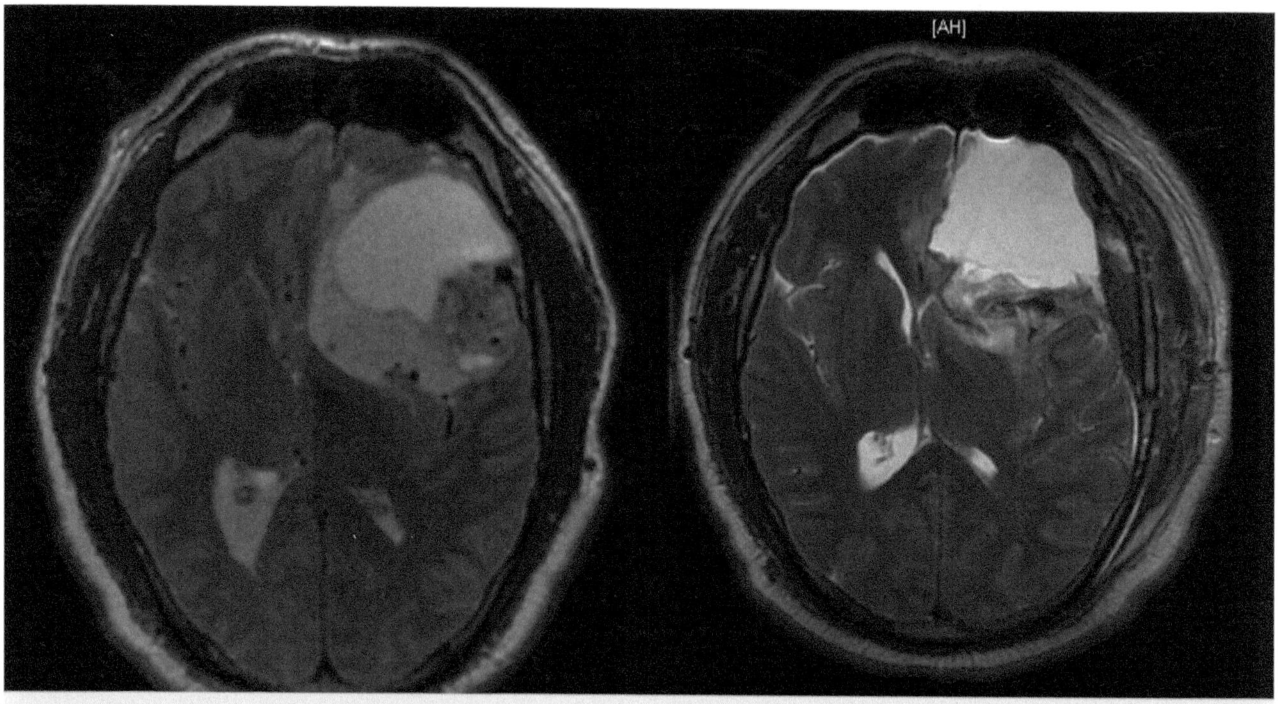

Fig. 9.6 The basic scheme of a lateral frontal disconnection.

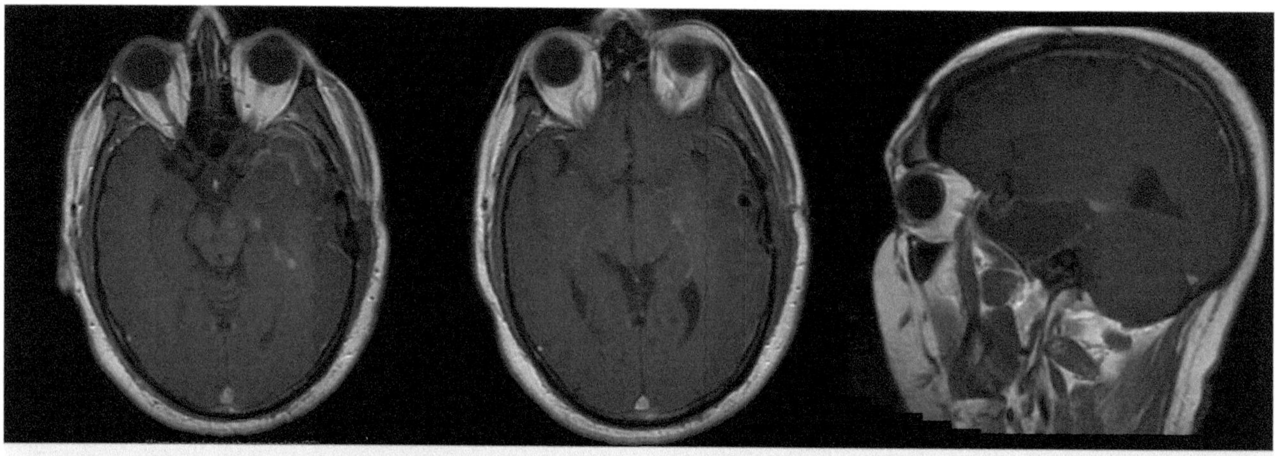

Fig. 9.7 The basic scheme of a posterior temporal disconnection.

anterior temporal lobe from the SLF posteriorly. It is taken into the temporal horn which is widely opened from anterior to posterior to separate the subinsula and IFOF from the specimen. STG removal provides access to the Sylvian fissure and insula, which with the temporal horn and medial temporal structures, provide key orienting landmarks.

Anterior Occipital (▶ Fig. 9.9)

This involves an anterior cut to separate the occipitotemporal region from the SLF anteriorly. It is usually an inverted L-shaped cut if the optic radiations are intact and can be saved. This L-cut is extended into the atrium and occipital horn. If desired, it is possible to address involvement of the medial temporal structures with this cut.

Medial Parietal (▶ Fig. 9.10)

This is a square shaped cut with the anterior cut separating the specimen from the sensorimotor region, the lateral cut paralleling the SLF the optic radiations, and sometimes portions of the IFOF (i.e., the lateral system), and the posterior cut respecting the visual system as much as is possible. All cuts connect in the atrium of the lateral ventricle, and extend medially to the falx.

Insula (▶ Fig. 9.11)

The insula is a challenging disconnection; however, this is not because the glioma involved insular cortex is critically eloquent (it's not), but rather because everything around the insula is. An insular disconnection is usually performed after a different

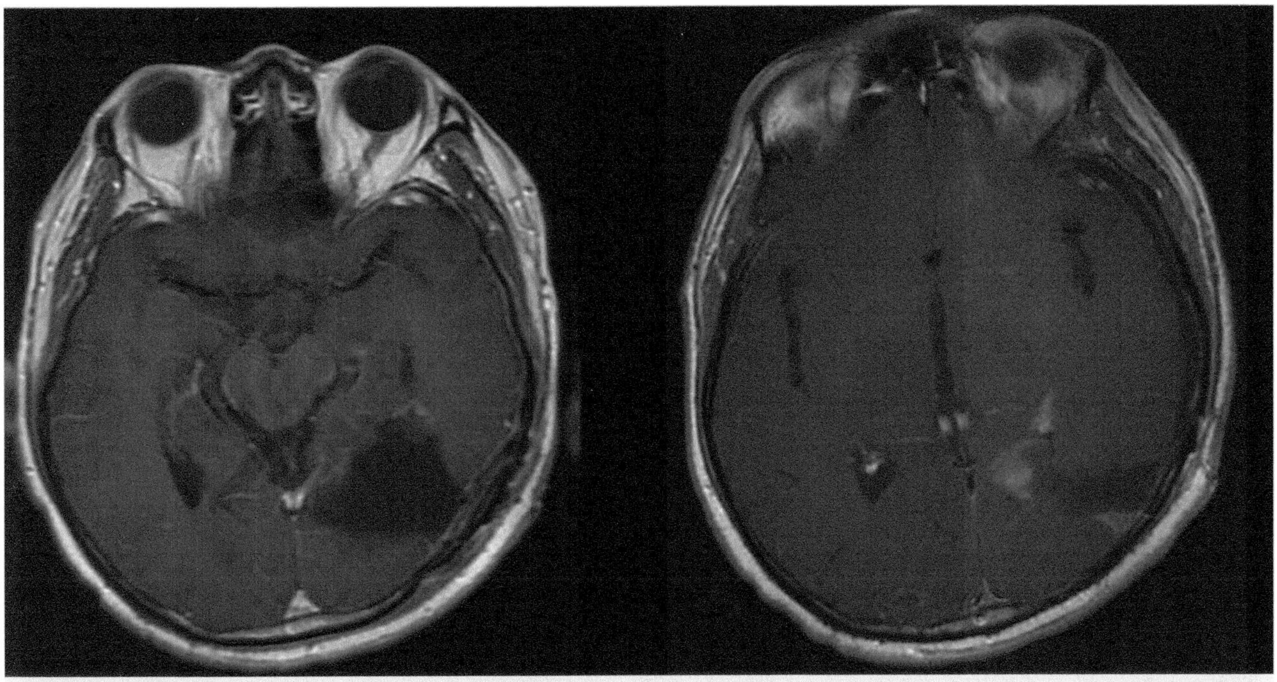

Fig. 9.8 The basic scheme of an anterior occipital disconnection.

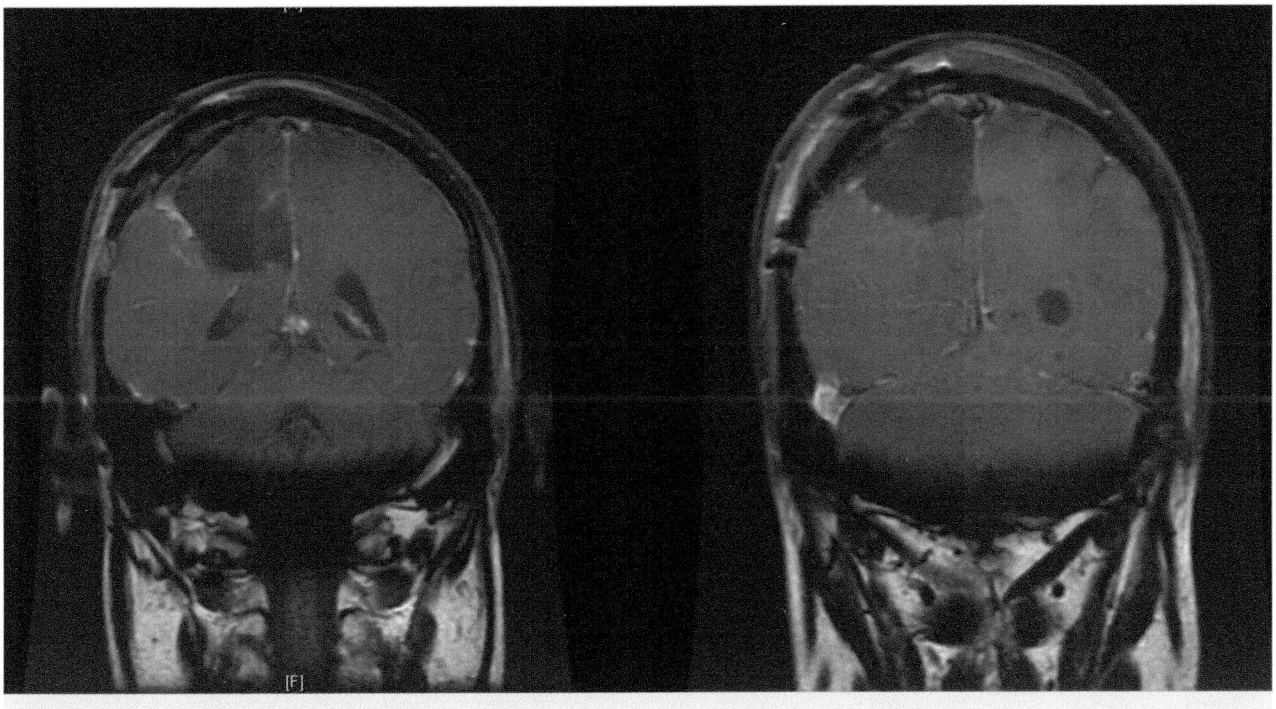

Fig. 9.9 The basic scheme of a medial parietal disconnection.

disconnection has been completed (most commonly temporal), to allow the insula and its boundaries to be properly visualized. The disconnection involves preserving the IFOF running in its inferior and anterior portion, the SLF on its superior border, and the motor fibers near the superior edge. The basal ganglia provide a deep landmark, and paralleling the hippocampus prevents you from heading too deep; however, it is important to note that the leg portion of the internal capsule often directly approach the insular cortex in its posterior aspect, and thus a deep cut on the disconnection should be mapped as well.

"Surrounded on All Sides"

This refers to a situation such as the in the temporoparietal junction, the motor region, or tumors deeply involving the speech areas. Often, these tumors are resected with all sides,

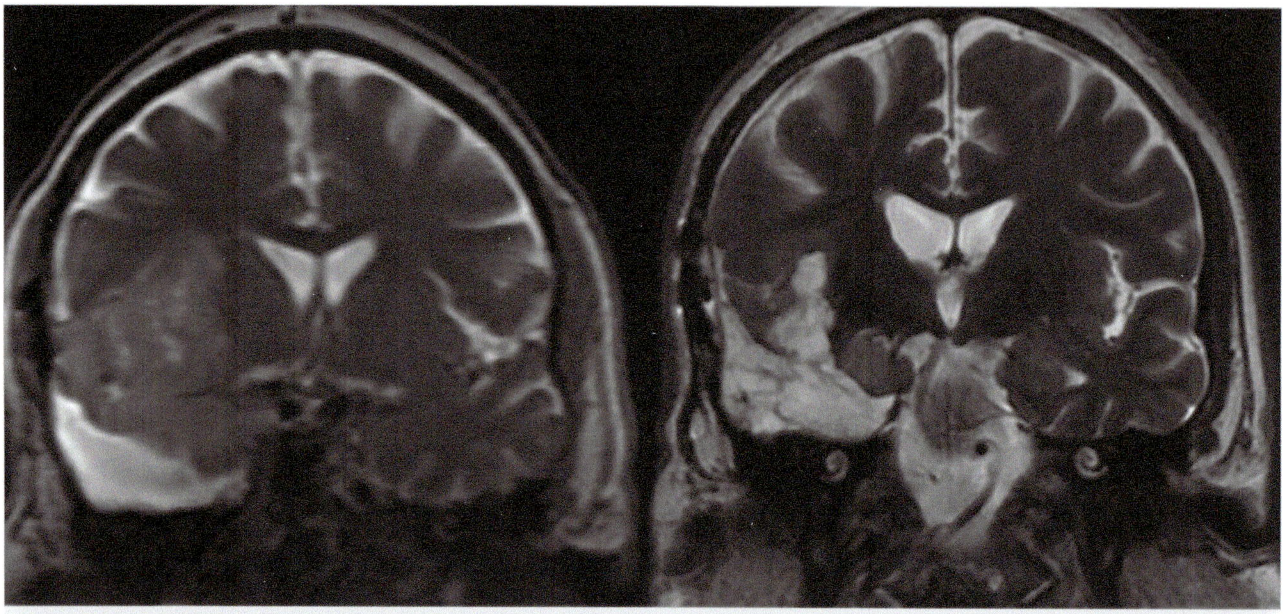

Fig. 9.10 The basic scheme of an insular disconnection.

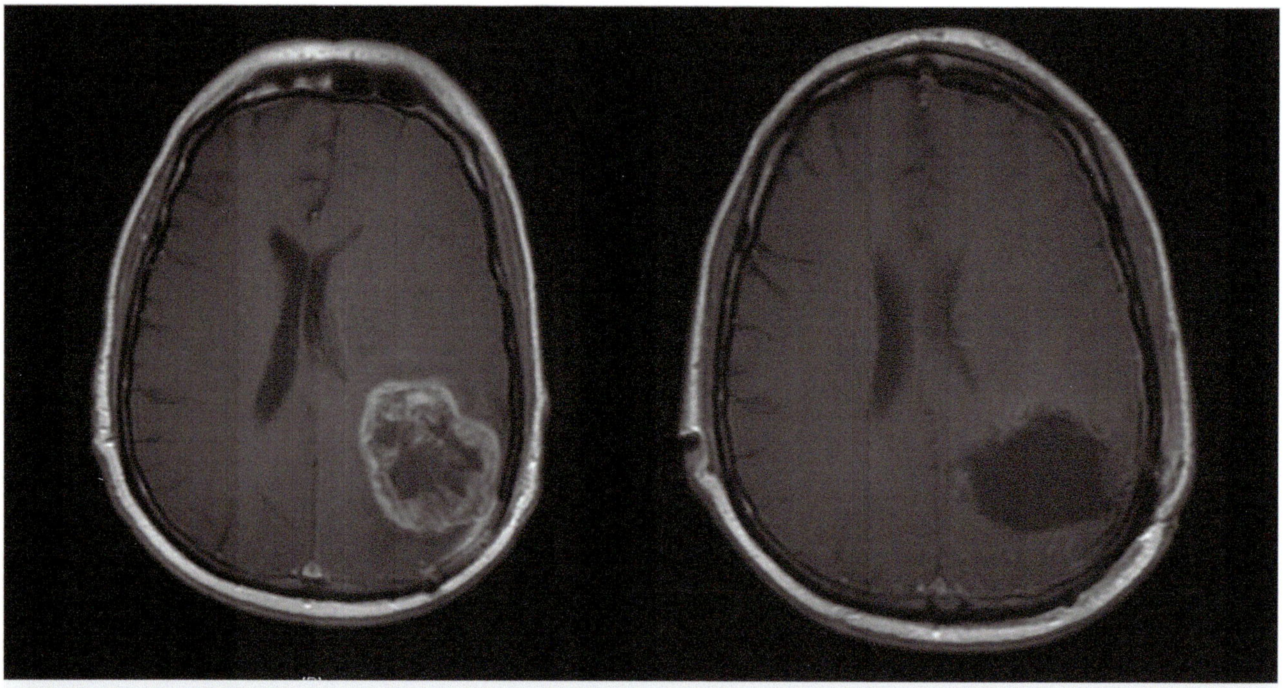

Fig. 9.11 The basic scheme of a surrounded on all sides disconnection.

including the deep side. Being viewed as an eloquent cut. Often an operculum or sulcus is the only anatomic landmark. Usually, when the "division" phase is done, the case is also done as there are no low risk parts of the case.

9.3.3 The "Destroy" Phase in More Detail

The "destroy" phase is an anatomic based resection of a newly non-eloquent brain region done with the patient asleep. Done correctly, the disconnection should remove eloquence issues from the operation, and this phase often involves workhorse maneuvers such as anterior temporal lobectomy, occipital or frontal lobectomy, subpial resection along sulcal boundaries amygdalohippocampectomy, and working within visible tumor boundaries.

In general, we have not found it necessary to extend our exposure to expose the entirety of tips of lobes, as non-eloquent brain does not require delicate microsurgery if the plan is to remove it. We generally focus our approach over our planned cut, leaving some space to maneuver if needed. However, if a lobectomy is performed, we make sure we can reach it under the bone flap. Thus, while you don't need to expose every millimeter, you have to be able to reach it.

Most other structures of interest are deep and thus are easy to reach without a big opening. The only additional thing we consider are key arteries which feed brain which is not in the specimen. For example, we do not advise a midline bone flap far from the sagittal sinus with a plan on pulling the medial frontal gyri inward to resect them after the disconnection, as this risks an injury to en passage ACA branches. We do not, however, take our bone flap across the sinus either. We just make sure we are close enough. There are numerous examples in the chapter on frontal lobe tumors.

9.4 Other Issues to Consider

Once we have an idea of the issues we will face taking this out, we begin to temper these thoughts with some key realities.

9.4.1 Preoperative Function

Patients with low grade tumors usually are neurologically normal or close to normal; however, this is not always the case with high grade patients. A patient with preoperative deficits may or may not recover with surgical resection, depending if the deficit is from invasion of the fibers or mass effect/edema. Either way they may be impossible to map, or at least less capable of doing it at a high level. While it is always best to save the function, I feel that the only thing worse than hemiplegia from a glioma is hemiplegia with the glioma still there. Sometimes we make the decision that a function is not recoverable based on the DTI anatomy, preoperative function, and duration of deficit, and in these cases, at least the patient have the tumor out, if the function cannot be saved.

9.4.2 Known or Expected Grade

High grade tumors are usually harder than low grades. They are bloodier, the patients are lower functioning, and they usually are a lot bigger. They also can densely encase arteries and invade their adventitia making their complete removal impossible or at least very dangerous. They also can grow through dural openings, like the tentorium and falx, and distort the anatomy.

When approaching a high grade, especially one encasing arteries, you need to have awareness of these issues and a plan for addressing them. Nothing complicates an insular disconnection more than bleeding from the MCA deep in a fibrous tumor portion.

9.5 Goals of Surgery

While a beautiful anatomic resection is the Platonic ideal of all glioma surgery, this is not always the right idea, or even possible. Sometimes the goal of a surgery is to trim a small enhancing area which is near a previously mapped eloquent area. Other times it is to get a massive tumor to a manageable size in the hope chemoradiation will have a prayer to work.

9.6 Conclusion

I plan every surgery in terms of the cut I think I can perform, what brain structures that cut will allow me to remove anatomically when it's completed, and temper this with how that makes sense in terms of the patient. The craniotomy is tailed to expose this cut, and to access the areas we plan on taking out as safely as possible.

10 Frontal Lobe Gliomas

10.1 Introduction

The frontal lobe (defined for this chapter as the parts of the frontal lobes not part of the motor or premotor cortices or their immediate white matter connections), has long been viewed by neurosurgeons as a "safe" place to operate. It is simple to explain why: this part of the brain has a great deal of parallel processing and redundancy, making minor transgressions into this lobe for tumors like brain mets and meningiomas forgiven, meaning that the patient lacks an obvious problem. It is unquestionable that minor incursions into the anterior frontal lobe to remove a non-infiltrating brain tumor are well tolerated.

Gliomas pose a different dilemma for the frontal lobe. They cover a larger area of the frontal lobe, especially if you consider the infiltration of tumor cells into the peripheral brain, and due to their nature, often mandate removal of a large part of frontal lobe. This brings frontal lobe functional concerns front and center, and this can often vividly teach you what the frontal lobe does, especially if you talk to patients and their care givers.

Having done numerous aggressive frontal lobe glioma resections, I have begun to respect the frontal lobe in a way I never anticipated. A hemiparesis is not good, but it does not change who you are as a person, leave you intolerable to friends or family, or make you unable to meaningfully interact with others: frontal lobe injury can do all of these. Ignore the frontal lobe and its anatomy at your own peril.

We do not entirely understand how the frontal lobe is wired up and how it works. Also in many patients, frontal lobe function is extremely redundant, and can tolerate a lot of alteration before problems arise, while others less so, and we do not know how to predict this or prevent problems. This is not to say that we can avoid all frontal lobe problems and still take out the tumor to a satisfactory degree: many of these tumors are massive, and as I have stressed repeatedly, leaving a bunch of glioma growing in the brain to save this function is unlikely to achieve this goal in the long term. Those who are willing to sacrifice tumor control for function often end up with neither in the long term.

This chapter is not going to solve these mysteries in 5 pages, but it provides a framework for more thoughtful planning of frontal lobe tumors, with the goal, as always, of balancing tumor resection with functional preservation. We cannot always prevent frontal lobe dysfunction, but we should base our trade-offs on rational decisions, instead of viewing the frontal lobe as the wild west where you can do anything you want with minimal consequences.

10.2 What Does the Frontal Lobe Actually Do?

The global functions of the frontal lobe are familiar to most physicians: judgment, attention, concentration, behavioral control, inhibition, higher executive control. Frontal lobe syndromes are also known: being "frontal" is used by many as a synonym for either being abulic, or being disinhibited, careless, rude, or unable to focus. But the functional anatomy and organization of the frontal lobe is less standard in neurosurgical curricula: partly because it is not well understood, and partly because the frontal lobe is relatively forgiving, so neurosurgeons have not spent the time passionately trying to find an answer to these mysteries.

The best neuropsychological and functional imaging data suggest the following classification of frontal lobe functions:

Medial frontal lobe: Motivation and attention.

Dorsolateral prefrontal cortex: Working memory and executive function.

Orbitofrontal cortex: Emotional regulation and judgment.

It should go without saying that these functions do not easily lend themselves to simple tests in the operating room, though we are actively evaluating adaptations of some more complex tasks to make this more easily testable.

A different view of the prefrontal lobe is as an organ of control or other brain regions. For example, the orbitofrontal cortex is involved in regulating emotional centers of the basal ganglia and other structures, but may not be a principle emotional driver itself. The medial frontal cortices are not motor areas, but are critical for controlling parts of the brain that are, i.e., turning them on. The dorsolateral cortices are not essential for memory formation, but help regulate areas that are.

10.3 Global Anatomy of the Frontal Lobe

Chapters 3, 5, and 6 spend a great deal of time on various aspects of frontal lobe anatomy and this section will merely summarize the key points to tie them together.

The white matter connections leaving the prefrontal gyri generally run roughly anterior-posteriorly to some degree, especially at the frontal pole. The more superior connections have a rostro-caudal component to their general anterior-posterior direction, and the lateral connections have some medial-lateral component in addition to their general anterior-posterior angle. A simpler way to view these connections is as somewhat pyramidal with the apex pointed at the key behavioral effectors of the central core, the basal ganglia and thalamus. Of course, not all tracts neatly fit this model, but many do.

The implications of these observations for rational frontal lobe surgery are significant. It is safe to say that most of prefrontal cortex function requires some anterior-posterior type connection with a distant effector structure (be it basal ganglia, thalamic, or other cortices), in order to manifest its activity in the form of an observable change in brain behavior. For example, it seems to me quite unlikely that the anterior superior frontal gyus can meaningfully change the function of other brain regions though a series of u-fibers to the MFG, then the IFG etc, after its principle apical outflow pathway has been cut (▶ Fig. 10.1). Thus, it is possible to disconnect and inactivate a great deal of the prefrontal cortices with a simple cut in the coronal plane (▶ Fig. 10.1). This is not to suggest that we avoid

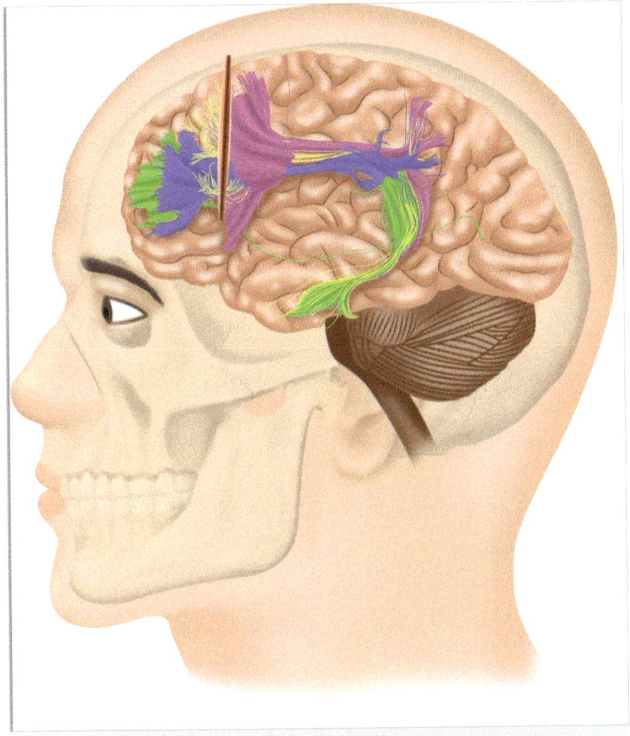

Fig. 10.1 This schematic demonstrates the effect of a deep cut across the back of the middle frontal gyrus on the connecting fibers leaving/entering this gyrus. Note that most of these connections run anterior to posterior, and that they would be disrupted by a cut in the coronal plane. A particularly large coronal cut would have the additional effect of disconnecting the neighboring gyri as well, further reducing the utility of the gyrus anterior to this cut.

this cut, because often it is the correct cut, but rather that if you have cut across the posterior part of a prefrontal brain region, that you have usually disconnected it from the rest of the brain, and it is basically non-functional. In glioma surgery, it does not make sense to leave non-functioning tumor involved brain in the head. If it is not meaningfully connected to the rest of the brain, it basically is like a meningioma or a met.

10.3.1 The "Back Wall" of the Frontal Lobe

Many of the key large pathways at the back of the frontal lobe and other key structures such as the basal ganglia, cumulatively form a conceptual boundary in the posterior aspect of the frontal lobe, which can be thought of as the "back wall" of the frontal lobe. This is roughly a coronal plane through the frontal lobe just anterior to the head of the caudate nucleus (▶ Fig. 10.2), but it is not perfectly planar and is warped somewhat near the frontal rami of the SLF, and near the premotor areas.

The structures of this posterior wall include the following (roughly from lateral to medial and superior to inferior):

1. Frontal rami of the SLF
2. Sylvian fissure
3. Frontal bend of IFOF
4. FAT
5. Anterior putamen

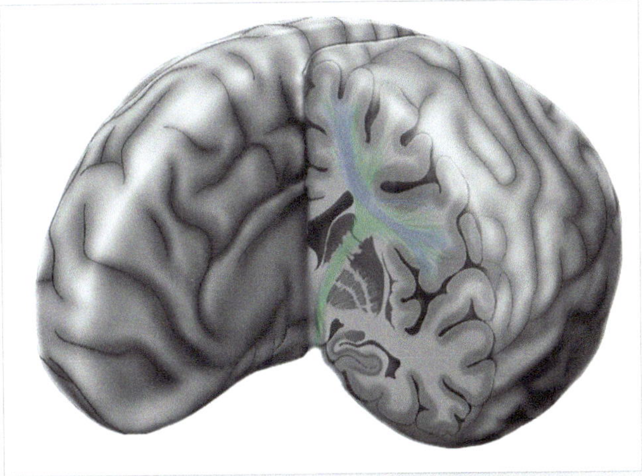

Fig. 10.2 This diagram demonstrates the "back wall" concept of frontal lobe disconnections. This wall is made up of the desending motor network, the basal ganglia, the FAT, the frontal ramus of the SLF, and the frontal connections of IFOF. The coronal cut of a frontal disconnection (medial or lateral) is usually limited and pushed anteriorly by this wall, and while all disconnections do not need to be made so far posteriorly, this is usually where the disconnection becomes difficult if this is necessary.

6. Descending fibers from motor and premotor areas
7. Head of caudate nucleus
8. Supplementary motor areas
9. Cingulum/default mode network

It is not an accident that the posterior frontal cut aims to navigate in front of these structures.

10.4 The Three "Ds" Applied to Frontal Glioma Surgery

10.4.1 Define

Preoperative Planning

It is well appreciated that the difficulty and risk of frontal lobe surgery increases as the work moves posteriorly. This is because posterior travel in the frontal lobe brings us in contact with structures such as the SLF, the FAT, the IFOF, the basal ganglia, and the motor and attention networks, which can have a major impact on circuits such as motor or language which are essential for the meaningful function of multiple other networks.

The principle question to ask when planning these cases is which systems and tracts are in the closest proximity with the desired cortical and subcortical cuts. The goal of brain mapping is to place a cut such that the networks that we wish to save are not in the specimen, and thus leaving an essentially non-eloquent brain tumor to be removed. The answer to this question not only involves the tumor's anatomy, but also the patient's preoperative function (there is no reason to try to save a damaged or unsalvageable system), the presumed tumor grade, and the goals of surgery (for example some cases have supramaximal resections as an option, while many don't).

By defining our goals, we can determine whether we need to focus our efforts on medial frontal disconnection or a lateral frontal disconnection, which in turn makes the sequence of mapping tasks, the location of the craniotomy, and the overall working angle more obvious.

Exposure and Cortical Mapping

Medial Frontal Disconnections

This is the more common disconnection in the frontal lobe and is useful for gliomas which are principally centered in the superior or middle frontal gyri. I personally prefer this angle of attack because it is less disorienting to me than the lateral disconnection, and this approach can be used to deal with most of the frontal lobe tracts.

Because the angle of attack is relatively superior to inferior, it is essential to try to get the apex of the head as high as possible in the operative field so that the remaining brain does not fall across your line of sight during the disconnection. In a sleeping patient, this is easily achieved by operating in the supine position. However, an awake patient should be on their side so they can see and interact with the examiner, so the position is a compromise achieved by tipping the apex of the head upward, and combining this with reverse Trendelenburg positioning of the bed (▶ Fig. 10.3).

Cortical mapping of the medial frontal lobe is often negative mapping, in part because many frontal lobe intraoperative tasks are still poorly localizable, and as we know, most of the center pieces of human brain functional networks (i.e., primary motor, speech etc.) are relatively posterior in the frontal lobe. The craniotomy (▶ Fig. 10.4) should be centered on the posterior most aspect of the planned resection as this is both the cut you are planning, and the area most likely to yield cortical findings (note that the keyhole principle predicts that the surface is the only area which cannot be easily reached by redirecting the microscope as needed, and thus, cortical surfaces which need to be mapped must be exposed). It should be planned so that you can reach the anterior pole, the midline, and the lateral extent of your cut, but these areas can be cheated and removed under the skull (▶ Fig. 10.5).

Medial frontal disconnections usually involve disconnection from more than one tract, and thus it is important to map motor and motor planning (which is posterior), but also speech, spatiotemporal function, and other tasks. For example, primary language planning areas are unlikely to reside in the medial frontal lobe, but speech arrest can be useful for finding motor planning areas like the SMA.

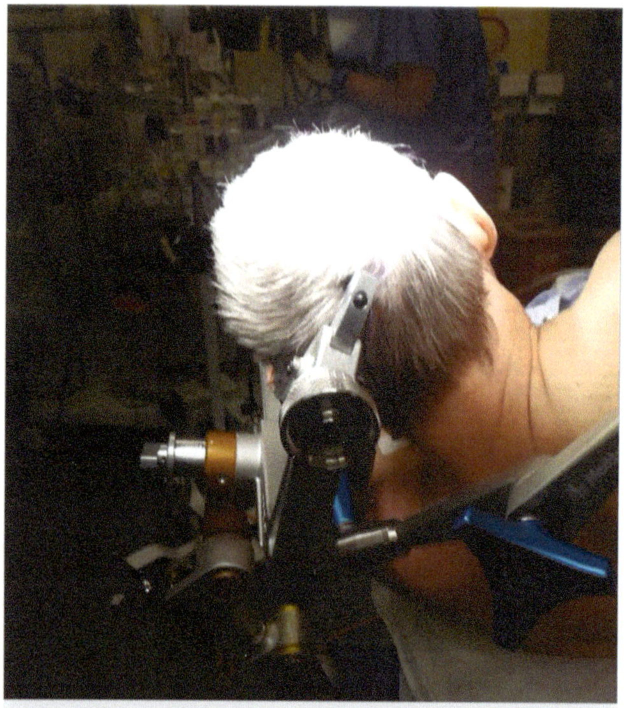

Fig. 10.3 Photos demonstrating patient positioning for frontal disconnections.

Lateral Frontal Disconnections

This disconnection is used when the principle goal is to separate the tumor from the frontal rami of the SLF, and when the medial frontal involvement is of lesser concern. In these cases, the head is not laterally flexed as in the medial frontal disconnection (▶ Fig. 10.6), and the craniotomy is centered over the surface involvement of the tumor. The DTIs are quite useful at predicting where the speech network is going, and planning the craniotomy accordingly.

There are two options that make sense to me: expected positive sites are either definitely in the field or definitely out of it (▶ Fig. 10.7). By this I mean, that if after looking at the tractography, I expect speech tracts to be densely involved, I want to be certain I know where they are, and this means extending the craniotomy to make sure I get a positive map. On the other hand, if they are not involved, I would prefer not to put them at risk by exposing them, and try to plan the craniotomy so they are not in the field.

I start by mapping the motor strip first, as it is the easiest to find and it helps to rapidly define the rest of the cortical map. Speech arrest is typically found just anterior to the face/tongue motor cortex (it is the motor planning area for speech). I also check naming here to make sure I know the network, and also

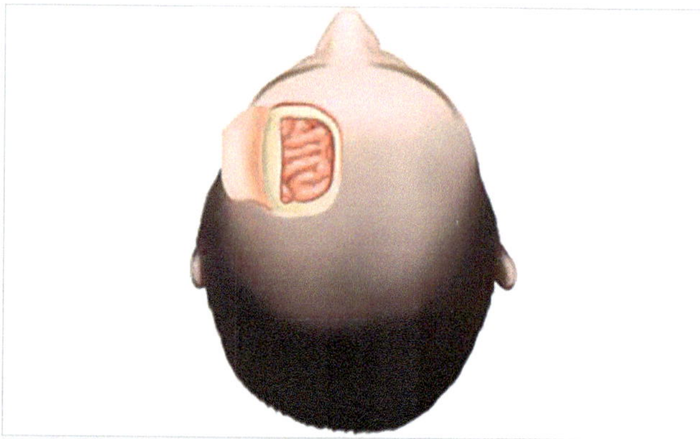

Fig. 10.4 A schematic demonstrating how to plan the craniotomy for a medial frontal disconnection type surgery. Note the following: First, the craniotomy is centered over the cuts. Second, it does not approach the midline sagittal sinus, but its medial edge is close enough to reach the midline comfortably. Finally, its anterior and lateral edges are far enough forward that the frontal pole and lateral opercula can be reached depending on the needs of the case. The craniotomy does not extend onto the forehead, as it is planned to be able to "cheat."

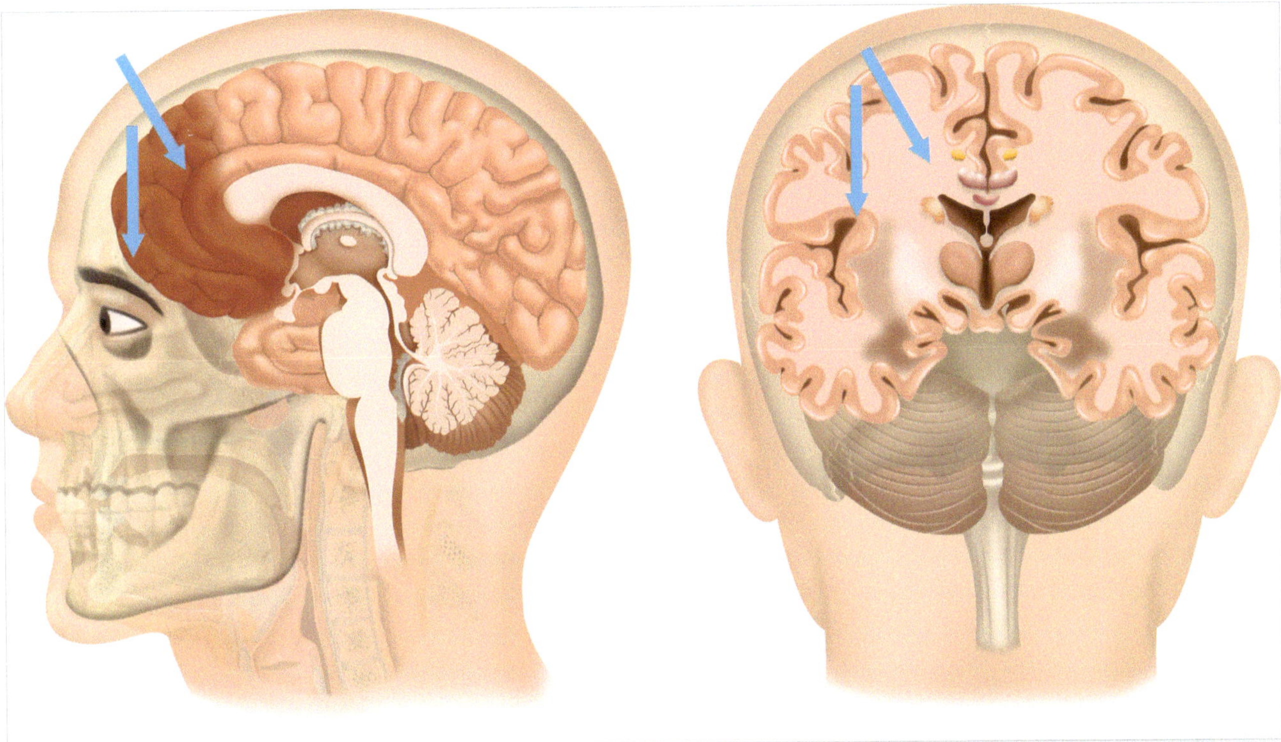

Fig. 10.5 The "downhill" principle of cheating in frontal lobe surgery. Cheating refers to the idea that we do not need to see the entire surface of a disconnected piece of the brain which is going to be removed anyway, as there is nothing that will be changed if it gets beat up by being pulled into the field. Thus, a cheated craniotomy is made so that we can reach the tip, but does not extend over its entire surface as this is unnecessary. In the frontal lobe, the frontal pole can easily be reached under the bone flap during the "destroy" phase, if the craniotomy is planned to use the downhill principle. In the sagittal plane (left), this means that we plan the anterior edge of the craniotomy so that it reaches the point at which the frontal bone angles superior-inferior (as opposed to anterior-posterior). When we do this, we can work superior to inferior down the long axis of our working angle ("downhill" so to speak) without too much trouble. In the coronal plane (right), we can use a similar principle to work superior to inferior and remove the frontal opercula, provided that in cases when we need to do this, that we extend the craniotomy lateral enough to access this bend in the skull.

to get the patient ready to double task. I then look for motor arrest to ensure I know where motor planning areas are. Finally, we have found neglect centers in this area, especially on the right (this is probably being an SLF mediated task), so I look for this as well

10.4.2 "Divide" Phase

Medial Frontal Disconnection (▶ Fig. 10.8)

This is an "L" shaped cut that separates the tumor from the motor system and SMA/FAT network posteriorly, the SLF and parts of IFOF laterally, eventually ending in the frontal horn of the lateral ventricle.

The lateral limb of this cut is always done first, typically with an arm/naming double task. This is because the posterior cut can lead to abulia or mutism, which can recover but will prevent you from meaningfully mapping speech functions to protect the SLF and IFOF. It is critical to get the angle correct, or you will greatly short change your resection in the depth. It is important to note that your natural angle of attack with the patient in the lateral position for brain mapping is angled medially towards the falx, and not on the superior to inferior as your brain generally thinks of it. Therefore, I start by subpially exposing the lateral sulcus of the most lateral gyrus I plan to resect (SFG or MFG), and keep this pia as a guide to the correct angle, which typically parallels the floor. I use a combination of the DTI and feedback from mapping to define my lateral borders. Initially, the goal is to separate the tumor from SLF, but inferiorly you can encounter IFOF, and realization of this caused me to begin to keep the patient awake until the lateral cut is down to the ventricle or orbital roof. Before switching to the posterior cut, I make sure I have an idea where the caudate head is, and that the anterior to posterior length of the frontal horn has been opened.

The posterior cut often involves a switch to motor based tasks, especially ones which require concentration as these can be used to protect the SMA/FAT and the medial networks such as the DMN. If not possible the double task is perfectly acceptable. The goal of this cut is to widely open the width of the posterior frontal lobe from the surface down to the medial-lateral aspect of the frontal horn from the midline until it joins the lateral cut. After subpializing the gyri on the surface, down to the bottom of the sulci, I start by finding the midline and continue the cut down to the falx. This allows me to find the cingulate sulcus, which is where I expect to find the attention networks. Depending on the surgical goals, I either remain lateral to the sulcus depths to stay out of the networks, or attempt to resect the cingulate cortices using repeated stimulations. Either way I try to find this early, so I am not encountering it in an

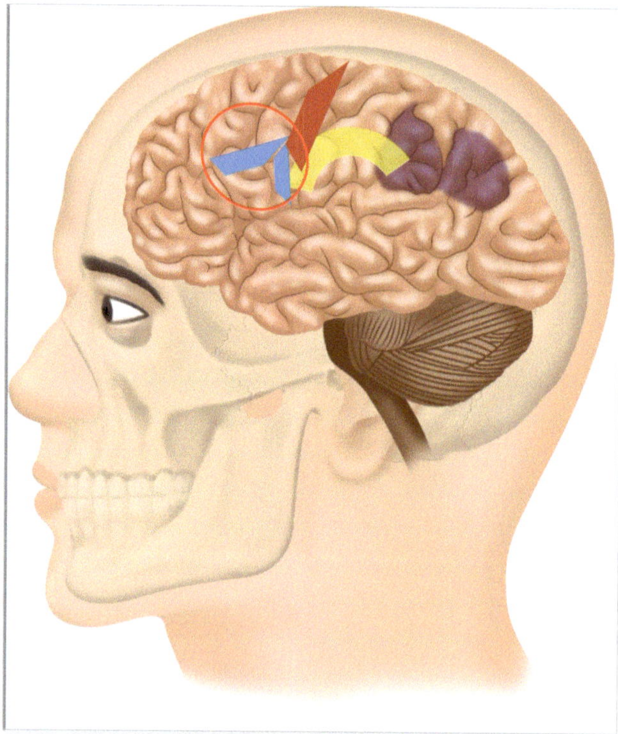

Fig. 10.6 This schematic demonstrates the craniotomy for a lateral frontal disconnection. The cuts are generally made with the SLF and IFOF posteriorly and the craniotomy is centered over these cuts and made superiorly enough to accommodate the needs of the case.

uncontrolled fashion in a deep hole. The rest of the cut follows the direction of the sulci as superior to inferior as possible, the goal being not to drift into the FAT or the descending communications with the basal ganglia/thalamus in the sub cortex. Once the L-shaped cut is down to the ventricle on all sides, the cut is complete.

Lateral Frontal Disconnection (▶ Fig. 10.9)

This is a J shaped cut that aims to parallel the ramus of the SLF and if needed, to remain in front of the caudate head. The IFOF is also at risk with this disconnection and should be considered in this approach.

I begin by subpially skeletonizing the relevant opercular cortices down to the pial bank of the Sylvian fissure. In a common theme for opercular tumors, I always want to know where the arteries and insula are as soon as possible. Sometimes, it is impossible or unwise to finish this step first when tumors are densely encasing the MCA vessels, so when I see this situation, I proceed to complete the cut to isolate the artery encasement, at which point the case becomes a meningioma type case with the anatomy made visible by the disconnection.

The plane of the cut is determined by the results of the mapping and navigating this path involves pushing your plane posteriorly, and being pushed back when your encounter function. Not all cuts need to be taken to the ventricle, this obviously depends on the tumor and your goals. After developing the plane along the "back wall," I convert this cut to a J by developing the superior plane before putting the patient to sleep.

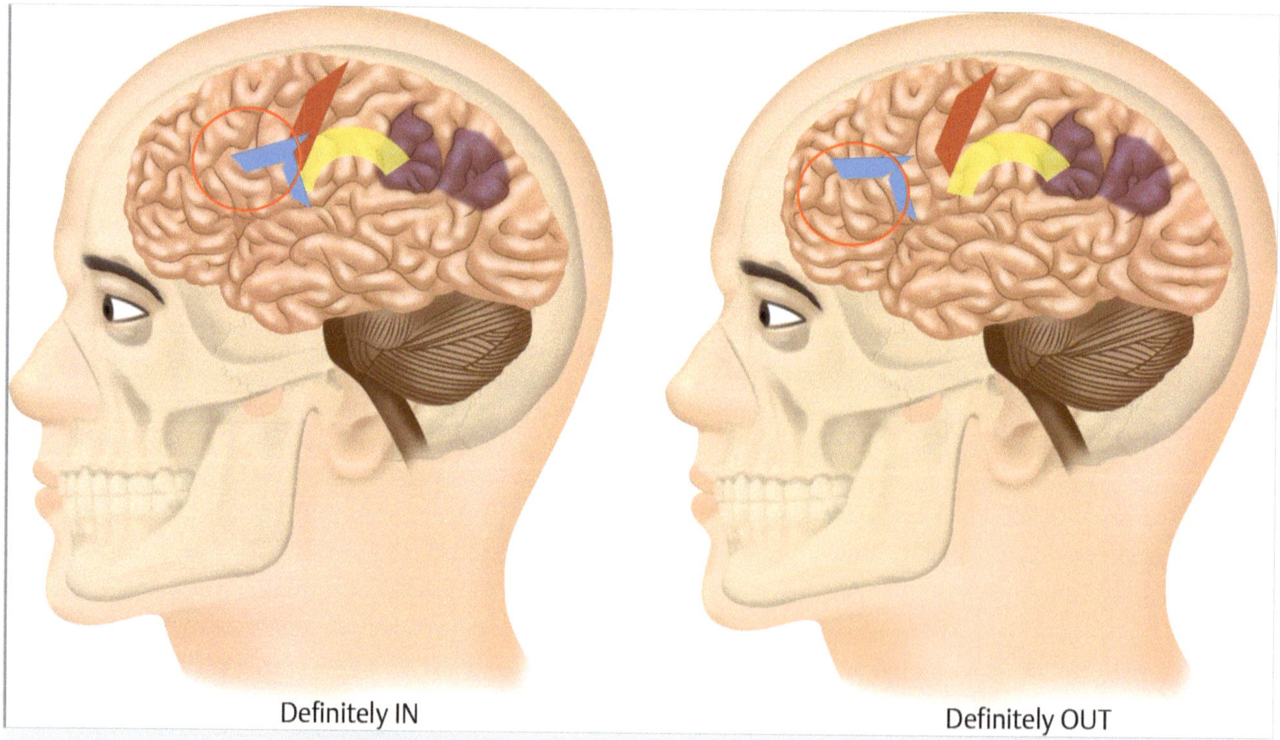

Fig. 10.7 A mapping craniotomy should have planned so that functional brain areas are either "definitely in" or "definitely out" of the field. If the tractography suggests that the tumor (left) is very close to tracts or functional areas, and you will need to spend time to separate them, then it is best to add a few mms of space toward these areas to ensure you get the best mapping possible. Alternately, my feeling is that if I don't need to be very close to the functional areas, I would rather not expose them and put them at risk. In this case (right), I want them "definitely out" of the field.

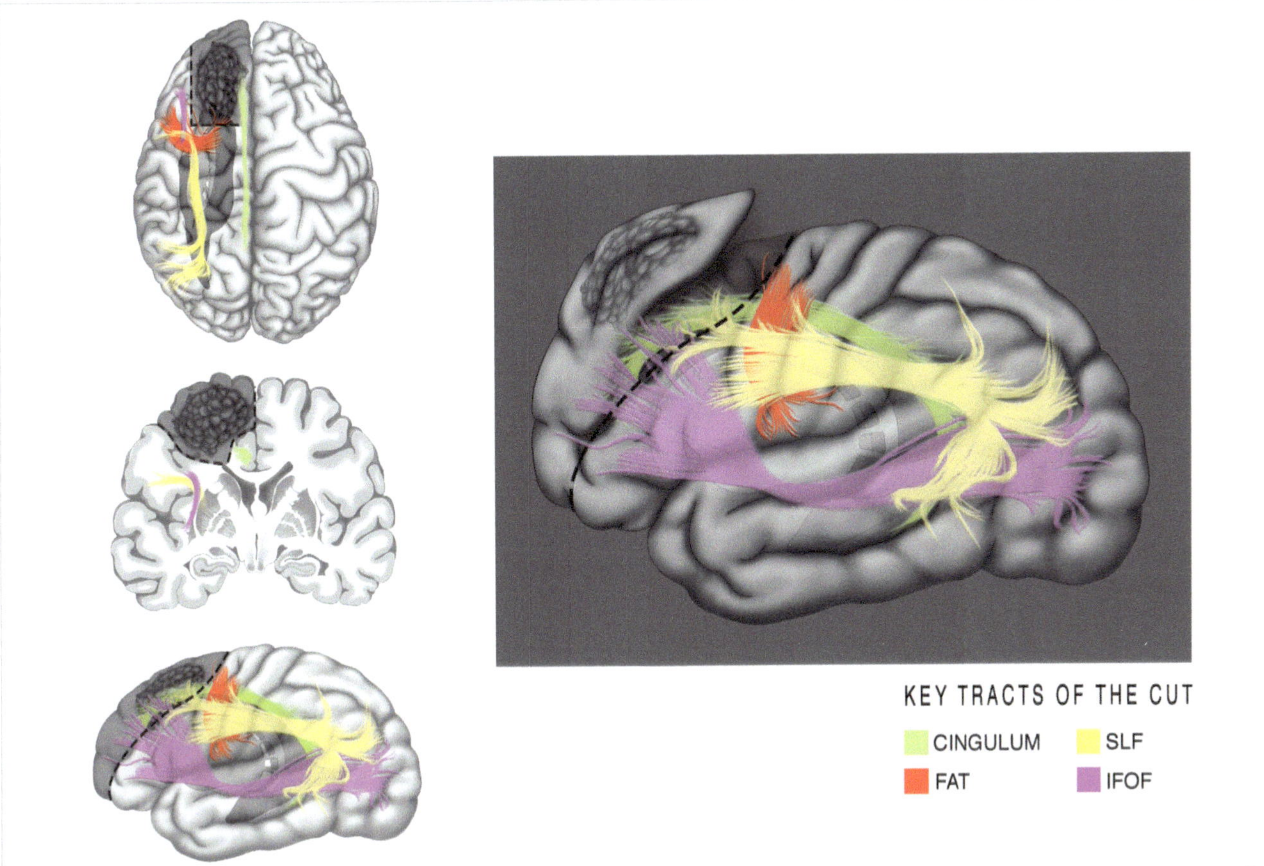

Fig. 10.8 The steps of a medial frontal disconnection: The cuts at the cortex form an L-shape. The sagittal cut (which is started first) runs along the lateral border of the resection and parallels the direction of the superior frontal sulcus. The goal of this cut is to separate the tumor from the SLF and IFOF. The coronal cut runs from the posterolateral border of the resection (defined by either the tumor or the functional boundaries) to the midline. The goal of this cut is to separate the tumor from the FAT and motor system. As the cut descends downward, it should be deflected to avoid two structures. First, it should move laterally to avoid the cingulate gyrus. Later, at its depth, it should move anteriorly to avoid the caudate head. Both cuts enter the frontal horn and open it widely until the cingulate, the caudate, and the motor system are free from danger.

10.4.3 "Destroy" Phase

The elemental frontal resection is a complete lobectomy, and more limited resections can be tailored from this one you grasp the steps of removing the entire lobe safely.

Frontal Lobectomy (▶ Fig. 10.10)

Once the cuts have been made and the patient is asleep, resecting the frontal lobe is a stereotyped process of finding specific landmarks in a predefined order which makes the subsequent step safe and maximally effective. This is true with most "destroy" phases, but surprisingly, few of us have been taught how to do this in an organized fashion.

The first order of business in removing the frontal lobe is to define the midline. The main thing to avoid at this stage is damage to the callosomarginal artery or any other ACA branch artery supplying brain you have left behind (it was presumably left there for a reason). This requires careful subpial work, and pruning branches when it is clear that they are feeding brain to be removed. If the cingulate gyrus is being spared (if it does not have tumor in it I always try to save it), then it will protect some of the main ACA trunks for you.

After defining the midline, the next step is to enter the ventricle and locate the head of the caudate clearly. Not only can caudate tissue be differentiated from normal by its appearance (reddish grey with faint white spots (▶ Fig. 10.11), but entering the ventricle makes its location obvious from its characteristic bulge into the frontal horn). Finding the caudate protects you against injury to the caudate, but also defines the coronal plane of the subcallosal gyri, basal forebrain structures, and septal nuclei. It also keeps you out of the anterior perforated substance, and protects you from the lenticulostriates. Caudate tissue is easily mistaken for gliomas (they look very similar, and both can bleed a fair bit), and if you don't know where to start focusing your eyes to look for the subtle features of caudate tissue, there is a reasonable chance you will resect it. The caudate also tends to be bloody and I do not make strong efforts to primarily hemostase it, but instead pack it off.

If you have committed to a full lobectomy, then it is safe to remove brain in front of and somewhat superior to the head without problems. At this point, I make a cut just anterior to the caudate head, and incise the pia of the orbitofrontal cortex from front to back down to the orbital room (▶ Fig. 10.12). I then take all the midline veins and free up the olfactory tract, and deliver the frontal lobe en bloc.

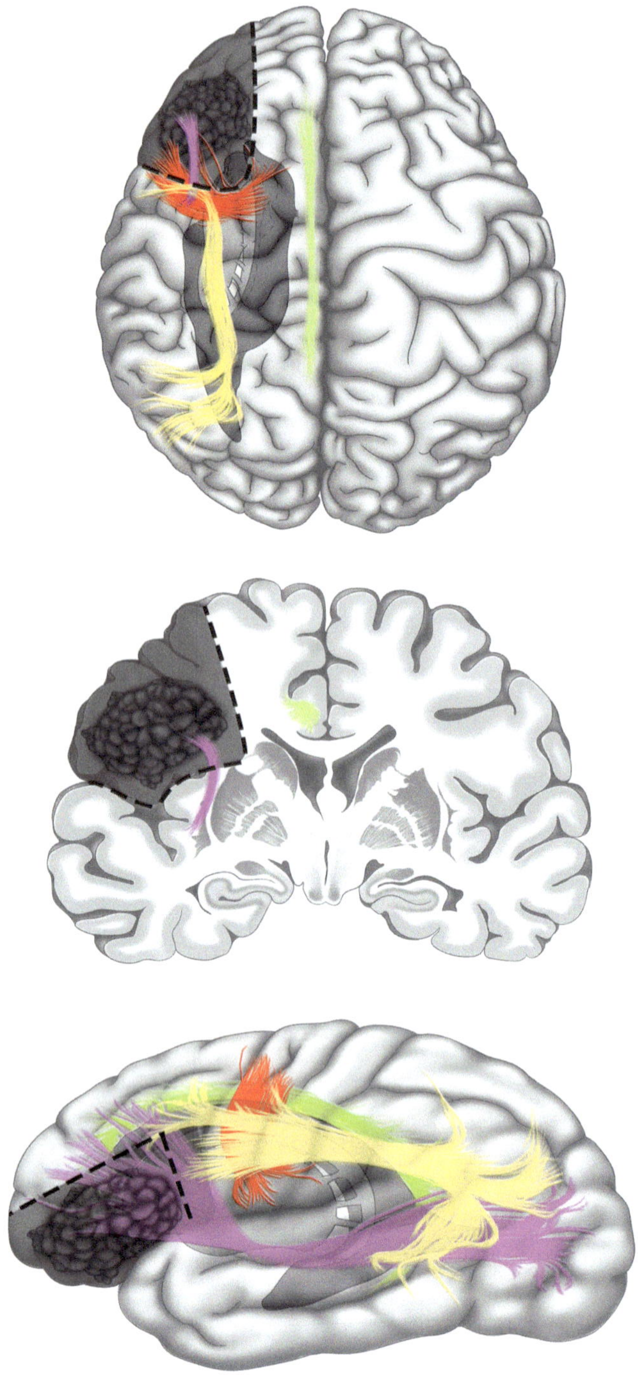

Fig. 10.9 Steps of a lateral frontal disconnection: This disconnection is designed to separate the tumor from the SLF, the FAT, and the IFOF posteriorly. It begins by skeletonizing the opercular vessels and finding the insula, which gives you depth perception regarding the likely location of critical tracts. The cut is then made in a J-shaped manner based on the mapping results, and this extends inward on the superior and posterior boundaries until the tumor is separated from the FAT and SLF posteriorly. Once its medial boundary is well deep to the tumor, then it hooks anteriorly to clear the deep margin.

Finally, I remove the rostrum of corpus callosum. There are two reasons for this. First, if you have entered the ventricle and removed the frontal lobe, then this part of the callosum has been sectioned, and basically is a bridge to nowhere. Second, this is a potential path of spread to the other frontal lobe, which usually spells the end for many patients, so it's unclear why leaving it behind if it has been cut is a good idea.

After the frontal lobe has been removed, I re-examine the ventricle. The corpus callosum is the front wall of the frontal horn and is all the white matter between the aca and the ventricle. I carefully resect this tissue until the ACA is floating and skeletonized, and until my exposure is widely biventricular (meaning I am all the way across). I am aware of the hydrocephalus risk of doing this, but again feel bifrontal tumor recurrence is a much worse problem.

Modifications

Not all frontal lobe gliomas need a full lobectomy. I believe marginal resections are a platonic ideal for glioma surgery, but there is always a line where this is neither necessary nor prudent, and a full lobectomy is overkill for many patients. Still,

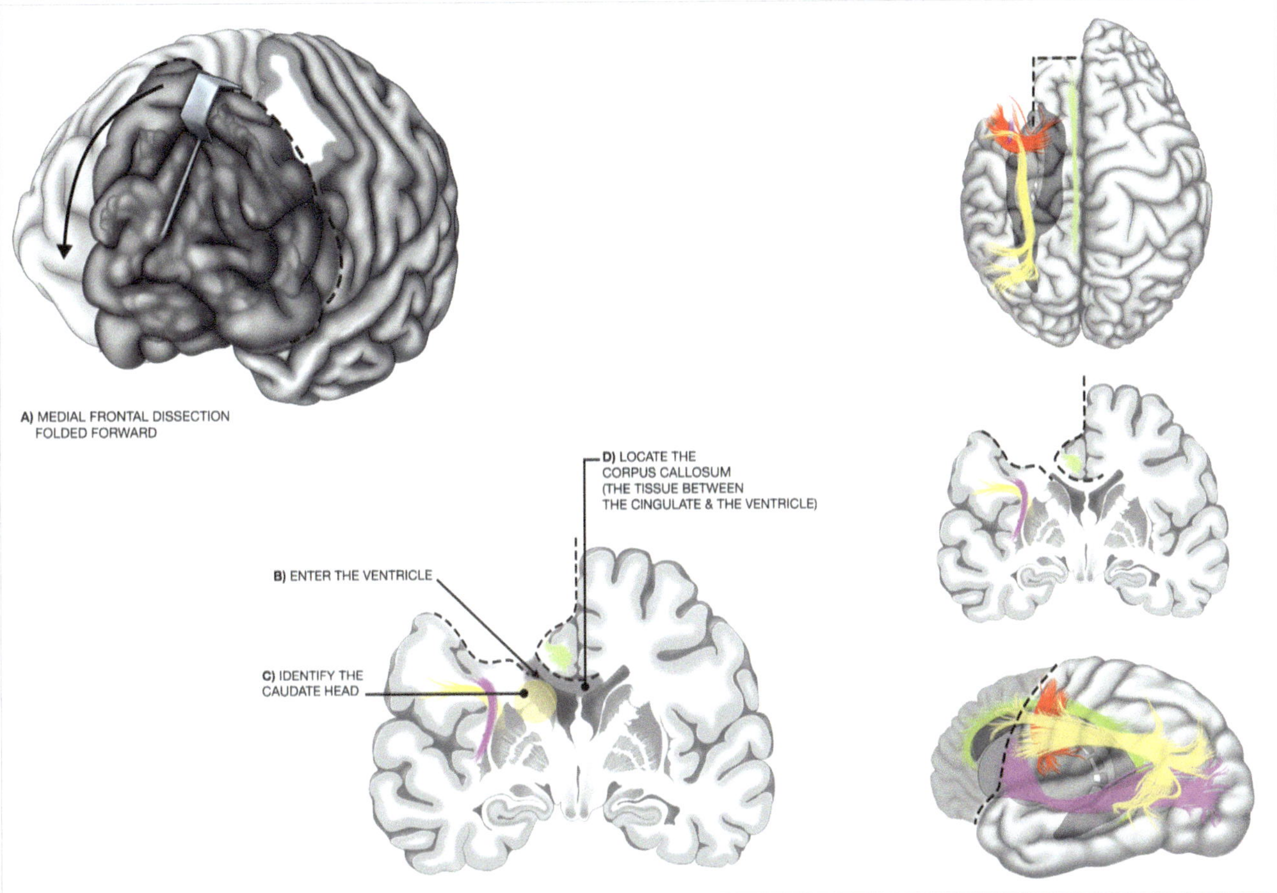

Fig. 10.10 Steps of a full-frontal lobectomy: Once the lobe is disconnected from the potential areas of function, the first step of completing the lobectomy (after the patient is asleep) is to address the midline. This involves subpially removing medial frontal lobe in front of the cut to identify ACA branches and follow them from origin to target. Most of these branches are going to the lobectomy, and can be sacrificed; however, it is important to avoid cutting callosomarginal or internal frontal branches headed to the SMA or motor strip. You continue this subpialization until you are in front of the cingulate, at which point you can fold the medial frontal pia in and divide this as far inferiorly as the orbital roof. You then need to lengthen the cuts anteriorly until you reach the orbital roof and divide the pia on the superior and inferior frontal lobe surface. This will allow you to pull the frontal lobe inward and remove it. By looking into the frontal horn, you can identify the location of the caudate by its bulge into the lateral wall of the ventricle, and the final freeing cut can be made down to the orbital roof just in front of the caudate. After the lobe has been removed, there is usually a bit of additional subpialization work needed to clean up the edges. At this point, if the plan is to remove the corpus callosum, you should identify the boundaries of the callosum in the frontal horn. Specifically, this involves identifying the callosal sulcus or ACA, which are the anterior and superior boundaries of the genu/rostrum, and the septum pellucidum, which is the posterior boundary. All tissue between these structures should be removed until your opening is widely biventricular.

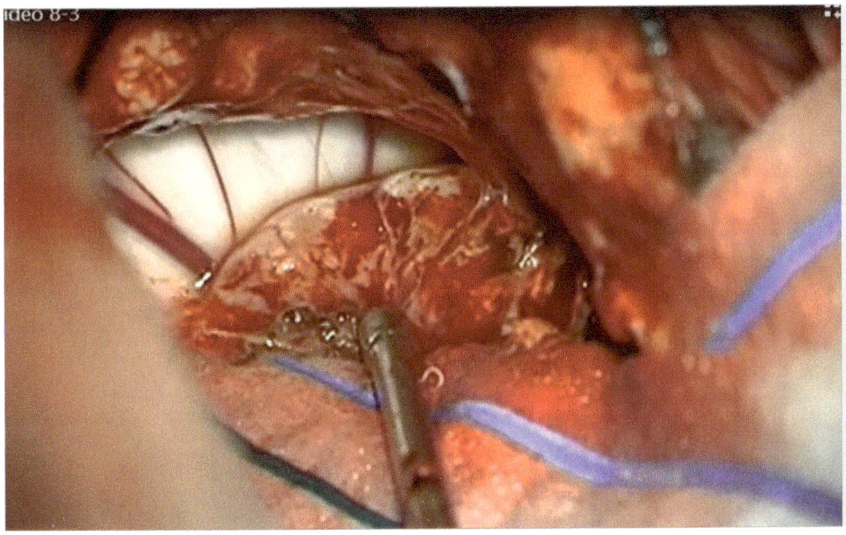

Fig. 10.11 Photo demonstrating the gross appearance of caudate and basal ganglia tissue under the microscope.

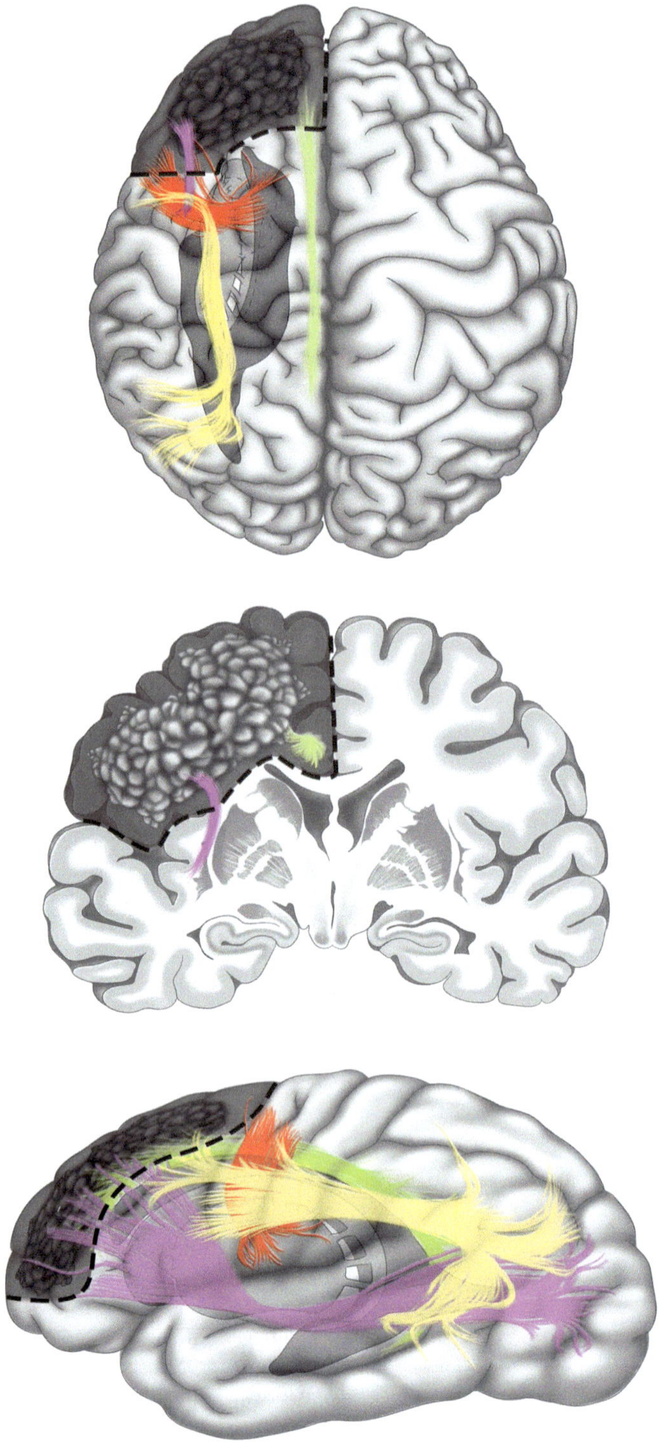

Fig. 10.12 This schematic demonstrates the modification of a frontal lobectomy to spare the orbitofrontal cortex. Note that the orbitofrontal cortex largely connects to a different network of white matter, and is frequently uninvolved. If it is clearly uninvolved, we try to spare it by modifying the lobectomy cuts as indicated.

more limited anatomic resections can be performed in these cases, and still achieve rational marginal resection.

Orbitofrontal Sparing (▶ Fig. 10.13)

As noted at numerous points in this book, the orbitofrontal cortex communicates with targets outside the frontal lobe via tracts which head anterior posterior and are inferior in the frontal lobe. In cases where the tumor is not especially near the orbitofrontal cortex, I try to spare it, to minimize problems with judgment and emotional regulation. To do so, after finding the caudate head, I make the inferior cut directly anterior paralleling the orbital roof, instead of cutting downward in front of the caudate head, which disconnects the orbitofrontal cortex from its targets.

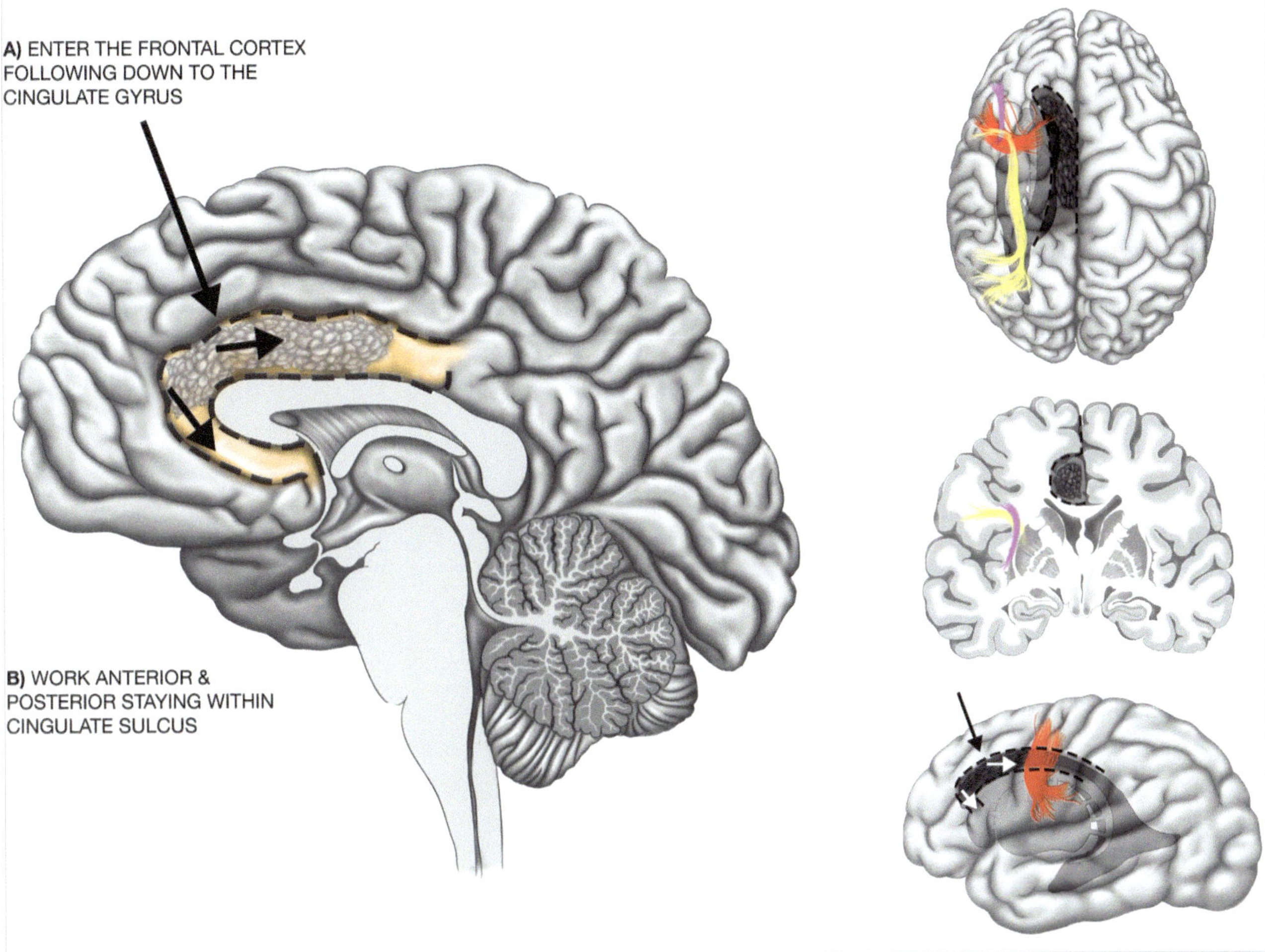

Fig. 10.13 This schematic depicts the steps of removing a tumor primarily focused in the anterior cingulate gyrus. A more limited medial frontal cut is used to access this tumor transcortically and to separate the tumor from the lateral and posterior frontal lobe. Following this, the cingulate sulcus is identified and everything between the cingulate sulcus and the corpus callosum is removed, at least as much as is tolerated. The resection continues from front to back as tolerated by the testing, ideally working under the motor strip to obtain a complete resection.

Anterior Cingulate Tumor Resection

Anterior cingulate gliomas can spread into neighboring frontal lobe, but they are fundamentally limbic tumors and preferentially spread in the limbic tracts. It may be tempting then to try to resect them using a fancy approach, such as an interhemispheric, transfalcine approach. I advocate for going through the superior frontal gyrus for several reasons. First, it is difficult to do brain mapping in an interhemispheric or transfalcine approach, as touching the dura is painful and unavoidable in these cases. Avoiding brain mapping is unwise, as I have found that the anterior cingulate is not silent. Second, by avoiding entering the superior frontal gyrus, you are failing to deal with the key pathway of spread of these tumors. Additionally, it is infinitely faster and easier to go through the SFG than the interhemispheric fissure, and there is minimal risk of damaging the uninvolved, contralateral cingulate. Finally, the angle for approaching these tumors via these approaches is wrong. The cingulate sulcus is deep laterally and an ipsilateral interhemispheric approach cannot reach out here. Further, a contralateral transfalcine approach weakens your ability to stop before going too deep, making it possible to disconnect the brain areas you were purporting to save by using an uncommon awkward approach. Note that the outflow of the superior frontal gyrus runs just deep to the cingulate sulcus and it is unclear how this is identified and not damaged. In short, these approaches are ideal for lesionectomy type approach (cavernomas, metastasis, etc.), but it is less ideal for cingulate gliomas, which are a totally different type of disease.

To remove a cingulate tumor (or a butterfly tumor), the initial steps are similar; however, the resection is limited to a portion of the SFG overlying the tumor and there is both an anterior and posterior cut to isolate this resected part of the gyrus. Note closely from Chapter 5, that the anterior portions of the SFG have outgoing tracts which are inferior and/or anterior to the trajectory, and these do not run through or under the planned path to the tumor. Thus, a limited approach to this tumor is probably best. Once you have encountered the tumor, developing the midline, and resecting the tumor follows similar steps to the analogous parts of a formal lobectomy.

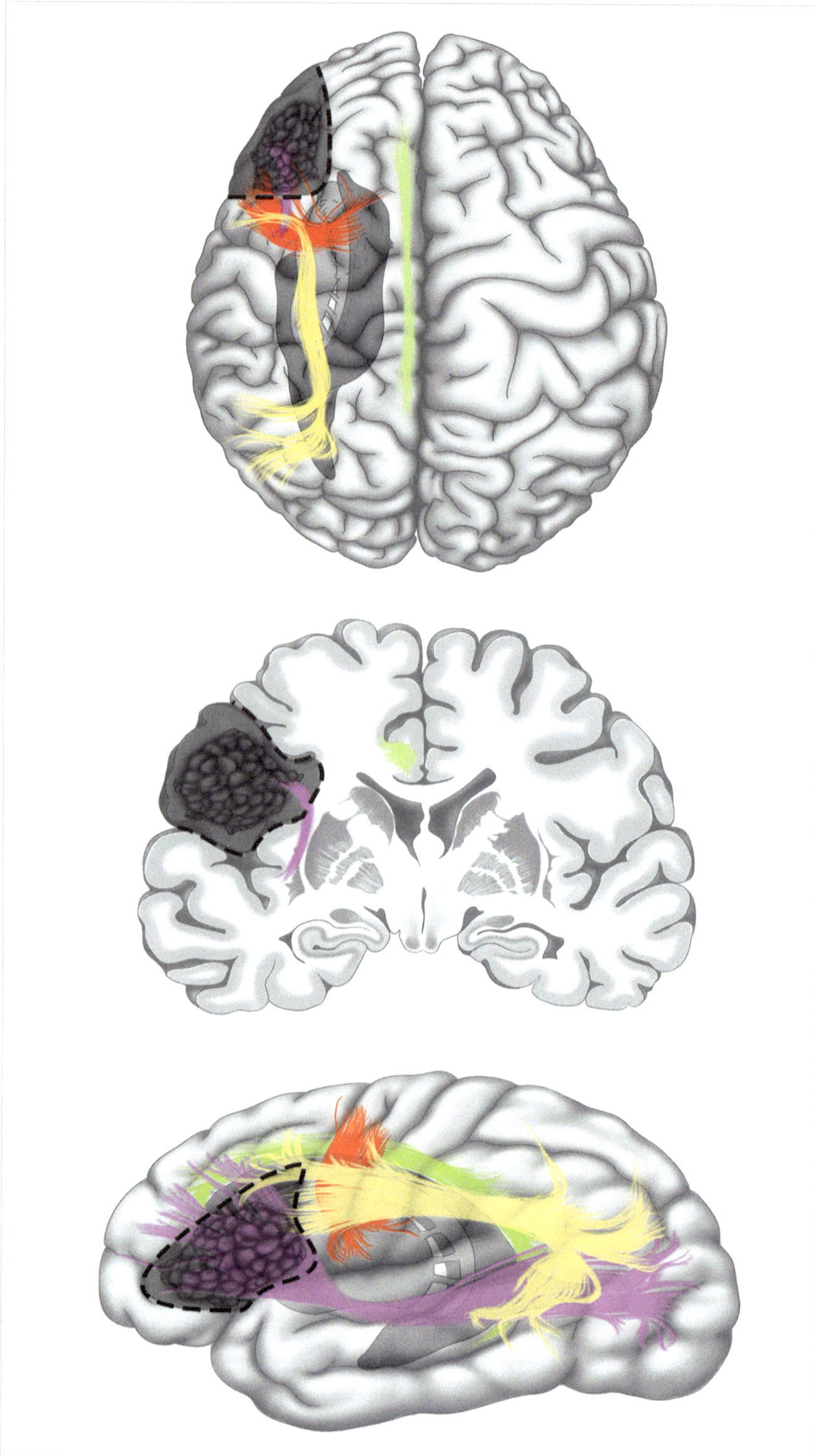

Fig. 10.14 In a limited lateral frontal lobe resection, we make our lateral frontal disconnection such that it is deep to the tumor, before hooking anteriorly, as opposed to performing a frontal lobectomy.

Limited Lateral Frontal Resection (▶ Fig. 10.14)

Not all lateral frontal disconnections require a full lobectomy. For one the tumor could be quite small making lobectomy overkill. Second, there is no point to do a massively supratotal resection if you are leaving gross tumor in a language area, for example, which often happens in these cases. Thus, it is generally wise to take some margin in these cases (otherwise you will often miss some gross tumor on the margin); however, there needs to be a limit. Finally, lateral approaches to frontal lobectomy are suboptimal at addressing the midline and the ventricle, and this limitation of angle takes away your greatest safety steps in this approach.

A limited lateral frontal resection follows the disconnection by arbitrarily determining a resection depth, and then directing the cut anteriorly paralleling the falx. It is important in these cases, however, to make sure the pars orbitalis of the inferior frontal gyrus is appropriately resected as it is probably disconnected in most lateral frontal lobe disconnections. The orbitofrontal cortices are not disconnected and should be spared.

10.4.4 Examples of Frontal Gliomas

Medial Frontal Resections

▶ Fig. 10.15 This case demonstrates a large predominantly medial frontal low grade glioma.

a) Two aspects of the preoperative scans are noteworthy. First, this tumor has undergone an open biopsy at a prior hospital which roughly crosses the left SLF with its trajectory, causing a preoperative aphasia. Second, the tumor is invading the basal forebrain structures through the diagonal band of Broca. Our plan in this case was to perform a medial frontal lobectomy, including the callosum and involved cingulate gyrus, and to leave the basal forebrain tumor for radiochemotherapy.
b) These images demonstrate the small craniotomy which is made just large enough to reach the "downhill" parts of the frontal lobe and is centered round the cut.
c) None.
d) The final images provided demonstrate that this migrating tumor often responds well to this approach, assuming the part in the basal ganglia is isolated by circumferential resection.

▶ Fig. 10.16 demonstrates a full medial frontal resection of a massive frontal glioma.

a) The tumor is filling the entire right frontal lobe including the orbitofrontal cortex. The initial goal when seeing this is to perform a formal frontal lobectomy if possible.
b) None.
c) The DTI demonstrate that the tumor boundaries are well anterior to the SLF and IFOF, and the SMA region does not seem to be involved.
d) The final result demonstrates a complete removal of the T2 changes obtained by an anatomic resection of the lesion.

▶ Fig. 10.17 demonstrates a grade 3 medial frontal glioma which has been treated elsewhere and which has enhancement and widespread T2 change. It has now transformed to GBM.

a) Looking at the preoperative films, one striking problem is that it is difficult to define the target precisely. The radiotherapy the patient had received in the past has clearly caused some leukoencepalopathy on the periphery of the lesion, but it is almost certain that the T2 changes around the enhancement are mostly non-enhancing parts of the tumor. Note that the conversion of a part of a low-grade tumor to high grade does not magically make the previously enhancing areas melt into edema, they are still there. My general approach in these cases is to resect the area up to anatomic and functional boundaries, but the principle mission to remove as much enhancing tissue as possible. There is no reason to perform a lobectomy for margin if you leave the bad stuff.
b) None.
c) Looking at the DTIs, it is obvious that this case is more complex than at initial glance. The SLF and motor network have shifted anterior to where we expect and this is a common event when a debulking has been done previously. The cuts here were challenging and SMA syndrome is a real risk. In fact, this patient developed mutism which improved in about 2 weeks.
d) The final result shows a good but not great resection. There are still some small enhancing areas in the SMA and a touch laterally. The T2 was aggressively resected but some areas remain in the premotor and motor cortices though these seem to be leukoencephalopathy. Note that we did not remove the orbitofrontal cortex here as this is not this tumor's most likely path of spread. This is the best we can do here, but highlights some of the challenges in operating on a case that someone has allowed to progress prior to our intervention.

▶ Fig. 10.18 demonstrates transformed low grade glioma treated at another center.

a) Reviewing the preoperative images, we see that the previous approach was trying to stay very frontal to enter the lesion. This has some value from a safety standpoint; however, this angle does not allow you satisfactorily to identify and protect the white matter pathways, notably the frontal rami of the SLF. In general, with all tumor surgeries, I try to avoid digging into a hole where at the bottom of the hole is something bad: it is slower, more nerve racking, and less effective than actively finding the structure I am worried about.

Further, given that this is a transformed low-grade glioma, the T2 should be removed to the extent possible. Our plan is to perform a frontal lobectomy with cuts to separate the lobe from IFOF and SLF.

a) The previous bicoronal incision forced us to perform an approach between my two usually attack angles. This frontal lobectomy focused on separating the tumor from SLF laterally, and performed the lobectomy from the side. This is somewhat disorienting to me as I typically perform frontal lobe resections from the top of the latter surface. When I recognize I am working at an unusual angle for me, I check my angles much more often with image guidance.
b) The DTIs look favorable, as the SLF frontal rami are far posterior to the back of this tumor. The IFOF frontal branches are in the tumor, but the important part of this tract for speech function is seldom in front of the caudate.
c) The postop scan shows an excellent resection. Of note, this patient survived for 19 months before recurring on the other side.

▶ Fig. 10.19 demonstrates a giant medial frontal lobe glioma (grade 3 oligodendroglioma, without 1p/19q codeletion) which has portions spilling into the frontal horn and tumor in the basal forebrain.

a) This is a complex and extensive lesion primary centered around the inferior frontal lobe, basal forebrain and corpus callosum. When it was first found on CT scan it was thought to be a skull base meningioma, as the patient presented with anosmia, and the cerebral arteries are encased in tumor. In addition to the obvious observation that this is spilling into the ventricle, a few other points. First, this tumor is spilling onto the other side of the head under the falx. This is because it is in the corpus callosum, but also because it has expanded the medial frontal lobe so much that it physically is herniating

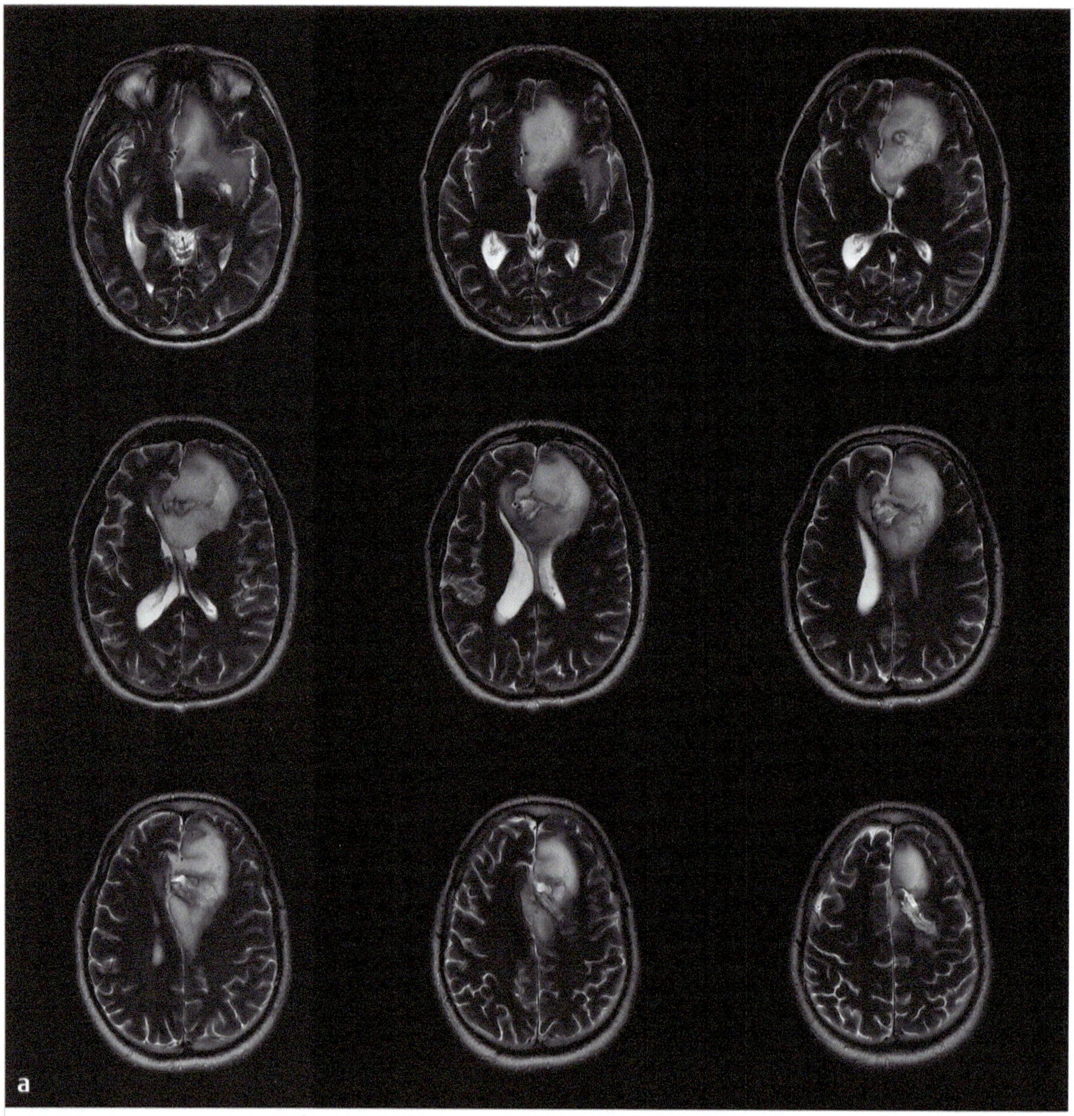

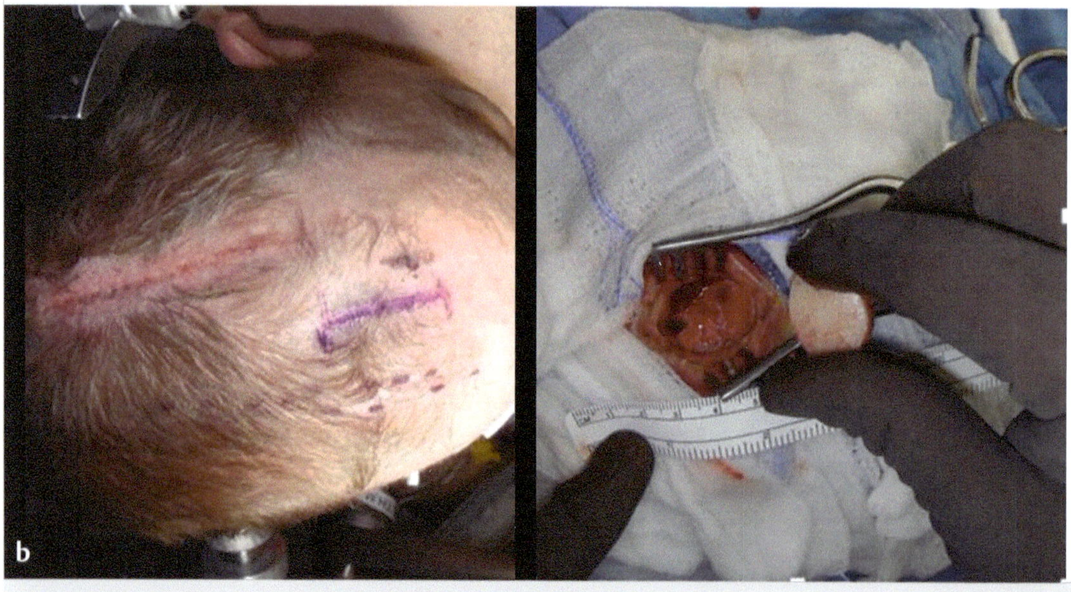

Fig. 10.15 Medial frontal resections; (**a**) preoperative images, (**b**) images of the approach.

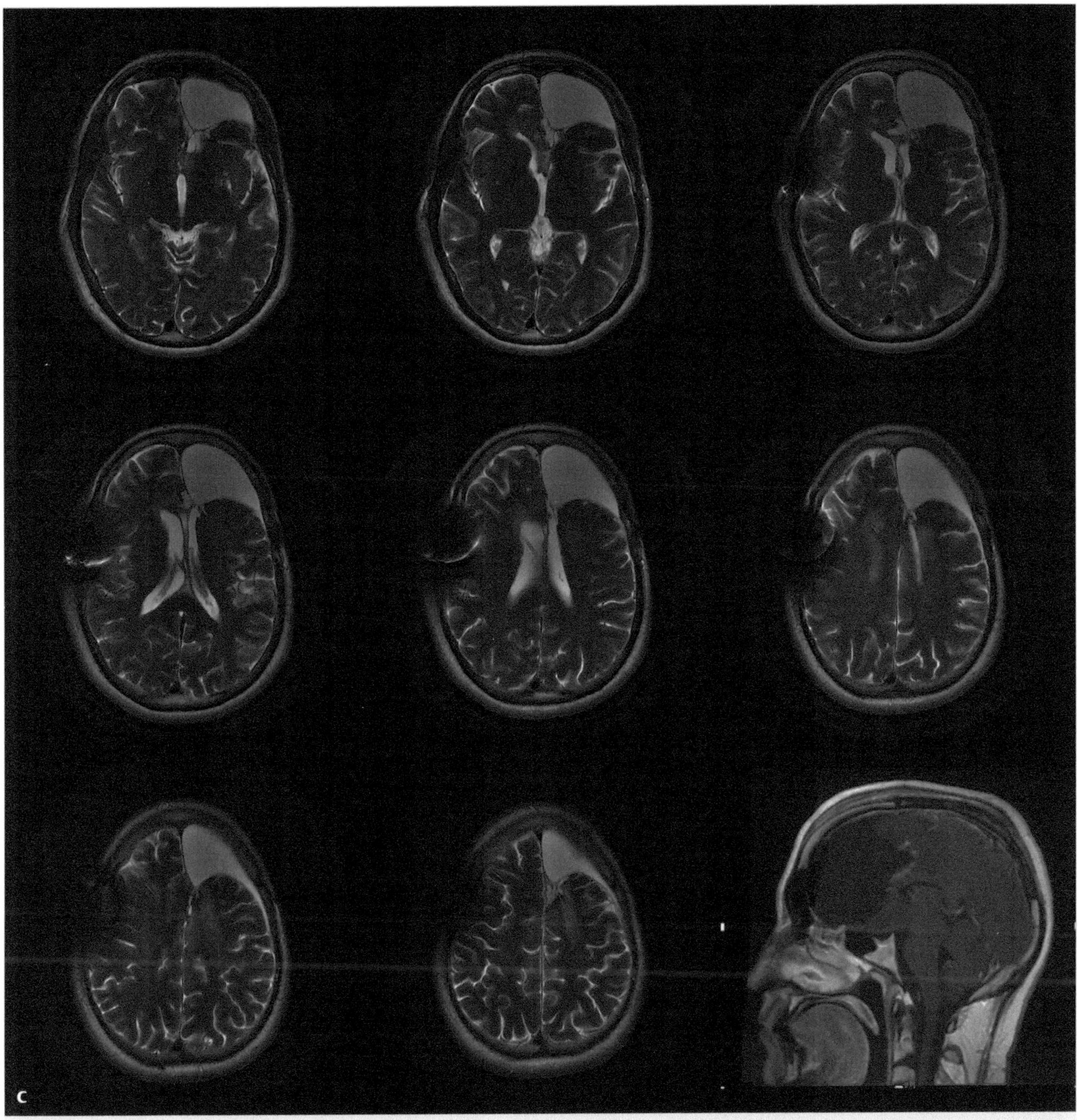

Fig 10.15 (*Continued*) (**c**) Postoperative images.

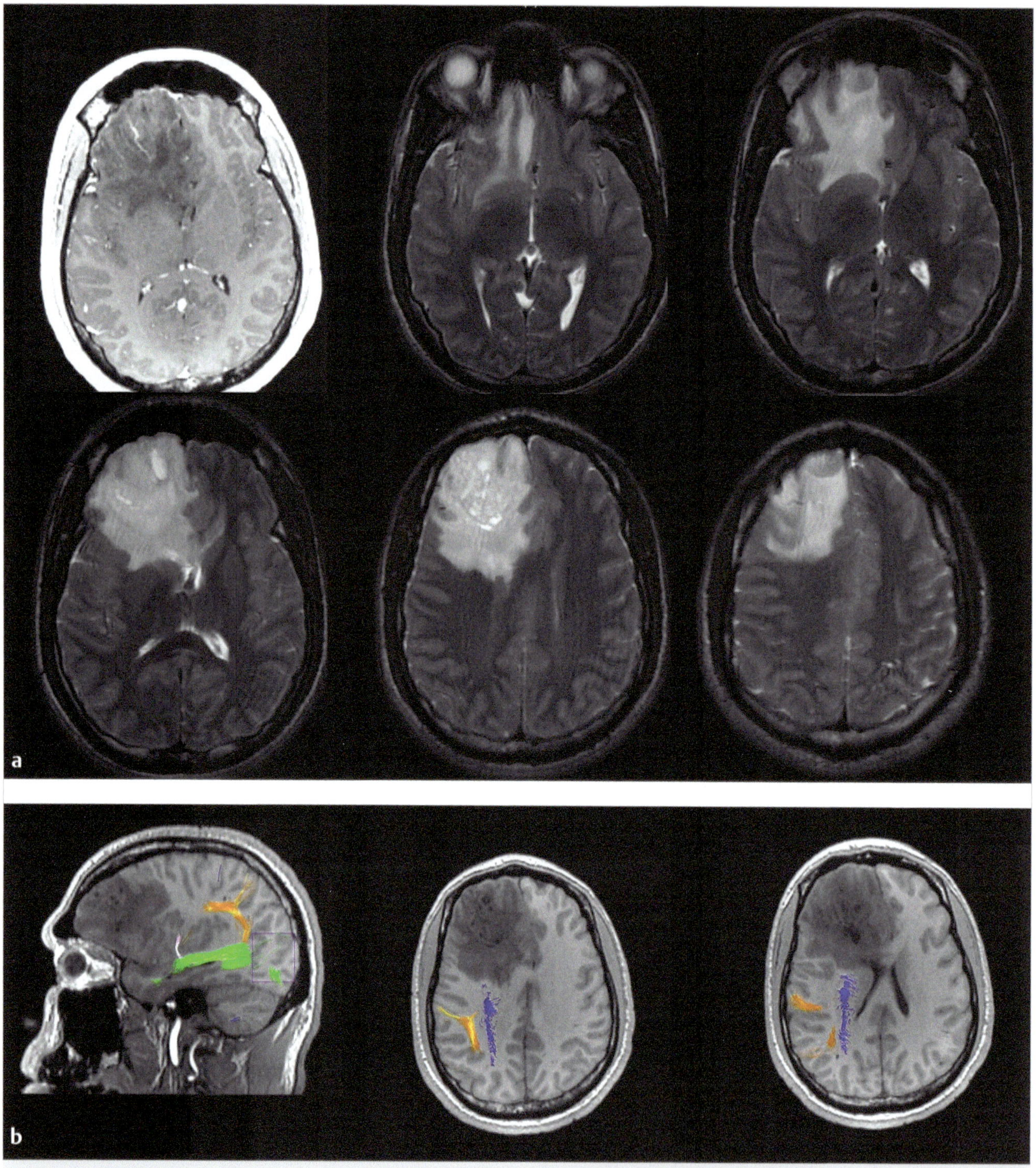

Fig. 10.16 Full medial frontal resection of a massive frontal glioma; (**a**) preoperative images, (**b**) images of the approach.

across the midline. This latter point is critical to note as the brain on the other side in cases like this is going to be distorted and the tumor may interdigitate between sulci of the other side. The other sided arteries, which are en passage arteries in many cases can also be encased in tumor. The key to dealing with this is to stay subpial, to recognize when you have reached the midline arachnoid, and to always consider that you might be looking at the other side.

The plan in this case was a medial frontal lobe resection beginning from an anterior starting point with conservative cuts. This does transgress some uninvolved superior frontal gyrus; however, any other approach (like some kind of pterional or skull base maneuver) has you working a disadvantaged angle to get to the top of this tumor, which is quite high. Those approaches also don't cut off the natural routes of spread that we can deal with from this approach. Finally, this is not an angle of attack into the

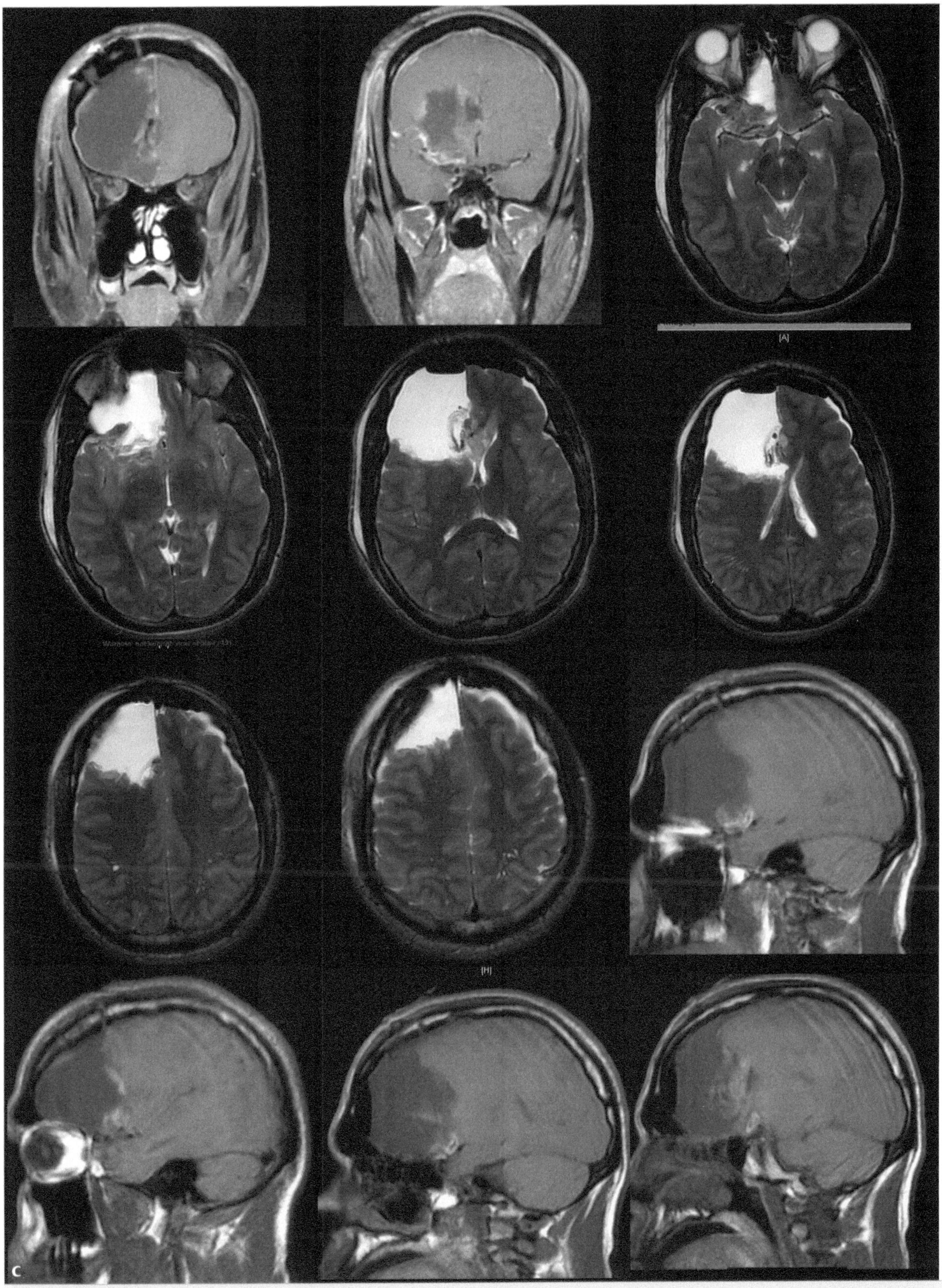

Fig 10.16 (*Continued*) (c) Postoperative images.

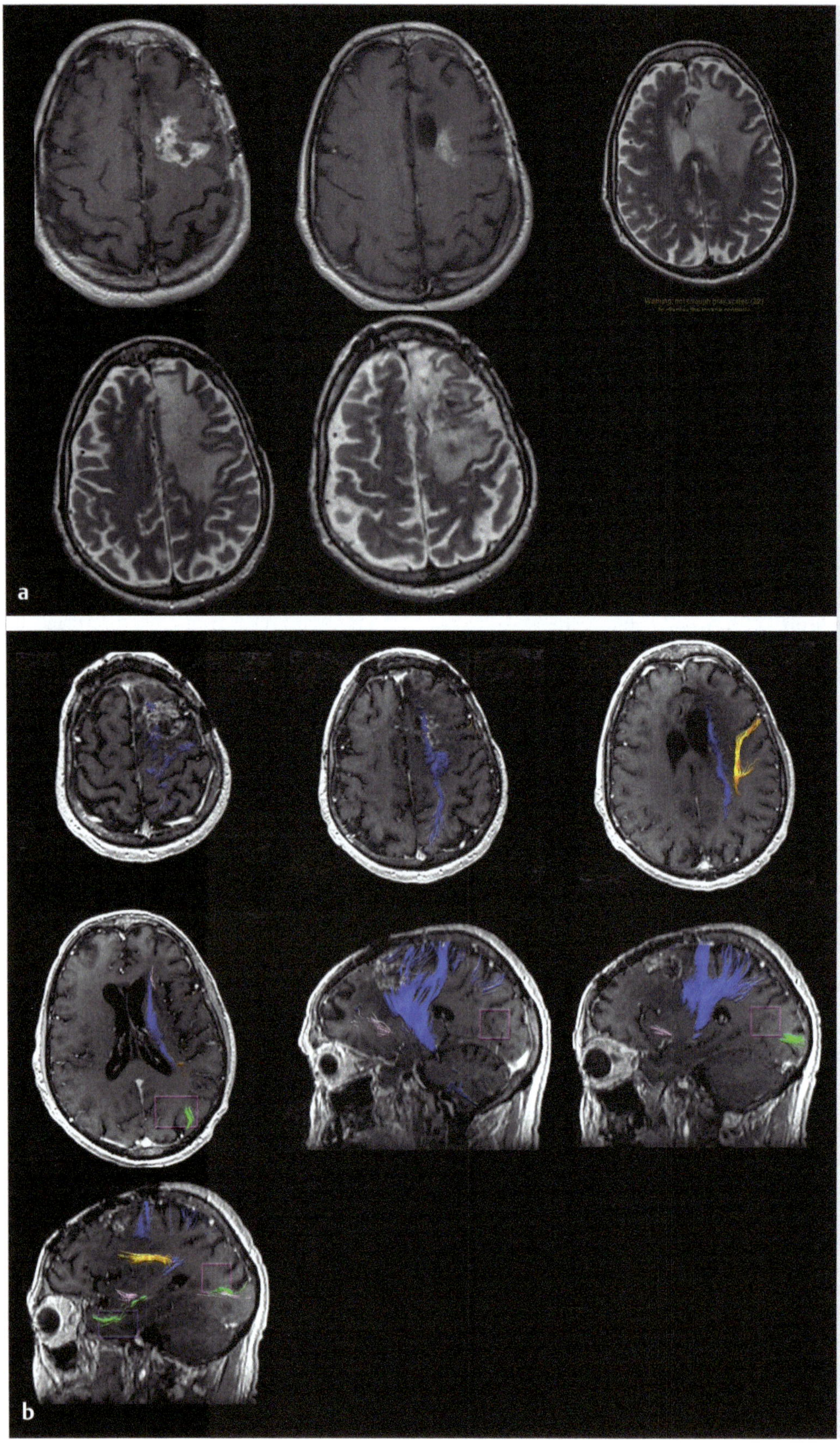

Fig. 10.17 A grade 3 medial frontal glioma which has been treated elsewhere and which has enhancement and widespread T2 change. It has now transformed to GBM. (**a**) Preoperative images, (**b**) images of the approach.

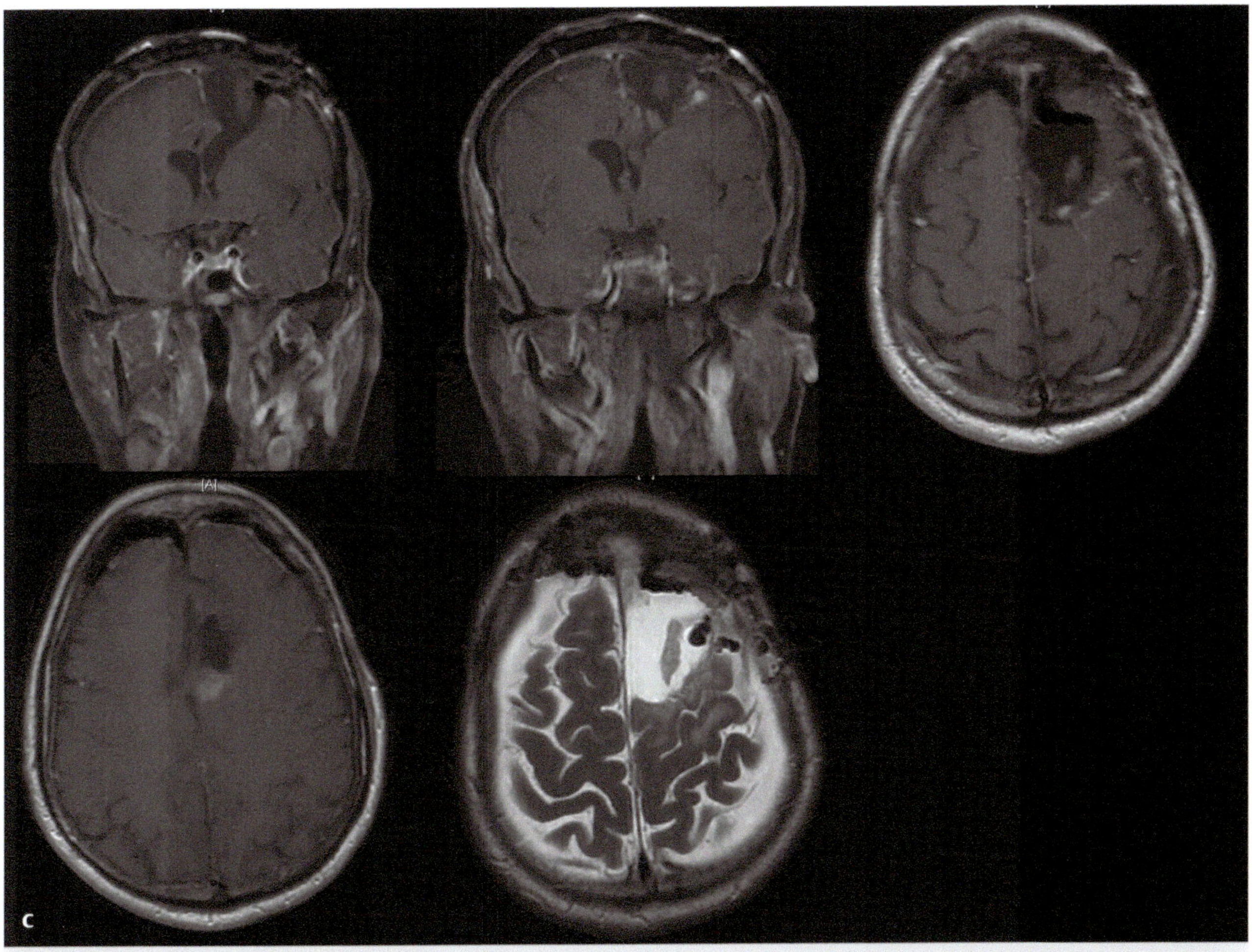

Fig 10.17 (*Continued*) (**c**) Postoperative images.

cerebrum that most of us have a lot of experience doing. This is an uncommon glioma, and trying to be flashy to "stay out of the brain" will usually end up with a big residual or you are getting lost. As I emphasize over and over, glioma surgery is not cavernoma surgery or meningioma surgery: the goals, techniques, and mandates are quite different.

a) This is an anterior incision for the medial frontal lobe resection. I have gone more recently to an incision at 45 degrees to this one for these surgeries, as I have seen some wound break down at the posterior margin of this type of incision, which suggests to me that it may be too far from the supraorbital artery.
b) None.
c) The postoperative scan demonstrates a good resection of the medial and orbitofrontal frontal lobe, as well as the corpus callosum. The residual is left in the subcallosal cingulate gyrus and basal forebrain structures.
d) The long term post-operative images also show an excellent response of the small residual in the basal forebrain to adjuvant therapy, despite not having favorable markers. I have noted this in several other cases, which is one reason I do not risk entering the basal forebrain when I see it involved.

Lateral Frontal Resections

▸ Fig. 10.20 demonstrates the resection of a lateral frontal glioma which was resected by separation from the language areas posteriorly.

a) This is a large cystic grade 2 glioma. Careful examination of the images suggests that this is principally located in the posterior MFG and somewhat the IFG. The motor cortex is pushed posteriorly. This mapping will focus on speech and motor planning.
b) None.
c) The DTIs are quite favorable as they suggest that the motor planning areas for speech and the motor cortex are pushed backwards by mass effect and seem to be terminating in an IFG which is smashed down and backward.
d) The postop imaging demonstrates that the bulk of the tumor lateral to the cyst seems to be well-resected. The T2 change on the medial bank of the cyst that I left, highlighted for me the importance of addressing all sides of the wall of a glioma cyst, even if it doesn't look grossly abnormal (unlike most tumors with cyst, the wall usually is tumor). As they will thicken when the cyst is drained. Some of the posterior residual was intentionally left behind when we encountered speech problems during that part of the resection.

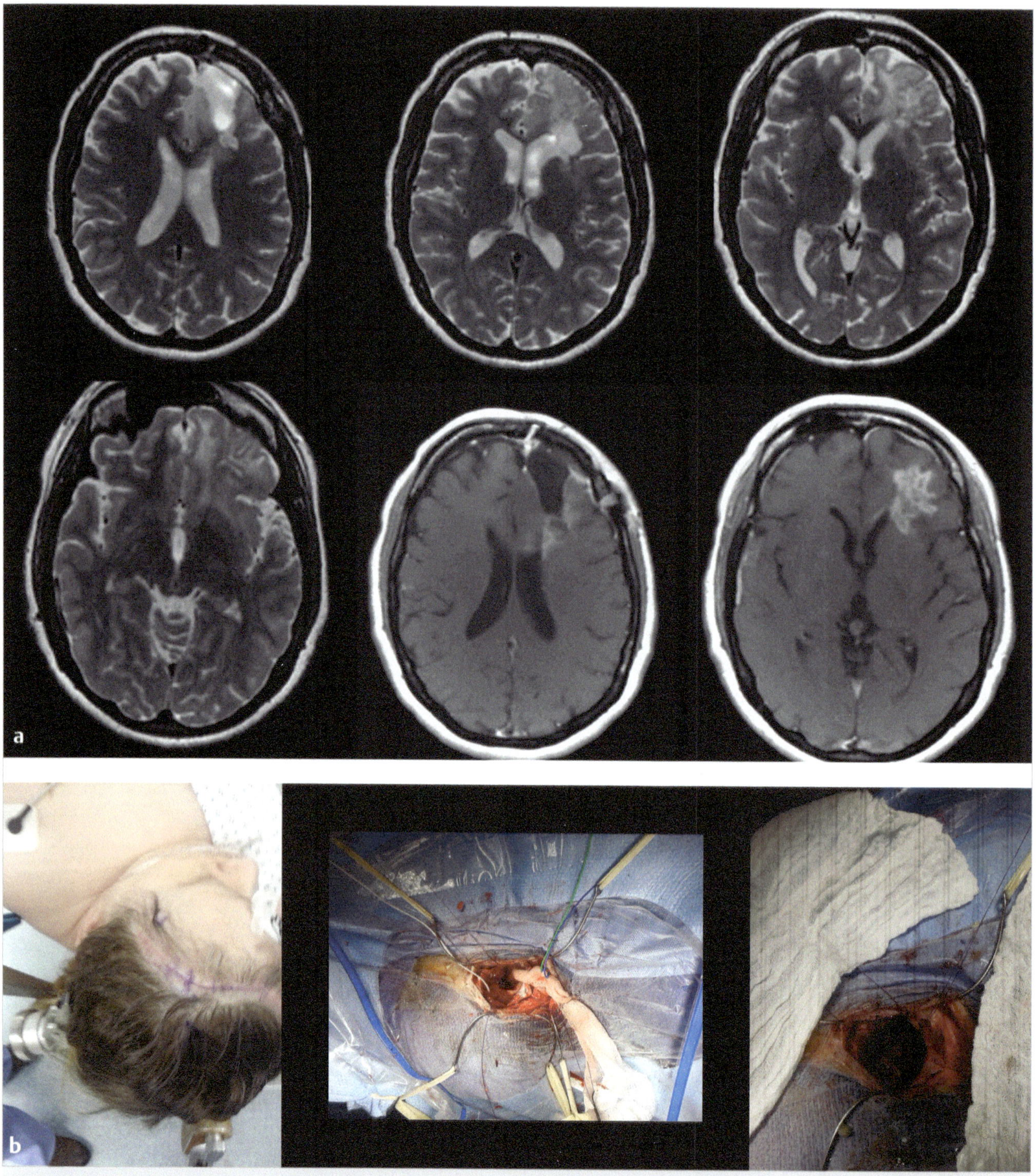

Fig. 10.18 Transformed low grade glioma treated at another center. (**a**) Preoperative images, (**b**) images of the approach.

▶ Fig. 10.21 demonstrates the interesting case of a glioblastoma in a young patient with marked reorganization of the language planning areas enabling an excellent resection of this tumor in Broca's area.

a) Review of the postoperative images demonstrates that the tumor is located in the IFG near the motor cortex. The coronal image demonstrates that it is principally opercular.
b) The images demonstrate a lateral frontal approach. Two areas of speech arrest are marked with the numbers and these lined up perfectly with the DTI for the SLF.
c) The DTIs in this case are quite remarkable as they suggest that the SLF does not terminate in the IFG anymore but instead to parts of the posterior MFG and the motor cortex. While it could be questioned whether this is real reorganization,

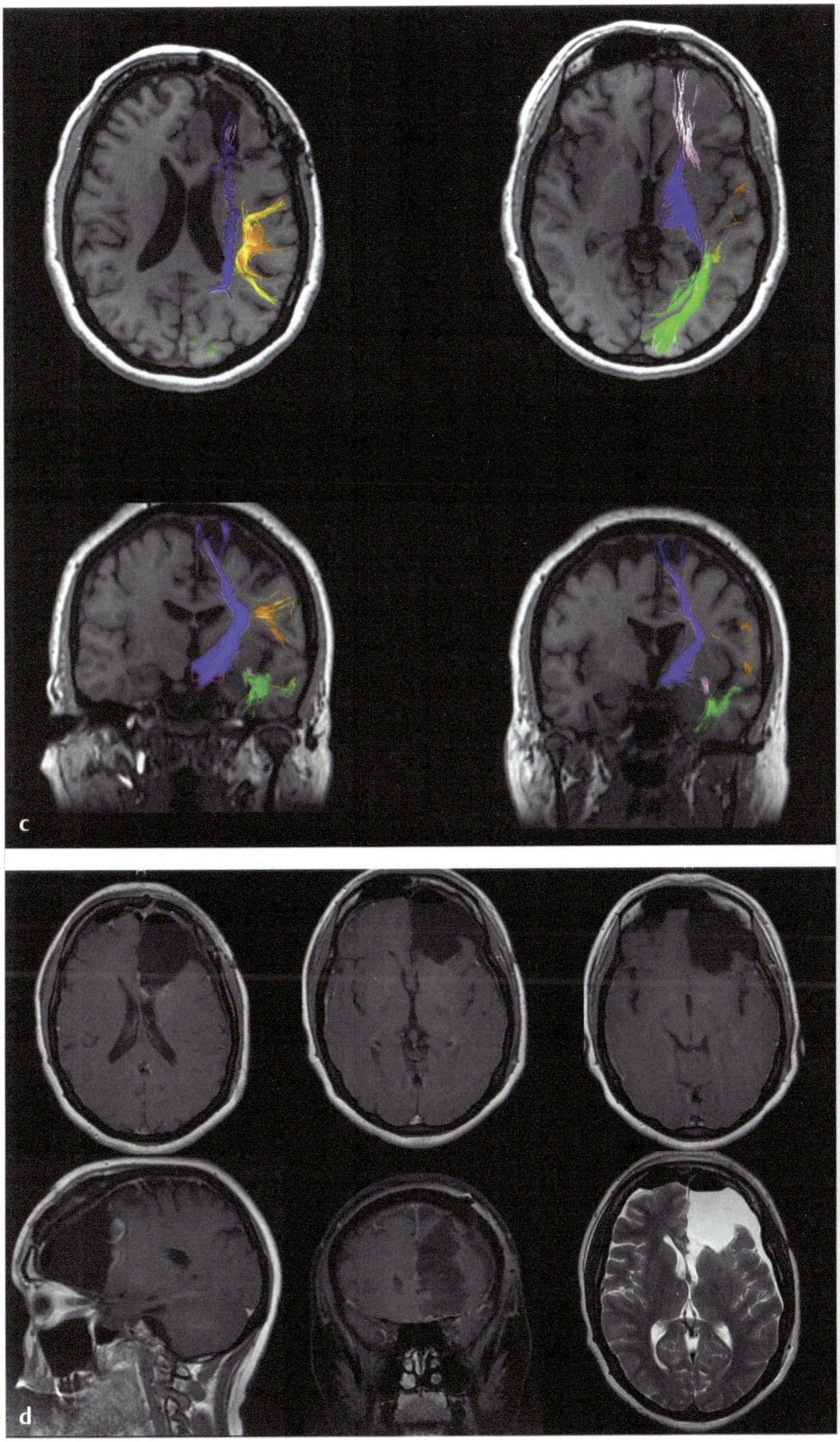

Fig 10.18 (*Continued*) (**c**) DTI tractography. (**d**) Postoperative images.

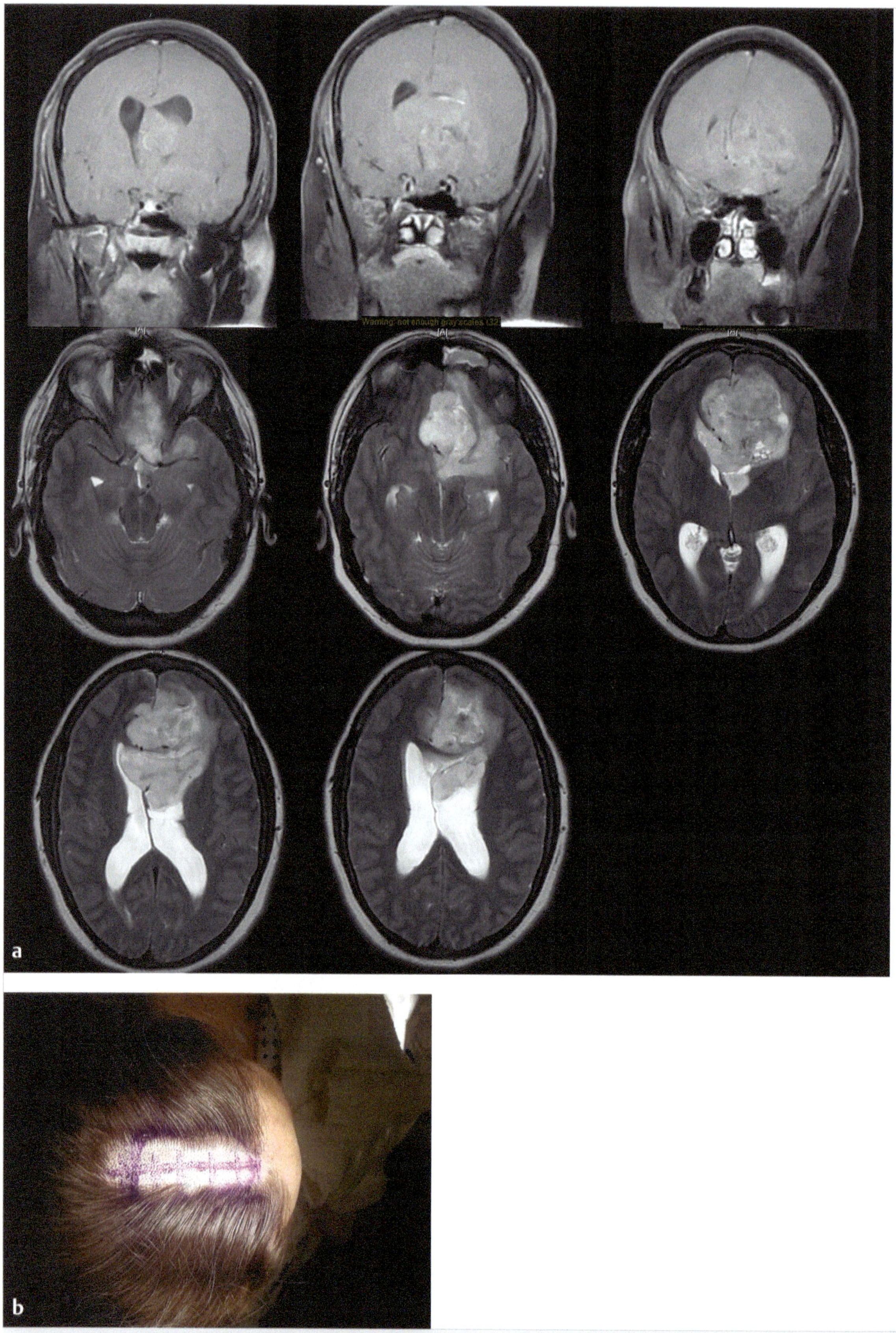

Fig. 10.19 Giant medial frontal lobe glioma (grade 3 oligodendroglioma, without 1p/19q codeletion) which has portions spilling into the frontal horn and a tumor in the basal forebrain. (**a**) Preoperative images, (**b**) images of the approach.

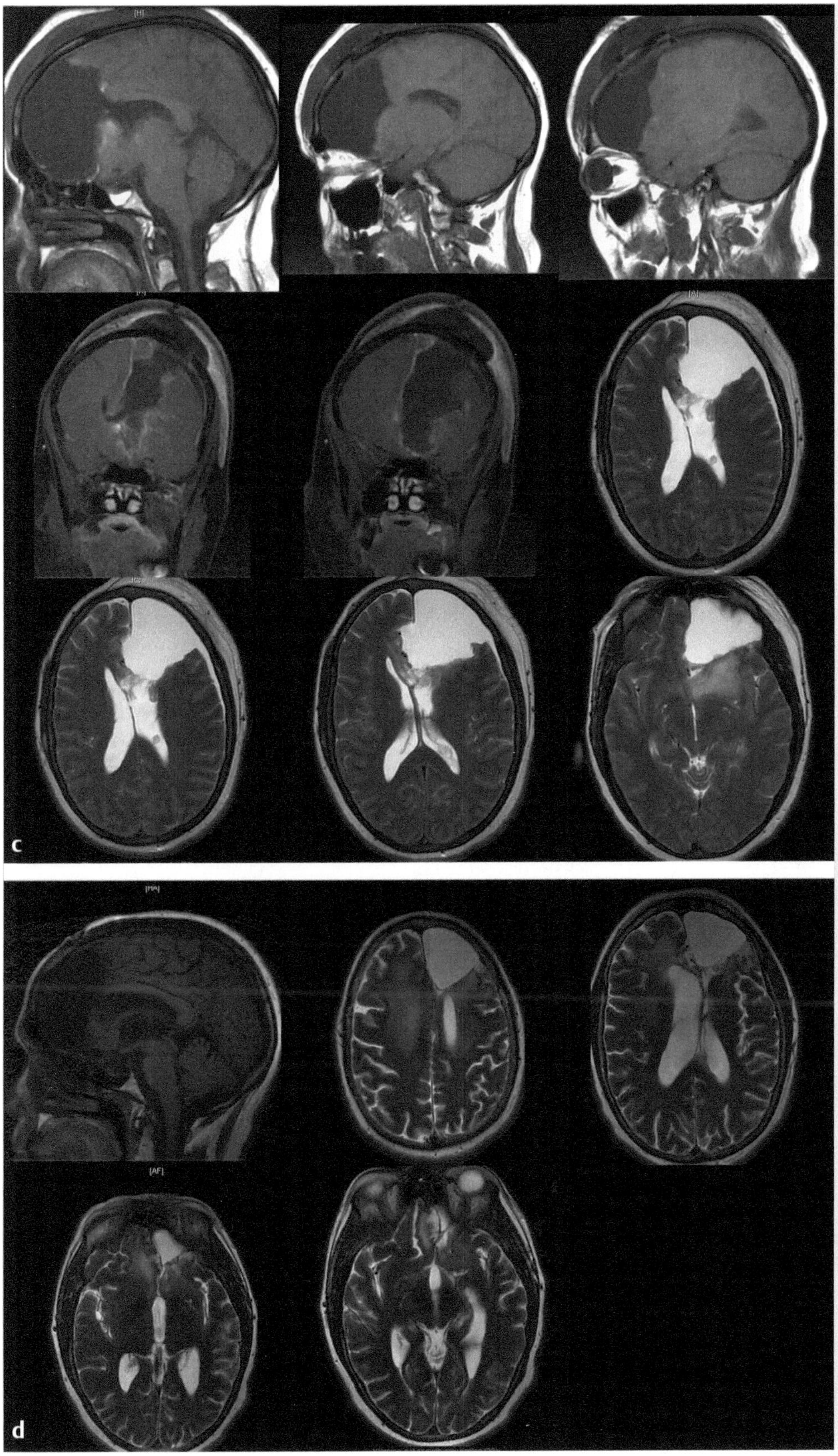

Fig 10.19 (*Continued*) (**c**) Postoperative images. (**d**) Long-term follow-up images.

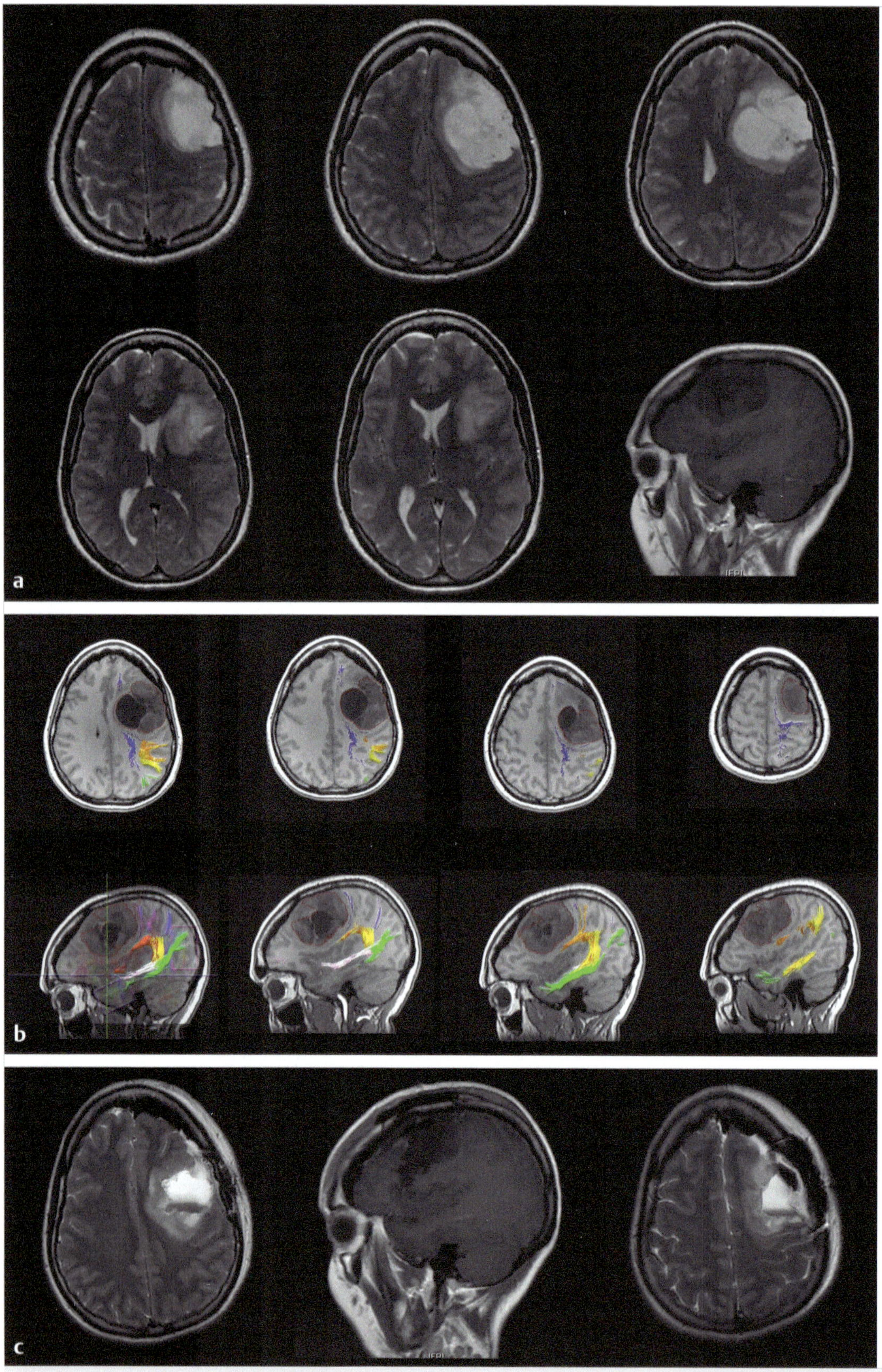

Fig. 10.20 Resection of a lateral frontal glioma which was resected by separation from the language areas posteriorly; (**a**) preoperative images, (**b**) postoperative images, (**c**) long-term follow-up images.

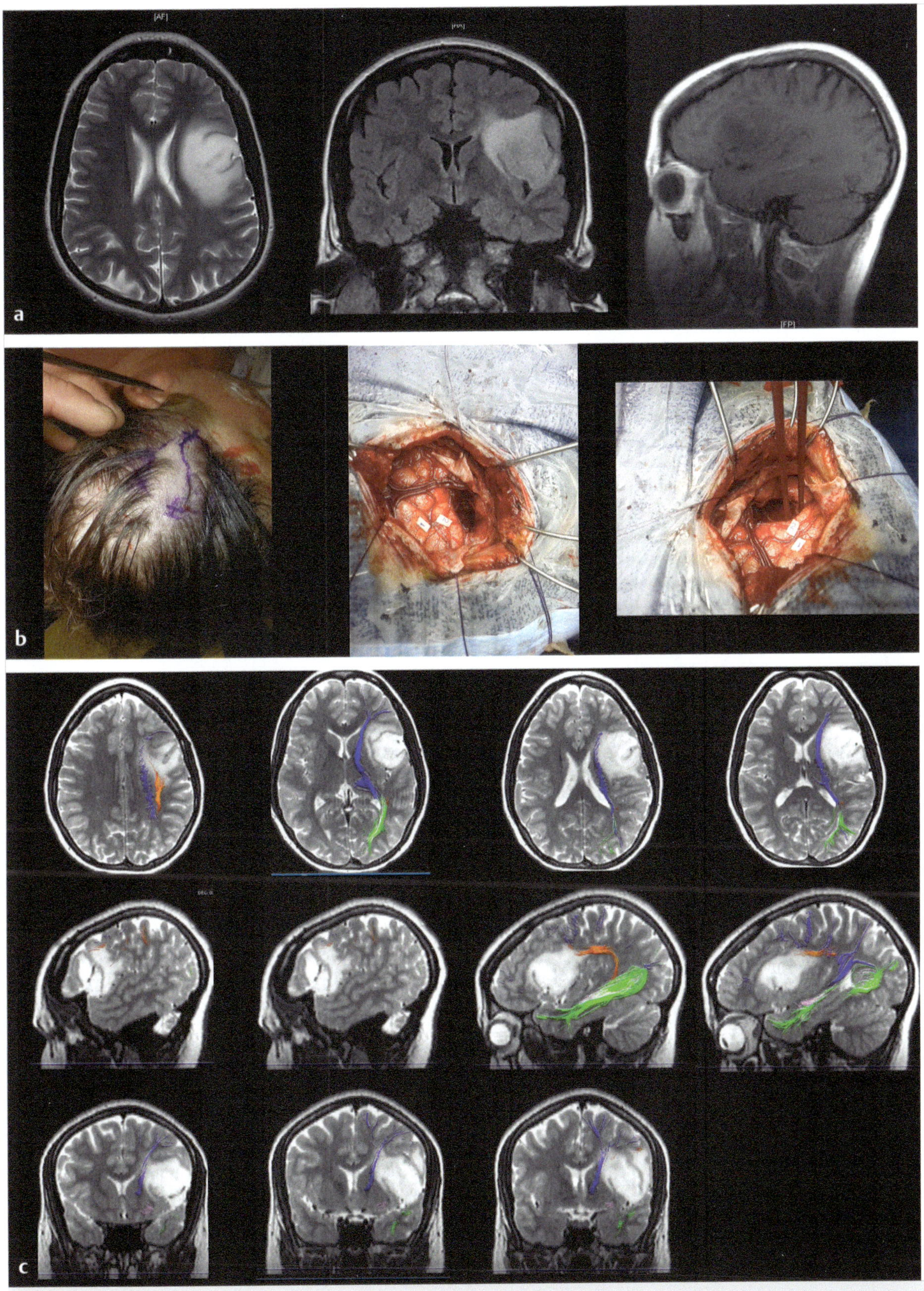

Fig. 10.21 Glioblastoma in a young patient with marked reorganization of the language planning areas enabling an excellent resection of this tumor in Broca's area; (**a**) preoperative images, (**b**) images of the approach, (**c**) DTI tractography. (*Continued*)

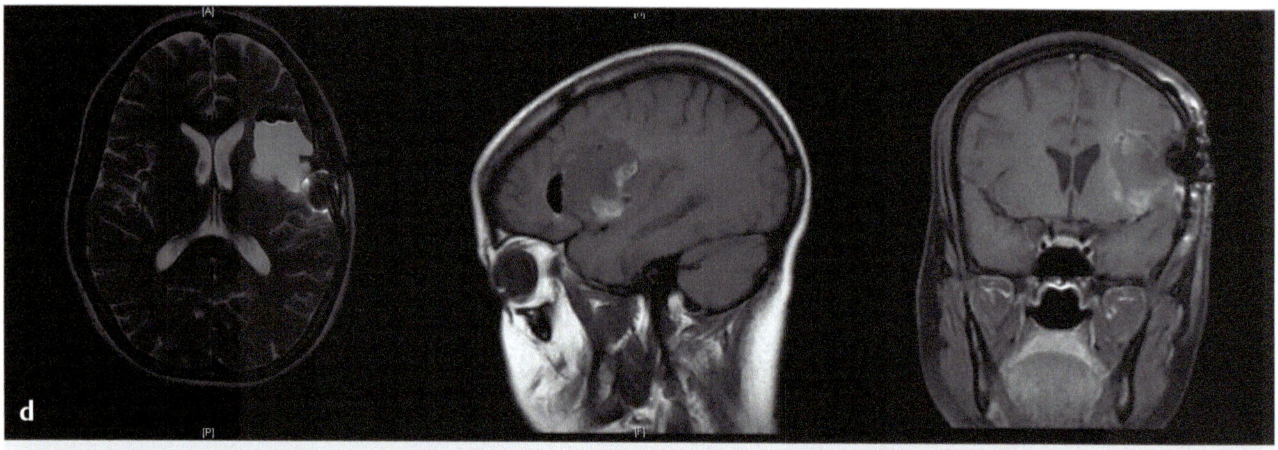

Fig 10.21 (*Continued*) (**d**) Postoperative images.

versus a technical issue with DTI and its ability to resolve fiber tracts in areas of T2 change, the fact that the mapping lined up perfectly with where the tracts come to the surface strongly suggests that the SLF has remapped. Also note that the IFOF is well clear of this tumor provided you remain lateral to the insula (see Chapter 14 where we discuss the use of insular cortex as a "depth gauge" to help stay out of the tracts during frontal opercular tumors.

d) This tumor was completely resected and the patient had completely normal speech throughout the postoperative period. This argues strongly that cortical anatomy predicts function in glioma patients far less reliably than network anatomy.

Limited Frontal Resections

▶ Fig. 10.22 demonstrates a large frontal resection of a glioblastoma which spares the orbitofrontal cortex. The patient was mostly mute and had severe abulia preoperatively; however, we mapped as much as possible given his poor function to permit our cuts with the SLF and FAT systems.

a) This is a massive tumor which fills most of the superior frontal lobe. Despite that, it is critical that we analyze what is not involved. The cingulate gyrus is compressed but not involved (meaning that we should try to spare it). The orbitofrontal cortex is uninvolved and the tumor is not especially close to it. Our goal was to try to spare it as this tumor's nature is probably not to spread to the orbitofrontal cortex which has different connections, mostly backwards towards IFOF, but instead to try to spread posterior into the premotor areas, and towards the other side. These are the connections of this area of the frontal lobe.
b) None.
c) The DTIs quickly point out the cause of his mutism: the FAT is smashed by the tumor and has to make a nearly 180-degree bend to get around it to its target in the motor planning areas (in fact it is in two colors because we had to map it in two parts to find the whole tract). The cingulum could not be resolved at all, not could much of the IFOF in the frontal lobe. This is a challenging case as we do not have much information from mapping (he can't do much) or DTIs (we can't find some of the relevant tracts) to keep us out of trouble. We must always go back to the idea that in these cases, the natural history without intervention is grim, that the tumor is trying to destroy these areas, and that we can only try to make things better.
d) Our resection spared the orbitofrontal cortex and cingulum, and this patient made a fantastic recovery within 2 days to nearly normal. This case highlights the importance of preserving the anatomic continuity of the FAT, but also of being aggressive when things get back. When in doubt, try to take the tumor out.

▶ Fig. 10.23 demonstrates a predominantly cingulate gyrus glioblastoma, and the limited resection through the superior frontal gyrus.

a) The first thought of many on seeing this scan, especially the T2 images in the upper left, is to guess that this is crossing the midline, but careful study shows that it is not. There is SFG overlying this lesion, and the corpus callosum is mostly uninvolved. This is a lesion of the cingulate gyrus. Note that while it is usually wise to stay out of the cingulate if it is uninvolved, it is usually reasonable to do if the tumor has done so, though they may get some abulia from this for a bit (they usually have some mild abulia preoperatively anyway if you ask). Most critical to note is that this tumor underlies the SMA and Motor cortex, and our goal is to remove some SFG as far posterior as the SMA and motor networks will allow us, identify the cingulate sulcus and corpus callosum, and remove everything between them.
b) The approach is similar to a medial frontal resection, with the patient in the lateral, head up position. The cortical resection of the SFG does not need to be especially big, but it does need to be somewhat farther back than is completely easy.
c) The DTIs show that there is some risk laterally with the tumor, but the key risk is obvious when we look at the blue motor fibers. This tumor is surrounded by the motor network. While we need to be aware of this, it also highlights that it is hard to do this case well without some risk to motor function.
d) The resection is good, but particularly informative are looking at the sagittal image This shows how far under the motor system you need to work to get to the back of this tumor.

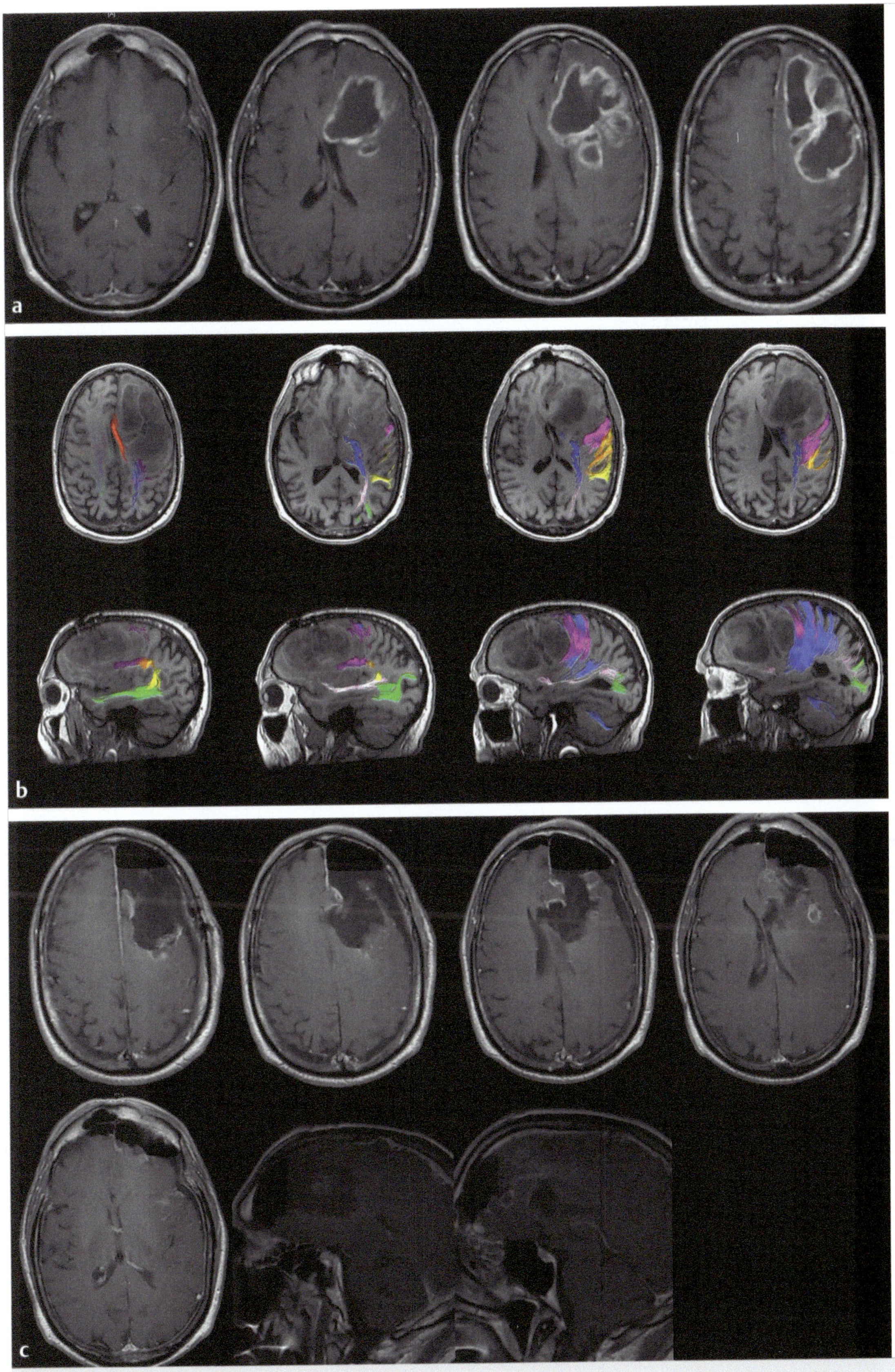

Fig. 10.22 A large frontal resection of a glioblastoma which spares the orbitofrontal cortex. (**a**) Preoperative images, (**b**) DTI tractography, (**c**) postoperative images.

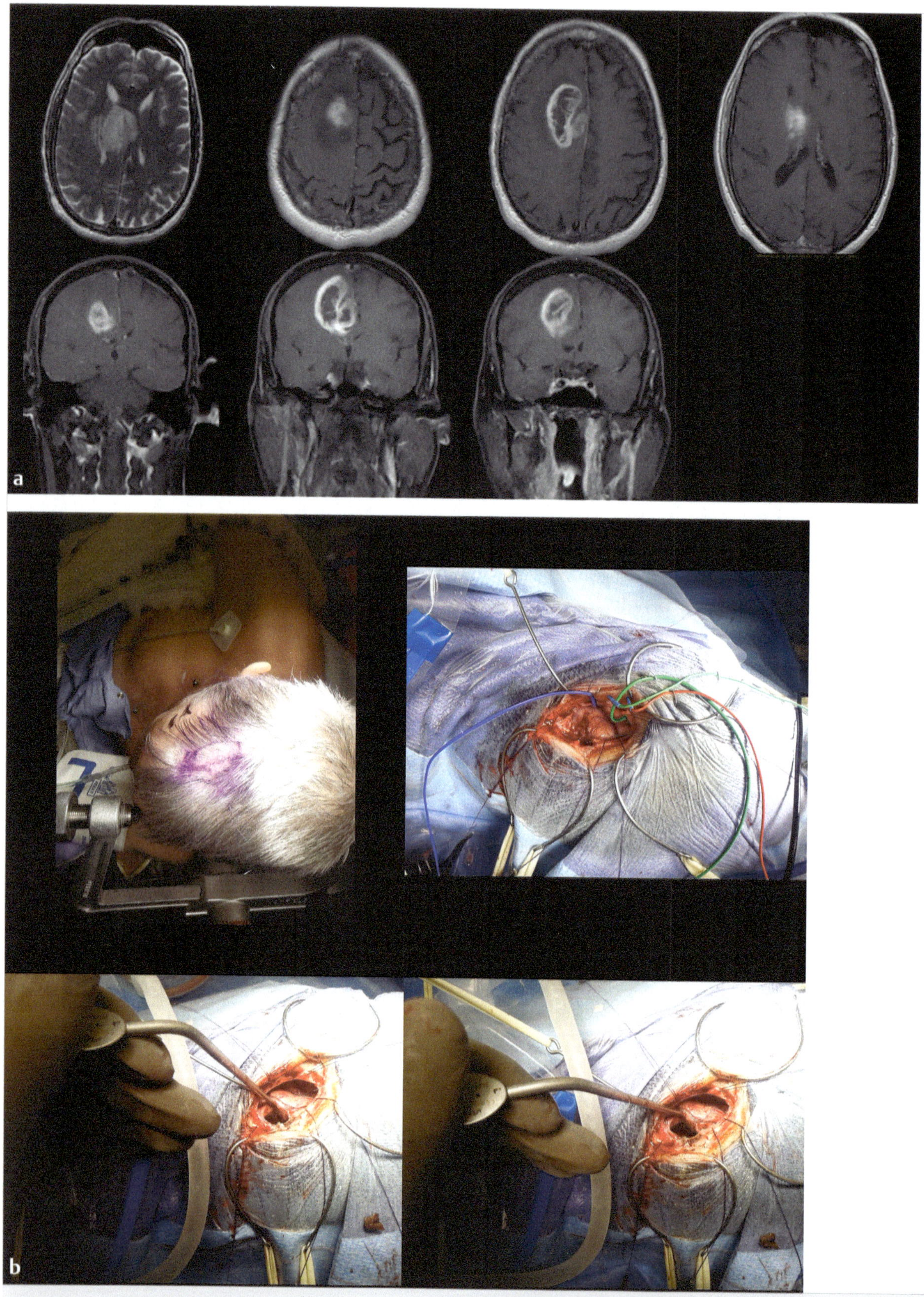

Fig. 10.23 A predominantly cingulate gyrus glioblastoma, and the limited resection through the superior frontal gyrus; (**a**) preoperative images, (**b**) pictures of the approach.

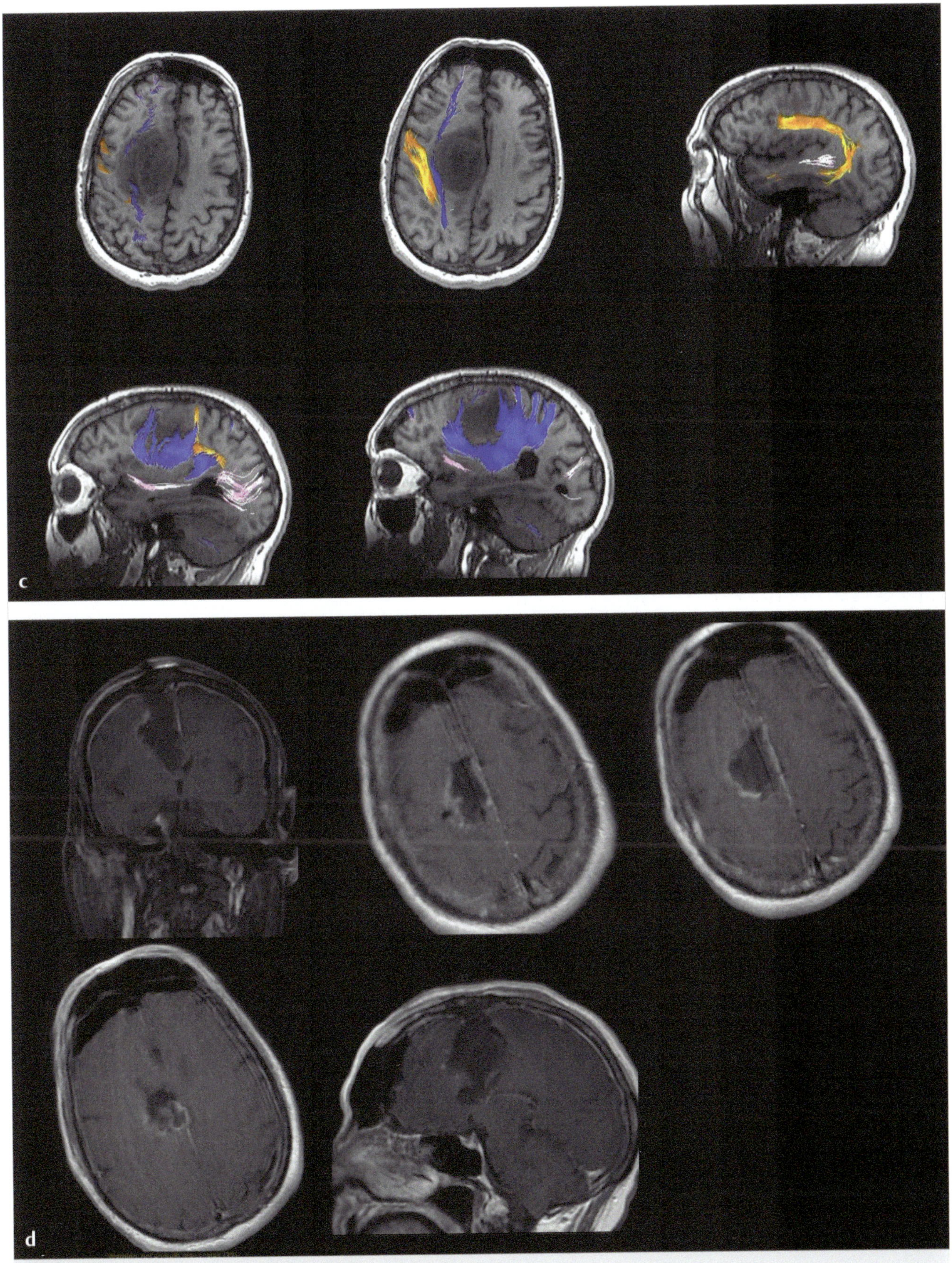

Fig 10.23 (*Continued*) (**c**) DTI tractography, (**d**) postoperative images.

11 Temporal Lobe Gliomas

11.1 The Importance of Temporal Lobe Gliomas

Temporal lobe glioma surgery is the foundation upon which excellence in glioma surgery elsewhere is built. In other words, if you want to be a great glioma surgeon, you need to start by mastering the temporal lobe.

In part this is because these tumors are common and they are defeated early in your learning curve. More saliently, learning the temporal lobe and how to not only stay safe, but also how to ensure a complete, aggressive resection teaches you a great deal about relationships with the rest of the cerebrum. Mastering a temporal lobe resection is mandatory before working in the insula, as the relationship of these two structures is complex, and necessarily intertwined. Further, knowing the anatomy of the temporal lobe provides you with a firm grasp of its relationships with the inferior frontal lobe, the anterior occipital lobe, and the temporoparietooccipital junction. This chapter is early in the sequence, because it's challenging to study the rest of this book without a firm handle on this chapter.

11.2 Overview of Temporal Lobe Anatomy

With two exceptions, the IFOF, and uncinate fasciculus, the white matter connections of the temporal lobe structures run posterior and to some extent superiorly in a "C-shape," which is what one would expect from the brain lobe at the embryologic end of the C-shaped cerebrum. The uncinate largely connects the temporal pole with the orbitofrontal cortex, and both it and the IFOF are largely running into the frontal lobe through the limen insula which is quite anterosuperior to most of the temporal lobe. Thus, most of the temporal lobe fibers are headed backwards to the SLF, the ILF, or the angular or parietal cortices. Thus, a posterior cut in the temporal lobe functionally disconnects most of the temporal lobe.

The most important anatomic observation is that most of key white matter tracts (SLF, IFOF, optic radiations etc) form a lateral system which overlies the atrium and posterior temporal horn. As previous chapters have made clear, the lateral system contains many of the most important connections of the human cerebrum, which comprise the speech, spatiotemporal, and visual networks. Also important is the observation that the medial temporal structures, the amygdala, hippocampus, and parahippocampal gyrus, largely lie in a distinct system medial to the temporal horn. Thus, one can safely follow the medial system using the temporal horn as a landmark, and remove brain structures almost back to the occipital pole, and around the back of the thalamus and brainstem without disturbing the lateral system (▶ Fig. 11.1). Indeed, this concept is the key to temporal lobe glioma surgery.

A few additional gross anatomic relationships are necessary to master for these cases (▶ Fig. 11.2). The STG is purely opercular, meaning that it only overlies the insula and Sylvian fissure. The second is that the insula in normal brains generally extends downward until it parallels the top of MTG. The MTG overlies the temporal horn, which is logical as this is just below the basal ganglia which are deep to the insula. The temporal tip

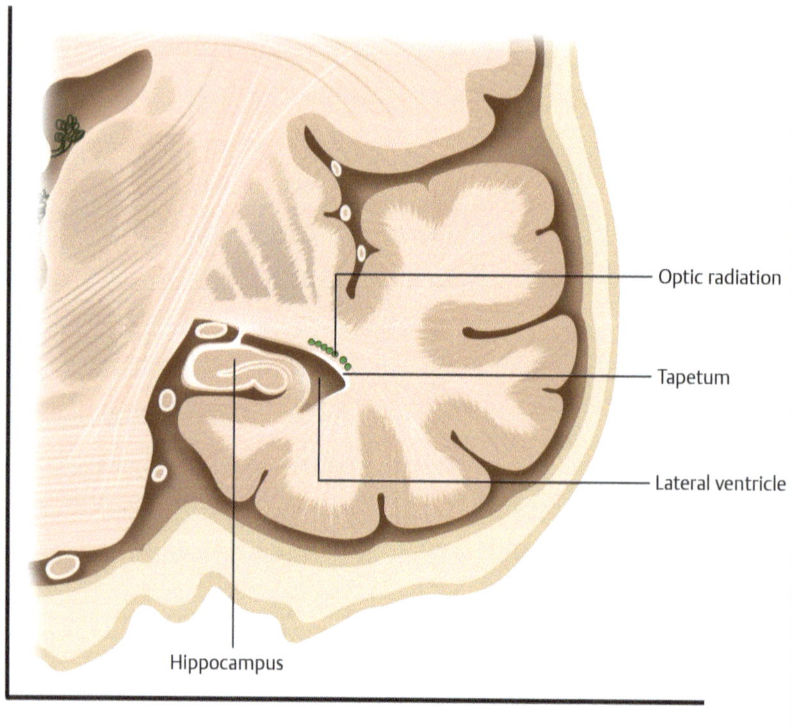

Fig. 11.1 This coronal section through the temporal lobe demonstrates the key relations between the medial temporal structures and the basal ganglia and internal capsule.

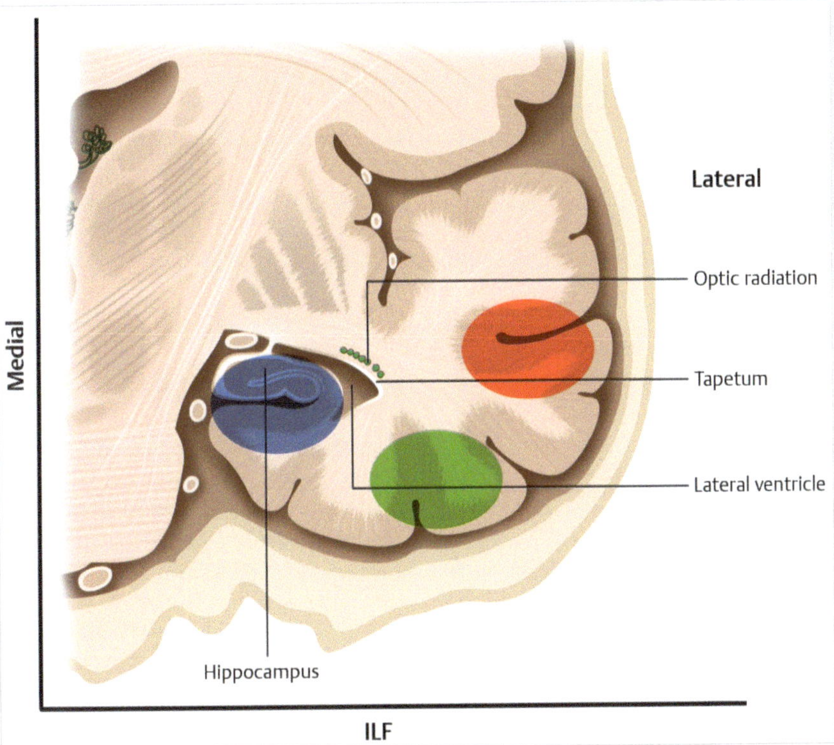

Fig. 11.2 This image depicts the three main systems of fiber pathways running anterior to posterior within the temporal lobe. The medial system involves the hippocampus, fornix, and cingulum. The inferior system involves the ILF. The lateral system involves a number of tracts including the SLF, the IFOF, the optic radiations, and the MdLF. Thinking about temporal tumors logically involves thinking of ways to address a system as relatively separate from other systems.

extends well in front of the limen insula and the uncus; thus you are not at the uncus in a temporal resection until you are behind the clivus, and over the tentorial edge, a common point of confusion for beginners.

Most critically, a firm grasp on the medial temporal structures and their relationships are of utmost importance (▶ Fig. 11.3), as they are commonly involved with tumor, are often distorted and grossly enlarged, and are full of traps for the unwary. The uncus/amygdala is anterior, superior and deep to the tip of the hippocampus, and is essentially always spilling over the edge of the tentorium. The hippocampus is the floor of the temporal horn, but it is not the medial bank of the temporal lobe which abuts the ambient cistern, the parahippocampal gyrus is. The hippocampus sits directly inferior to the putamen, which is perhaps the most important anatomic landmark to store in your memory for glioma surgery. While the fornix enters the atrium to course around the thalamus, the PHG bifurcates to join the isthmus of the cingulate gyrus and the lingula.

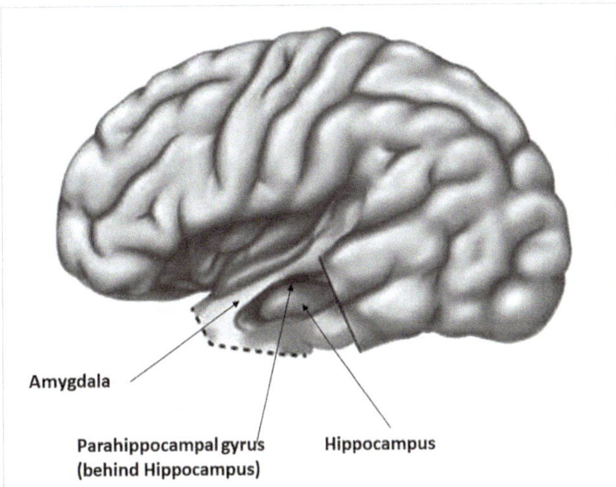

Fig. 11.3 This diagram highlights the relationship between amygdala, the hippocampus, and the parahippocampus gyrus. The hippocampus lies within the temporal horn. The amygdala is anterior, superior, and medial to the tip of the hippocampus. The PHG is largely medial to the hippocampus and abuts the ambient cistern.

11.3 The "Define" Stage

11.3.1 Preoperative Planning

First, put the epilepsy book away. Temporal lobe glioma surgery is foundationally based around the temporal lobectomy, which was first mastered in epilepsy, but glioma surgery is not epilepsy surgery any more than meningioma surgery is. Epilepsy surgery aims to disconnect the epileptic focus from the rest of the neural circuit, and the trend has been to cause this lesion in an increasingly targeted way, such as selective amygdalohippocampectomies, radiosurgery, and more recently laser ablation. This trend not only makes sense from a phenomenological perspective, but also from a goals of care perspective: epilepsy patients are usually not going to die of their disease in a short time frame, and thus minimization of mild cognitive and memory problems makes sense with in this mandate.

While targeted methods and avoidance of mild cognitive problems make sense within that framework, I would argue that they are completely illogical in a disease with a fatal natural history, and that sacrificing tumor resection for attempted preservation of subtle functions usually ends in the long-term effect of accomplishing neither. It makes little sense in performing a trans-Sylvian selective amygydalohippocampectomy for a disease that cannot be accurately defined by the naked eye or imaging, but that we know has spread to the surrounding brain. Glioma is an area of the brain, and not a discrete lesion, and it is foolish to ignore the fundamental nature of this disease and allow tumor to recur in easily expendable brain. Further, a selective amygydalohippocampectomy was mastered for a limited resection of the hippocampus, and not for following the hippocampus to the isthmus and behind the thalamus, which is often necessary to completely remove gliomas extensively following the hippocampus. In short, glioma surgery has different goals, and trying to avoid an overwhelming attack on the tumor, often is not doing the patient a favor.

Temporal lobectomy is the best tolerated lobectomy and is highly effective at guaranteeing an excellent resection (there is no chance of leaving residual disease along the temporal floor after a lobectomy for example). Most cuts on the back of the temporal lobe disconnect the most of the temporal lobe circuits from the rest of the brain anyway, so in most cases it is best to just maximize the amount of tumor cells being removed.

11.3.2 Types of Temporal Lobe Gliomas (▶ Fig. 11.4)

While there can be overlap of these subtypes, especially at more advanced stages of the disease, most temporal gliomas can be classified as one of six principle types.

1. Anterior: These tumors are the most common and are centered within the anterior temporal lobe without major invasion of the SLF. They can spread into the insula via the uncinate fasciculus or into the medial temporal structures.
2. Hippocampal: These are also common, and involve the medial hippocampal structures. Their preference is to follow the Papez circuitry and extend backwards along the forrix into the ventricle, or into the cingulum and isthmus. They can follow the diagonal band of Broca into the basal forebrain and contralateral amygdala, or the ventral amygdalofugal tract into the hypothalamus. They generally do not spread to the lateral system until late stages.
3. Inferior: There are uncommon and are based in the fusiform gyrus and preferentially spread along the ILF into the occipital lobe, though they may invade the medial structures as well. The "pull-through" approaches described in Chapter 16 were designed to address these tumors when they become extensive.
4. Lateral: Thankfully, these tumors are relatively uncommon, but are usually bad news. They invade the lateral system, and preferentially follow the SLF. Many times, very little can be removed due to functional concerns. The hippocampus is generally spared (as we would expect with the lateral vs. medial tract distinction), and I generally try to leave the hippocampus in these cases if it is normal, as the recurrences do not commonly occur there.
5. Junctional: These are the worst of the bunch. They are fundamentally lateral temporal tumors, extend along the junctional anatomy of Hescl's and/or supramarginal gyrus, into the posterior insula and abut the internal capsule. The right-sided ones can be resected with patients, but the left-sided ones are often impossible to make much progress with if they are small and in the SLF or internal capsule. In essence, they combine all the bad parts of a lateral temporal case, with the risk of injuring the back of the internal capsule. Oh, and the arteries at the back of the insula can also be headed to the motor strip, speech areas, or TPO junction.
6. Anterior occipital: These are better classified with occipital lobe tumors, but they can invade the medial temporal lobe, but do so largely behind the SLF, instead of in front of it. I discuss this more with occipital lobe tumors, as the anterior occipital cut is a key part of occipital glioma surgery and these cases fit better in that discussion.

11.3.3 The Approach

Unlike frontal gliomas, the decision is relatively simple as there are two major tracts at risk, the temporal ramus of the SLF, and the IFOF. Further, with the exception of lateral and junctional cases (which are a "surrounded on all sides" type cut), the division will be either a posterior temporal or an anterior occipital cut, depending on the tumor's relationship to the temporal ramus of the SLF. The IFOF is a deeper tract, and while it is critical not to disconnect temporal gyri from this tract during the subcortical work, its exact position does not determine the position of the craniotomy significantly as it is not on the surface.

The craniotomy (▶ Fig. 11.5) is placed over the planned portion of the STG and MTG where I anticipate the SLF and its termini to be based on the DTI. The bone flap is made large enough to be able to move a bit if I find essential parts of the speech network (this movement is almost always anteriorly). I make sure I can reach the "corner of the temporal lobe" (i.e., the part of the STG which intersects with the bridging vein to the sphenoparietal sinus, which is the STG which lies anterior to the limen insula). I also make sure I can reach the temporal floor under the bone flap. There is no need to elevate the entire temporalis muscle and take bone down to the middle fossa floor, as I have never had trouble doing the temporal lobectomy under the bone once the cut is finished.

In anterior, inferior, or hippocampal temporal lobe gliomas, it is almost always smart to drop the tip of the head downwards (▶ Fig. 11.5) as the difficult angles are typically looking from inferior to superior over the patient's shoulder under the Insula or the lateral system, or upward into the atrium. For hippocampal gliomas which extend so far posterior that they are in the atrium, a slight ipsilateral head rotation can be helpful for looking under the lateral system, but this can be disorienting and it is better to achieve this largely by rotating the bed, as opposed to overly rotating the head position from the ideal.

11.3.4 Cortical Mapping

As always I start the mapping with motor, motor planning, and speech arrest, but it is basically a warm up as these functions are not usually found in this part of the brain. I generally do not expose the supra-Sylvian opercula in these cases. Naming and reading are critical here, especially on the left side. I also perform neglect tasks, on either side, but it usually is mostly right sided and localizes to the SLF. These are cases in which we generally find something, and the cortical mapping is usually not negative.

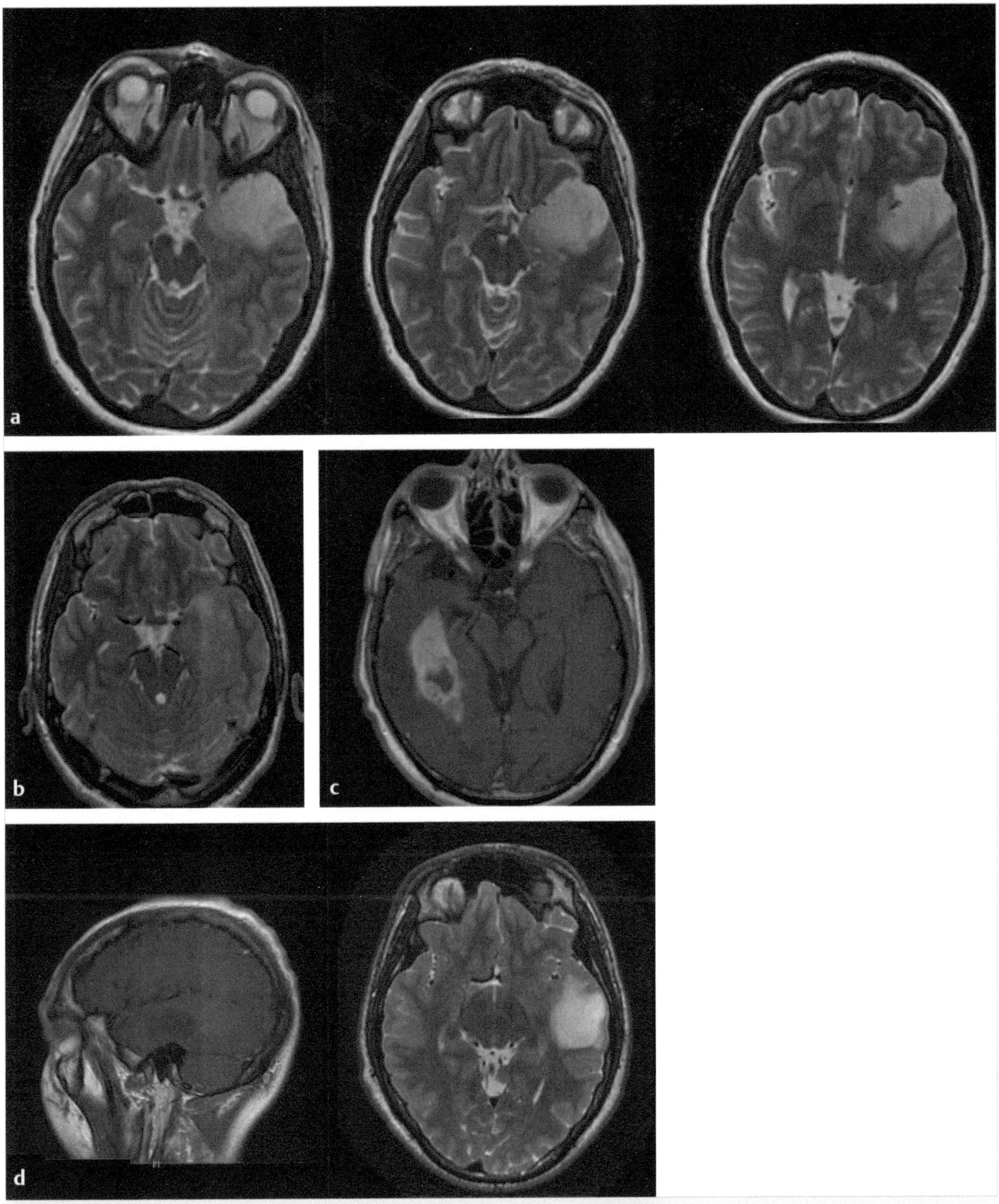

Fig. 11.4 These images demonstrate examples of (**a**) anterior, (**b**) hippocampal, (**c**) inferior, (**d**) lateral. (*Continued*)

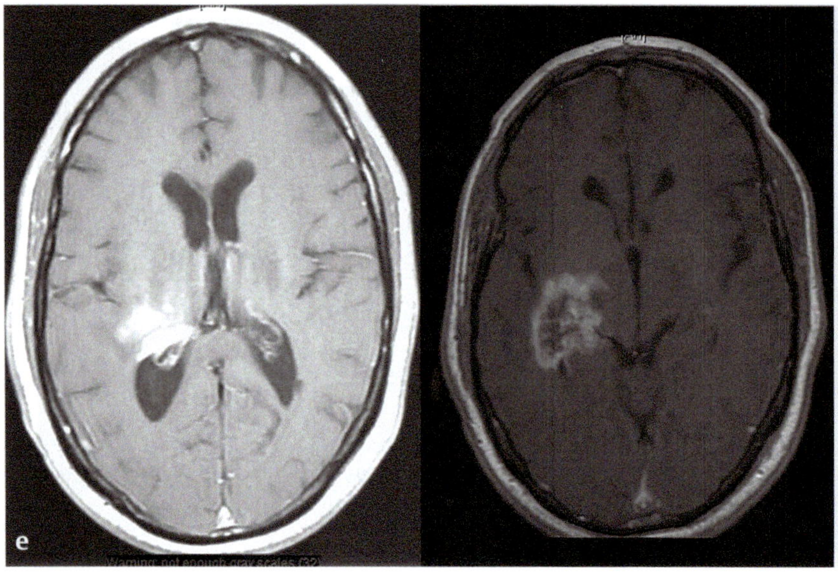

Fig 11.4 (*Continued*) (**e**) Junctional temporal lobe gliomas.

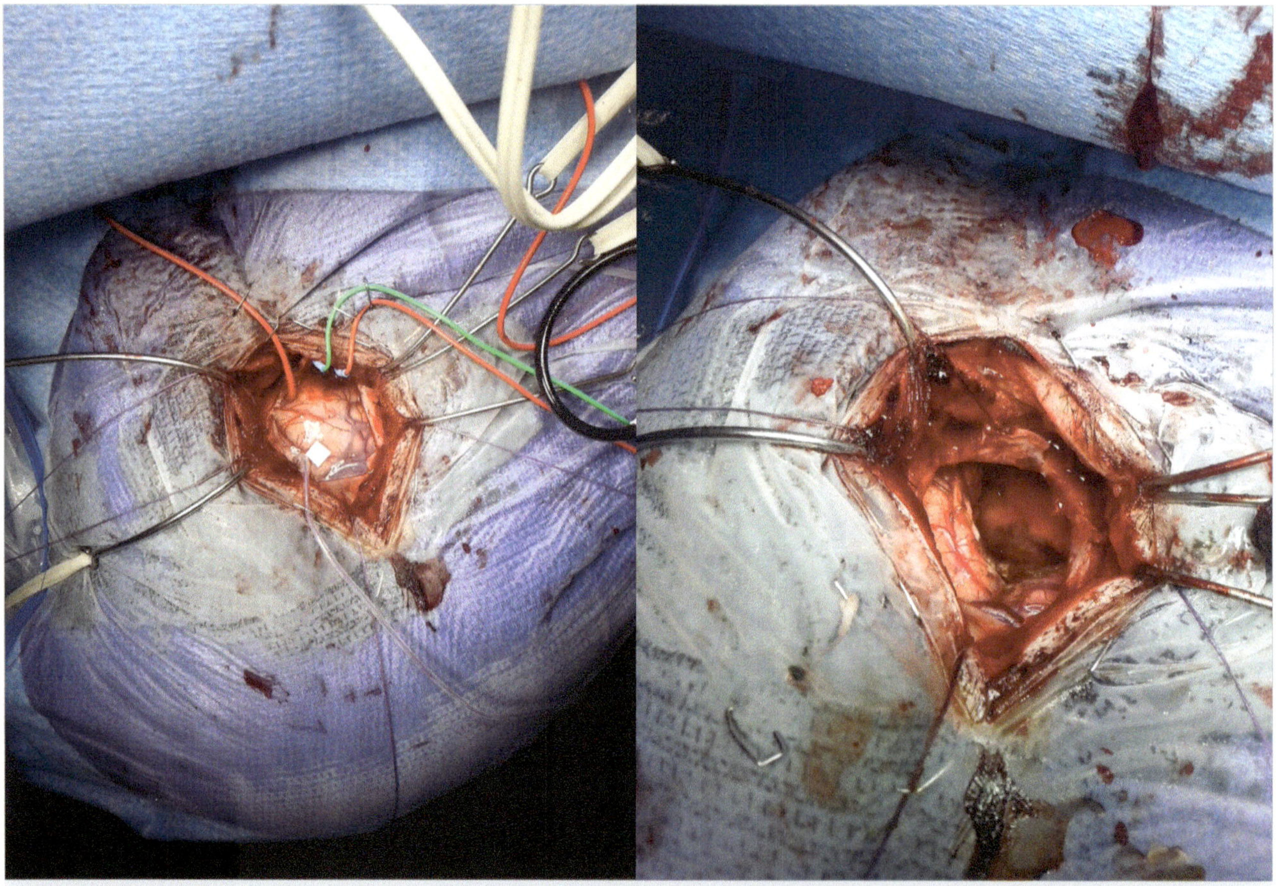

Fig. 11.5 This diagram demonstrates the craniotomy for most temporal lobe glioma surgeries. The cut is planned to separate the temporal lobe from the SLF posteriorly, and to address as much of the STG, and supramarginal gyrus as needed (this is obviously more for lateral and junctional tumors). The craniotomy is centered over this cut, and is made large enough to reach the anterior superior "corner" of the temporal lobe, and the temporal floor. The anterior inferior tip does not need to be exposed.

11.4 The "Divide" Stage

11.4.1 Posterior Temporal Division (▶ Fig. 11.6)

This is an L-shaped cut which seeks to separate the anterior temporal lobe from the SLF, IFOF and the subinsular region using the temporal horn as a landing site. In general, the further posterior the cut is angled posteromedially under the lateral white matter system into the temporal horn, the easier resecting the medial structures will be, which is especially important in extensive hippocampal gliomas, where an inadequately posterior cut can make reaching under the lateral system to reach involved fornix or isthmus impossible (▶ Fig. 11.7). The challenge with putting the cut very posteriorly is you encounter the semantic networks, which on the left are naming sites and the right are neglect sites. The subcortical work involves balancing the need to push the cut backwards, versus the functional need to push the cut anteriorly.

The first order of business with performing this cut is to find the Sylvian fissure and insula by taking down the STG from front to back. If you have mapped the cortex well, then it is safe to remove the STG anterior to any naming sites found, as the STG's output is largely headed posteriorly. It is essential to identify the "artery of death" exiting the posteroinferior fissure and try to manuipulate this as little as humanly possible. A stroke of this artery will often injure the entire semantic network and on the left side this is devastating to language. Taking down the STG first teaches you the orientation of the temporal lobe, shows you where the bottom of the insula is, and frees the temporal lobe anteriorly and superiorly for en bloc removal.

One the STG has been removed, I make the posterior cut. I generally use an arm movement and naming double task for the posterior part of this cut. It is proceeds superior to inferior and it is best to try to find the temporal horn as soon as possible as this tells you where the IFOF is running (always above the horn), and the horn is the anchor that the rest of the cut is based around. I then continue the cut inferiorly until I am close to the temporal floor. At that point, I work in the temporal horn from inside out to extend this cut anteriorly below the insula. Once I am roughly anterior to the limen insula, the temporal lobe is disconnected, and the patient is put to sleep as the work on the middle fossa dura is painful and does not need mapping.

11.4.2 Lateral Temporal and Junctional Disconnections (▶ Fig. 11.8, ▶ Fig. 11.9)

These are challenging the sagittal cut runs from t cases. In lateral cases the disconnection is the entire case, as you are potentially disconnecting on the posterior, inferior, anterior and medial surfaces, with the only safe boundary being the pia of the Sylvian fissure. Here, I stimulate often, work slowly, stay subpial as much as possible, and use sulcal boundaries as thoughtfully as possible. At some point, the subcortical mapping, or concern for a tract on DTI will cause you to stop dissecting deeper, and the lower boundary is arbitrarily defined. Occasionally you can make it to the ventricle in these cases.

Junctional disconnections are more complex as they involve two phases (as do all insular disconnections). The first involves exposing the involved deep structures by resecting STG or SMG as much as possible permitted by the mapping. This is slow and deliberate as there are multiple arteries at risk, including the "artery of death." While the STG is best thought of as a tube sitting on the insula, the SMG is more complex, and can be confusing the first few times you subpially remove it. Essentially it is best thought of as a wide mouthed ice cream cone, with the apex pointing at the back of the insula and the atrium Once you have made the best window into the tumor possible, you

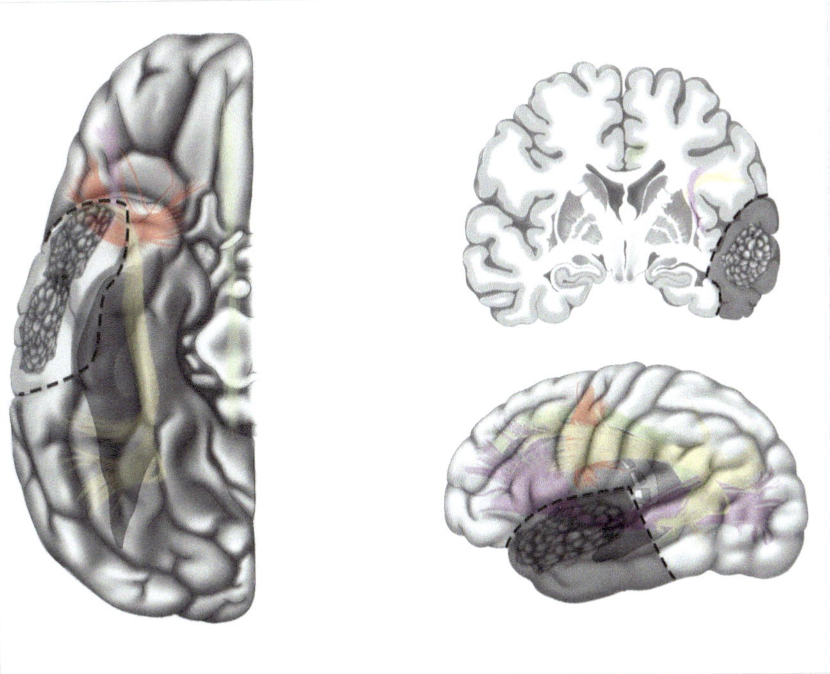

Fig. 11.6 The posterior temporal disconnection is the workhorse of temporal lobe surgery and is depicted here. The cut is an upside down L-shaped cut, with its principle limbs paralleling the STG, and dividing the back of the temporal lobe from superior to inferior. The principle landing site for these cuts are the temporal horn and the middle fossa floor. First, the STG is removed subpially from front to back to identify the insula, to identify and free the arteries, and to get an idea of the exact orientation of the temporal pole. This subpialization continues into the "corner," i.e., the anterior superior part of the STG which lies in front of the limen insula. Following this, the temporal horn is located by cutting the MTG and beginning the posterior limb just inferior to the location of the posteroinferior insula. Once this is opened, this opening is continued anterior to posterior along its length to clear the tumor from the IFOF from back to front. Finally the posterior cut is continued until it roughly reaches the temporal floor and is down to the depth of the temporal horn. At this point, the SLF is clear, and the disconnection is complete.

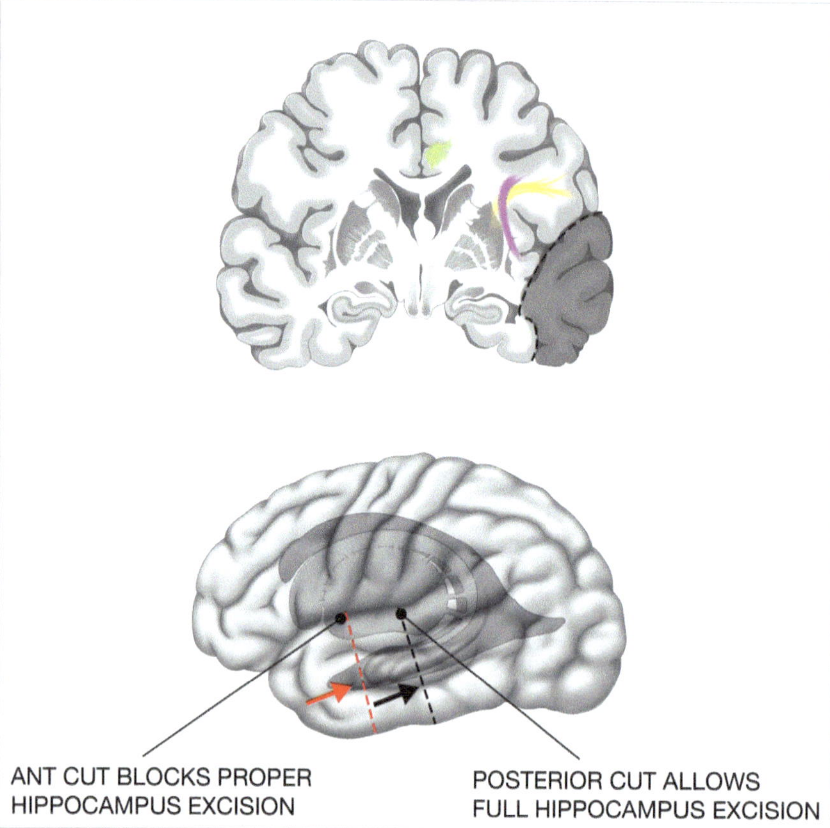

Fig. 11.7 This diagram demonstrates the importance of placing the posterior temporal disconnection as far posteriorly as possible in a case with substantially posterior hippocampal involvement. The goal in hippocampal gliomas is to reach under the lateral white matter network to remove the medial temporal structures underneath them. If you do not get the cut as far back as possible, the lateral system will limit access to the posterior medial temporal structures, and make it difficult to reach into the atrium.

should identify the surface of the insula (which may be small this far posteriorly, and if possible enter the atrium, which provides excellent orientation to this area (most of these patients already have field cuts and even if they don't it is unlikely you will avoid it and still take a tumor like this out). In some cases, a lesser version of a posterior temporal cut, or even a temporal lobectomy may be warranted based on the anatomy. One you reach the deep part of the work, it is wise to switch your mapping to monitoring the leg, as this is what is at greatest risk.

I usually do not stop the subcortical mapping for these cases until the tumor work is done.

11.5 The "Destroy" Stage

11.5.1 The en Bloc Anterior Temporal Lobectomy (▶ Fig. 11.10)

Most temporal gliomas of the type which have an asleep portion (i.e., the anterior, hippocampal, and inferior), can be best managed with a temporal lobectomy. Usually an amygdalohippocampectomy is indicated as well as these patients usually have some medial temporal lobe involvement, often have seizures, and medial temporal lobe involvement gives the tumor access to an effective path to distant places including the other side of the brain.

If you have performed the cuts described above, then the remainder of the temporal lobectomy can be done in a few minutes. This involves a lazy "c" shaped cut along the inferior temporal lobe and pia, which extends from the part of STG abutting the anterior Sylvian fissure, continues anterior to posteriorly along the temporal floor running just lateral to the hippocampus then hooking laterally parallel to the superficial parts of the posterior temporal cut until the cut joins the inferior portion of the cut, after which the bridging veins are cut, and the lobe is removed in one large piece. This typically takes me about 10–15 minutes in a virgin case.

The first steps of developing the anterior-superior part of the cut take a bit of subpial dissection and sacrifice of the anterior temporal artery, until you clearly see the sphenoid wing and Sylvian fissure. It is essential to define the "corner" as otherwise it is easy to leave tumor up there which is not connected to the rest of the brain. The rest of the resection flows from this quite easily.

11.5.2 The Medial Temporal Structures (▶ Fig. 11.11, ▶ Fig. 11.12, ▶ Fig. 11.13, ▶ Fig. 11.14)

I always save the hippocampus for last as this is the key orienting landmark for the rest of the medial structures. The uncus, hippocampus and, PHG should be removed subpially to prevent injury to the cisternal structures, but in most cases (the exceptions being large radiated high-grade gliomas with a large uncus where you should be more careful, as discussed in Chapters 2 and 17), in a glioma case this requires much more persistence than an epilepsy case. In hippocampal tumors especially, the uncus can be quite large, as can the hippocampus, and this requires you to keep going with the resection until you

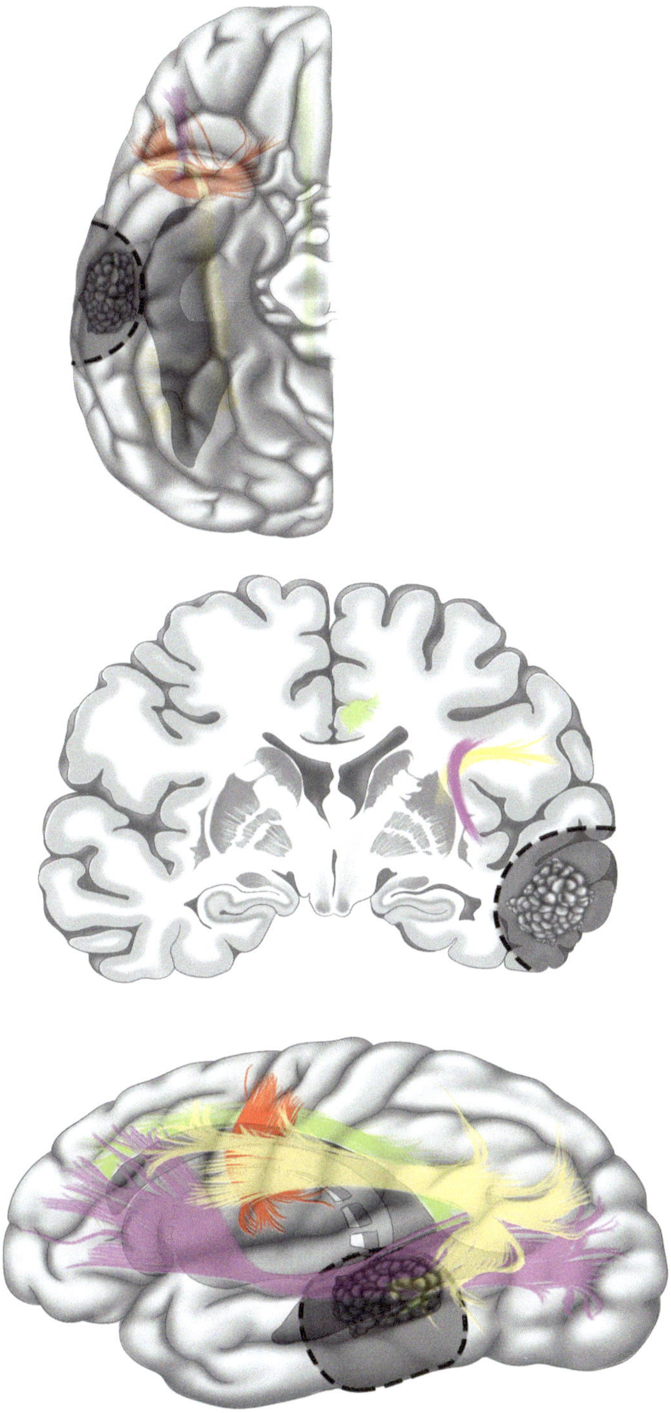

Fig. 11.8 Schematic demonstrating a lateral temporal disconnection. Tumors of the lateral system involve finding the SLF and sematic network, and slowly trimming tumor from the front or back of the networks as tolerated by mapping.

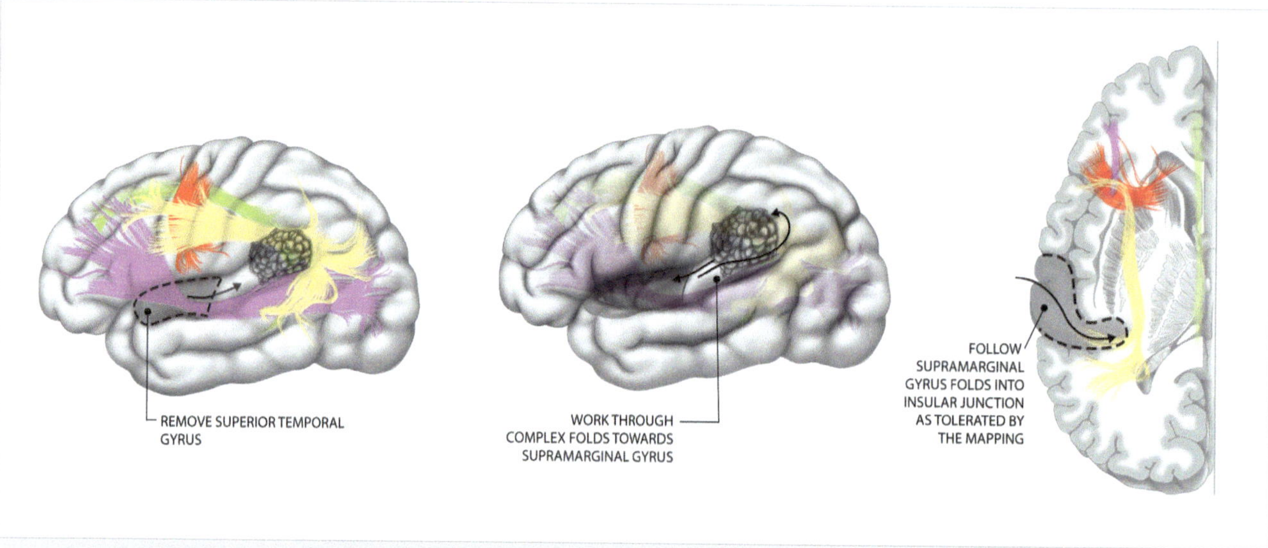

Fig. 11.9 Junctional tumors of the temporal lobe present the difficult challenge of not only involving the lateral networks, but also following the fibers of the SMG into the deeper structures which puts the posterior internal capsule and basal ganglia at risk. The disconnection proceeds in two phases, similar to an insular glioma. In the first phase a lateral disconnection is performed to remove as much of the STG and SMG as tolerated by the mapping. Note that the subpialization in this area is very complex and patience is key. The second phase involves, following the tumor into the back of the insula and resecting this as tolerated.

have clearly seen the boundaries of the structure, otherwise you are likely to be disappointed by your resection.

Subpialization is a fundamental aspect of safe glioma surgery, especially in the medial temporal lobe, and this is a major reason I do not use ultrasonic aspirators. It involves gentle repeated suctioning on the surface to pull the brain out from under the pia. It is unwise to bipolar extensively on the pia as the heat can conduct through and injure arteries and nerves below the pia, but occasional light bipolar bursts can loosen up the brain and allow it to suck away from the pia. You should resist the urge to use the bipolar to stop artery bleeds in this area, however.

The uncus should be resected first as it shows you the depth of the medial pial bank and defines the tentorial incisura for you. Subpialization continues until you see four major boundaries (1) the inferior sulcus: which lies on the tentorial edge and is encountered first, 2) the anterior sulcus, 3) the posterior sulcus: which is just in front of the hippocampus, and the 4) superior sulcus: above which is the optic tract and internal capsule. You should also be able to see the third nerve and the ICA, and usually the PCA through the pial bank by this pointin the resection, and it should cause you to rethink your completeness of resection if you can't see them. Being able to see this high under the insula is a major reason one should tip the head downward for these cases. No matter how uncomfortable it makes you to continue resecting a large uncus, if you have not seen your landmarks, there is still uncus remaining.

When working posteriorly, it is critical to know whether the tumor follows the fornix, the cingulum, or neither. If the tumor is following the fornix into the atrium and around the thalamus, I remove the hippocampus first and follow this into the atrium and address this part first, as it prevents disorientation. It is important to pad the lateral tract system when you do this, as you are retracting and working underneath them. Following the temporal horn back into the atrium along the plane of the hippocampus allows you to remain in the correct and safe angle. You generally know when you have cleared the atrium when the cyst of the atrial choroid plexus descends. This can be a challenging angle, and is impossible if the temporal lobe is still in place, or the posterior temporal cut cannot be made far enough posteriorly due to functional anatomy.

Once the hippocampus is removed, everything remaining directly medial to the resection cavity is PHG. This can be removed by following the pia backwards from the uncus until the side of the brainstem is visible though the ambient cistern. This will eventually take you behind the midbrain at the isthmus if you keep following it and it is possible to go much further in some cases.

Finally, it is important to preserve arteries deep to the tentorial incisura, but there are many arteries crossing the incisura at right angles to supply the hippocampus, PHG etc. These are always sacrificable once their identity as such is clear, as they are supplying brain you are removing. Even the anterior choroidal is no longer sacred once it turns laterally to enter the ventricle, as it is just a choroidal artery at that point. It is best to deal with these arteries before they avulse off their more important parent arteries in the cistern.

11.6 Example Cases

11.6.1 Anterior and Hippocampal Tumors

▸ Fig. 11.14 demonstrates a prototypical anterior temporal glioma. The cut was placed along the posterior temporal lobe and the craniotomy is centered. A temporal lobectomy was performed.

a) This is a repeat surgery for a GBM which was partially resected previously. The majority of this tumor is anterior

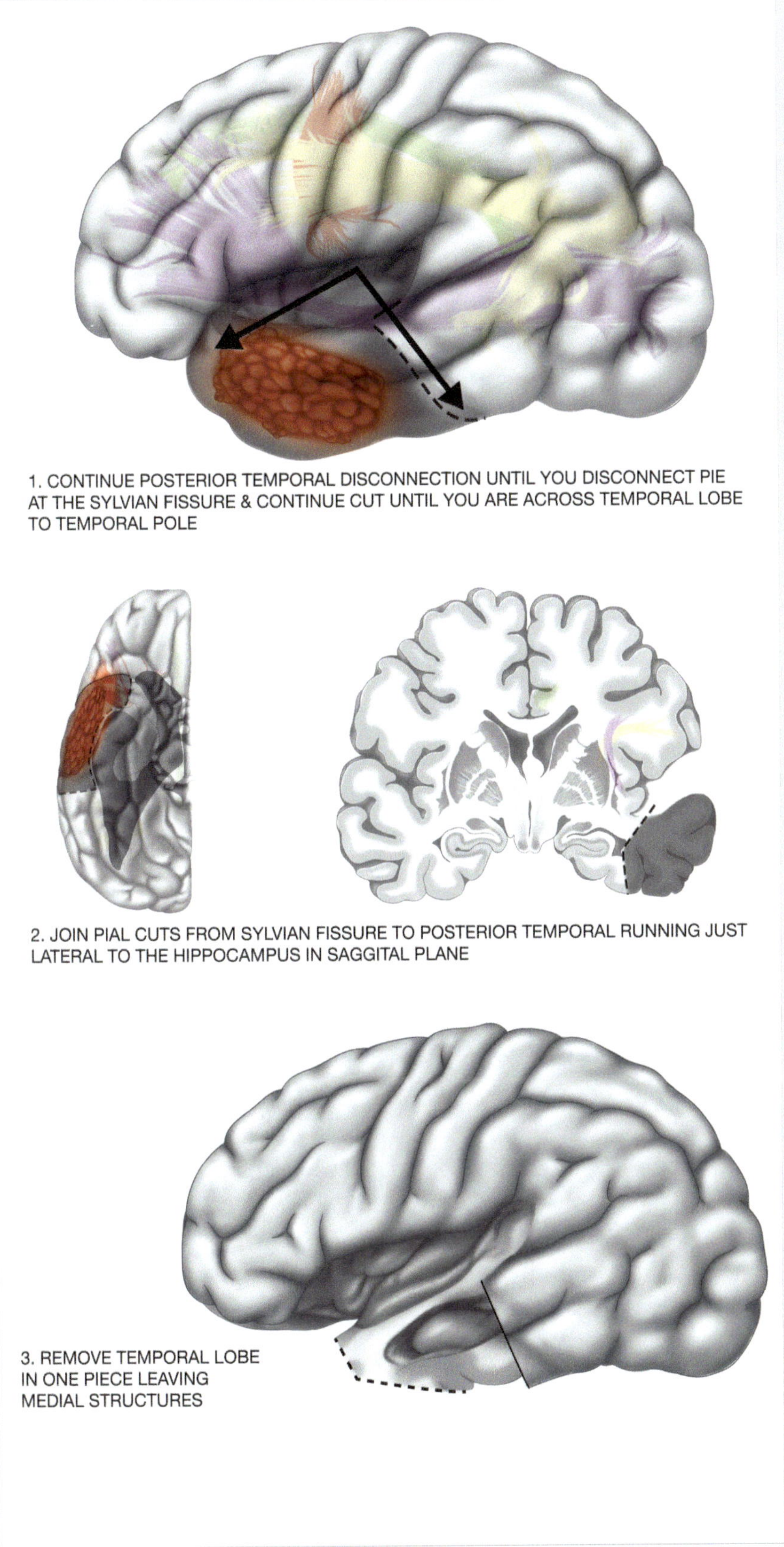

Fig. 11.10 Steps of an "en-bloc" temporal lobectomy. The rationale for an en-bloc resection of the temporal lobe has nothing to do with oncologic benefit (as with en-bloc resections for other cancers), but instead its benefit is that it is faster, more complete, and I would argue, safer, than the traditional method of trying to subpialize your way from lateral to medial until you encounter the uncus. Once the disconnection is complete, the brain is subpialized from the anterior-superior corner, and the pia is cut and divided just below the sphenoid wing. The pial cut continues from anterior to posterolateral running just lateral to the hippocampus until it curves laterally to join the posterior limb of the disconnection. The temporal pole is then folded inward and the bridging veins are sacrificed and the lobe is removed in one piece.

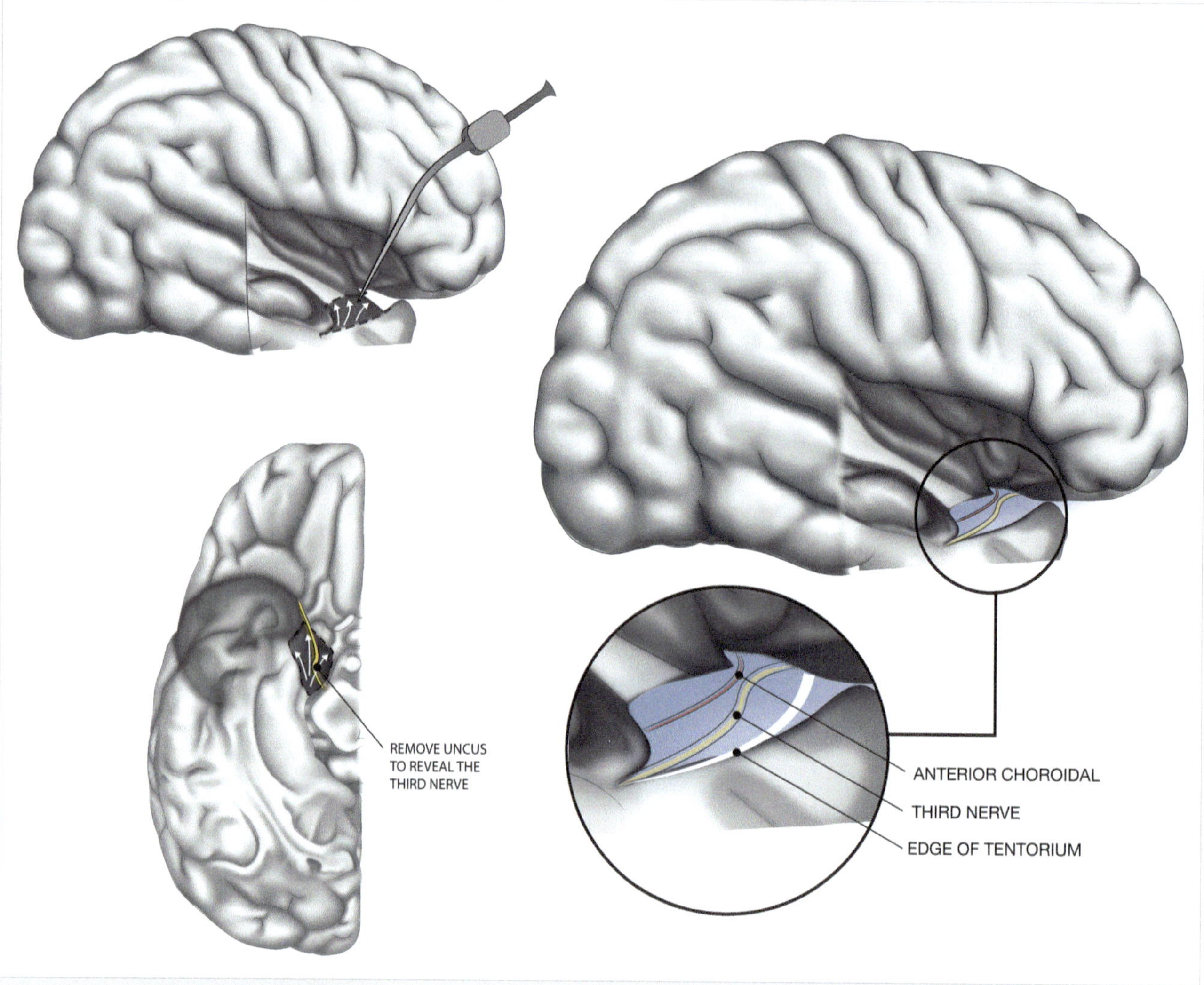

Fig. 11.11 Removal of the uncus. The uncus is identified as the tissue lying just anterior, superior and medial to the hippocampus, which extruded over the tentorial incisura. The uncus should be removed subpially, and this should continue until you visualize all four sulcal boundaries of the uncus, and until the third nerve and carotid are visualized through the pial bank.

temporal though some spread into the atrium can be observed. The fact that the enhancement extends to the floor of the middle fossa raises the possibility that the tumor might invade or be stuck to the dura and it was in this case.

b) The craniotomy is small and focused on the posterior temporal lobe, namely MTG and STG. The large incision from the previous craniotomy is incorporated to a limited extent.

c) None.

d) The resection is good. There is a small amount of blood visible in the region of the hippocampus and uncus, and this is due to my cautiousness with stopping bleeding in this area, especially in repeat, radiated GBM cases.

▶ Fig. 11.15 demonstrates a GBM predominantly sitting within the temporal horn extending backwards. A posterior temporal cut was performed in order to reach backwards into the posterior temporal horn and to take a marginal resection around this tumor with temporal lobectomy.

a) This GBM has an unusual appearance and is in a patient with familial adenomatous polyposis, which first raised the possibility that it was a metastasis. In appears to be sitting in the temporal horn. This raises the point of what do you do when the diagnosis is in doubt. You certainly do not want to do temporal lobectomy for a metastasis, or worse a non-neoplastic diagnosis like multiple sclerosis. At the same time, it would be best to complete most of these patient's surgery in one stage, and not biopsy all likely gliomas at a separate first surgery, just to avoid the uncommon GBM mimic. Doing a needle biopsy for this tumor additionally risks intraventricular hemorrhage. I negotiate this balance by performing awake surgery on all patients who I think might have or likely have a glioma. I perform a frozen section guided by the DTIs and send this specimen before the cortical mapping begins. This allows us to back out prior to irreversible steps, other than the biopsy have been performed and using the DTIs minimizes the risk of entering eloquent brain prior to mapping it; however, in cases where all possible paths into the tumor could pass through an eloquent brain, I will wait until I have completed the cortical mapping prior to taking the biopsy and will sit and wait for the results.

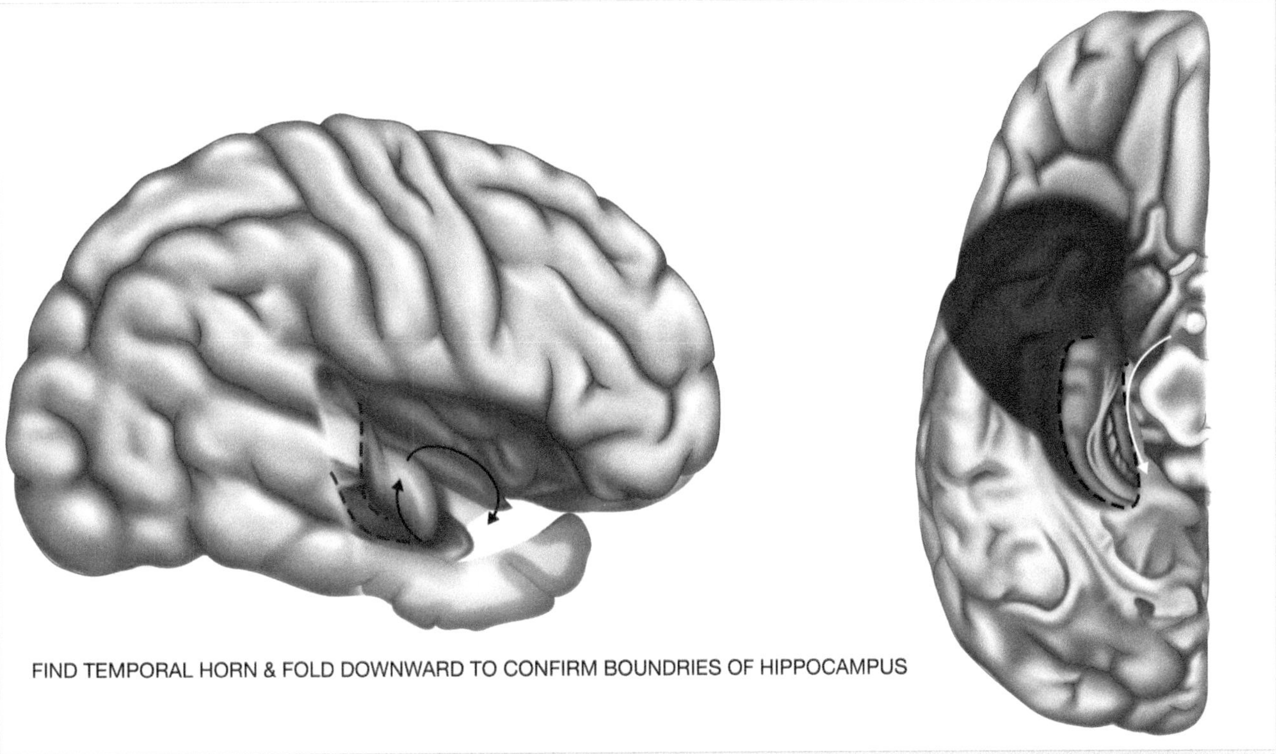

Fig. 11.12 Removal of the hippocampus. This step is always done last, as the hippocampus is an excellent landmark. It is essential to continue to work until you clearly see the ependymal boundaries of the hippocampus within the temporal horn, as the hippocampus can be massive in these cases. After removing the hippocampus, further subpialization over the edge of the tentorium will remove the parahippocampal gyrus as far back as needed, until the edge of the brainstem is visible through the pia.

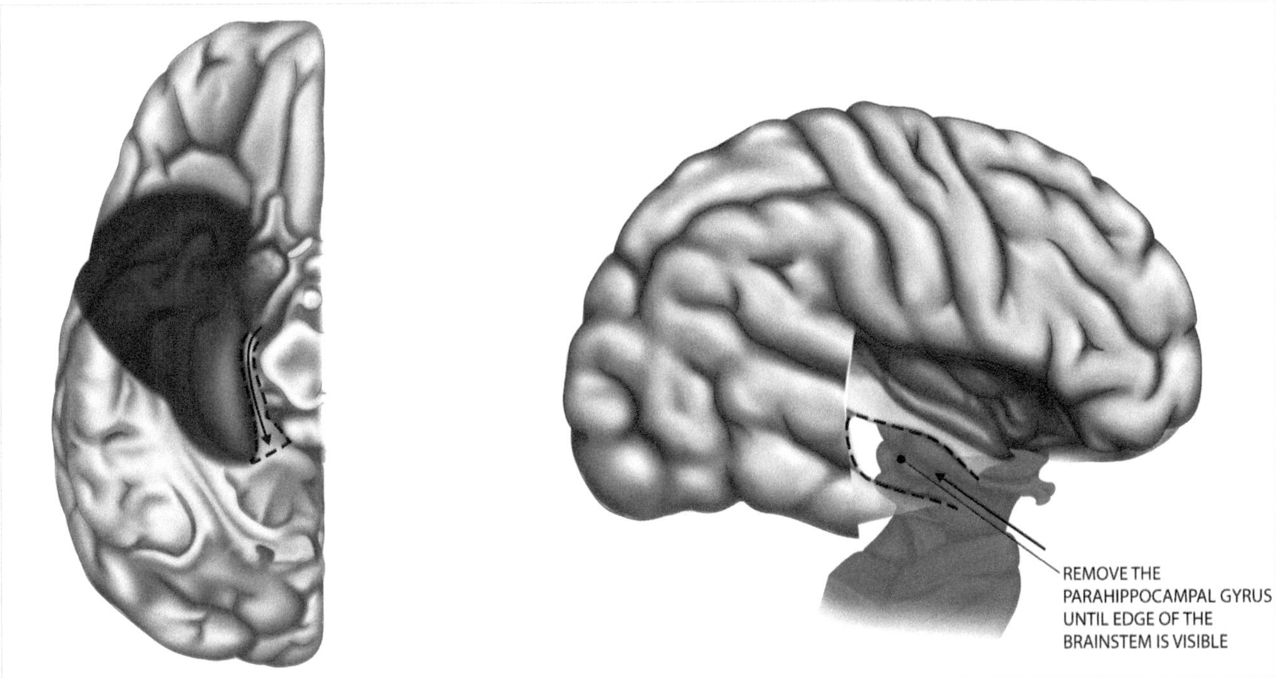

Fig. 11.13 The removal of the parahippocampal gyrus.

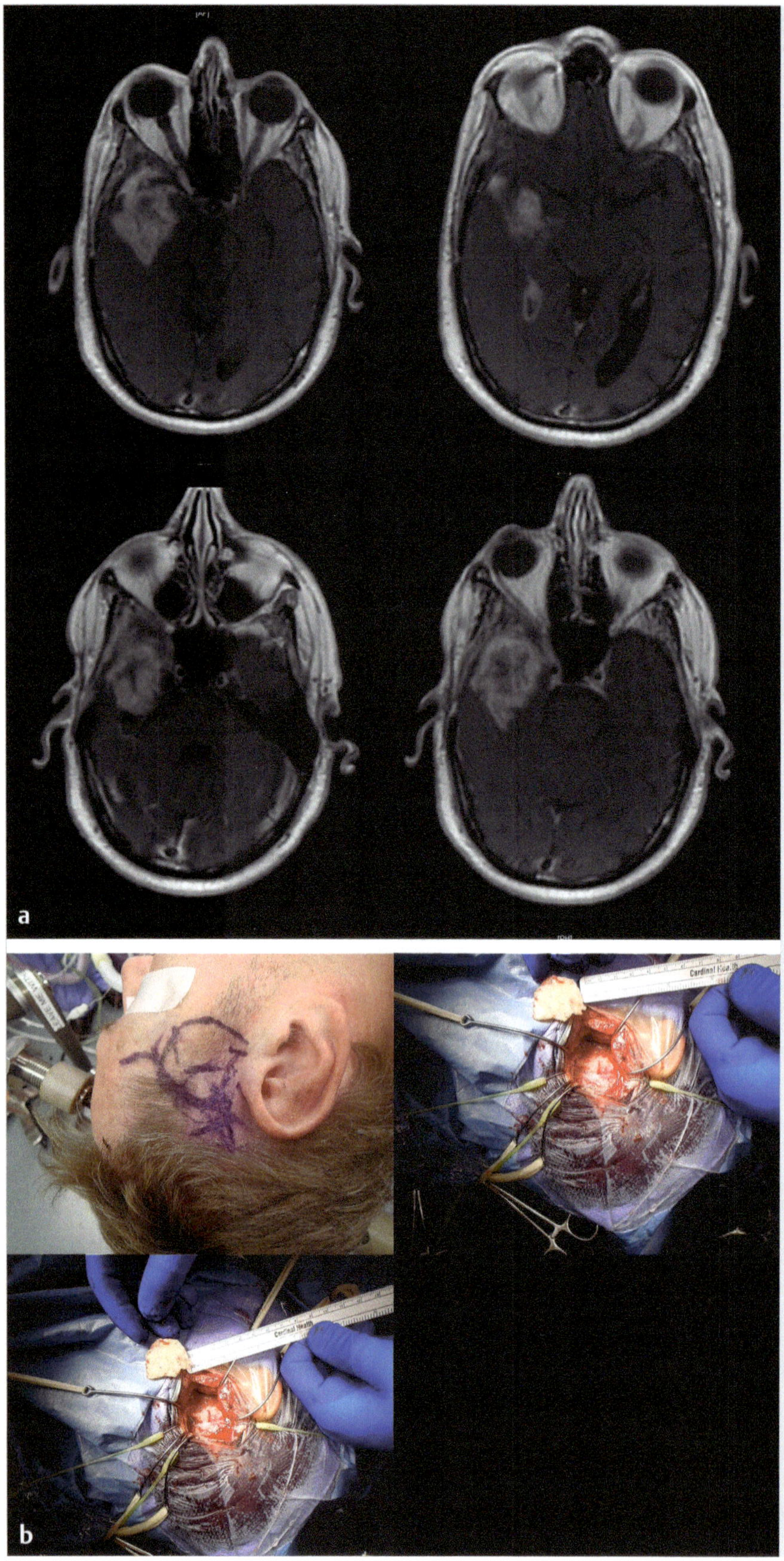

Fig. 11.14 A prototypical anterior temporal glioma. The cut was placed along the posterior temporal lobe and the craniotomy is centered. (**a**) Preoperative images, (**b**) images of the approach.

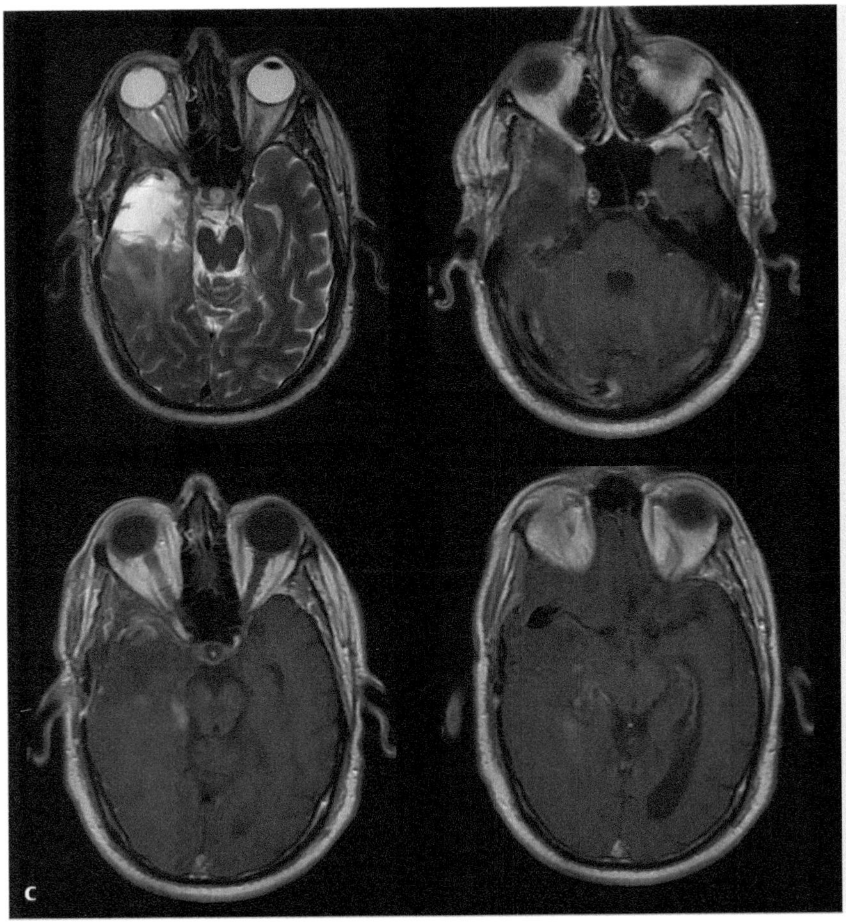

Fig 11.14 *(Continued)* (**c**) Postoperative images.

Notably, I have only had the frozen section be revised in two of the previous 500-plus cases I have approached with this strategy (both were lymphomas and neither patient was hurt). I have only once had to abort a surgery I approached using this protocol (an old infarct in a young patient), though I have found several metastases, which caused be to alter our approach to a non-anatomic type lesionectomy surgery.

a) None.

b) None.

c) The resection is good. Of note this patient did well for about 2 years. He then developed a small spot of new enhancement in the junctional white matter. I was hesitant to operate there and was talked into radiosurgery as the benefit of this small amount of cytoreduction was probably outweighed by the risk of operating in the junctional white matter. MR perfusion and SPECT suggested recurrent tumor. This expanded dramatically in about 2 months after radiosurgery, and he lost some speech function and control of his leg. We re-operated at that point, and this was all radiation necrosis. Eventually, despite avastin, the radiation necrosis continued to expand and cost him his life. While we cannot prove that the initial spot was radition necrosis, this case provides a serious caution towards treating repeat gliomas with radiation without tissue. Advanced imaging presently cannot reliably differentiate them, and treating radiation necrosis with more radiation can be devastating.

▶ Fig. 11.16 demonstrates a large right hippocampal glioma in a patient who presented unable to walk. This is a common presentation of hippocampal gliomas when they become large and this is probably due to superior compression of the descending motor pathways running over the top of the temporal horn. We made our posterior temporal cut as far posteriorly as possible as this hippocampus was large, and we needed to reach posteriorly under the lateral white matter system as far back as possible to ensure we could reach all of this tumor. The critical step in a case like this with a massively enlarged hippocampus is that you need to visualize the ependymal surface to ensure you are removing all of the medial structures. You are likely to be disappointed if you don't.

This patient began walking again shortly after surgery and made an excellent recovery.

a) The key to figuring out that this is a hippocampal glioma is to look at the coronal images. The axial images can give you the false impression that this tumor is invading the internal capsule, and in a patient with a weak leg and unable to walk, this can seem like it all fits. But the coronal clearly shows that this tumor in principally in the hippocampus, that the deep structures are pushed upward, and not likely invaded (there is no clear connecting path of spread between the hippocampus and the internal capsule as gliomas generally spread via white matter tracts and not by crossing fissures, sulci, or ventricles). Invasion of the internal capsule is more of a tendency of junctional and lateral type temporal gliomas, highlighting the fact that they are different white matter systems.

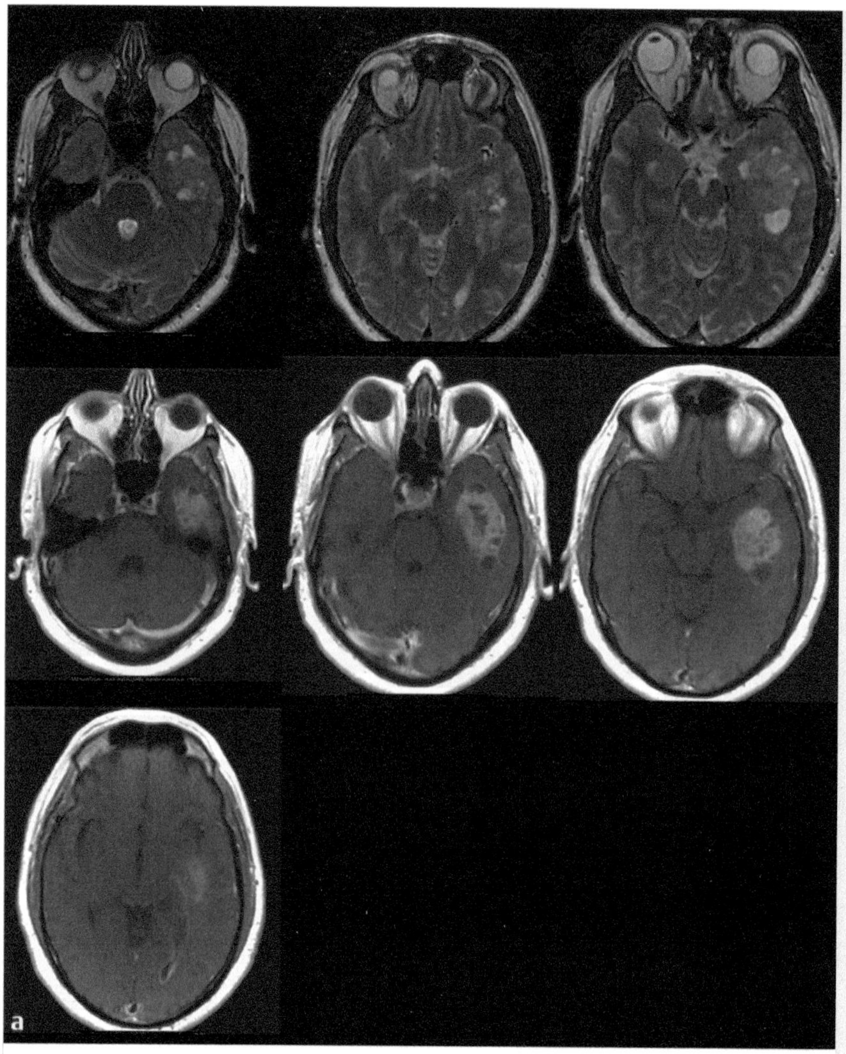

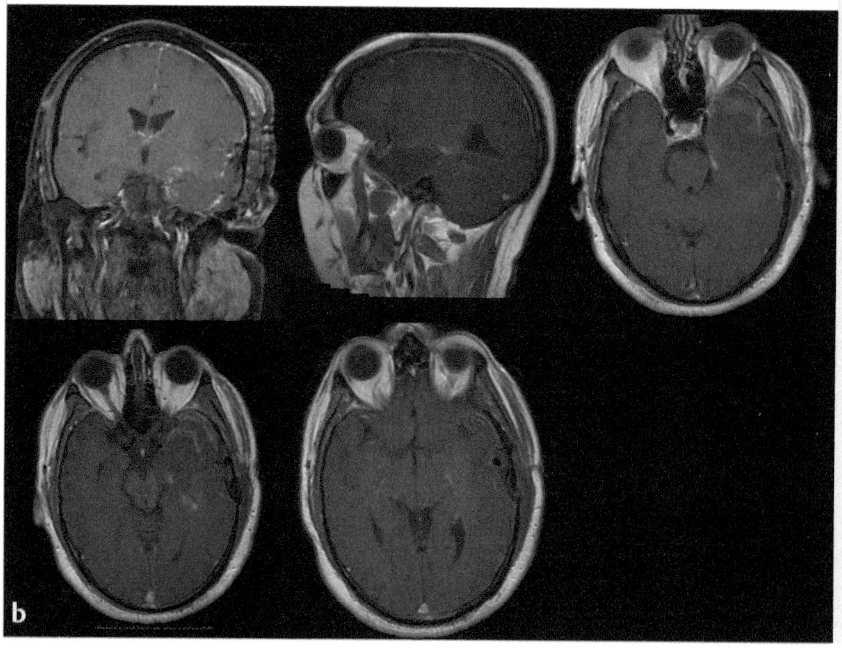

Fig. 11.15 A GBM predominantly sitting within the temporal horn extending backwards; (**a**) preoperative images, (**b**) postoperative images.

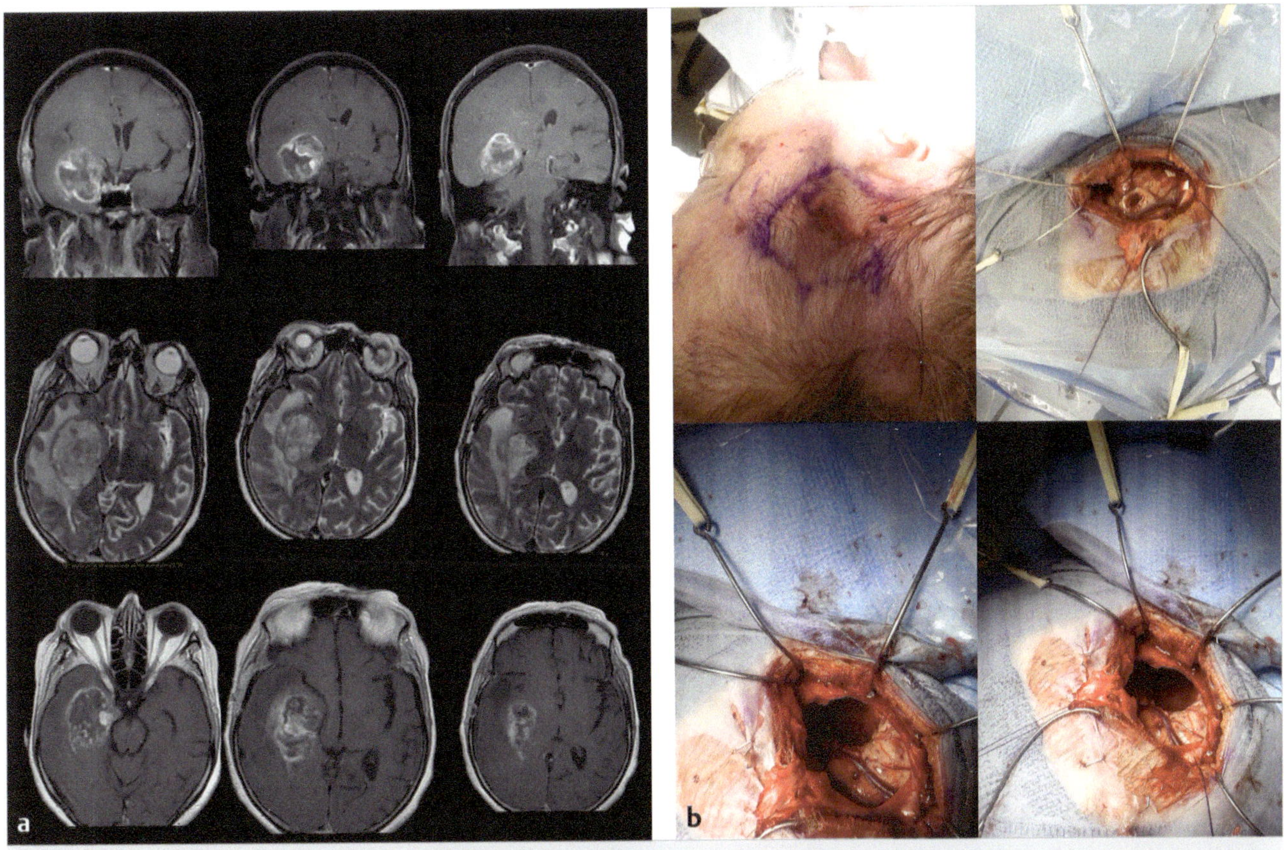

Fig. 11.16 A large right hippocampal glioma in a patient who presented unable to walk. (**a**) Preoperative images, (**b**) images of the approach. *(Continued)*

b) A keyhole brain mapping approach is slightly bigger than the smallest possible approach, as you need more room to maneuver, especially if you find positive sites in the middle of the field. Using DTIs to plan the case can make this unpleasant event somewhat less common, but you need to be ready for it. We have found that a slight S-shaped incision can greatly increase the cortical exposure, without meaningfully lengthening the incision, or compromising the vascular supply in the way a question mark incision will.

The biopsy is obtained through the anterior MTG can be seen. Two small white squares indicate sites of neglect measured on target cancellation which line up with the SLF on DTI.

a) The first thing notable here is that the internal capsule and descending motor fibers are completely uninvolved, which confirms that this is a hippocampal tumor. The SLF is displayed relatively posterior to the best posterior cut needed. This may be due to edema from the tumor, but it is promising.
b) Note after complete resection the capsule has descended in the coronal plane. I expect these patients to recover significant function very quickly after surgery for hippocampal gliomas.

▶ Fig. 11.17 demonstrates an extensive left hippocampal tumor which follows the fornix into the atrium of the lateral ventricle. This was initially sent to us as a thalamic tumor, but close inspection reveals that this is not in the thalamus, but instead is in the fornix and is sitting on the thalamus. Part of this should be obvious given the absence of direct connections between the thalamus and the hippocampus and the absence of tumor in the junctional temporal lobe (which can spread to the deep structures and para-thalamic regions.

How far posteriorly you can follow a tumor like this is entirely dependent on the anatomy of the lateral white matter system, especially the positions of the SLF and the IFOF, which in turn determine where your cut can go and how far posteriorly you can reach underneath them to access the lateral system. In this case, we were able to follow this fairly posteriorly into the atrium. Gradient postoperative images show blood products in the tumor posterior to the thalamus, thus demonstrating how far up it is possible to reach with a good posterior cut and a temporal lobectomy.

a) When this case was sent to see me, it was described to me as a thalamic tumor extending into the temporal lobe. It is only possible to conclude this if you think of the enhancement as the only thing that matters in these tumors. This is really a very big hippocampal glioma which has followed the fornix and is now is wrapped around the back of the thalamus. This is a challenging case, as it requires us to perform as posterior of a cut as the speech networks will allow, but it is not a thalamic glioma.
b) I made the opening slightly larger than other cases as I am performing this cases as a "definitely in" type case. By this I mean I plan on having speech areas in the field, finding them,

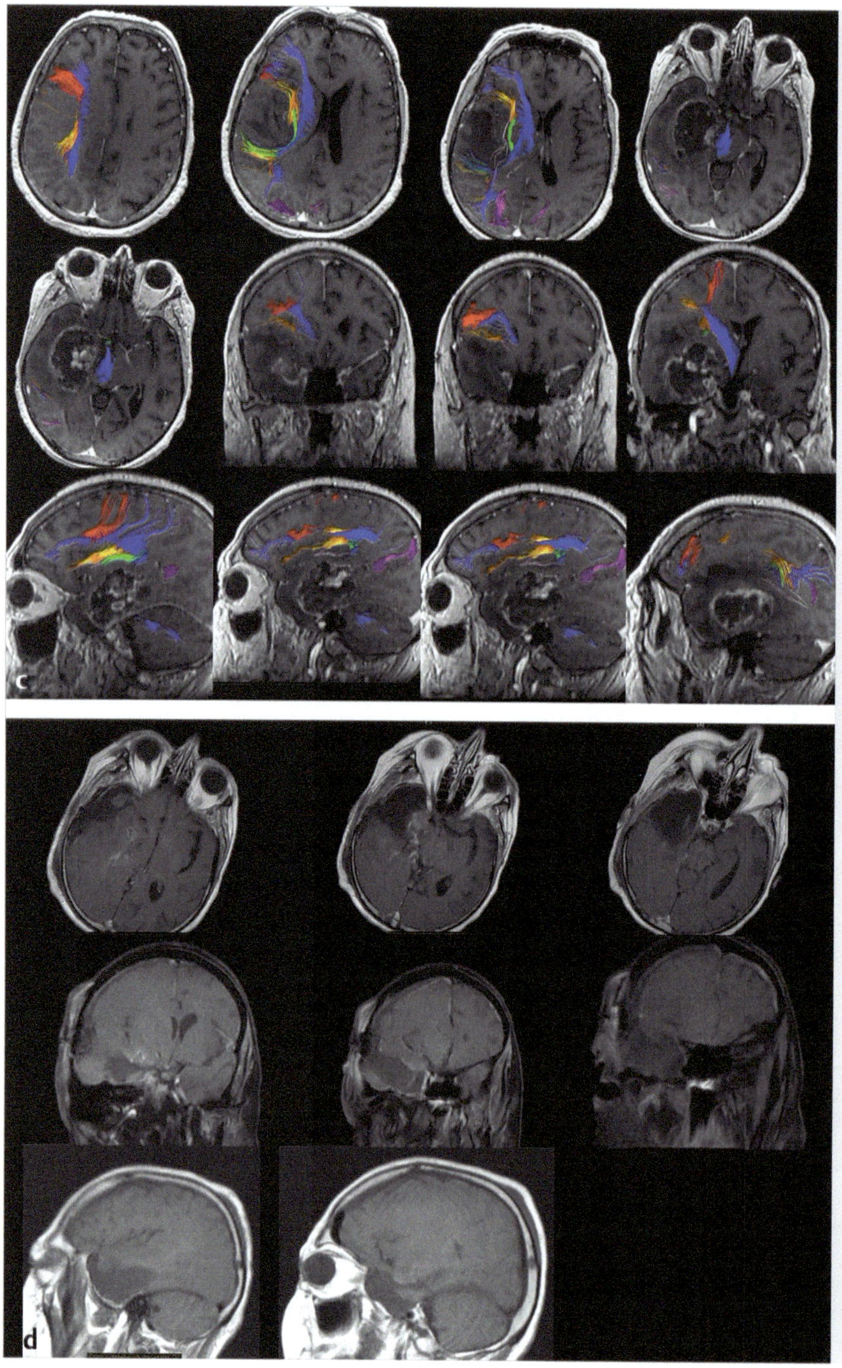

Fig 11.16 *(Continued)* (**c**) DTI tractography, (**d**) postoperative images.

and cutting right next to them. For more anterior temporal gliomas, I prefer not having speech areas in the field if this is possible. Note that we found a naming site and cut just anterior to it. What the final images fail to demonstrate is that the cut works posteriorly underneath the speech network quite a bit. The final cut entered the ventricle at the atrium, which requires patient subcortical work to spare the speech network.

c) A few things are notable. First, the SLF and IFOF seem to converge at a promising posterior point and the speech networks do not seem to head very anteriorly into the temporal lobe. Eventually, the IFOF will limit our access to the atrium, but I expect to be able to get a fairly posterior cut from these DTIs. Additionally, the optic radiations are at serious risk in this case, as we will have to reach quite a bit under them to get into the atrium.

d) Note on the sagittal postoperative images how well the posterior aspect of this cut lines up with the predictions of the DTIs. I was able to debulk the enhancement in the highest reaches of this tumor, but could not get high enough to safely visualize and remove all of the enhancement. Otherwise, this is an excellent resection of this tumor.

▶ Fig. 11.18 demonstrates a giant holotemporal low grade glioma. The craniotomy needs to be tailored to account for this.

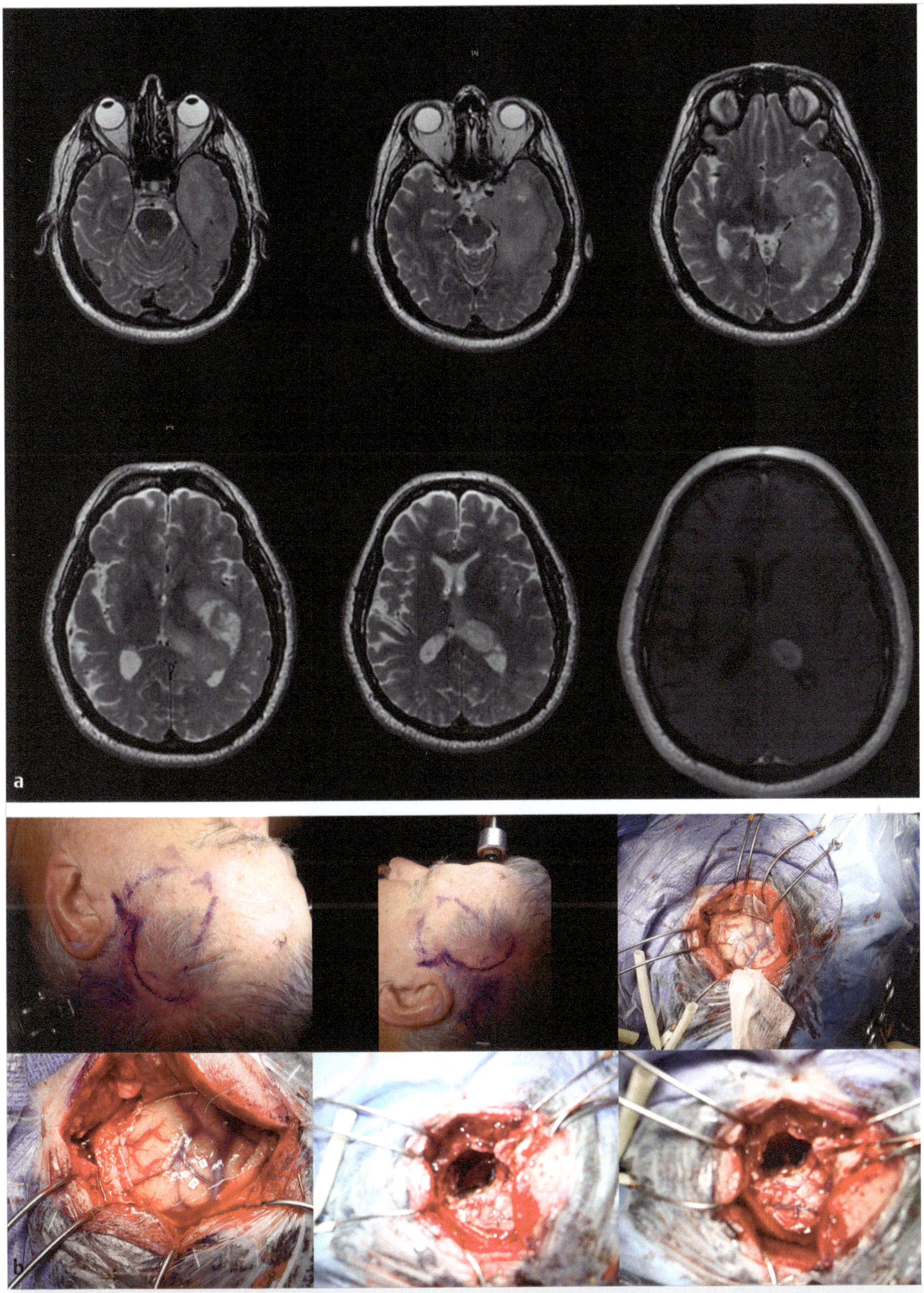

Fig. 11.17 An extensive left hippocampal tumor which follows the fornix into the atrium of the lateral ventricle; (**a**) preoperative images, (**b**) images of the approach. (*Continued*)

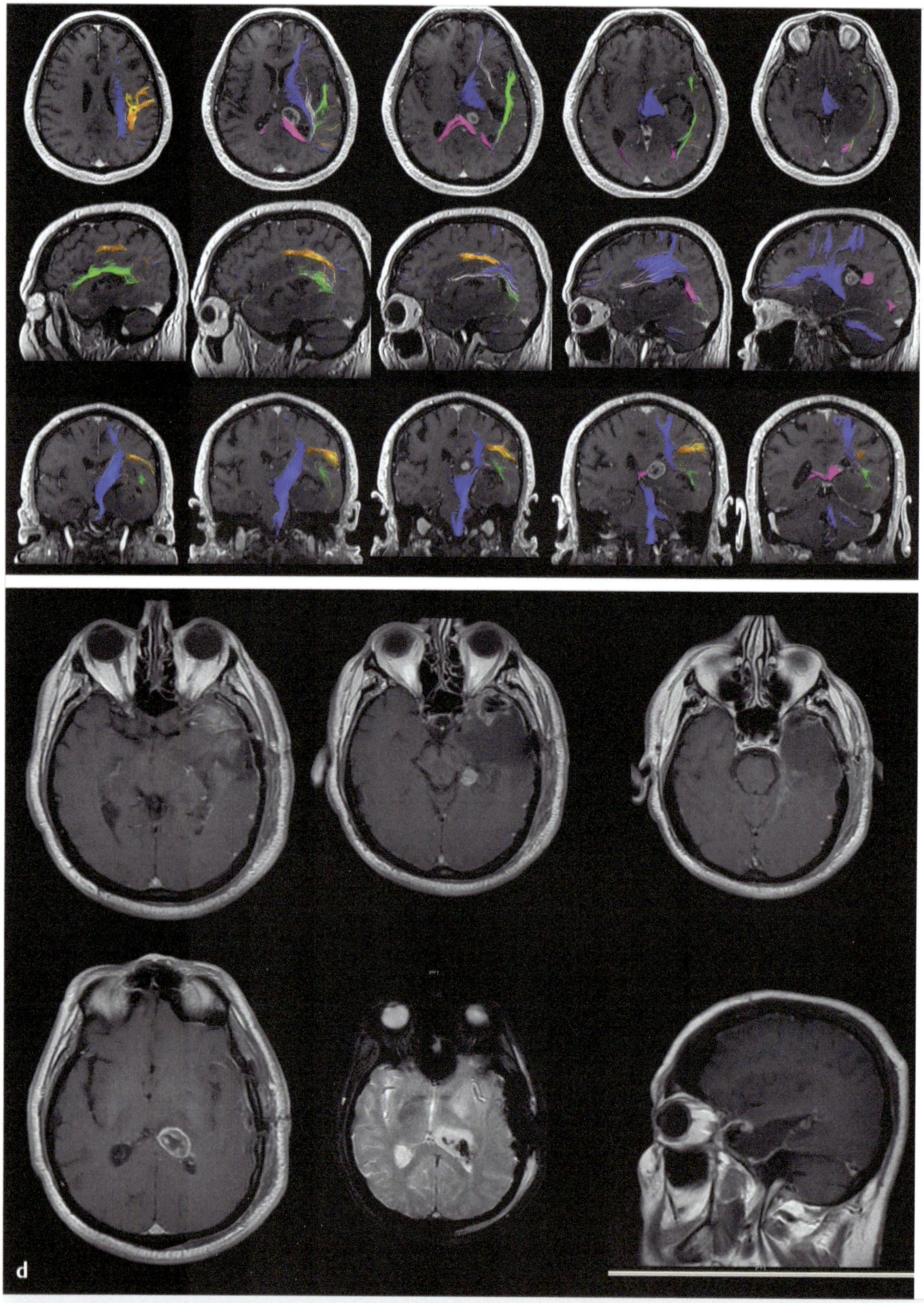

Fig 11.17 (*Continued*) (**c**) DTI tractography, (**d**) postoperative images.

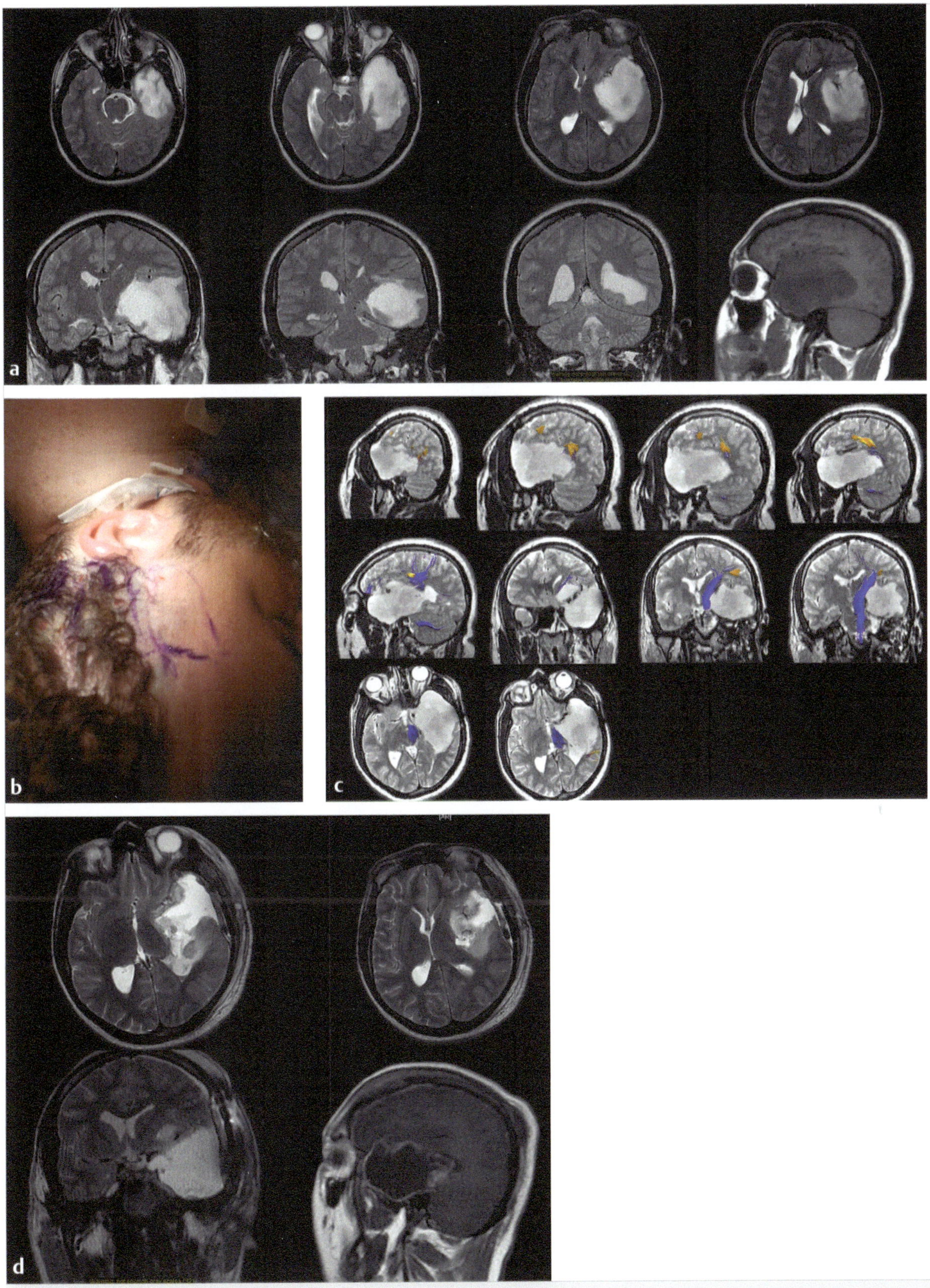

Fig. 11.18 A giant holotemporal low grade glioma; (**a**) preoperative images, (**b**) images of the approach, (**c**) DTI tractography, (**d**) postoperative images.

The resection is good; however, some tumor was left in the lateral system as it was found to be part of the language pathways.

a) This tumor is quite large, but it is important to ignore its size and stick to fundamentals. Its most favorable aspect is that is seems to be displacing, but not involving, the lateral system. This means that a posterior cut which clears out a lot of tumor is probably possible. The MCA and insula are largely pushed up, though some tumor invades the inferior insula and puts the IFOF at risk.
b) A slightly larger craniotomy is necessary, but again note that we do not need to expose the entire temporal lobe. Speech is not located at the temporal tip.
c) The DTIs look like a case where you should try to go for glory. The SLF largely terminates very posteriorly. Concerningly, we cannot visualize the IFOF on tractography.
d) The resection shows we had to leave some tumor in the inferior insula and a small piece in the lateral system, in both cases because of speech arrest when we tried to approach these areas.

11.6.2 Inferior Temporal Gliomas

▶ Fig. 11.19 demonstrates a low-grade glioma primarily centered around the fusiform gyrus with some involvement of the medial temporal structures. The best clue that this is an inferior glioma is the relatively long anterior-posterior distance this covers, implying that it is primarily following the ILF. The absence of lateral involvement and minimal enlargement of the amygdala and hippocampus are also clues. The craniotomy needs to be posteriorly centered to get this cut as far back as possible, as the more lateral fusiform is harder to follow under the lateral system than the more medial limbic structures.

a) This is predominantly an inferior temporal glioma, but it also involves the medial structures to an extent. The principle challenge in these cases is getting far enough back on a relatively more lateral tumor than a hippocampal tumor (where it is relatively easy to do this). The long axis of this tumor takes you through the orbit or the occipital pole. I have heard of people doing a skull base approach, like a pterional or similar approach, to get this angle (the occipital angle is undesirable due to the visual concerns). I would argue that this is much more easily dealt with by going through the anterior temporal lobe. It is basically inhumane to do a pterional type approach in an awake patient (so brain mapping is sacrificed) and it is also disorienting (it is easy to angle a few degrees superior into the basal ganglia from this angle, and most of us do not do intra-axial tumors of this type through this angle very often). The anterior temporal lobe is likely full of glioma cells in this case, and anterior temporal lobectomy with mapping is well tolerated and familiar. Any other approach (such as coming from the side and doing a lesionectomy through the middle temporal gyrus) is off axis, and is likely to miss tumor, usually at the back.
b) The craniotomy is planned for a very posterior cut, and aims to stay relatively lower than for a more anterior temporal tumor. The craniotomy is elongated in the anterior-posterior axis. The cut is quite far posteriorly and aims to enter the ventricle at the atrium if possible.
c) The SLF is primarily a parietal-frontal system in this patient, though the small temporal rami have moved relatively far posteriorly in this patient. There is no edema in the lateral system to otherwise explain this, suggesting that this has reorganized. The IFOF is at risk at the top of the tumor, but this is addressed by remaining below the ventricle. The DTIs suggest that we can make a very posterior low cut without causing neglect.
d) The post-operative images demonstrate an excellent marginal resection of this tumor. Despite the large amount of temporal lobe removed, this patient returned to a high functioning profession job and is recurrence free at 4 years. The secret in this case was to make the disconnection as far posterior as possible.

▶ Fig. 11.20 demonstrates an inferior GBM which is mainly sitting in the temporal horn. Again, it probably involves the hippocampus to some extent, but the key to recognizing this tumor for what is, is the anterior to posterior spread, which contrasts with spread into the cingulum, the lingula, or the fornix seen with hippocampal tumors. As with the previous tumor, making the cut as far posteriorly as the mapping allows is key to success.

a) While the enhancement is focused in the inferior lobe, the entire temporal lobe has T2 change, suggesting that a lobectomy is probably warranted for oncologic purposes, in addition to the need to remove this in order to reach effectively under the lateral system to get to the back of this tumor.
b) The linear incision from the previous surgery done elsewhere demonstrates that this incision is a bit anterior to our desired posterior temporal cut. This can be addressed by lengthening the incision slightly (as we did here), or putting a small posterior T at the top of the incision. I try to avoid horseshoe incisions and T-ed incisions like the plague as I think they are usually unnecessary and they heal worse. The mapping for the neglect along the posterior cut was negative and we performed an aggressive division.
c) The SLF does not appear to be in our way for the necessary disconnection, though caution as always should be utilized interpreting DTIs in the presence of an edematous lobe. The patient already has a field cut, and this can be expected to worsen after this approach.
d) The post-operative images emphasize the value of being able to get a very posterior temporal cut. In this case, we were able to work almost to the occipital pole without causing neglect, simply by padding and working under the lateral system.

11.6.3 Lateral Tumors

▶ Fig. 11.21 demonstrates an extensive holotemporal non-enhancing GBM. The difference from ▶ Fig. 11.18 is the prominent lateral temporal involvement. This is a remarkable case of probably the most reorganized speech network I have ever encountered or seen reported.

a) This tumor is quite extensive and the basic plan is for a temporal lobectomy. The challenge here on initial view is that the speech networks are usually located in the region that the T2 changes are sitting, meaning that we should expect to encounter language areas in this patient. Additionally, note that there is tumor in the cingulate gyrus, meaning that you need to also address the medial temporal structures.

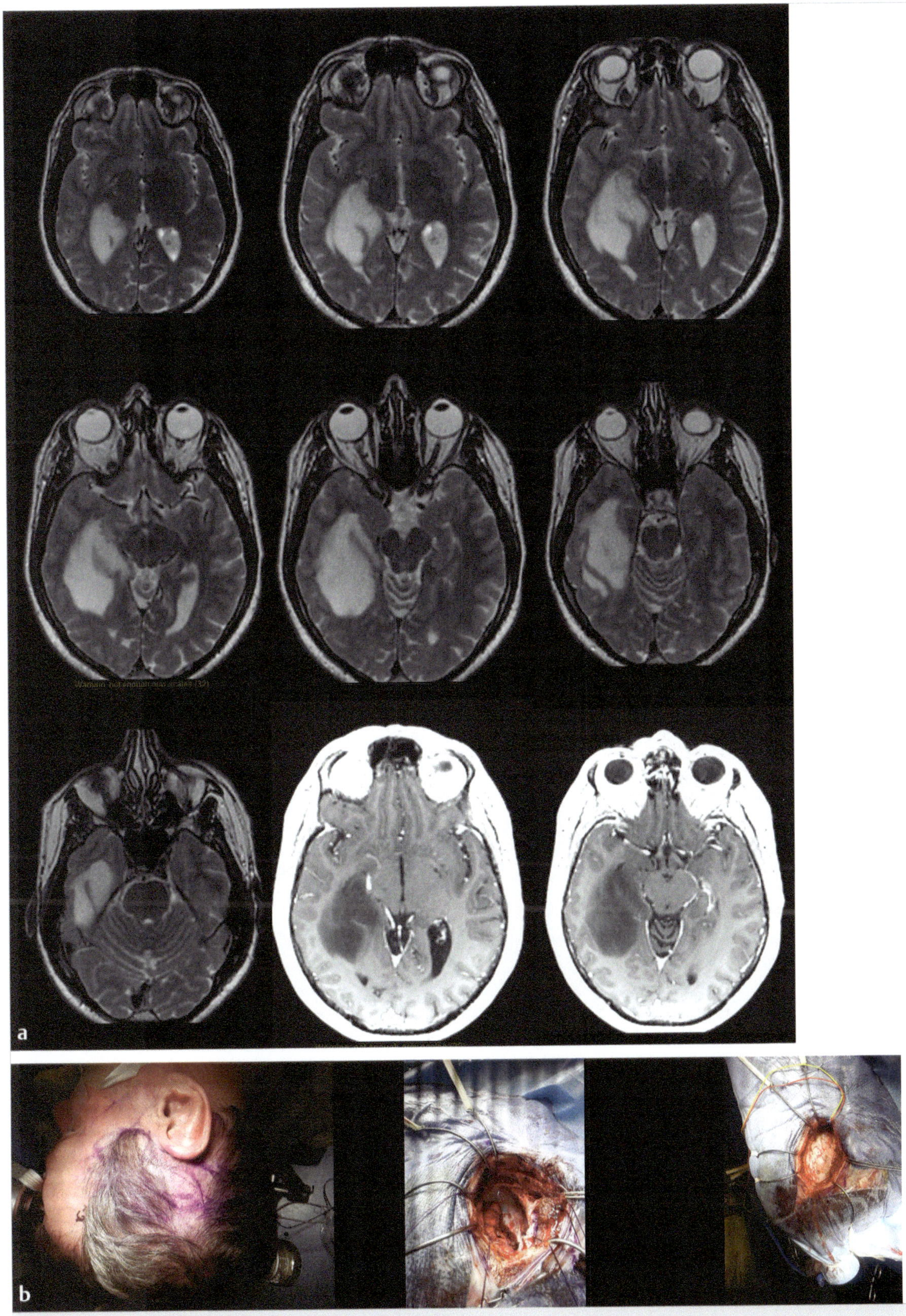

Fig. 11.19 A low-grade glioma primarily centered around the fusiform gyrus with some involvement of the medial temporal structures; (**a**) preoperative images, (**b**) images of the approach. (*Continued*)

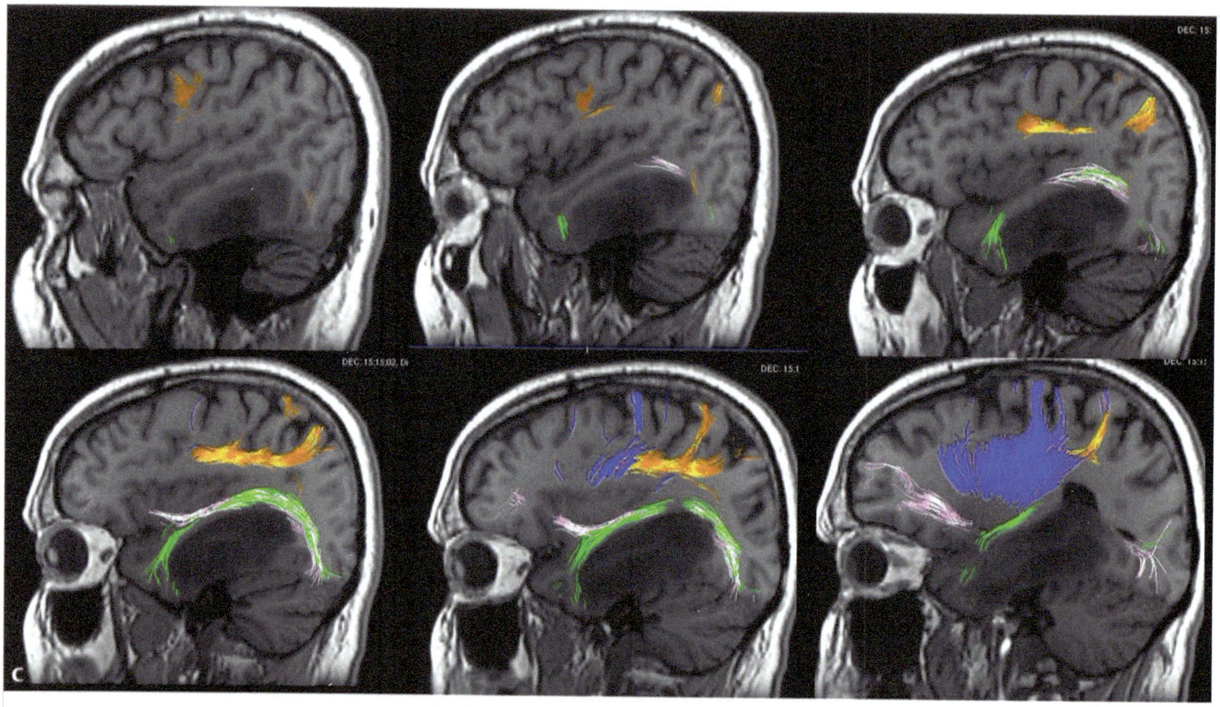

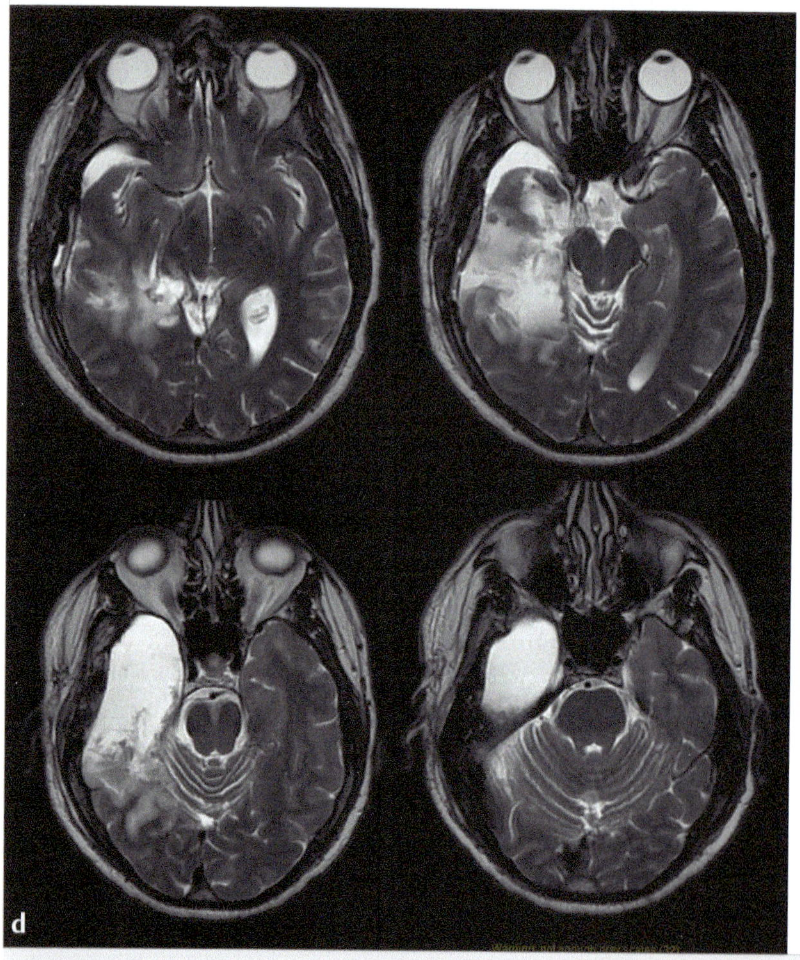

Fig 11.19 (*Continued*) (**c**) DTI tractography, (**d**) postoperative images.

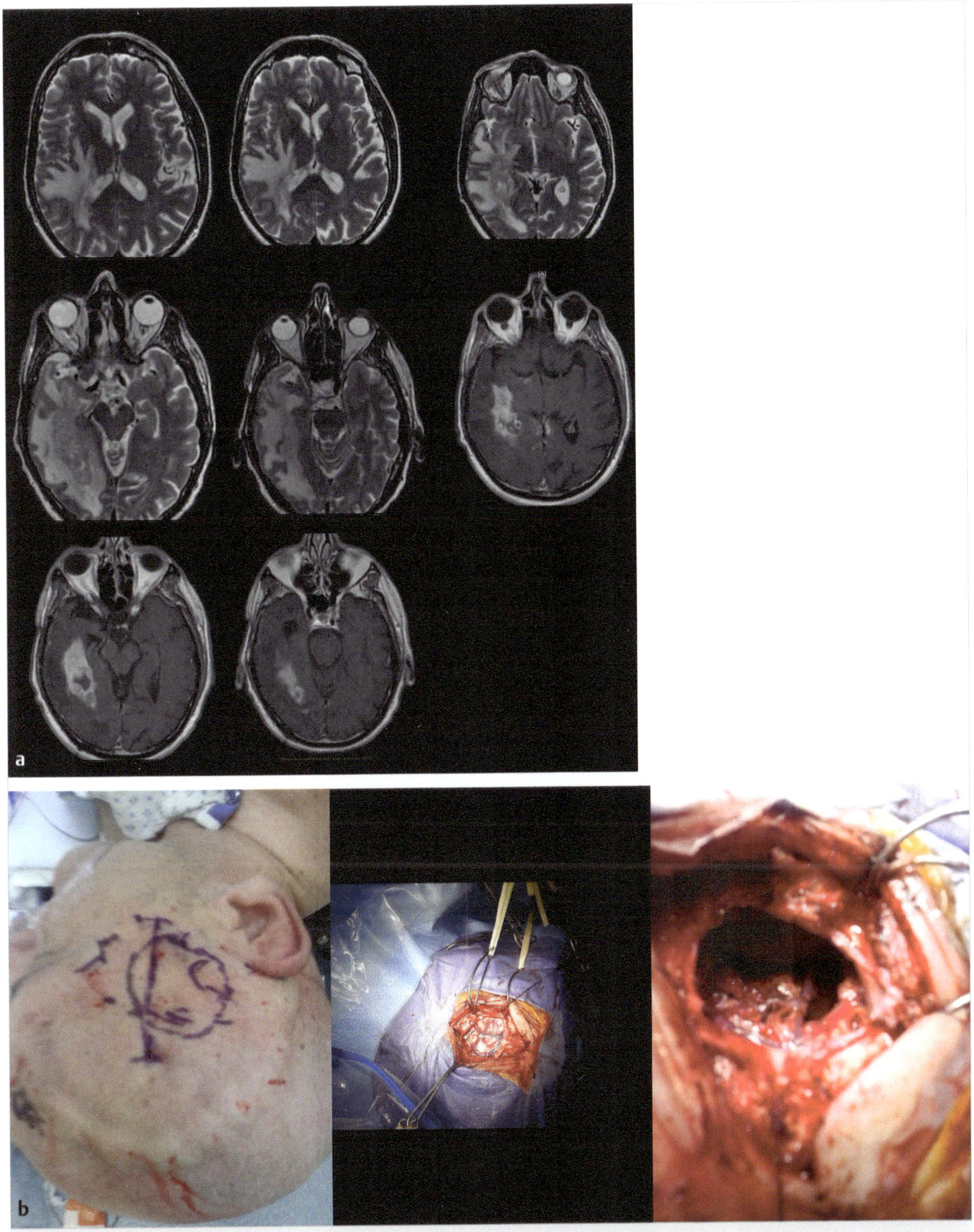

Fig. 11.20 An inferior GBM which is mainly sitting in the temporal horn; (**a**) preoperative images, (**b**) images of the approach. (*Continued*)

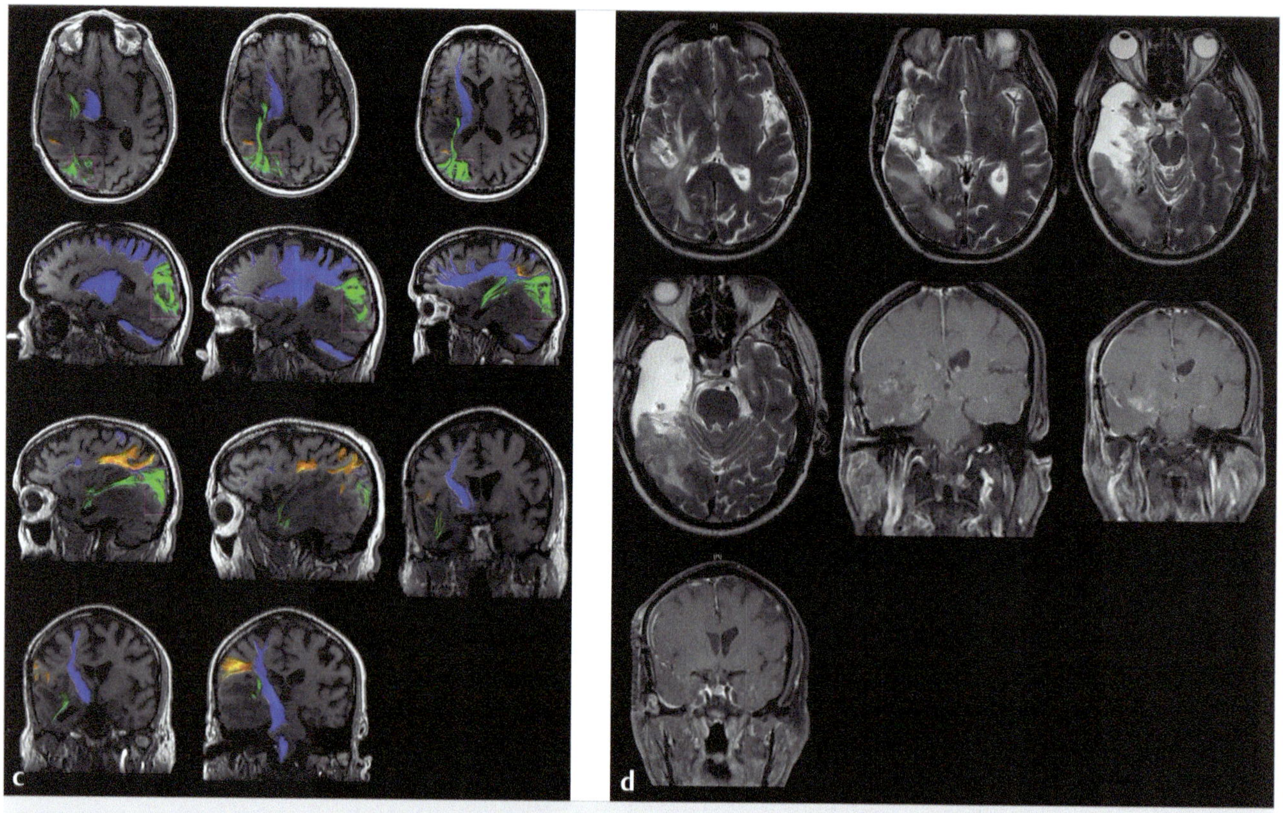

Fig 11.20 (*Continued*) (**c**) DTI tractography, (**d**) postoperative images.

b) Thus, while a temporal lobectomy is planned, the craniotomy needs to be planned and centered like a lateral temporal tumor, which is a battle on the surface more than it is a posterior temporal cut. This, is why despite having a previous pretragal incision, we made a much larger posterior exposure to ensure we have enough posterior temporal access. Note the similarities with a case like this, and an inferior temporal tumor.
c) This is a remarkable case in that the tractography demonstrated the SLF terminating in the parietal lobe without a temporal ramus. This is consistent with our experience in this case, as it was possible to obtain an aggressive resection without any speech problems in this patient.
d) This patient never developed even temporary speech problems after this surgery. After about a year, he developed a small recurrence in the area indicated by the DTIs which caused significant speech problems: the network can't run forever.

▸ Fig. 11.22 demonstrates a small but unresectable lateral temporal glioma. This small tumor is sitting in the SLF and IFOF, and despite our patient efforts to try to get something out, we had to settle for a biopsy alone which revealed grade 2 histology.

a) This small tumor had been diagnosed elsewhere and treated as multiple sclerosis until it progressed and perfusion images suggested glioma. It is small but dangerous.
b) None.
c) The tumor is located in the junctional white matter. This is not usually safe to resect without deficits and mapping confirmed this.
d) None.

▸ Fig. 11.23 demonstrates a massive right lateral temporal glioblastoma. Note the general absence of medial temporal involvement, and the encasement of opercular MCA branches on the T2 scan. This is a dangerous case, and it forced us to leave some tumor on the Sylvian vessels, which slowed the patient's recovery by exacerbating the swelling. Eventually, he made a good recovery.

a) This tumor involves almost the entire temporal lobe. The most concerning part of this tumor is that there is enhancement in the Sylvian fissure. It is almost certainly not invading the frontal lobe from this path but it can (and this case did), invade the MCA adventitia.
b) As you can see, the temporal lobe is massive, and the tumor presents to the surface.
c) The DTIs are favorable, as the SLF appears to be posterior to the tumor.
d) There is still enhancing tumor on the MCA branches. Efforts to try to separate them made it obvious that this would cause a stroke if we pushed further. This can recur, but it lacks a clear path to the white matter, which at least limits its ability to spread.

▸ Fig. 11.24 demonstrates a deceptively difficult lateral temporal GBM. It is small and relatively inferior; however, you should never underestimate a lateral temporal tumor until it is in the trash, especially on the left. Mapping demonstrated that there were language sites involved with the semantic networks extending almost down to the middle fossa floor. We were

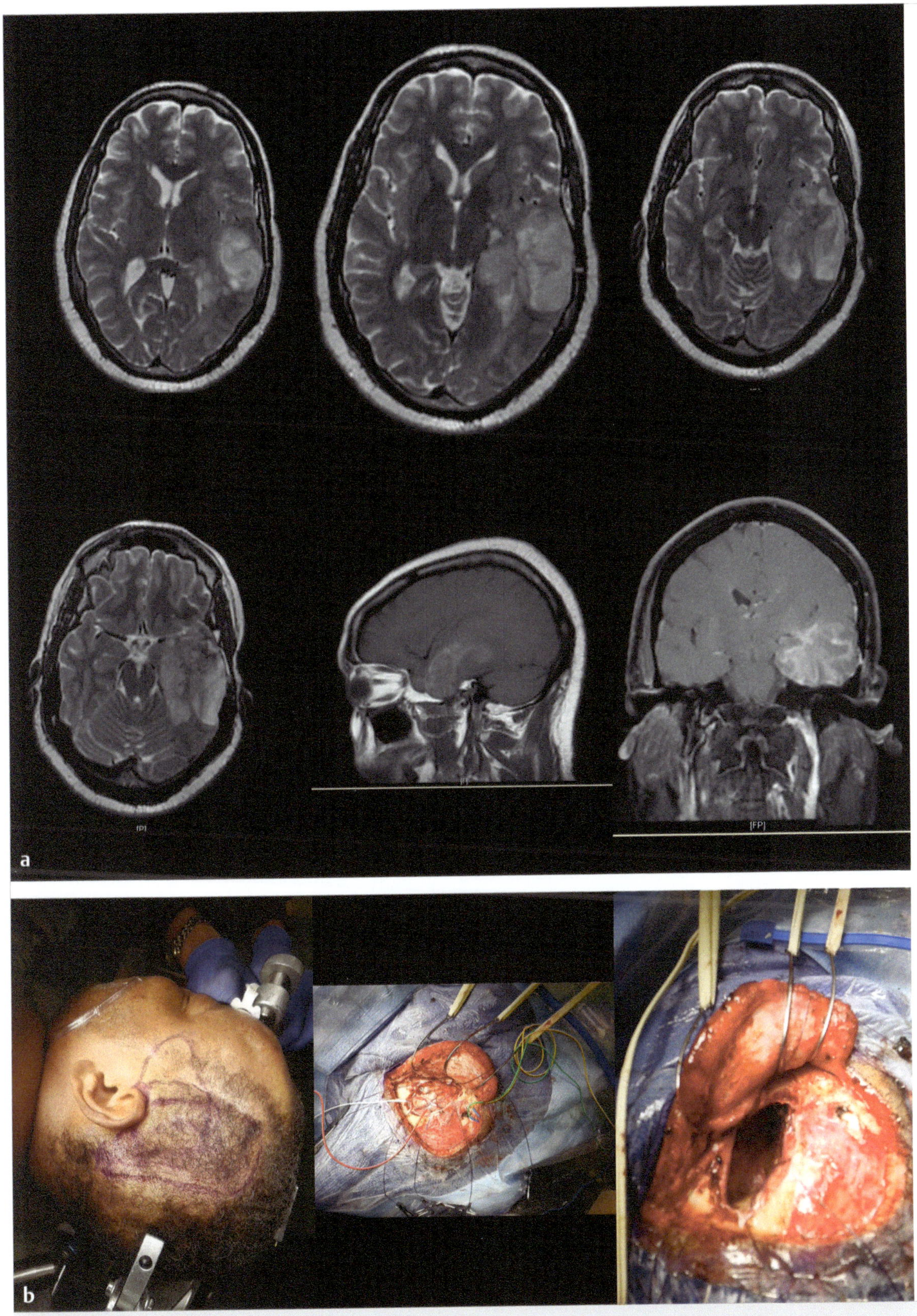

Fig. 11.21 An extensive holotemporal non-enhancing GBM; (**a**) preoperative images, (**b**) images of the approach. (*Continued*)

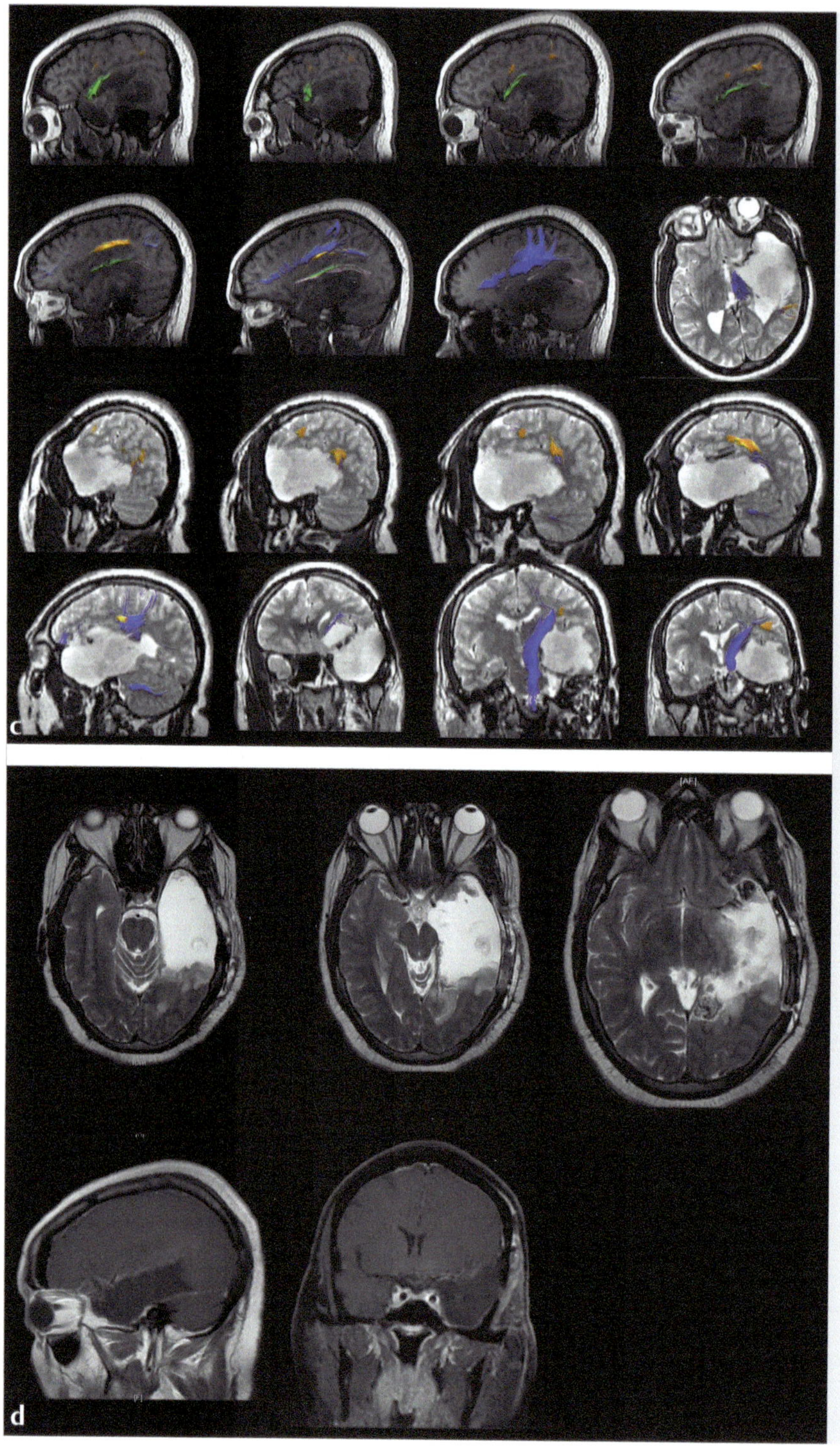

Fig 11.21 (*Continued*) (**c**) DTI tractography, (**d**) postoperative images.

happy to safely obtain a lesionectomy in this case. (**a**) The tumor is small and relative low, but importantly it is lateral in the temporal lobe. Size matters a lot less than location in neurosurgery, and this is a key example. (**b**) We performed a small craniotomy over the lesion. You can see the speech areas extend nearly to the floor of the temporal fossa and this means that the network directly overlies this tumor. (**c**) The DTIs make the challenge of this case obvious. The SLF network runs low into the temporal lobe (the semantic areas seem to be centered around and fibers are terminating in the temporal lobe nearly at the floor of the middle fossa. The tractography suggests that if we encounter speech in the way, our best bet is to move anteriorly. We did encounter speech in the way, and had to move anterior to get this tumor out. This required extending the craniotomy with a few kerrison bites after the mapping demonstrated how difficult this would be. (**d**) The resection is good but note how far inferiorly we had to enter the temporal lobe compared to many other cases in this chapter. Networks in glioma patients are complex and often unpredictable, which demonstrates how valuable tractography can be in cases like this.

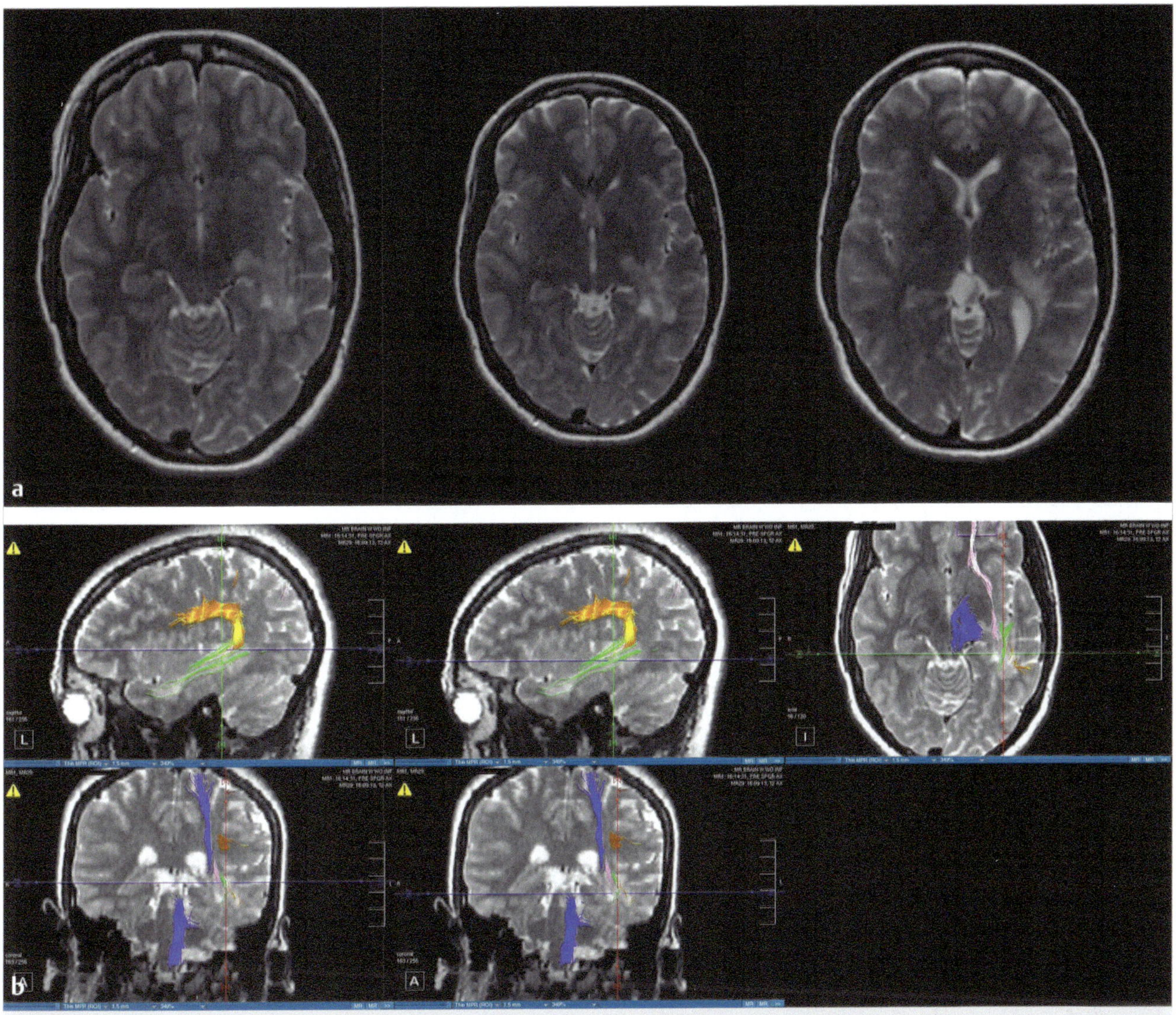

Fig. 11.22 A small but unresectable lateral temporal glioma; (**a**) preoperative images, (**b**) DTI tractography.

▶ Fig. 11.25 demonstrates what appears to be a multifocal GBM involving the lateral temporal lobe and the right temporal junction as two sites. (**a**) This patient came to me for a second opinion after being told that her tumor was multifocal and inoperable (radiochemotherapy was given without a biopsy). Close inspection of the T2 images demonstrate that the entire temporal lobe is probably involved. (**b**) We planned the craniotomy over the junction (i.e., SMG and STG), and first performed a posterior temporal cut, and then followed the SMG into the junction. Note that it is critical that junctional cases expose the junction, which is usually right above the pinna, as this kind of surgery will likely find eloquent areas (we found neglect sites which lined up with the SLF on DTI). We then slowly advanced our resection into the deep tissue of the junction and the back of the internal capsule monitoring the patient with attention tasks alternated with lower extremity motor tasks. (**c**) The DTIs predicted that we would have a narrow window into the junction, and that neglect considerations would form the posterior bound of the cut. However, examining the relationship between the capsule and the tumor, this suggests that there are capsular fibers somewhat anterolateral to this tumor, arguing that we need to enter the deep white matter as far posterolaterally as possible. This means that in addition to taking whatever parts of the STG and SMG possible, we also need to mobilize the opercula to get a clearer view into the insula. (**d**) There is residual disease in the junctional white matter, which we left as the patient began struggling with leg motor function, but in general the resection was as extensive as possible. This patient lived progression free for about a year with good quality of life until recurring.

(**a**) An inexperienced eye might mistake this case for a somewhat easier tumor, it is small and near the surface. This is obviously not true as this tumor is probably in the junctional white matter (SLF, IFOF, MdLF, crossed semantic loop, optic radiations, posterior thalamic peduncle). (**b**) The craniotomy is small and located in the safest plane I could find based on the DTIs. (**c**) While the inferior foci of this tumor may be possible to address, the superior foci are in the worst possible place. It may be tempting to over interpret the DTIs as saying that there is a small window into this tumor in the anterosuperior angle

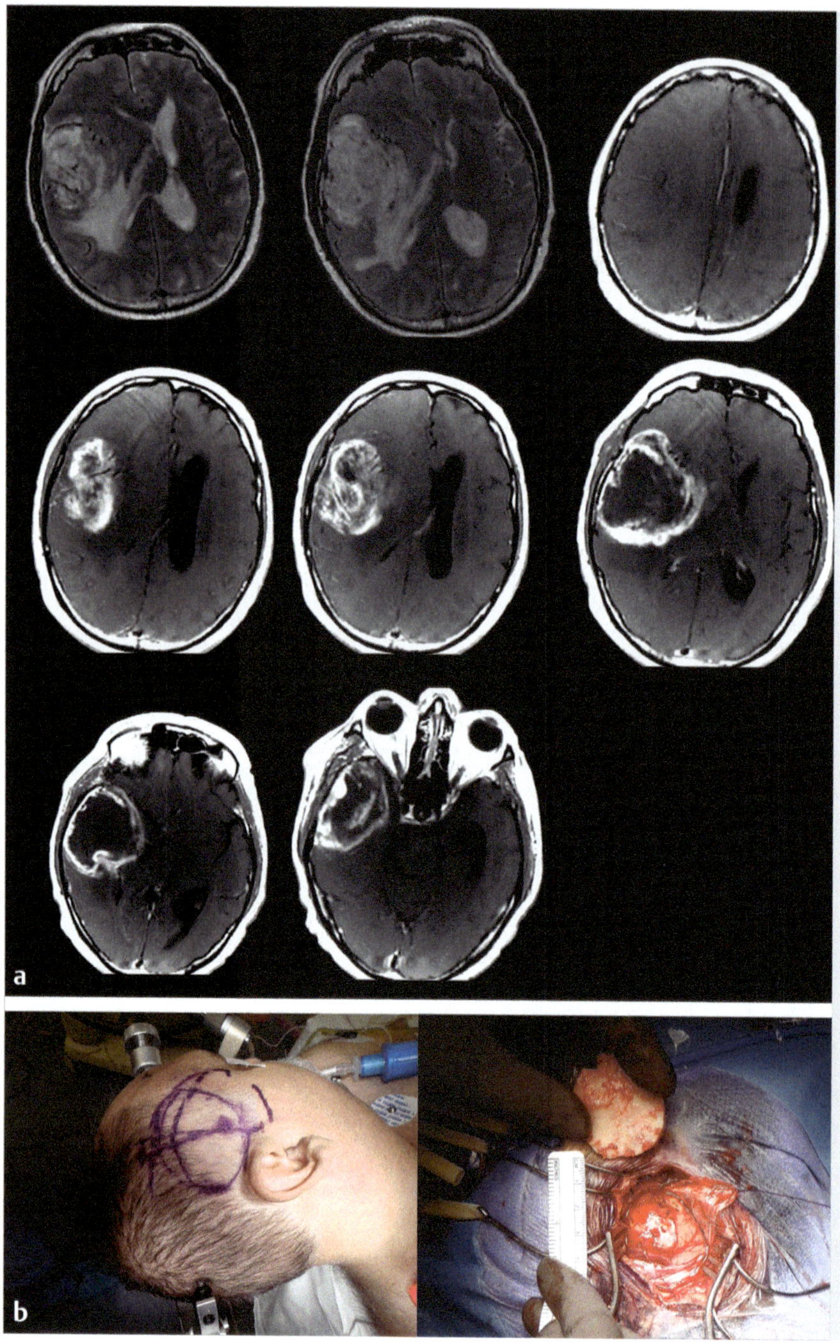

Fig. 11.23 A massive right lateral temporal glioblastoma; (**a**) preoperative images, (**b**) images of the approach.

between SLF and IFOF, but this involves a substantial overestimation of the anatomic detail provided by DTIs. There are numerous small fibers entering and exiting these tracts from the surrounding semantic cortices, and these are not shown on DTI as they are too small, and involve crossing fibers, which DTI fails to resolve well. Remember, tracts are a bus route not an airplane flight: if you try something too aggressive like this, you will eliminate some important bus stops along the route because you cannot visualize them. It may be possible in some cases to do something like this, but you shouldn't base your entire plan for the case around being able to do this. (**d**) The postoperative scan demonstrates that we were able to work under the tracts to a limited extent to get some of the enhancement out, but this was with great struggle and there is a fair bit of the tumor left.

▶ Fig. 11.26 is another small tumor which sits in the left temporal junction. Due to involvement of the tumor in the SLF, we could only perform a minor resection of this tumor.

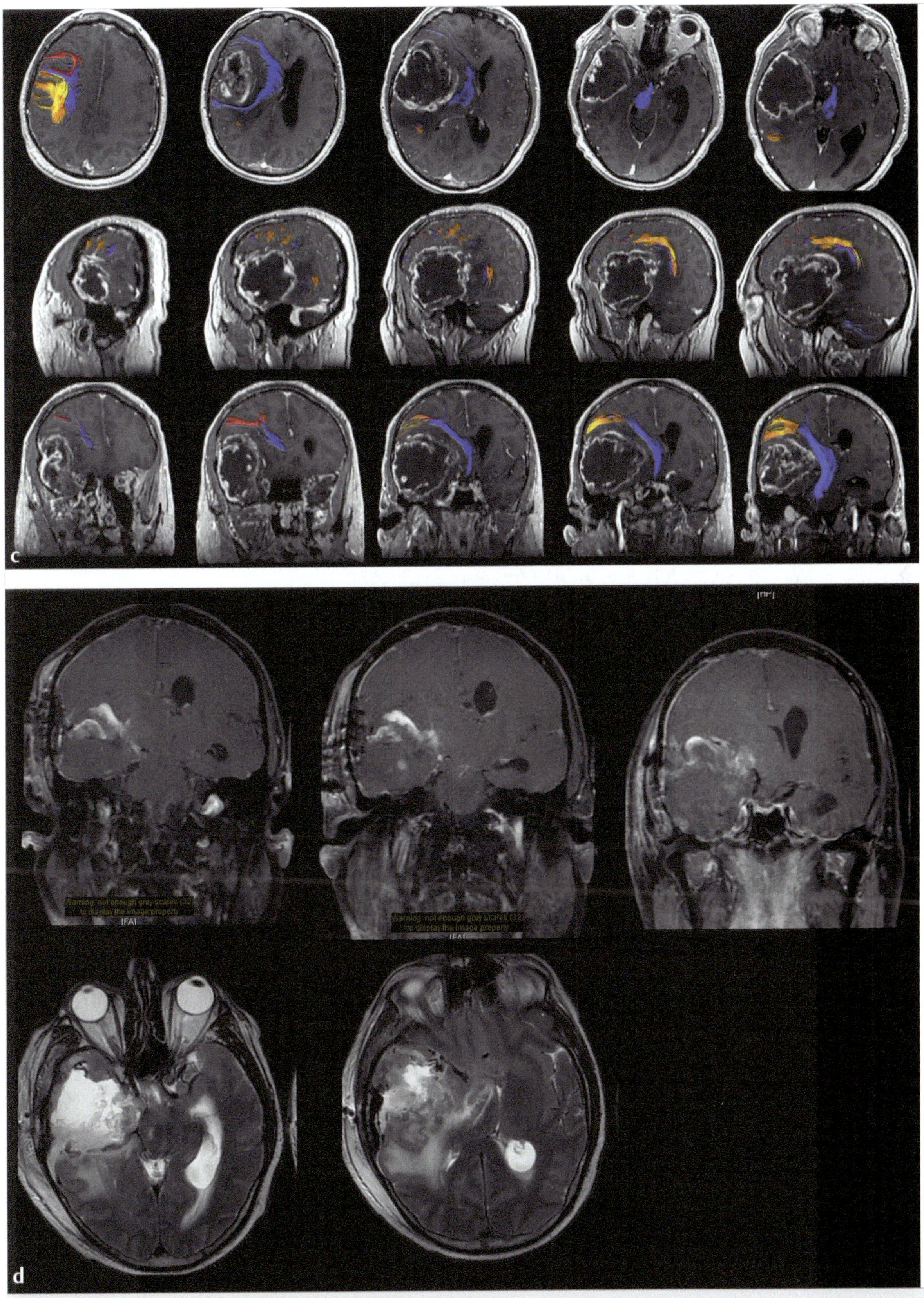

Fig 11.23 *(Continued)* (**c**) DTI tractography, (**d**) postoperative images.

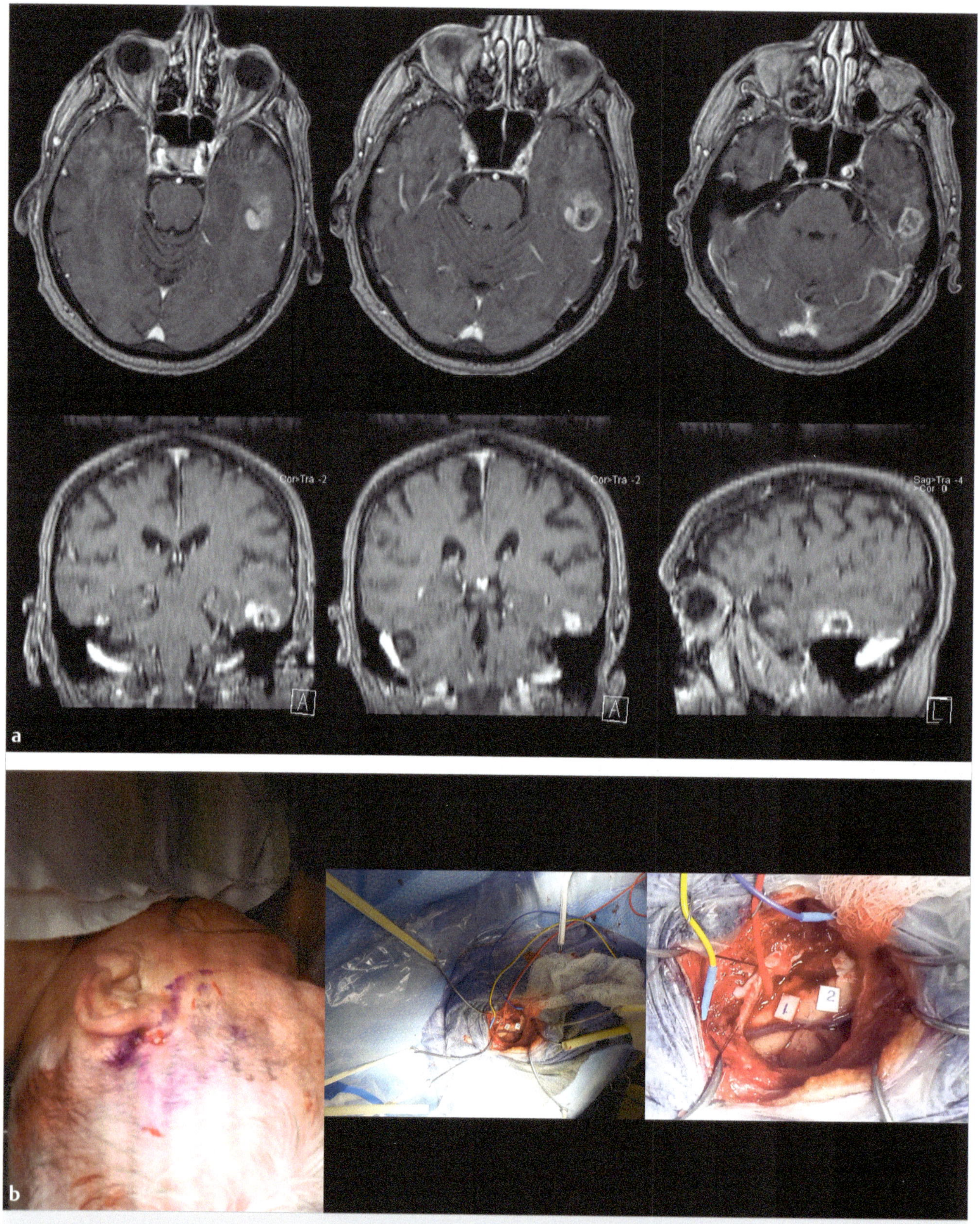

Fig. 11.24 A deceptively difficult lateral temporal GBM. (**a**) Preoperative images, (**b**) images of the approach.

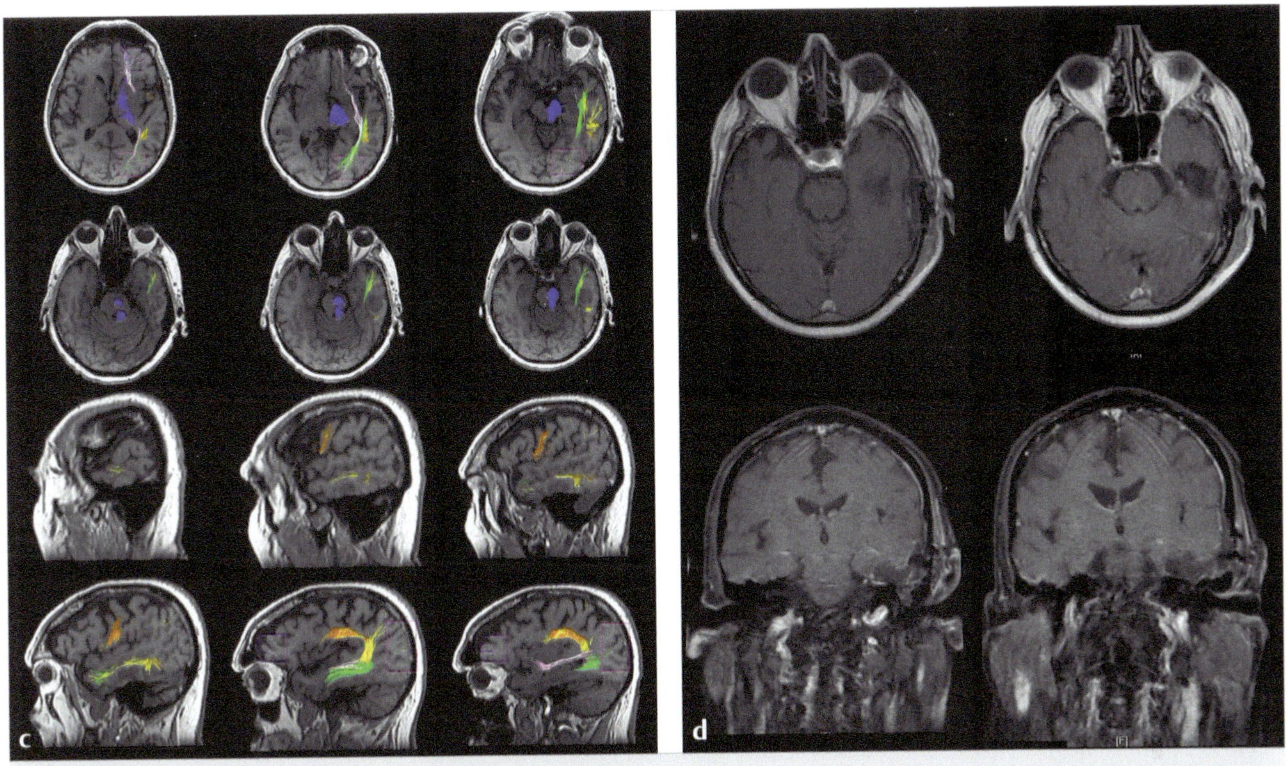

Fig 11.24 *(Continued)* (**c**) DTI tractography, (**d**) postoperative images.

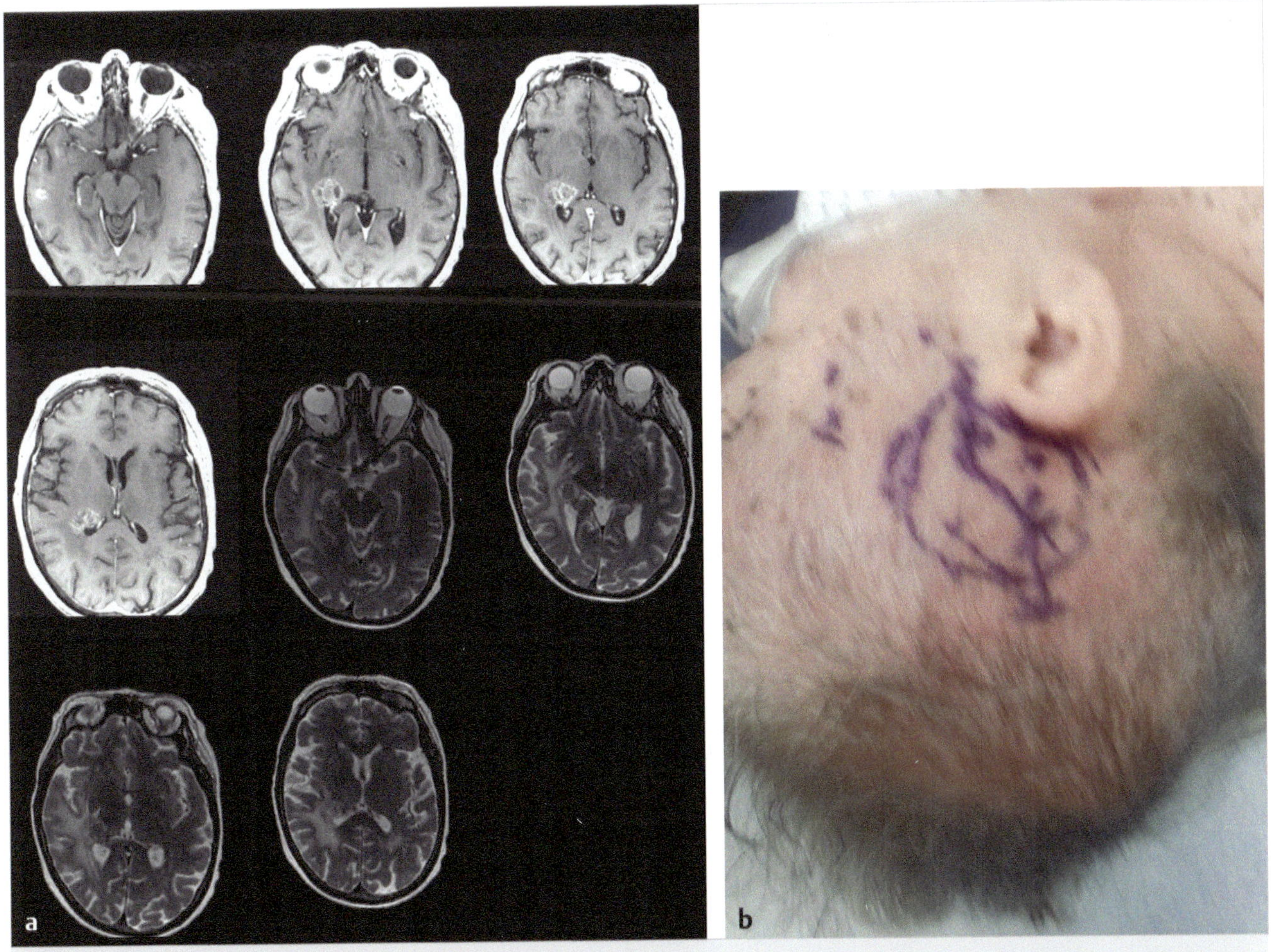

Fig. 11.25 Demonstrates what appears to be a multifocal GBM involving the lateral temporal lobe and the right temporal junction as two sites; (**a**) preoperative images, (**b**) images of the approach. *(Continued)*

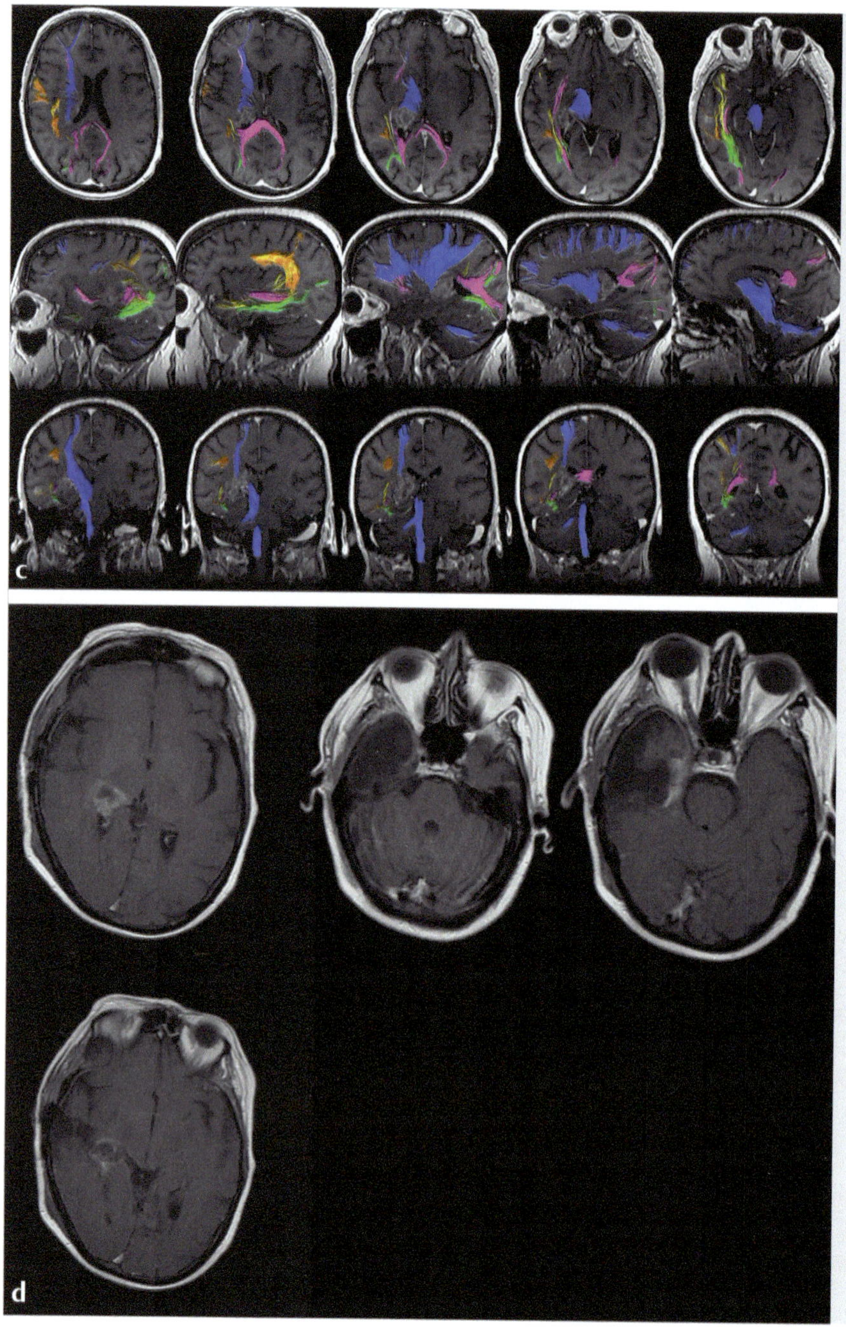

Fig 11.25 (*Continued*) (**c**) DTI tractography for that case, (**d**) postoperative images.

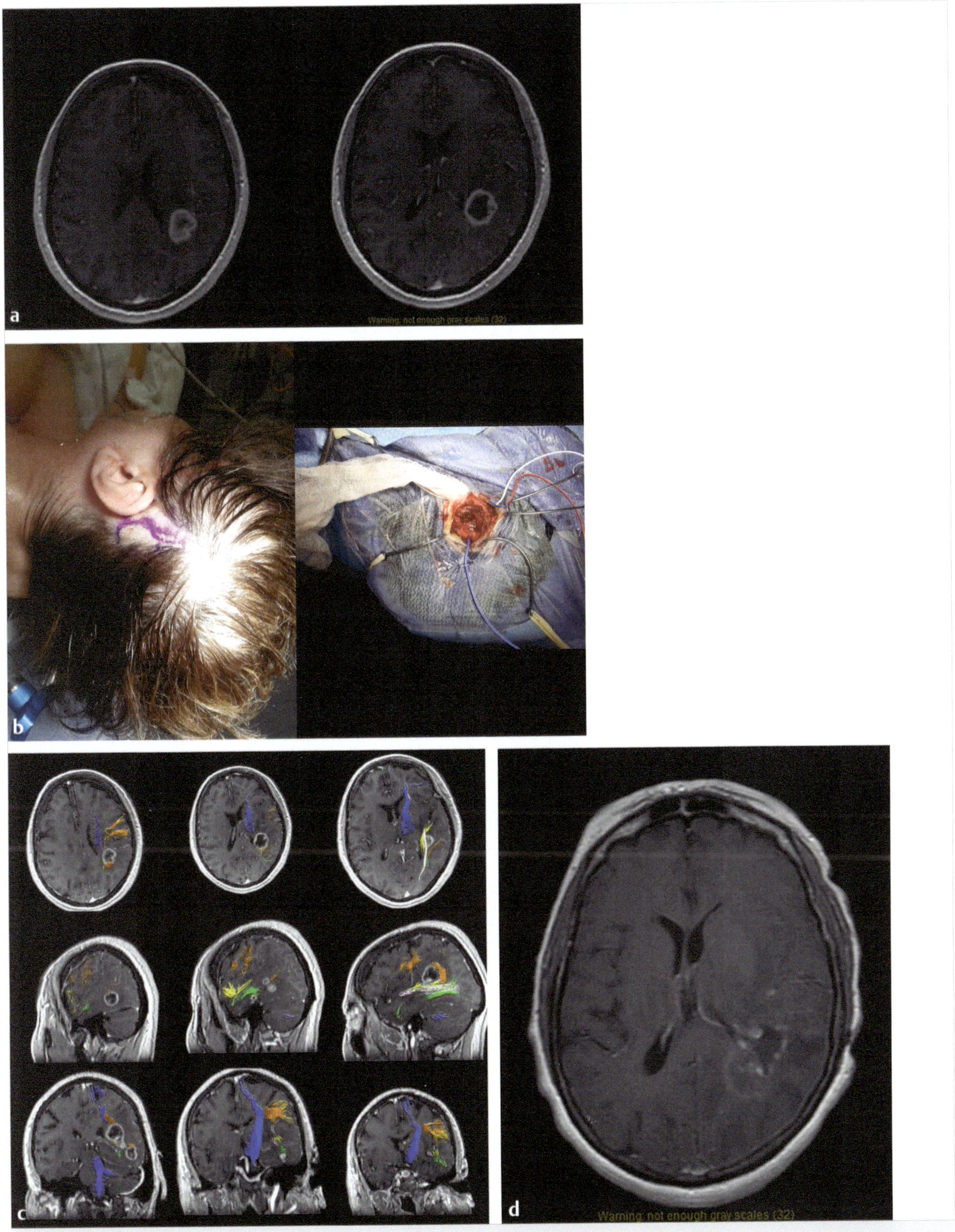

Fig. 11.26 A small tumor which sits in the left temporal junction; (**a**) preoperative images, (**b**) images of the approach, (**c**) DTI tractography, (**d**) postoperative images.

12 Insular Gliomas

12.1 Climbing the Mountain

Insular gliomas have a long learning curve. While I was learning to do these surgeries, I found many of the resources for learning how to take these tumors provided inadequate insight and detail to successfully achieve excellent results every time. I estimate it took me about 40 cases before I had one truly satisfying case (meaning complete resection without neurologic problems).

There are a fair number of facts one must understand about the insula, its anatomy, and techniques for safe and effective resection. Despite these challenges, insular gliomas are a tumor which you can consistently achieve good results if you adhere to a disciplined pattern of attack which builds on the groundwork we have set forth in previous chapters.

What follows is a guide I wished I had had during my learning curve.

12.2 Fundamental Anatomic Relationships of the Insula

What follows is a list of facts about insular anatomy which are essential to success in these cases:

1. The insula is roughly a right triangle with its right angle under the frontal operculum and its hypotenuse running from the parietal operculum to the Sylvian vallecula (▶ Fig. 12.1). This means it is not rectangular, and it extends more posteriorly on the parietal side than the frontal side.
2. The insula is completely covered by opercula cortices. You cannot see the insula without either removing them or splitting the Sylvian fissure, mobilizing and retracting them.
3. The insula extends significantly beyond the immediate boundaries of the Sylvian fissure (▶ Fig. 12.2). The circular sulcus runs roughly parallel to the top of MTG inferiorly, and the top of IFG and SMG superiorly. A significant part of the insula is covered by the face/tongue sensory and motor cortices.
4. The MCA branches run over the surface of the insula. This means the insula must be removed between the MCA branches.
5. The insula is bounded by a sulcus on all sides (the circular or marginal sulcus) outside of which the white matter folds over onto the opercular cortices. This means that if you have not seen the circular sulcus, there is still more insular tissue under the operculum in the direction you are looking. The circular sulcus also provides an excellent idea of where the white matter tracts are running.
6. The putamen is the deep boundary of the insula. It is roughly superior to the hippocampus in the coronal plane as I have pointed out several times in the book. When people ask me how I know how deep to go and when to stop, this is what I tell them.
7. The SLF and IFOF roughly frame the boundaries of the insula (▶ Fig. 12.3). The SLF dominates the posterior and superior boundaries, while the IFOF runs in the inferior and anterior boundaries.
8. Deviating out of the insula accidentally in two places can put the motor fibers at risk (▶ Fig. 12.3). One of these places is superiorly above the circular sulcus under the motor opercula. The other is at the posterior aspect of the insula, where the leg portion of the posterior limb of the internal capsule extends laterally at the junction.

12.3 The "Define" Phase

12.3.1 Preoperative Planning

It is important to note that most insular gliomas are not limited to the insula, but are multilobar, as pure insular gliomas are an uncommonly found, early stage of disease. Pluralities of these tumors are primarily temporal, some are primarily frontal, and occasionally they are both. It is critical to understand how these tumors have left the insula, so that these tumor extensions can be addressed in addition to the insula.

Common ways tumors leave the insula are as follows:

1. Inferior extension into the medial temporal lobe: This is the most common type of spread, this can also be spread to the anterior temporal lobe.

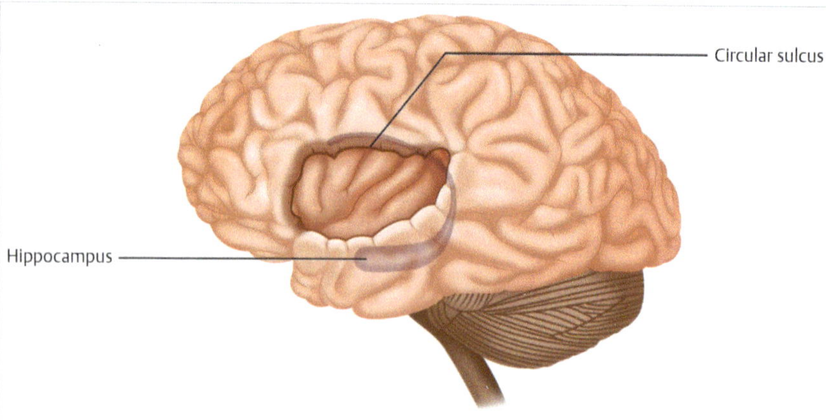

Fig. 12.1 This image demonstrates the irregular right triangle shape of the insula.

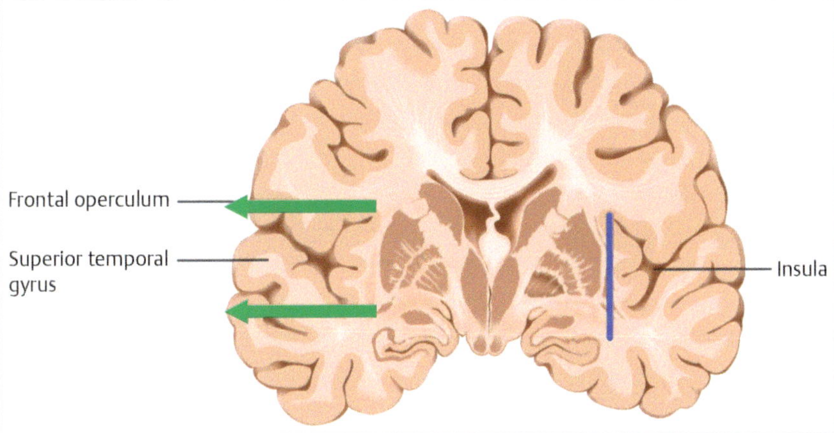

Fig. 12.2 This image depicts the position of the insula relative to the opercular cortices which overlie it. Note that the bottom edge of the insula rests roughly at the top of the middle temporal gyrus, and that the top of the insula runs to the top of the SMG, the MFG, and under the sensorimotor cortices. This highlights one of the main advantages of the transopercular approach to the insula.

2. Spread to the orbitofrontal cortex via the uncinate fasciculus: Also common. This is usually best removed during the insular resection by following the tract under the frontal lobe.
3. Spread upward into the premotor regions: Less common, but it is the worst form of spread.
4. Spread into parahippocampal gyrus and cingulum: Usually occurs with spread to the medial temporal lobe.

12.3.2 Transopercular versus Transsylvian Approach

I have tried both approaches, and have strongly sided on the side of basing my insular surgeries on the transopercular approach to the insula. The reason for this is a matter of access. The insula extends well beyond the Sylvian cleft under the opercula both frontally and temporally. By limiting to your exposure to that which can be reached by mobilizing the opercula, you are increasing the difficulty of a difficult case by working under lips of brain to see the circular sulcus.

More critically, the insula is bounded by tracts on all side by large white matter tracts. It is difficult or impossible to map the IFOF along its length by reaching under an entire gyrus, and equally difficult to work along the posterosuperior portions of the insula without working blindly near the SLF. By taking off the STG, you get an excellent view of the inferior insula and can map and protect it.

Finally, it is uncommon that a glioma is entirely confined to the insula, and by trying to conceptualize these complex, multilobar tumor merely in terms of the insula, you will tend to underaddress the tumor elsewhere. Insular gliomas are typically a much bigger problem than just the insula. This is human nature: to fixate on the unusual and to ignore the more typical. Most insular gliomas need more than just an insular resection, and the temporal lobe often needs to come out as well, making the transopercular approach necessary for more than just access.

By taking off the operculum, it's much easier to see what you are doing, to define the boundaries of the insula, and to protect the white matter tracts. Again, gliomas are big tumors and require big resections. Clever and precise approaches make for good videos, but are not always the easiest way to take out a glioma reliably effectively. Perhaps some people can do insular gliomas through a split Sylvian fissure, but you are much more likely to hit the target approaching transopercularly.

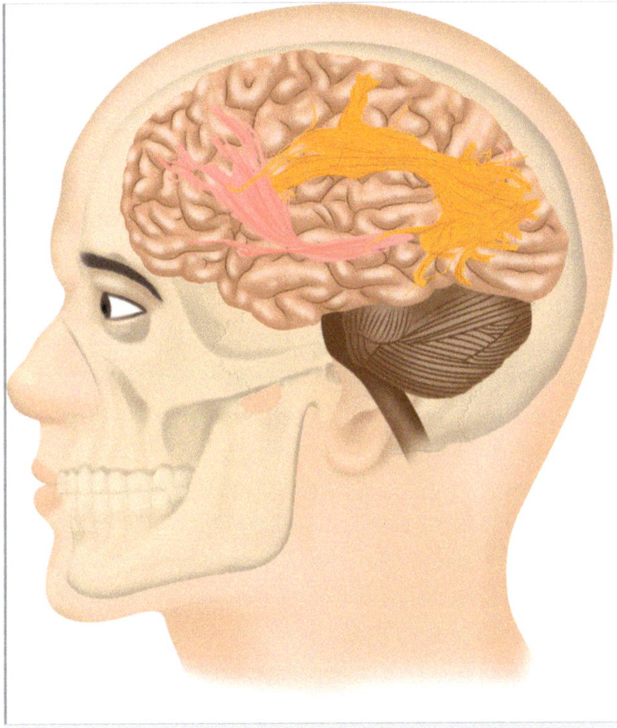

Fig. 12.3 This diagram highlights the relationship the insula and the SLF, IFOF, MdLF, and descending motor fibers. The SLF and IFOF, most notably, form a frame around the insula, a fact which dominates insular glioma surgery.

12.3.3 Frontal versus Temporal Approach

The key decision to make in the planning phase is which side of the insula to approach the insula by removing the temporal or frontal opercula. This is generally obvious in most cases. For example, if a temporal lobectomy is planned for part of the tumor resection, then the temporal approach is the obvious choice. If frontal operculum or premotor areas are significantly involved, then a frontal approach is needed as it is challenging to just work beneath the frontal operculum. When it is unclear, I approach from the temporal side, as the frontal side can be more limiting due to premotor, motor and speech areas in the frontal

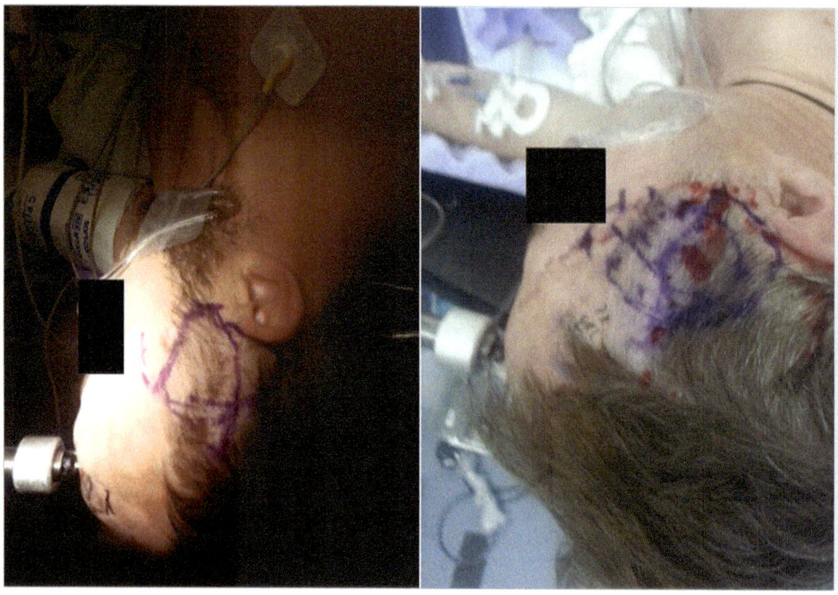

Fig. 12.4 These images demonstrate the head position for (**a**) approaching from the temporal side, (**b**) approaching from the frontal side.

operculum. The STG usually can be resected over most of its length in most patients. Massive tumors and tumors encasing the MCA complex might need an approach from both sides.

As could be expected from the positioning described in the previous chapters, a temporal approach should be positioned with the slightly tipped head down, and a frontal approach with the head tipped up to provide a good angle on the insula (▶ Fig. 12.4).

12.3.4 Intraoperative Definition

In an insular glioma case, the aim of cortical mapping is principally to take off the operculum to provide good access to the insula for mapping and resection. This is in addition to the needs of any other parts of the case, such as temporal lobectomy, medial temporal resection, or lateral frontal disconnection. If they need to be done, additional cortical mapping and disconnections need to be added to the insular case as described in other chapters.

What mapping tasks to focus on, obviously depends on the angle of the attack and what else is involved. For example, a left-sided temporal approach is dominated by language considerations, and a right temporal approach by neglect system of the STG. Supra-Sylvian mapping involves language, and motor planning anteriorly. As always, DTI tractography is helpful at predicting the location of the networks to guide your mapping; however, note that the connections between the semantic areas of posterior temporal lobe and the IFOF are often not visible on DTI tractography, as they cross and intermix with the temporal ramus of the SLF. The temporal ramus is usually located in the immediate proximity of the semantic areas though.

12.4 The "Divide" Phase

An insular glioma is a complex two phase resection, which can take some time to complete. Phase one involves removing or mobilizing the opercula in order to visualize the insula, and phase two involves defining and removing the insula.

12.4.1 Phase 1: Exposing the Insula

From the Temporal Side (▶ Fig. 12.5)

A large fraction of insular gliomas co-inhabit the medial and/or anterior temporal lobes, and thus a large percentage of these cases will involve a temporal lobectomy. It is critical to note that I generally do not use the valuable time during mapping to complete the lobectomy. A patient will only map for so long, and you should use this time to focus where you really need to map. Plus, you will bump the dura multiple times taking out the lobe which causes pain, which in turn is distracting.

The initial phase of a temporal approach involves making a posterior temporal cut as described in Chapter 11. This involves first removing the STG from the posterior limit of the cut forward until you reach the anterior corner (i.e., the front of the Sylvian fissure) in front of the limen insula. This shows you where the insula is located, defines the vessels of the inferior Sylvian fissure, and helps locate the IFOF. In this phase, there are two key mistakes to avoid. First, the "artery of death" is usually leaving the Sylvian fissure and heading to the posterior temporal lobe, and this can completely undo a speech mapping case. Second, you want to keep an open mind regarding the short communications between a mapped site (especially language sites) and the IFOF or SLF as DTI tractography may not demonstrate these small fibers well and they can arc gently anterior or just dive directly medially. You should resect the STG as far posteriorly as the mapping will allow, as the posterior insula is both dangerous and easy to miss unless you make a concerted effort to find it. A fair bit of insula is tucked into the temporal junction.

At this point, you should extend the cut inferiorly across MTG towards the middle fossa floor. Once you know where the insula is, then finding the temporal horn is easy. This cut is complete once it extends into the ventricle or to the floor across the entire length of the cut.

Once the temporal lobe is out of the way, the next step is to elevate the frontal opercular cortices. I let the patient rest during this period. I do this by gently retracting the opercula off of the insula bluntly, i.e., by padding the cortex then sweeping to pull

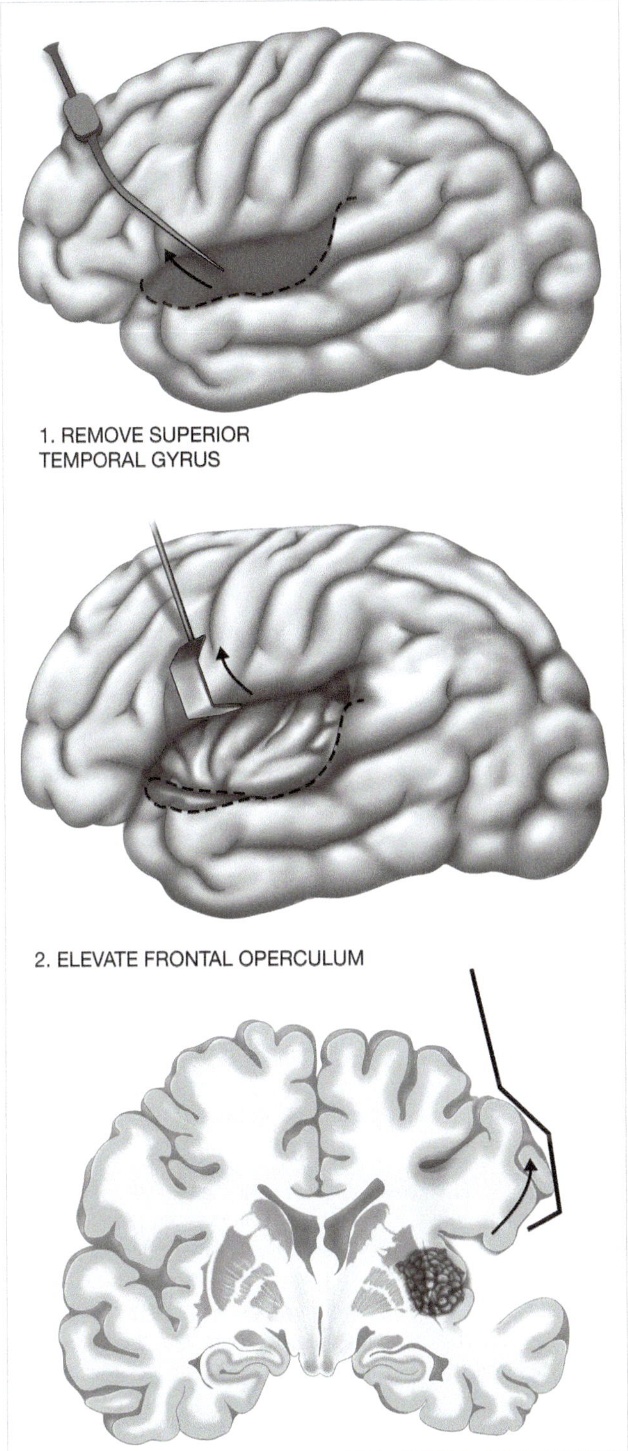

Fig. 12.5 The transopercular approach to the insula from the temporal side. This diagram demonstrates the first stage of an insular glioma operation when the tumor anatomy or preference dictates a temporal angle. The STG is first resected as far posterior as allowed by the mapping. This can be combined with a temporal lobectomy, as described in Chapter 11, if warranted. Once the inferior insula is identified, the frontal opercula are swept upward gently to identify the superior boundary of the circular sulcus.

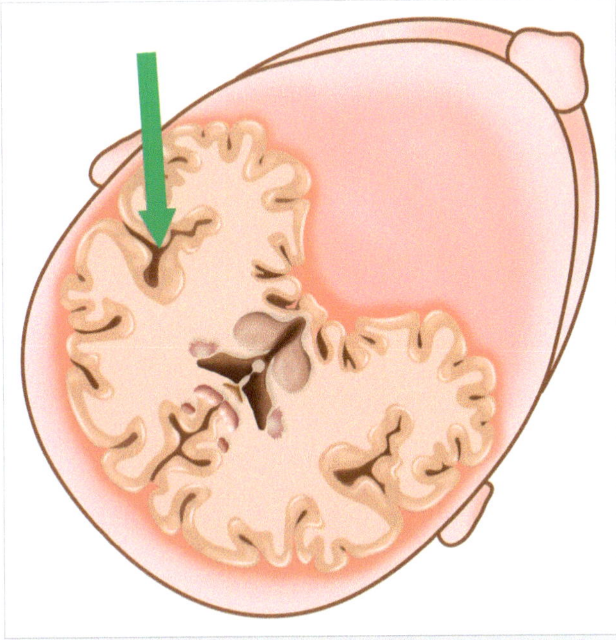

Fig. 12.6 This diagram demonstrates the angle that a temporal approach gives you into the insula. It is critical that you do not view the angle you are working at as purely inward, as you will misjudge the direction you are working at.

apart the arachnoid of the Sylvian fissure. You should be careful to not over retract across the plane of an artery leaving the fissure; however, with care this maneuver is usually safe and effective. You should continue doing this from anterior to posterior until you clearly see the circular sulcus on all sides. If you have not seen the sulcus and its groove where the opercular cortices turn back on themselves to overlie the insula, then there is a very high chance you will miss a fair bit of the insula. Of particular importance, is the need to see the posterior superior and anterior superior portions of the circular sulcus, which are much higher underneath the frontal opercula than you think. If you cannot see them then you will either miss a great deal of tumor, or you will be blindly sweeping near the SLF or corticospinal tract, both of which are suboptimal ways to operate in the insula.

You should be aware that approaching from the temporal side, your attack angle is running slightly parallel to the cortical surface, with a medial angle, which you should take into your calculations as you descend into the insula (▶ Fig. 12.6). The angle is more medial inferiorly and more flat as you progress superiorly.

From the Frontal Side

This is the less desirable approach, as it requires you to tangle with potential speech and motor sites, which adds to the risk. However, if those opercula are involved and are spilling into the insula, then there is no way to adequately address these tumors without a frontal approach. Also tumors which a large superior extent are often very difficult to tackle from the temporal side alone, and sometimes adding a frontal approach is the only way to get a good exposure.

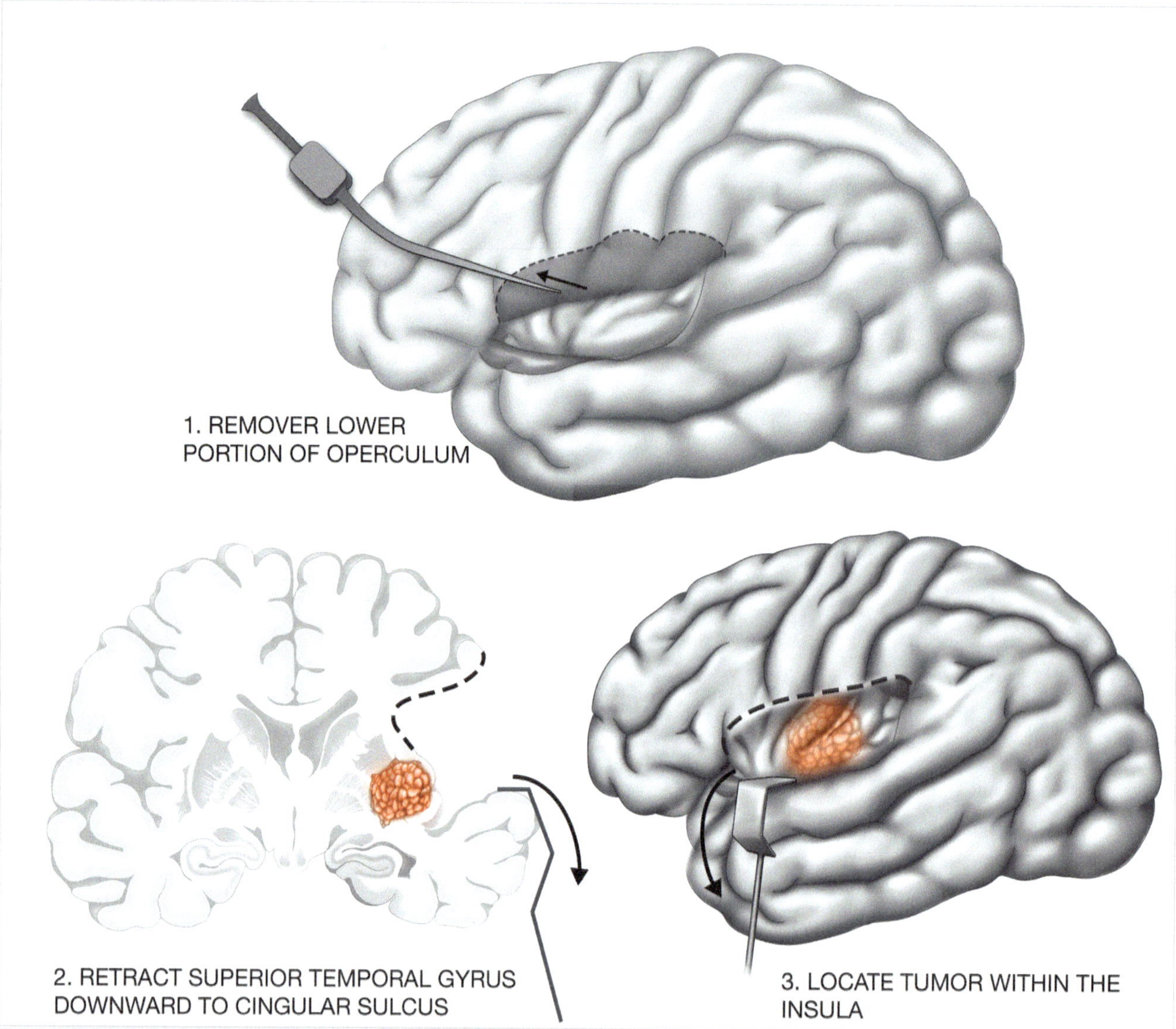

Fig. 12.7 The transopercular approach to the insula from the frontal side. This diagram demonstrates the first stage of an insular glioma operation when the tumor anatomy or preference dictates working in the frontal lobe or working from a frontal (or parietal) angle. The upper Sylvian opercula are first resected as much as allowed by the mapping. This can be combined with a lateral frontal lobe disconnection, or limited frontal lobectomy, as described in Chapter 10, if warranted. Once the upper insula is identified, the temporal opercula are swept downward gently to identify the superior boundary of the circular sulcus.

The frontal approach (▶ Fig. 12.7) involves slow, subpialization of the opercula as dictated by the mapping and tumor anatomy. Usually, if a cortex has mapped negative during the define phase, then it can be resected down to the level of the insula. It is also acceptable to resect portions of the subcentral and lower sensorimotor cortices if absolutely needed (they are bilaterally represented and well tolerated). There are numerous arteries intertwined with these cortices, and many of them are going to the motor cortex, speech, motor planning, and other critical sites.

Uninvolved opercula (i.e., ones which are being removed for exposure but not for tumor resection) do not need to be gross totally resected, but instead need to be sequentially trimmed from bottom to top until you can see their pial bank curving into the circular sulcus. A debulked sulcus is often enough to mobilize the pia and arteries and get them out of the way.

An analogous sweeping of the STG off of the insula is then performed with the caveat that the "artery of death" may limit how much you can do this, and you may need to remove some STG as well to get enough room.

Note that while the attack angle of the frontal approach also parallels the insular cortex, it is more consistently parallel than the temporal approach (▶ Fig. 12.8). In other words, you are often looking at the side of the insula, instead of directly medial to lateral as your mind thinks of it.

From Both Sides

Obviously, there are numerous possible permutations depending on the size and anatomy of the tumor and the functional brain anatomy. In most combined cases, I do the temporal side

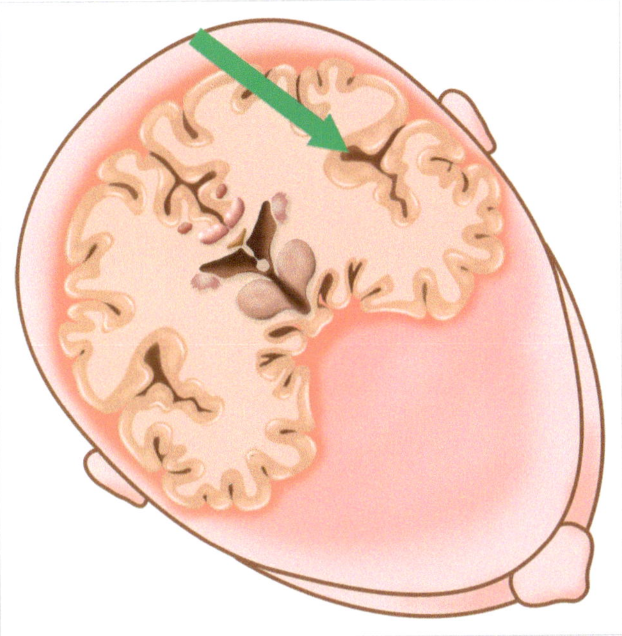

Fig. 12.8 This diagram demonstrates the angle that a frontal approach gives you into the insula. It is critical that you do not view the angle you are working at as purely inward, as you will misjudge the direction you are working at. Note that you are working nearly parallel to the insular cortex.

first, because it makes a lot of room quickly, and this shows me where the insula is which assists with the other portions.

12.4.2 Phase 2: Removing the Insula

The insular cut is a concept (▶ Fig. 12.9), as it is probably not possible to remove the insula in one piece. Rather, you are using mapping to separate the insula from the tracts which frame it, the SLF above and posterior, and the IFOF which runs somewhere in the subinsular stem and which hooks forward in the medial limen insula. There is also a deep cut which separates the tumor from the basal ganglia and the posterior limb of the internal capsule which is fully laterally exposed in the posterior portion.

The value of the transopercular approach is particularly evident when trying to find the IFOF. Stimulation mapping with continuous subcortical monitoring will allow you to determine what parts of the inferior insula can be safely resected and when to stop.

The superior cut risks the SLF as well as the descending motor fibers. You should utilize the fact that you are largely angled parallel to the insular cortex whether you are coming from the temporal or frontal side to prevent yourself from overshooting into these tracts. The circular sulcus is the critical landmark, and you should not veer far superior to this into the deep white matter.

If the tumor is following the uncinate fasciculus into the frontal lobe, it is important to stay within the insula as you head anterior-superior into the orbitofrontal region. You can also enter this by removing the pars triangularis, but this risks disorientation, as having the frontal lobe cortices in place is a good safe guard against taking wide angles into important white matter tracts.

12.5 The "Destroy" Phase

I never stop mapping the patient while I'm removing the insula, so there isn't a true asleep phase saves from a temporal or frontal lobe resection which is described in other chapters.

But there are some aspects of insular resection which are uniform, and not altered by brain mapping, which are discussed below.

12.5.1 How Do You Know How Deep to Go?

This is a common question I am asked, which should have an obvious answer by now, if you have been paying close attention. If you have entered from the temporal side, there is a reason the hippocampus is always left for last (▶ Fig. 12.10), as it sits directly inferior to the basal ganglia in essentially all patients. The insular resection should continue until it is flush with the basal ganglia. Thus, I resect the insula until the lateral aspect of the resection cavity is roughly parallel with the hippocampus in the sagittal plane. Obviously, this is a judgment call, and you should also be continually looking for tissue characteristics suggesting that you are in the putamen (putamen tissue looks like the caudate head tissue grossly), as it can look deceptively like tumor and you can remove a fair bit of putamen before you realize you are in it.

There is a less obvious reason for keeping the hippocampus in place until the insula work is finished: it prevents disorientation when working on the inferior surface of the insula and central core (▶ Fig. 12.10). Medial-to-lateral orientation is easy to lose when there is nothing preventing you from working on the undersurface of the central cerebral core, and it is easy to drift into the wrong plane, and into trouble. The presence of the hippocampus prevents this from occurring, and serves as a depth gauge.

If you have approached solely from the frontal side, you lack this depth gauge and it is harder to tell how deep to go. Obviously, subcortical monitoring is one source of this information, and the appearance of putamen tissue is another, but also the angle of access to the insula in the frontal transopercular approach parallels the cortex, meaning heading too medial is not usually a natural maneuver (usually you have to force yourself medial or you will be inadequately resecting tumor. Another trick is to use the STG and/or MTG width as a guide of about how deep to take the insular resection below its cortical surface (you are looking down on both of them at the same angle). If part of the STG has been removed you also can use the medial base of MTG to estimate the approximate site of the hippocampus.

12.6 Rules of Working in Insular Windows

The insula is removed between branches of the MCA by making small windows in the insular cortex between these arteries, and then connecting those windows underneath the arteries. This sounds simple enough, but there are a lot of pitfalls you need to avoid in order to do this effectively which are summarized below (▶ Fig. 12.11).

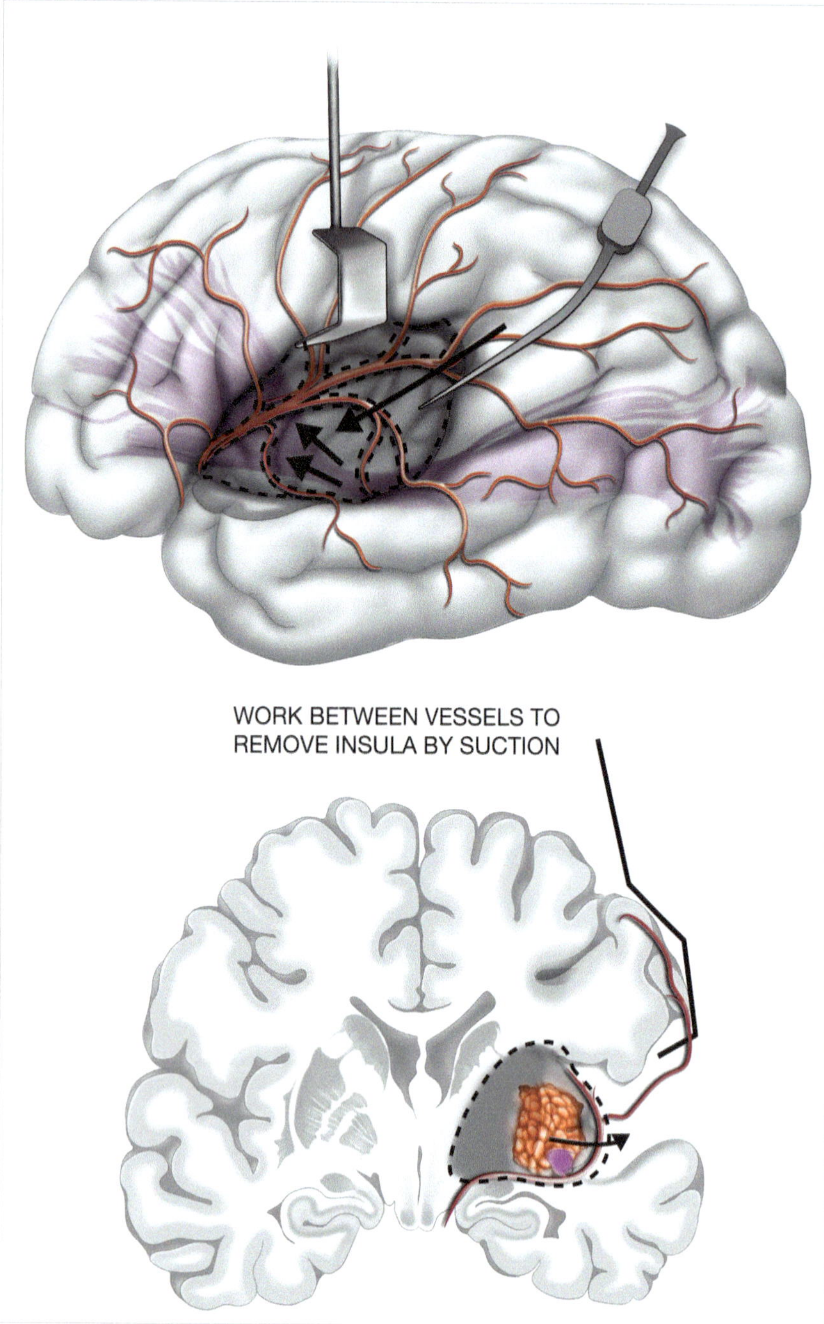

Fig. 12.9 Removal of the insula. Once the transopercular approach is complete, removal of the insula involves identifying the windows between the MCA branches and sacrificing the circumflex arteries which supply the insular cortex. Following this, involved insula is removed until the depth of resection roughly parallels the hippocampus and temporal horn, meaning that it is approximately down to the level of the basal ganglia. The windows are then connected underneath the MCA branches until the branches are floating freely. The resection is performed with care taken to identify and save the IFOF, and the mapping portion of the case does not end until this is completely clear from front to back.

Rule 1: Don't work in any windows until you have exposed all windows and all relevant boundaries of the insula. It is easy to become disoriented in the insula, and as soon as you start removing tumor, you begin to destroy the anatomy, making it very hard to re-orient yourself.

Rule 2: Work in all possible windows. This is a logical extension of subsequent rules, but remember that it is a lot easier for parts of the insula to hide behind arterial complexes than you think. Even with the opercula off, you don't have a panoramic view this deep in the brain

Rule 3: Connect all windows. There is a lot more hiding under the arteries than you think there is. When you are done, you should see the entire MCA trunk floating in space. This will be unnerving the first time you do it, but this is what resecting the insula means.

Rule 4: Kill the circumflex arteries before they kill you. The insula has a blood supply, and that blood supply comes from the MCA via small circumflex arteries which come off the MCA trunks and branches. These small arteries need to be sacrificed and divided from the MCA trunk at the earliest point possible, as they are prone to avulsing off the MCA branches leaving a hole in the artery which needs to be closed.

Rule 5: Do not take more than a window will allow. This is perhaps the most important rule. It is easy to find a nice space between MCA trunks which seems easy to work in and to try to continue to resect the insula in that window indefinitely. You must discipline yourself to not do so, and to follow rule 2, even

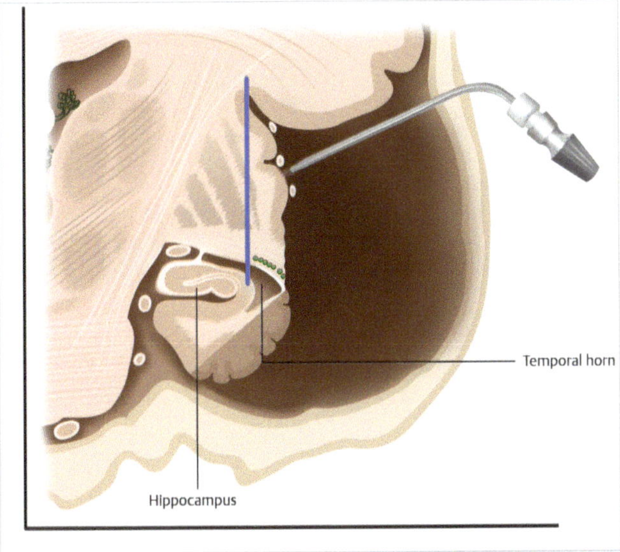

Fig. 12.10 This figure reiterates the role of the hippocampus as a landmark and depth gauge during insular resection. Not only does it indicate the approximate depth of the basal ganglia, but it also prevents you from entering the basal ganglia from below when it is present.

if that means working in a less comfortable window. You have to manipulate the arteries and gently retract them in order to do this case, but if you get too greedy with a window, you can tear a main trunk at its branch point, which is dangerous and unpleasant. If you are working far under an artery, even if you think you can keep going, you should explore other windows and work towards using all of your spaces instead.

Rule 6: Beware retraction at arterial bifurcations. Bifurcations are great places to overstretch arteries, as often one branch is often leaving the fissure and is tethered to the operculum. You will often have to work inside a tight bifurcation, but you should strongly consider only doing so long enough to detach the brain immediately in the "V" of this bifurcation, and then use this new mobility to work on both sides of the "V" which is usually roomier.

Rule 7: Maintain orientation. It's very easy to get on a roll in this case, but you should always make a conscious effort to slow down and reconsider what angle you are working at. You can't go back and put white matter or putamen back in if you get lost and go too deep at the wrong angle.

12.7 Case Examples

12.7.1 Temporoinsular Tumors

▸ Fig. 12.12 demonstrates a large residual insular glioma after a minor resection in the anterior temporal lobe done elsewhere. A temporal lobectomy was performed as part of a transopercular resection of the insula. This is an excellent photo of the expected final product of an insular resection: the MCA should be floating in the air. This is also visible on the post-operative MRI. There is residual disease in the pre-motor regions.

a) The lateral part of the anterior temporal lobe has been removed but the insula is quite large, the hippocampus is full of tumor, and the tumor extends into the premotor areas. The plan is to perform a temporal lobectomy, remove the STG, and use the inferior angle to reach under the opercula to reach the top of the insula.
b) This image demonstrates the final resection appearance which demonstrates the MCA branches are floating freely. This will seem overly aggressive if you have never done this before, but it is well tolerated if other anatomy is respected. Of note, we utilized the previous incision, which was larger than I would normally do.
c) The DTIs demonstrate that the upper portion of this tumor involve the motor planning networks. Note that there is tumor in the FAT and anterior contributions to the motor planning networks. This is the most challenging thing insular gliomas do, and you have to decide if it's worthwhile to try to remove frontal opercula and go after it. I decided not to (it was earlier in my series; today I probably would try under the idea that it may be difficult).
d) Overall the tumor resection is good. Obviously there is tumor intentionally left in the premotor areas. Unintentionally left was a small area of involved medial temporal lobe. The reasons this was missed were likely two-fold. First, it was early in my experience, and I wasn't as confident chasing an enlarged medial temporal lobe as far medial as I do today. Today, I continue until I see the carotid, third nerve, and PCA clearly, no matter how much this seems uncomfortable (the exception being radiated recurrent glioblastoma. Second, it is easy to not position the patient correctly for these cases, and in an insular case, if you approach from the temporal side and you don't drop the head downward a bit, you will be slicing the uncus in the sagittal plane and will miss the top of it as I did here.

▸ Fig. 12.13 demonstrates a large right-sided temporoinsular glioma. Spatiotemporal mapping limited the posterior cut, slightly but despite this, this was a complete resection.

a) The obvious approach in a case like this is to approach this from the temporal lobe side as a lobectomy is warranted. The sagittal and coronal images show a C-shape of this tumor which is following the uncinate into the orbitofrontal cortex. This should usually be followed upward and anterior into the frontal lobe through the insula.
b) None.
c) The tractography is very favorable: IFOF is pushed medially, the SLF network is fairly far posterior, and the FAT is not directly threatened by the top of this tumor.
d) The resection is excellent. Note that with continuous subcortical monitoring, we took this resection right up to the internal without deficit.

▸ Fig. 12.14 demonstrates the interesting case of a small left insular glioma which deflected the IFOF medially. This does not always occur, but luckily for this patient we were able to get an excellent resection of this tumor due to this deviation of IFOF in the subinsular space.

a) Note that the primary pathway of spread for this tumor is down into the temporal lobe, but it also involves junctional SMG folds. On the left side, a tumor which straddles the subinsular space and involves the SMG usually spells trouble on two fronts, IFOF and SLF/semantic networks. Also it is

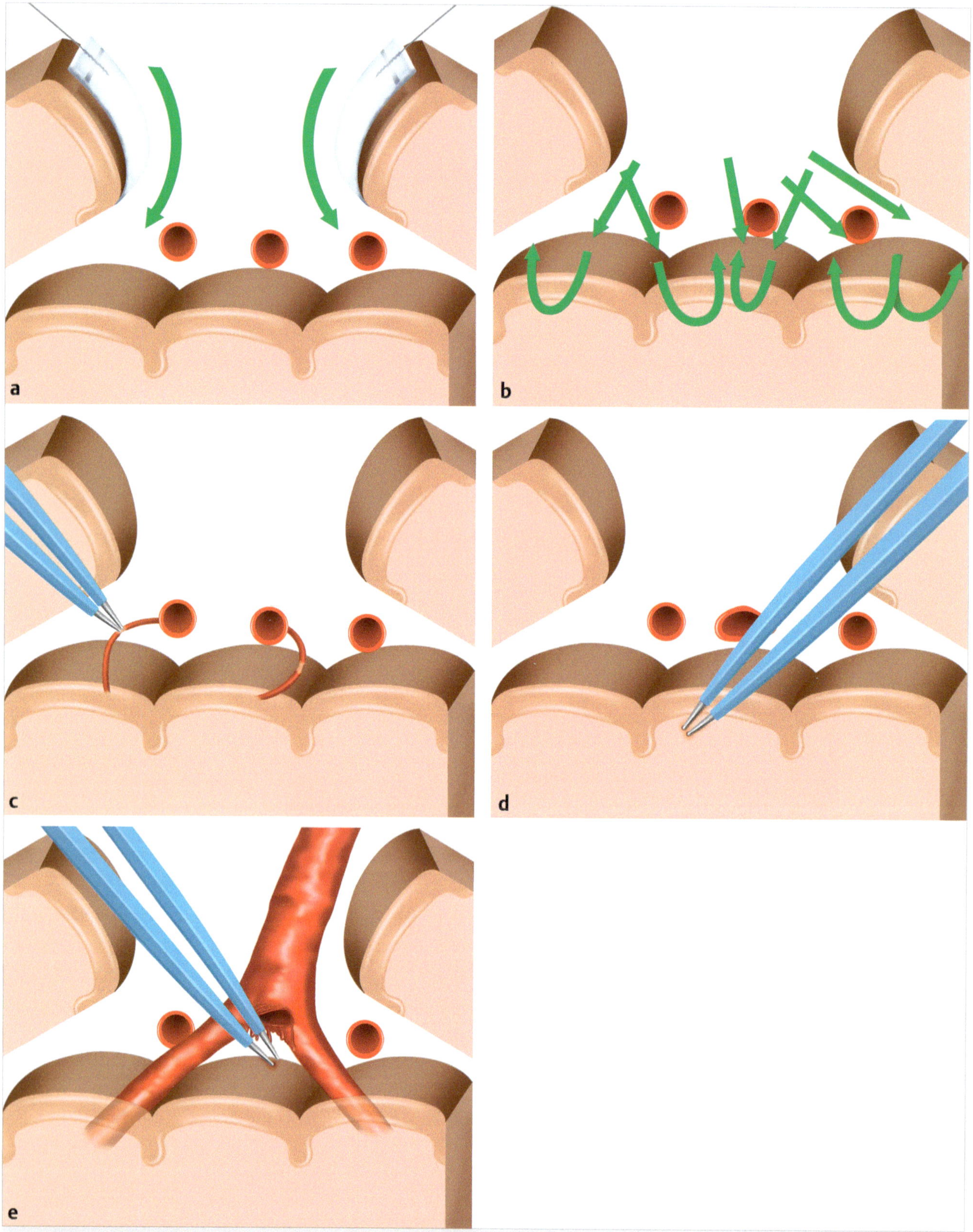

Fig. 12.11 These figures demonstrate the rules working safely in insular windows. (**a, b**) Rules 1–3 in the text describe the need to maximize the use of windows in a systematic way. (**c,d**) Rules 4–6 describe ways to avoid injury to the MCA, and these issues are depicted in this figure. (**e**) Rule 7, specifically the consequences of disorientation in the insula, is depicted in this figure.

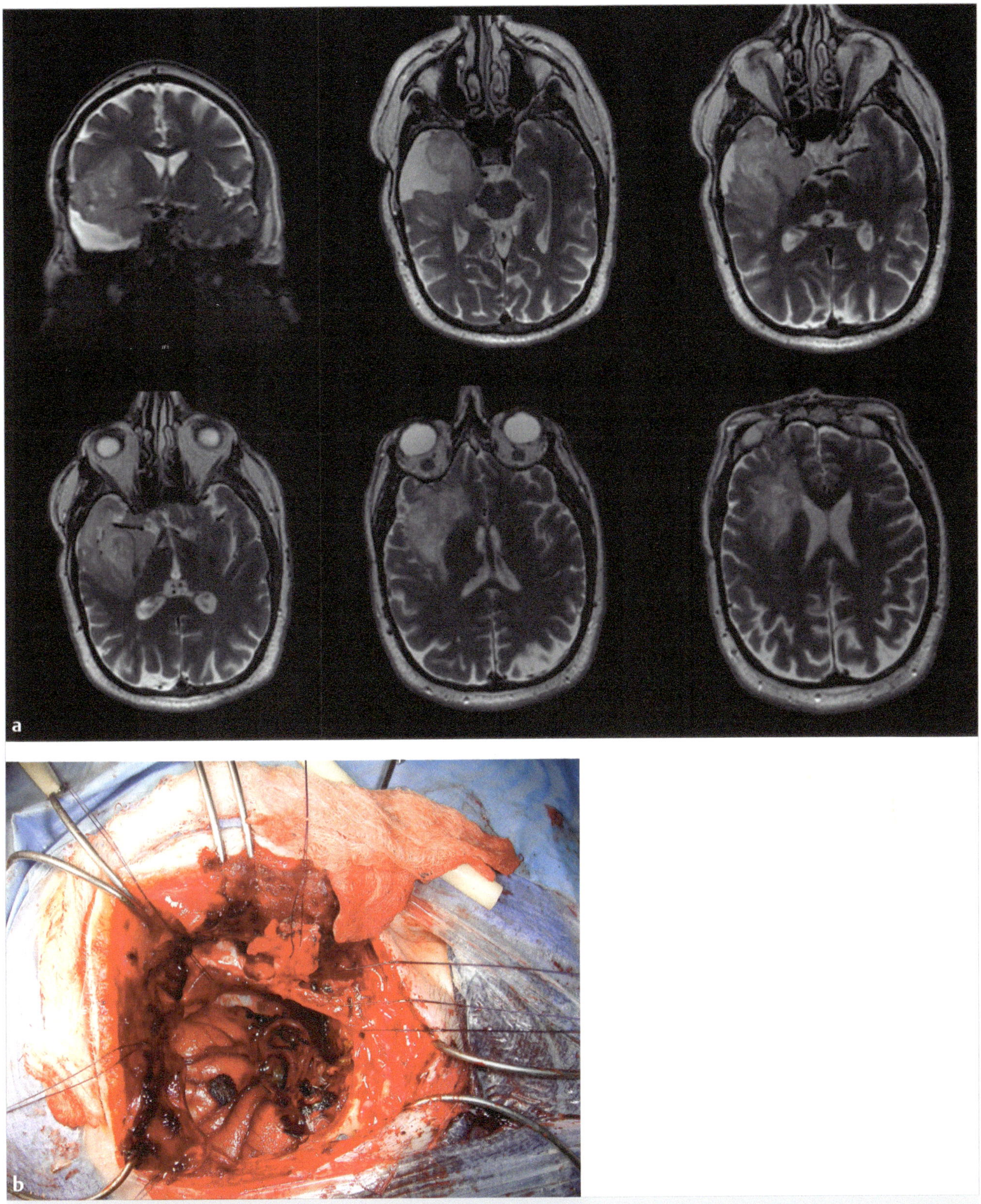

Fig. 12.12 A large residual insular glioma after a minor resection in the anterior temporal lobe done elsewhere. (**a**) Preoperative images, (**b**) images of the approach. (*Continued*)

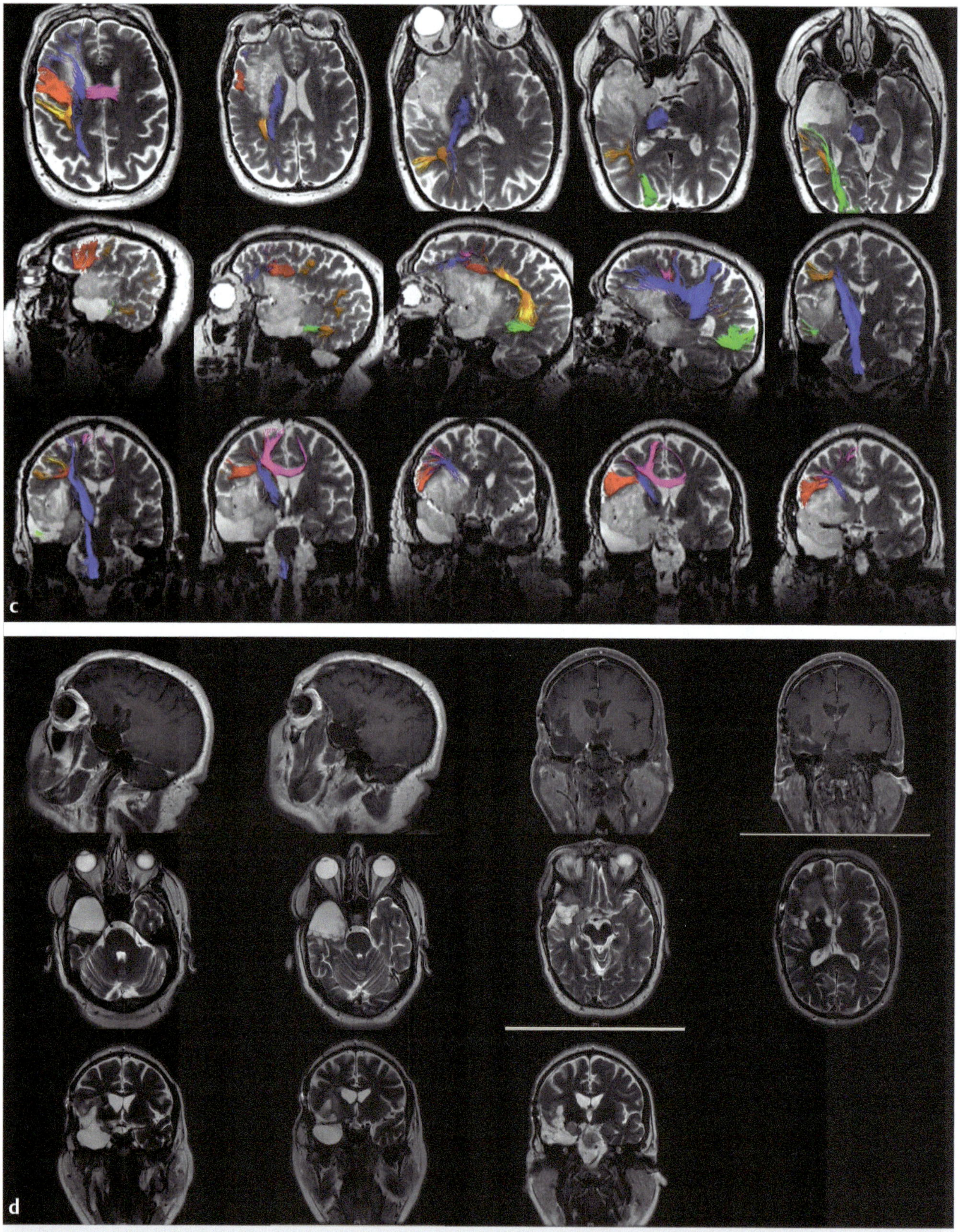

Fig 12.12 (*Continued*) (**c**) DTI tractography, (**d**) postoperative images.

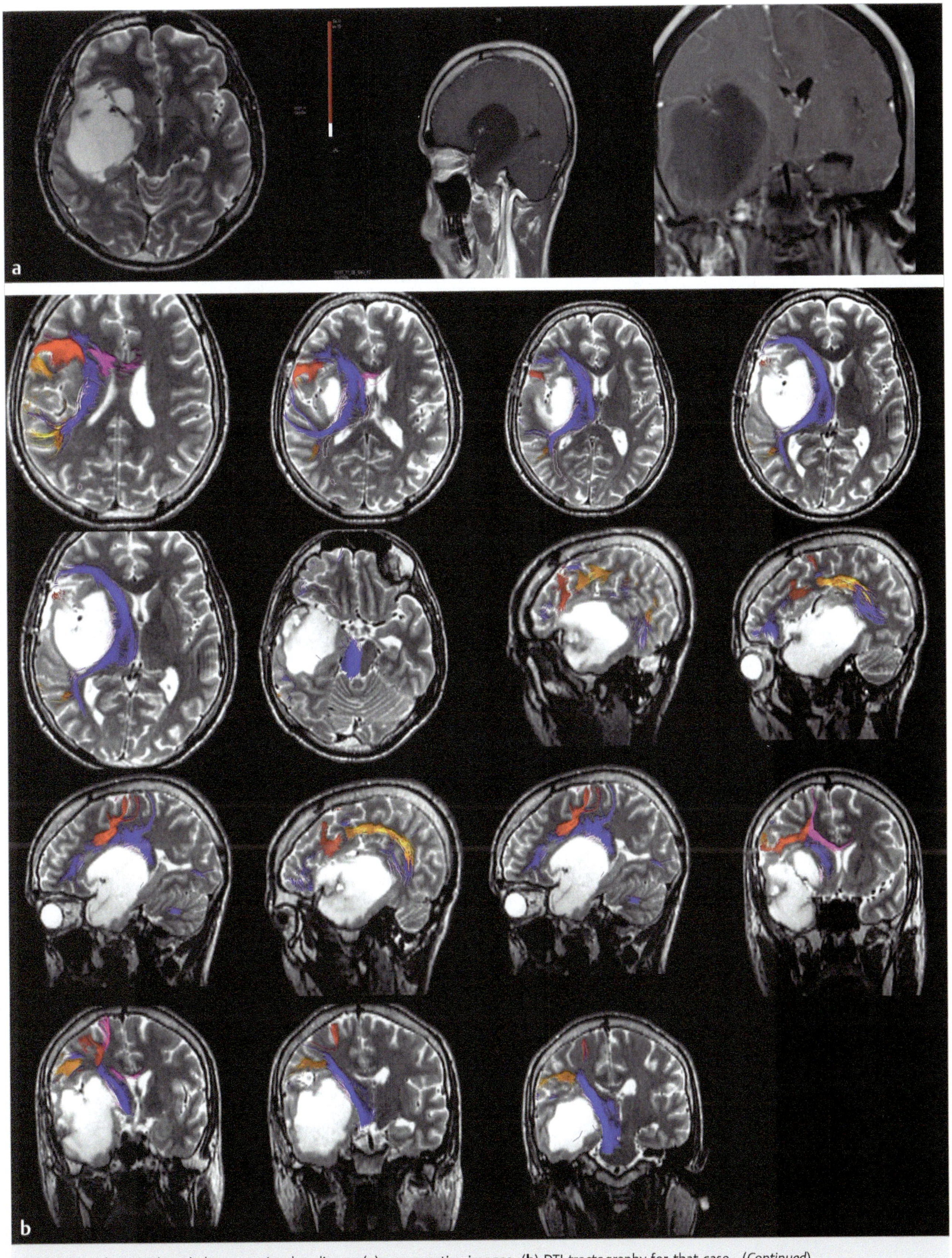

Fig. 12.13 A large right-sided temporoinsular glioma; (**a**) preoperative images, (**b**) DTI tractography for that case. *(Continued)*

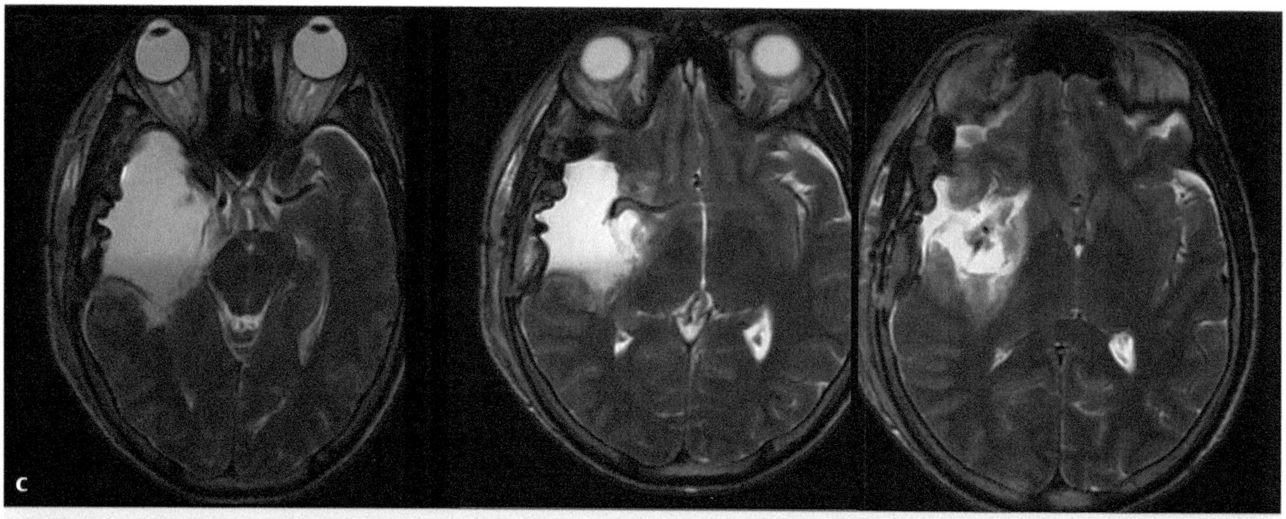

Fig 12.13 (*Continued*) (**c**) Postoperative images.

important to note that there is signal change in the pulvinar. I have seen this at least 15 times in various insular gliomas and have never seen this area progress without treatment once, even when followed for a few years. I suspect that this is some kind of Wallerian degeneration involving some aspect of the posterior thalamic peduncle as I have followed the signal change on multiple cuts in these cases and have never seen one which directly connects the insula and pulvinar with signal change and have never seen one of these combos cross the internal capsule to get there. It could always be spread on a microscopic level, I acknowledge; however, until I see one progress in the thalamus, I will continue to leave the thalamic part alone in these cases.

b) Given the DTIs which show an unfavorable SLF, and the small amount of temporal tumor, we planned for a limited temporal approach. This involves STG resection and focusing our efforts around the insula and temporal junction as much as possible. If possible (namely if the DTI of the IFOF was real), we would address the small part in the temporal lobe by following the tumor downward from the insula. We were ready for this to be a challenging case. Finding a naming site in the STG didn't make this easier.
c) The DTIs were extremely important in understanding this case. The IFOF, fortunately made a nearly 90-degree medial bend at the back of the tumor and remained there throughout its course, which was a big help. The SLF, in contrast was far anterior in the STG (and this was accurate at surgery). This caused us to change our approach to a more anterior and limited approach than we would normally do, as it was clear he had not reorganized to any significant extent.
d) The resection was surprisingly good and we managed to clear out the subinsular space and temporal lobe due to the displaced IFOF.

▸ Fig. 12.15 demonstrates a sizeable left temporoinsular tumor aggressively resected. Tumor was left in the temporal junctional areas due to speech considerations.

a) This tumor is so large temporally that tumor has herniated over the tentorium and is compressing the midbrain. Most of this is temporal, and the correct approach is clearly from the temporal side, but the insula needs to be accounted for. This is probably best done by removing the STG and working in the insula.
b) Despite the large question mark incision from a previous debulking done outside, we ignored this and put a linear incision in the middle of it which healed fine. Generally, as much as possible, I try to do my surgery as if the last surgery never happened. I strongly recommend not allowing someone else's decisions in a previous operation to change your decisions in the present one. Thus, I almost never reopen the entire previous incision, or remove the old bone flap. I put my incision and bone flap where I think it needs to be unless absolutely forced.

Note that this tumor extends very far posteriorly in the medial temporal system. The cut needs to be angled as far posteriorly under the speech networks as possible. Note that we found an anomia site which limited our posterior extent of the cut, but we angled underneath this and turned the bed to be able to work as far back as possible.

a) The SLF is terminating at a favorable site. The IFOF is faint but can be seen on the coronal sections. It is running through the medial and inferior part of the insular tumor. From this, we expect to be able to put our cut posteriorly enough to reach back and remove the medial temporal lobe quite well. The IFOF will cause some problems, however, as we address the insula.
b) The postoperative scan overall looks good, but there is tumor still in the posterior junctional white matter, obviously left there to protect the IFOF. There is also a small bit of tumor in the fornix. Neither of these have progressed at 3 years of follow-up to date.

▸ Fig. 12.16 demonstrates a right temporoinsular tumor which involves the basal ganglia also. Invasion of the basal ganglia is uncommon in insular tumors; however, in my experience, resecting the insula and temporal lobe, and treating the basal ganglia component with chemoradiation is often able to make the basal ganglia portion regress. It did in this case.

a) This tumor is centered in the medial temporal lobe and insula, but concerningly in this case, it appears to be in the

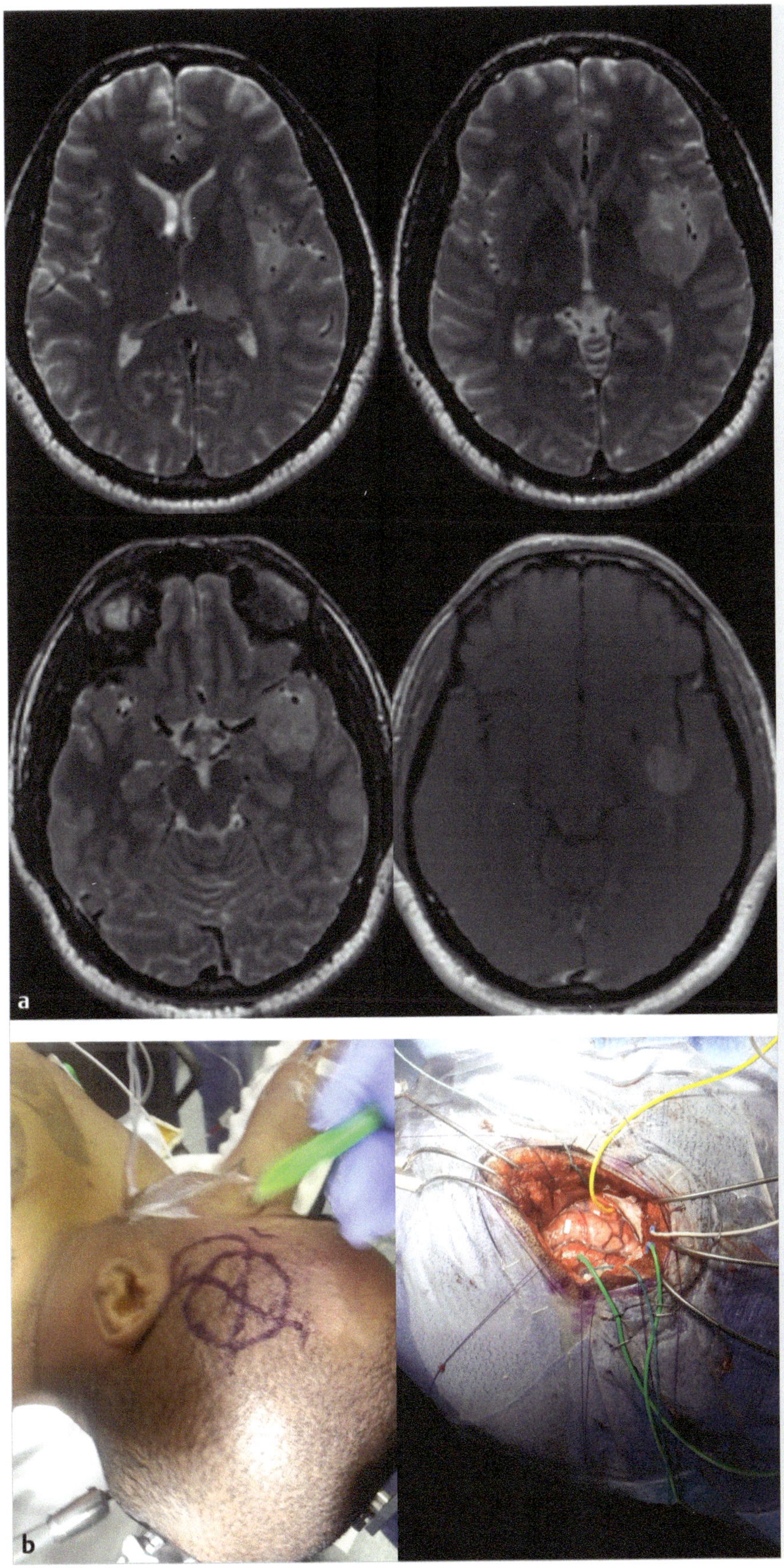

Fig. 12.14 An interesting case of a small left insular glioma which deflected the IFOF medially; (**a**) preoperative images, (**b**) images of the approach. (*Continued*)

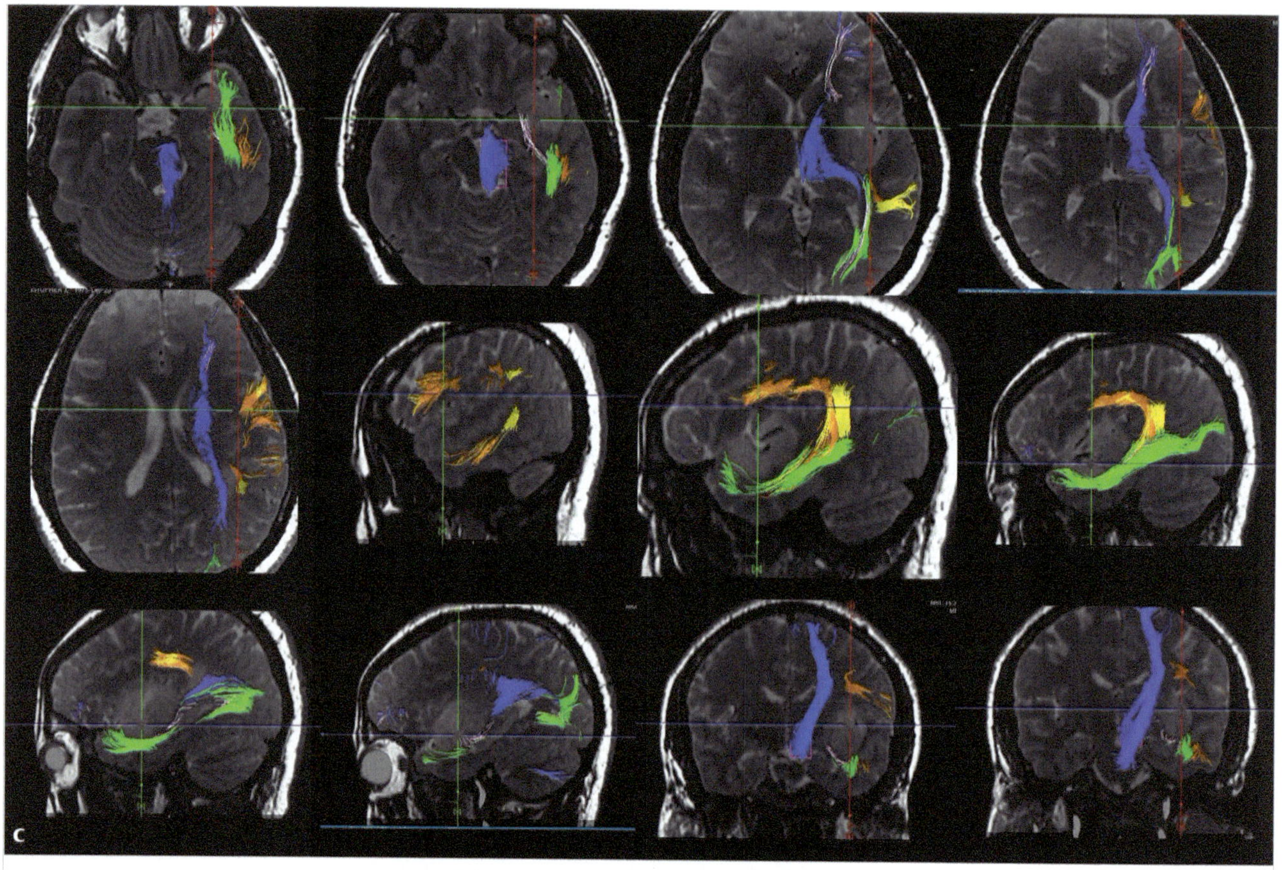

c

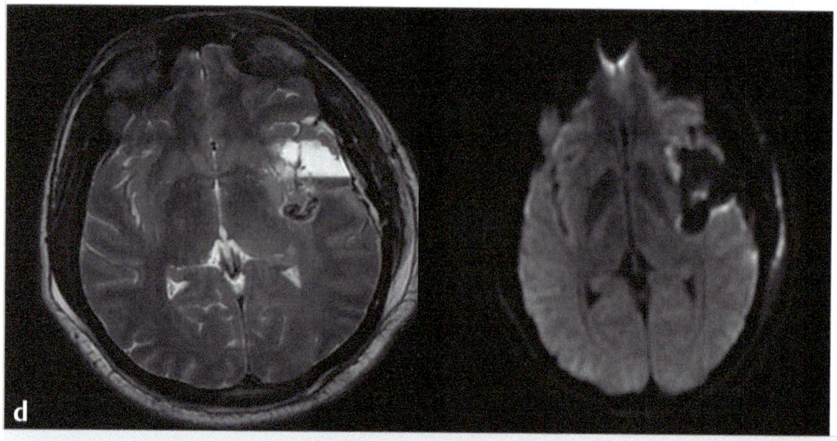

d

Fig 12.14 *(Continued)* (**c**) DTI tractography, (**d**) postoperative images.

subthalamic regions, and has the anterior commissure running through parts of it. Our goal in this case is not complete resection, but rather to isolate the bad parts by dealing with the majority of this tumor.

b) The craniotomy is centered on the back of the Sylvian fissure and the STG/MTG. This allows us to understand the right semantic network and preserve it. The temporal lobe is removed under the bone flap and the insula (whose anterior edge is quite posterior to the temporal tip) is centered under this flap. The right panel shows the skeletonized MCA in the resection cavity.

c) The IFOF is somewhat at risk at the top of this tumor, but is mostly deflected superiorly and medially. The SLF is quite favorably posterior.

d) Note that after removal of the insula and temporal lobe, there is still T2 change in the putamen, and subthalamic region.

e) This 1 year post-treatment image demonstrates regression of the tumor from the deep structures. I have found that this often happens.

▶ Fig. 12.17 demonstrates a large recurrent glioblastoma involving the temporal lobe and insula which encases the lenticulostriates. I am cautious medially with this high risk artery situation, but resected the rest, leaving some tumor medially.

a) This tumor is filling the temporal lobe resection cavity, filling the insula, and following the uncinate fasciculus. The coronal images suggest that this tumor might be on top of and

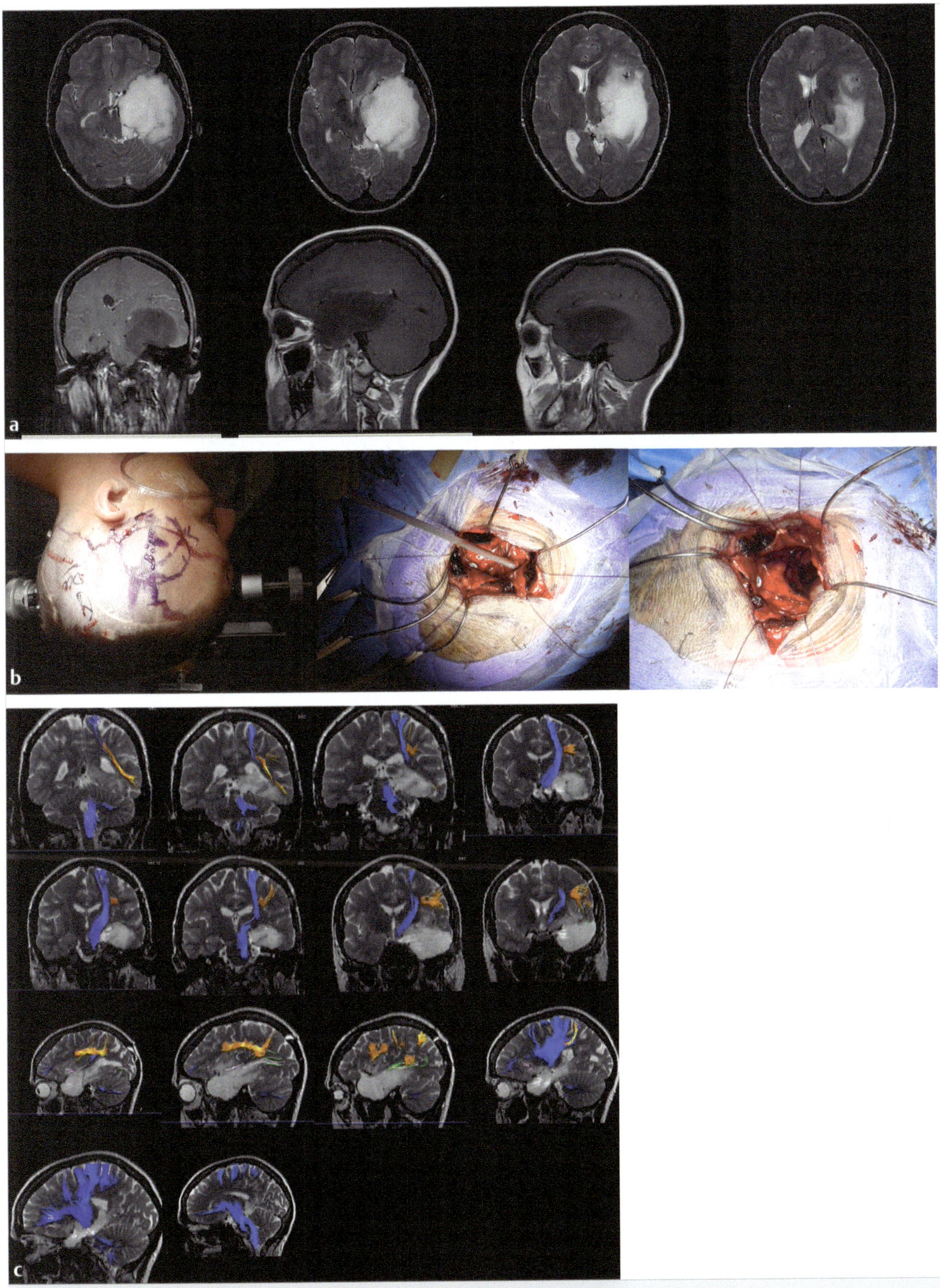

Fig. 12.15 A sizeable left temporoinsular tumor aggressively resected; (a) preoperative images, (b) images of the approach, (c) DTI tractography for that case. (*Continued*)

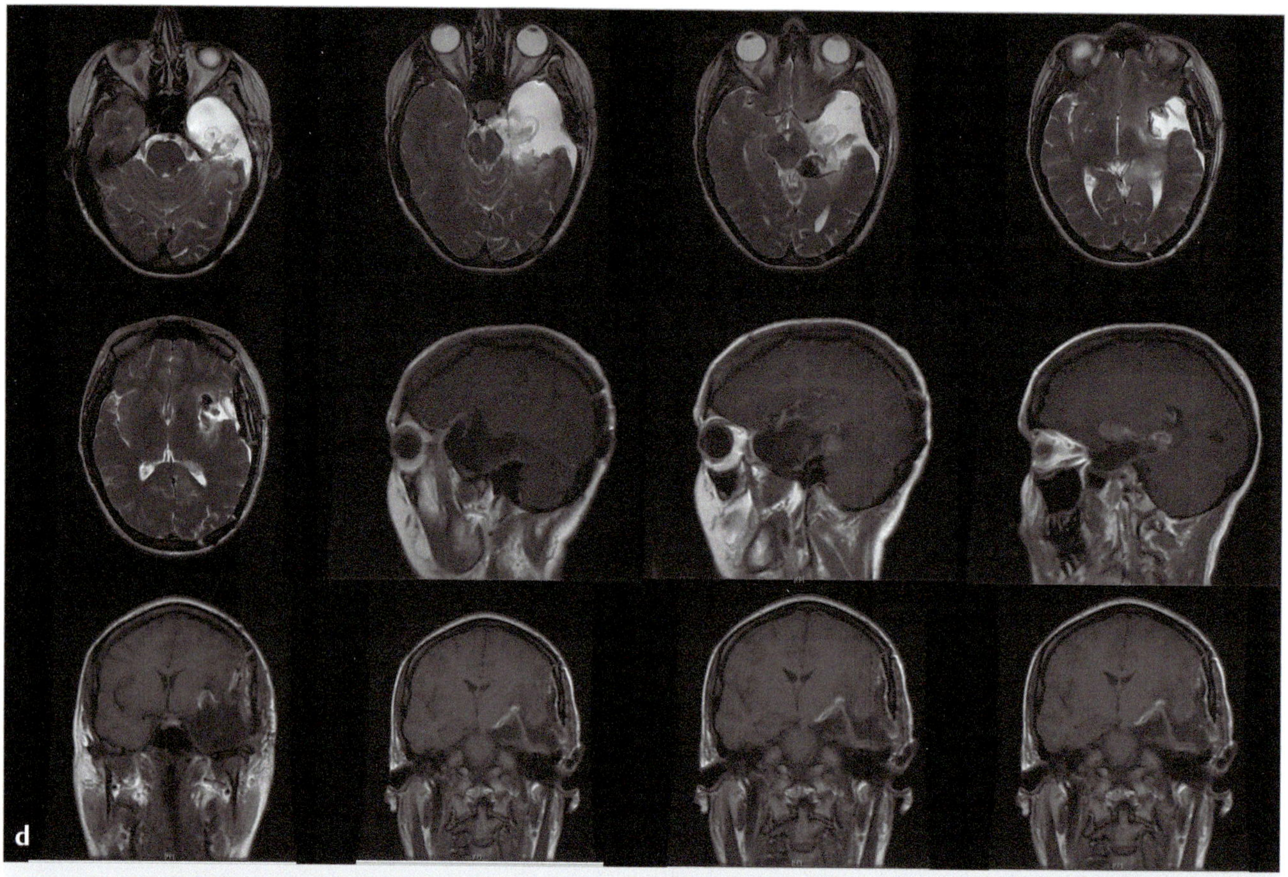

Fig 12.15 (*Continued*) (**d**) Postoperative images.

behind the M1, and the T2 images suggest that there are small arteries within the anteromedial parts of the tumor. We should have realistic goals with cases like this.

b) The large question mark incision of the previous surgery, left us unable to totally ignore it and make a vascularly acceptable skin incision. Thus, we opened the bottom of the incision and folded it forward. The cuts were made in the usual locations.

c) The IFOF, SLF, and descending motor fibers look like they are pushed well away from the tumor, which left us optimistic that we should be able to aggressively resect the temporal lobe and insula with acceptable risk. The temporal lobe cut was a kind of J-cut, as described in Chapter 15, to re-establish a posterior temporal division plane.

d) Note that while there is a small rim of enhancement near the deep structures, that we will removed the temporal lobe, insula, and followed the tumor medially. Having a goal of less than gross total resection doesn't open the door to leaving tumor where it is safely removable, it just means we stop. This is still a very good cytoreductive surgery, despite not being 100% complete resection.

▶ Fig. 12.18 demonstrates a temporoinsular recurrence of a previous anterior frontoinsular glioma. The resection involved a temporoinsular type approach, using the anterior resection cavity as a guide to know when we are anterior enough. Despite the massive resection cavity, this patient remained quite functional.

a) This patient had previously undergone two surgeries with Professor Yasargil for a frontal low grade glioma, which explains the large resection cavity. He now has progression in the insula and temporal lobe years later. Note that the basal ganglia are pushed, not invaded. The plan is for a temporal insular glioma which ends in the previous resection cavity.

b) There was a previous pterional type incision, which we used the bottom half of to expose the temporal lobe and insula.

c) The SLF is primarily a parietal system in this patient with minimal extension into the temporal lobe. Looking at the axial images demonstrates that the IFOF hooks quite medial around the tumor and runs just medial to the resection cavity.

d) The resection cavity is quite large but was very well tolerated. Interestingly, the ultimate site of recurrence after this surgery was not the edge of the resection cavity, but the diagonal band of Broca and basal forebrain. The amygdala is a pathway of spread to the other side and into unresectable areas, and this should give pause to anyone who leaves involved amygdala behind to prevent "mild memory problems."

12.7.2 Frontoinsular Approaches

▶ Fig. 12.19 demonstrates a GBM centered in the anterior insula which encases portions of the MCA. This approach involved an anterior temporal lobe resection, but our work focused on the

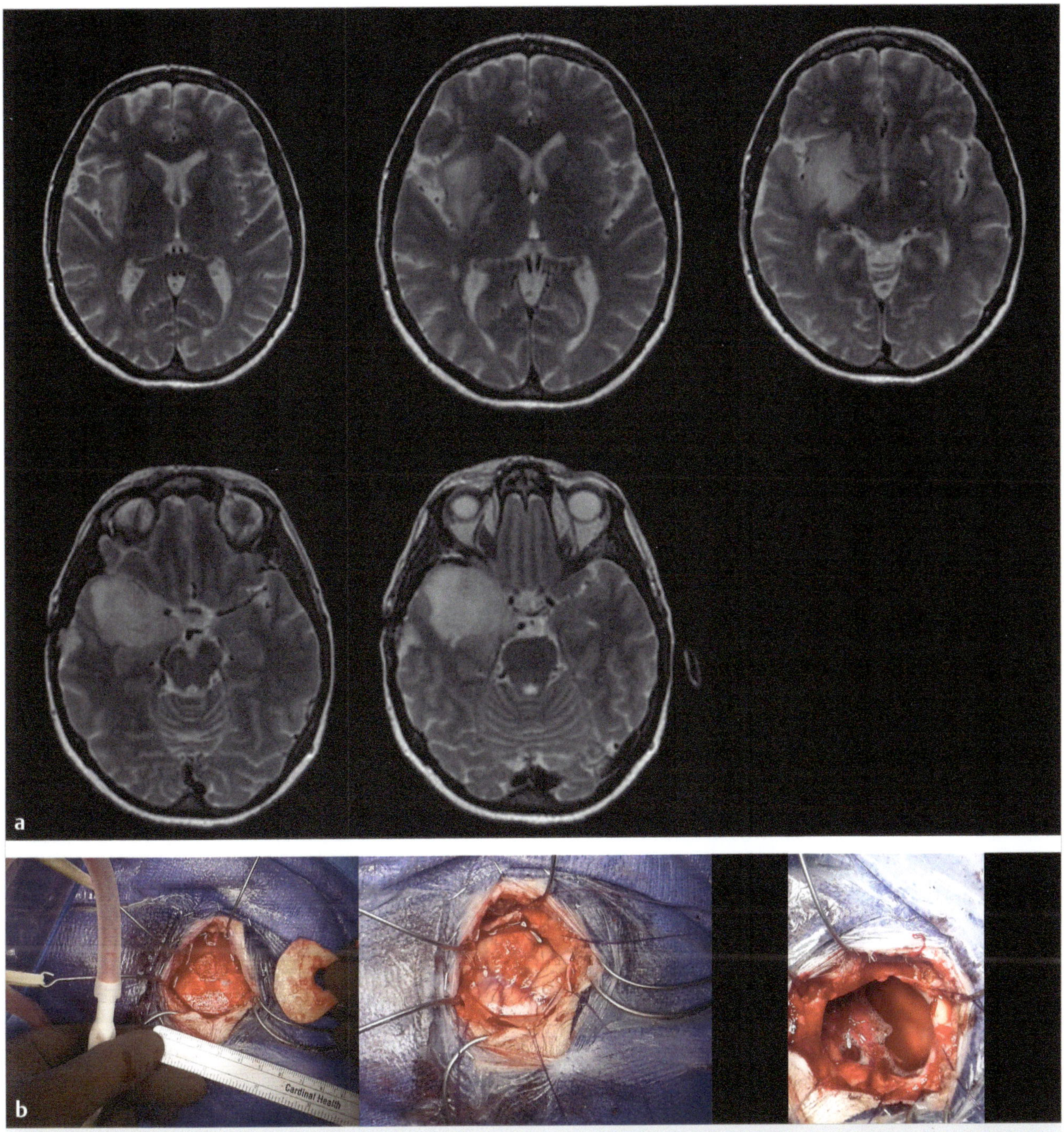

Fig. 12.16 A right temporoinsular tumor which involves the basal ganglia; (**a**) preoperative images, (**b**) images of the approach. (*Continued*)

frontal side to get access. By making a lateral frontal type cut to separate the tumor from the SLF, and resecting the anterior insula behind the tumor, we were able to isolate the tumor from the cerebrum, allowing us to dissect this tumor from the vessels under direct visualization, similar to a meningioma.

a) The anatomy of this tumor is interesting. It is in both temporal and orbitofrontal cortices, implying that it is in the uncinate fasciculus or less likely IFOF. The critical detail in this case is that the MCA and Sylvian cleft is entirely pushed backward by this tumor, suggesting that most of the insula is behind the tumor (though it has to be in the insula to some limited extent to be following the uncinate). This means that the secret to this case is view this case like it is a lateral sphenoid wing meningioma, that it is mostly anterior to the MCA, and that our job is to separate it from the MCA trunk. The goal of mapping in a case like this is to cut it out of the frontal and temporal lobe so it is basically a sphenoid wing meningioma. Obviously the difference is that part of this tumor will be in the insula, but much of this is anterior to the insula.
b) Note the typical surface mapping of the insula and opercula. This craniotomy is made far more anterior than other ones based around the thought that we are mentally dealing with something similar to a sphenoid wing meningioma.

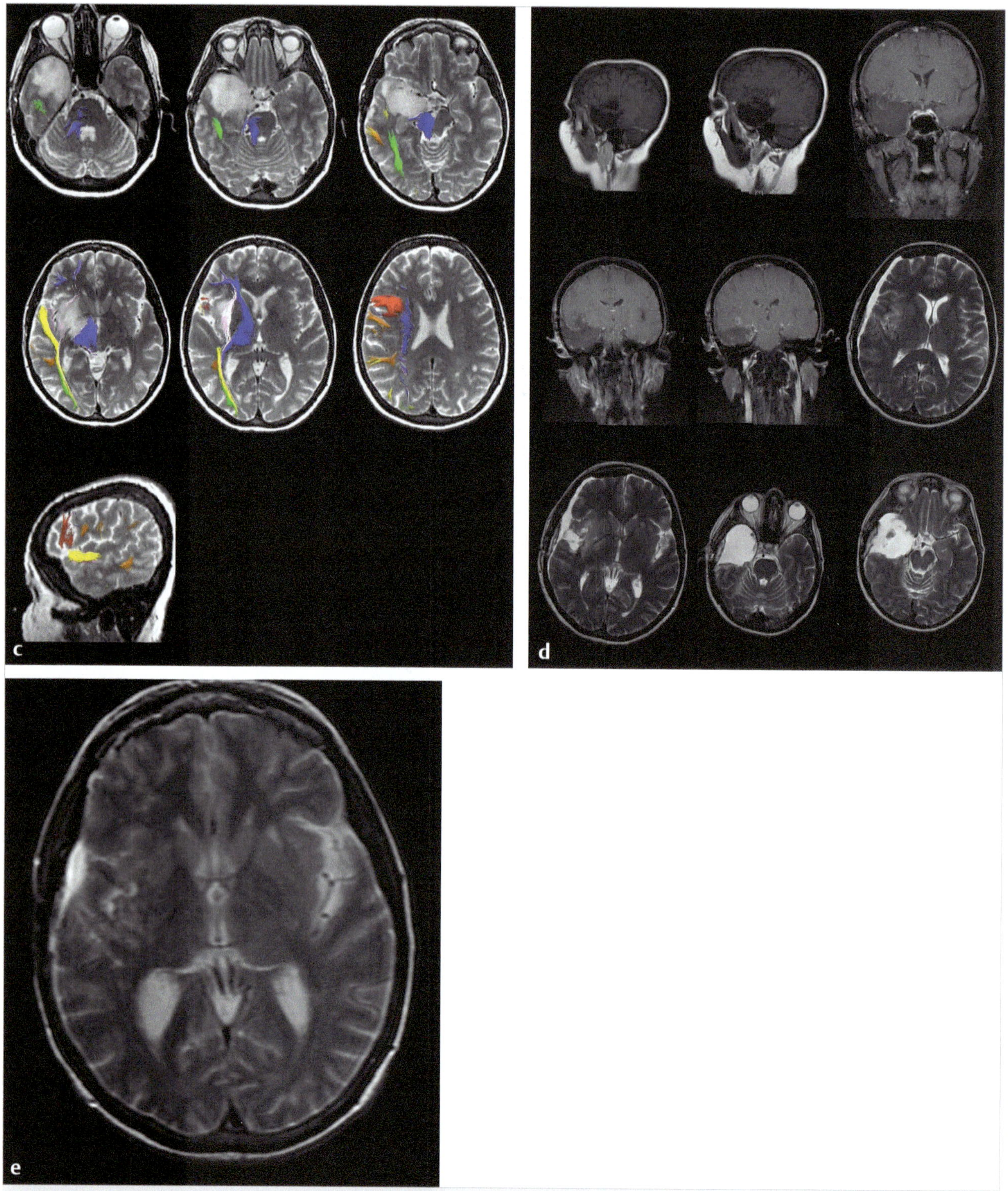

Fig 12.16 (*Continued*) (**c**) DTI tractography, (**d**) postoperative images, (**e**) long-term follow-up image.

c) The DTIs indicate that the SLF and FAT are far posterior to this tumor, and this is favorable in our goal to separate this tumor from the motor planning areas. As seen in the operative images, we were able to make an aggressive lateral frontal cut which made the boundaries of the tumor clear.

d) Note that on the postoperative images that the enhancement has been completely removed. Blood products surrounding branches of the MCA indicate that in addition to removing the enhancement, I have also removed parts of the insula and the anterior temporal tip to remove as much of the T2 changes as possible.

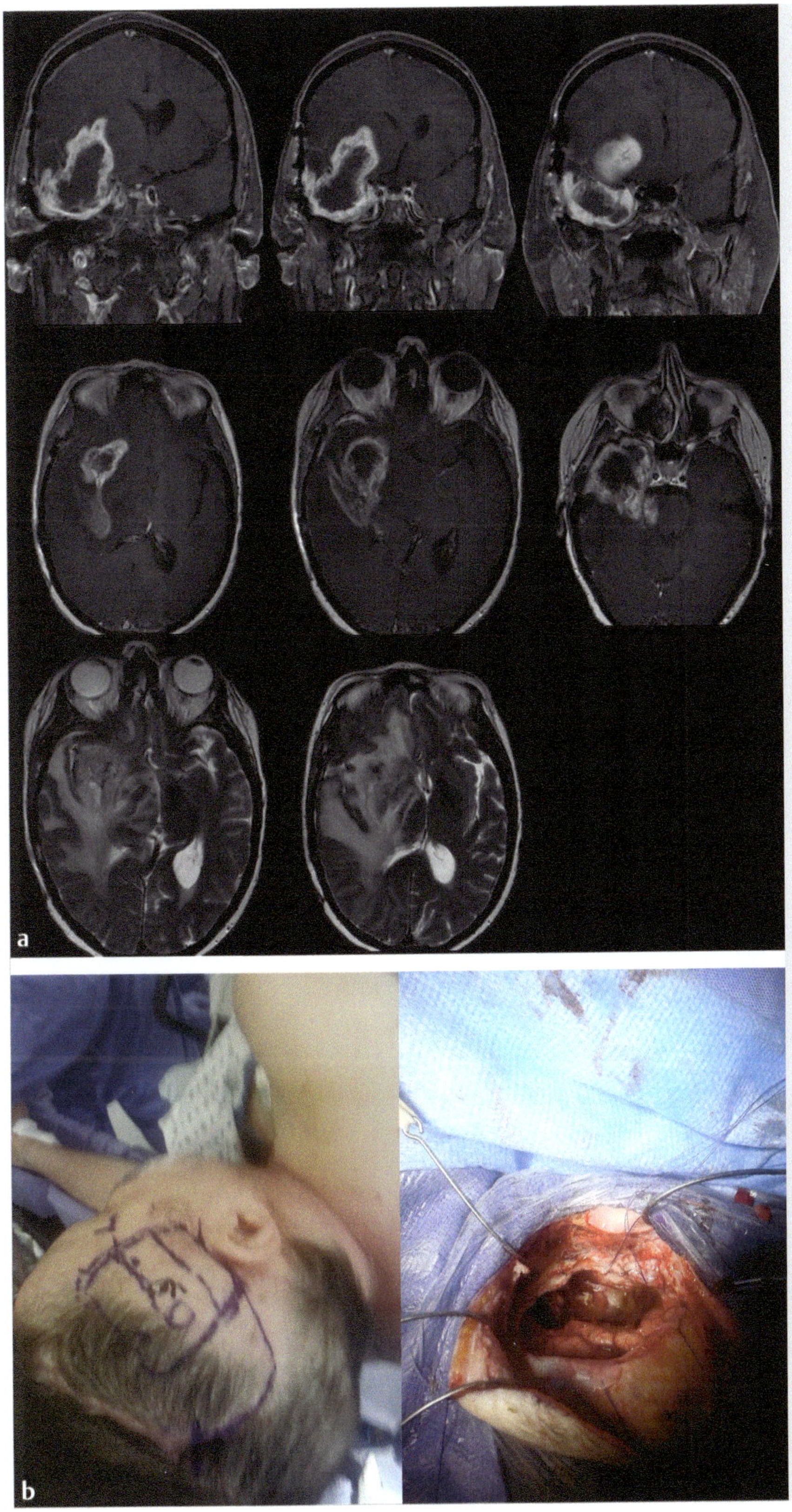

Fig. 12.17 A large recurrent glioblastoma involving the temporal lobe and insula which encases the lenticulostriates; (**a**) preoperative images, (**b**) images of the approach. (*Continued*)

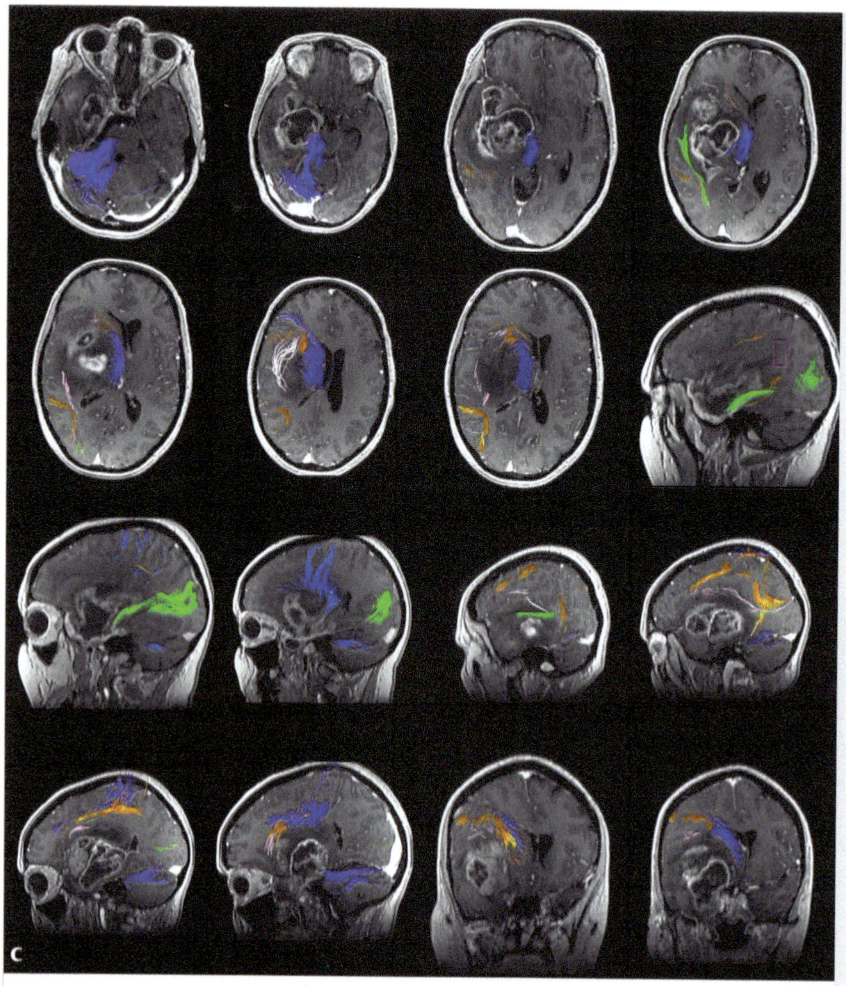

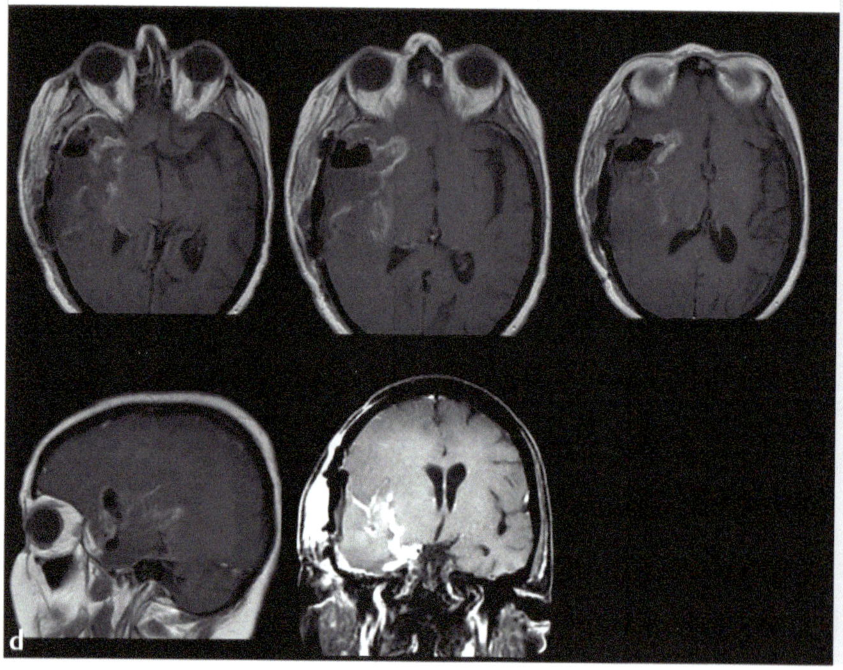

Fig 12.17 (*Continued*) (**c**) DTI tractography for that case, (**d**) postoperative images.

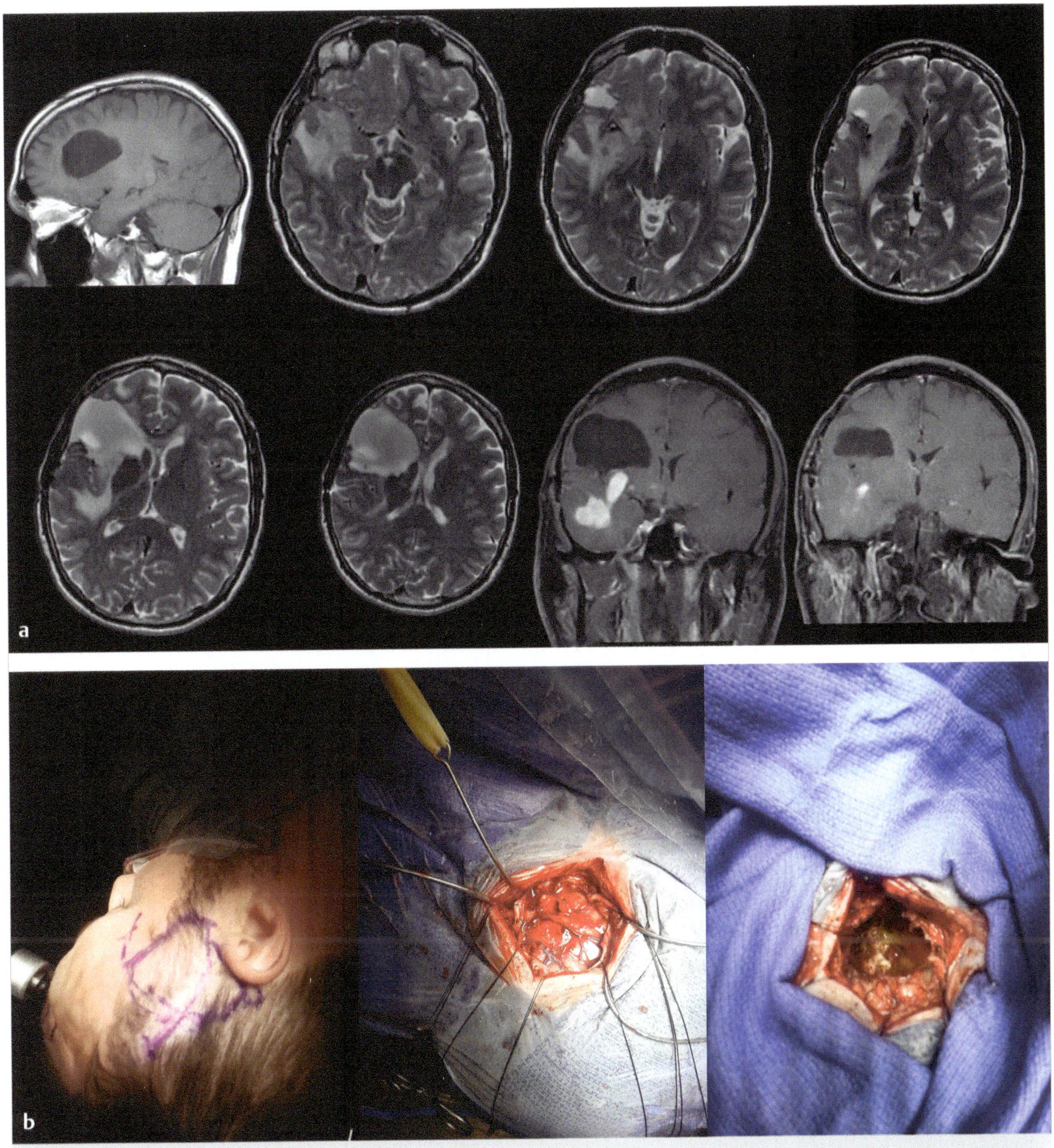

Fig. 12.18 A temporoinsular recurrence of a previous anterior frontoinsular glioma; (**a**) preoperative images, (**b**) images of the approach. (*Continued*)

▶ Fig. 12.20 demonstrates a sizeable insular glioma resected via a combined above and below approach. The frontal opercula were removed so that we could reach as superior as possible and to address as much of the premotor and motor region tumor that the functional anatomy would allow under direct visualization.

a) This tumor involves the temporal lobe, but the axials clearly demonstrate that there is a major extension of this tumor superiorly into the motor network. It would be unwise to try to do this all from the temporal side, as this would involve blindly sweeping tumor from the motor network blindly under the frontal opercula. To deal with this tumor, we need to get some of the frontal opercula off and see what we are doing.

b) Note the diagram drawn on the side of the head. This shows the boundaries of his insula and its relationship to the temporal lobe. I do this exercise in every case to ensure that I have a clear idea of which opercula need to come off to

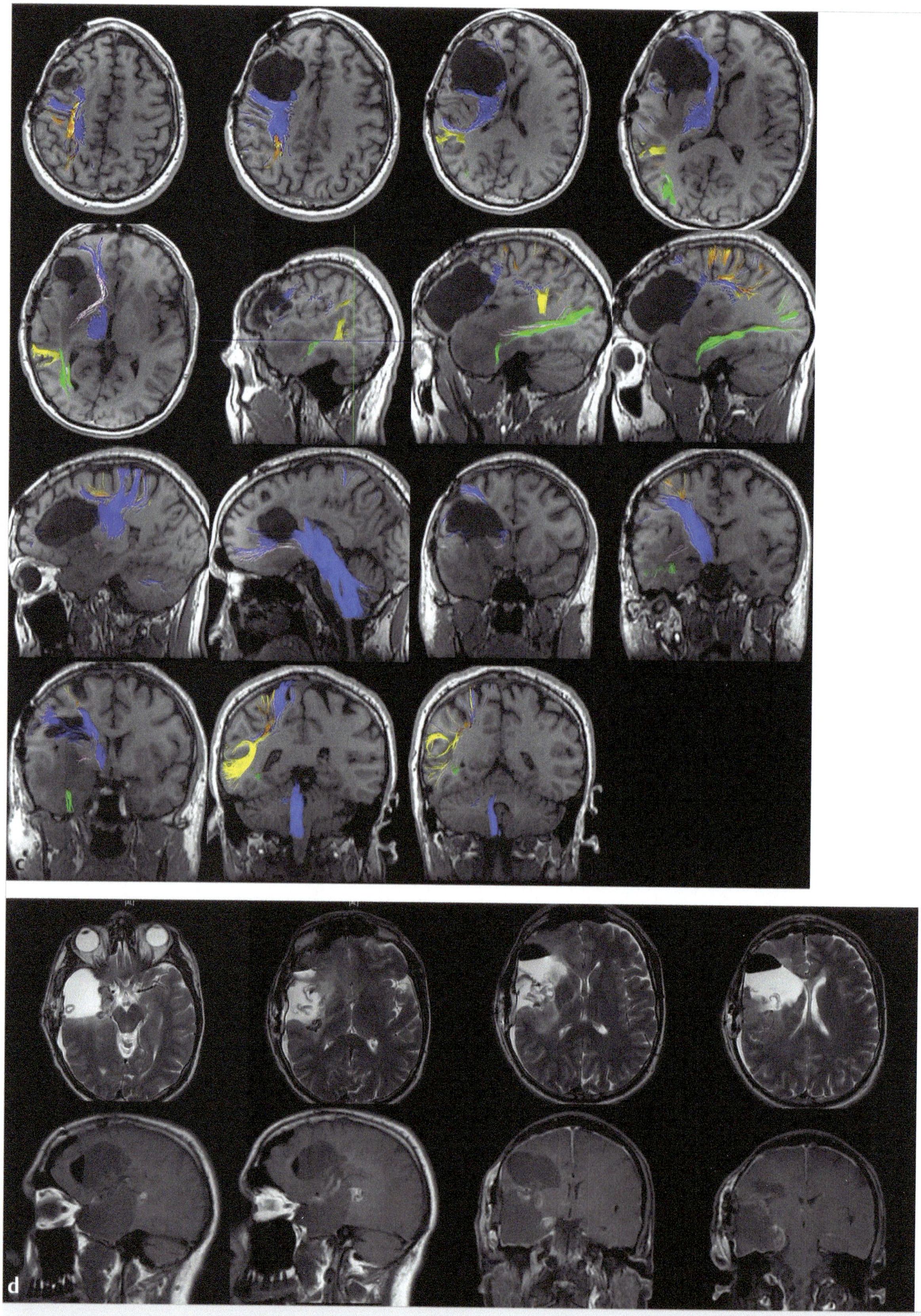

Fig 12.18 (*Continued*) (**c**) DTI tractography, (**d**) postoperative images.

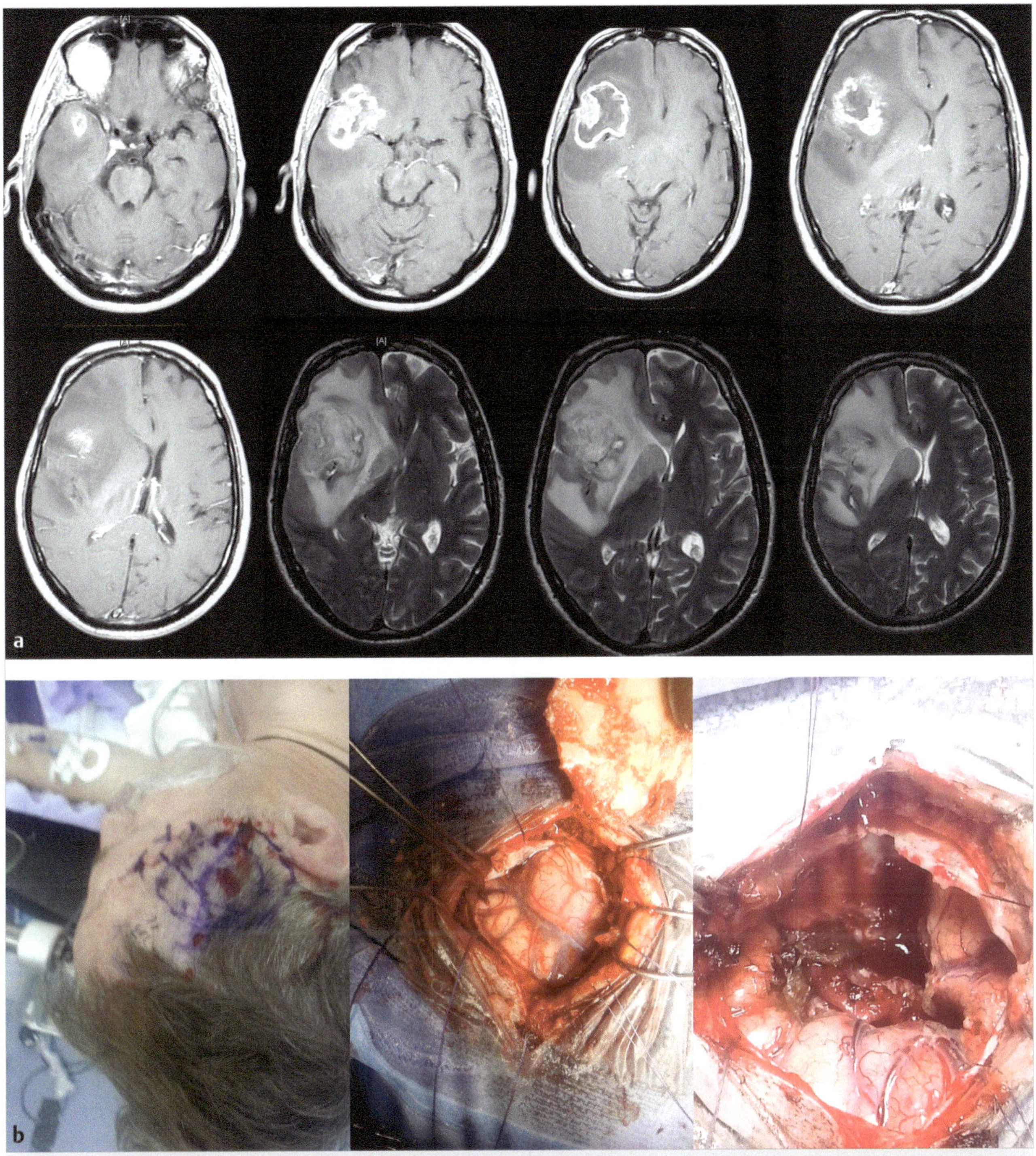

Fig. 12.19 A GBM centered in the anterior insula which encases portions of the MCA; (**a**) preoperative images, (**b**) images of the approach. (*Continued*)

expose the circular sulcus boundaries and where the critical opercula are so I expose them. An above and below keyhole approach will often involve a reasonable sized craniotomy which resembles a more traditional opening. Again, it all depends on the anatomy.

The two markers note two neglect sites, in the STG and the inferior frontal gyrus, both lining up with the SLF tractography. Note that that I have undercut this gyrus slightly on its inferior surface, despite the fact that it mapped positive slightly superiorly. This is possible because the tracts are coming from superior (FAT) and posterior (SLF) to this point, meaning that removing a small amount of opercular lip is not going to disconnect this network. This was well tolerated in this patient.

a) The majority of tracts are deflected by this tumor. The most notable finding is on the coronal imaging where the top of

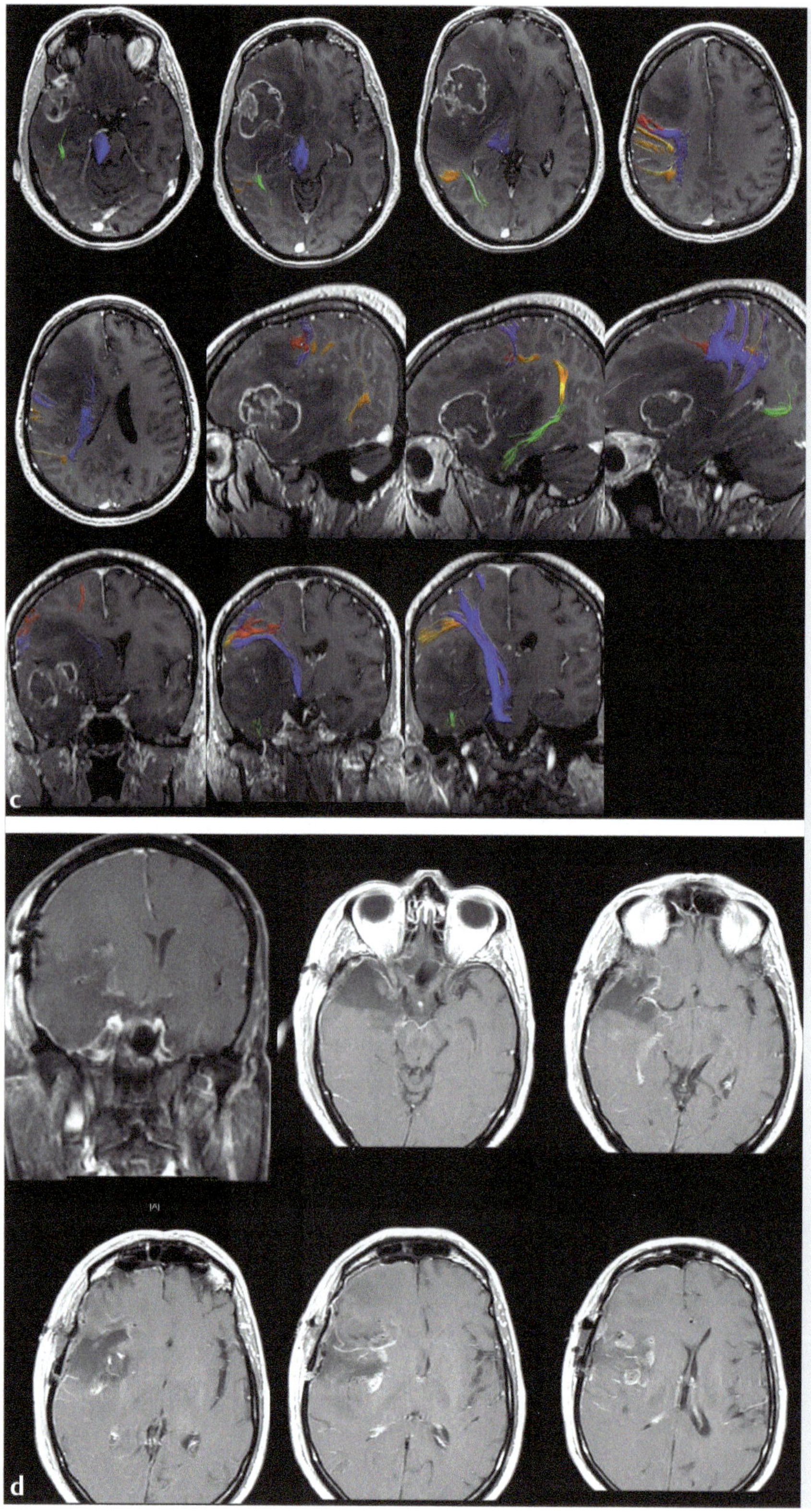

Fig 12.19 (*Continued*) (**c**) DTI tractography, (**d**) postoperative images.

this tumor is clearly abutting or invading the descending motor fibers.

b) Functional considerations forced us to stop at the top and back of this tumor. The superior pole had to be left to spare motor function and the posterior insular part was left due to neglect considerations placed by the SLF as the subcortical SLF fibers which run near the posterior superior border (aka, the hardest border to reach) and the cortical sites of neglect limited our opercular resection and access in this region. Also note that a bit of medial temporal lobe is also left and this is

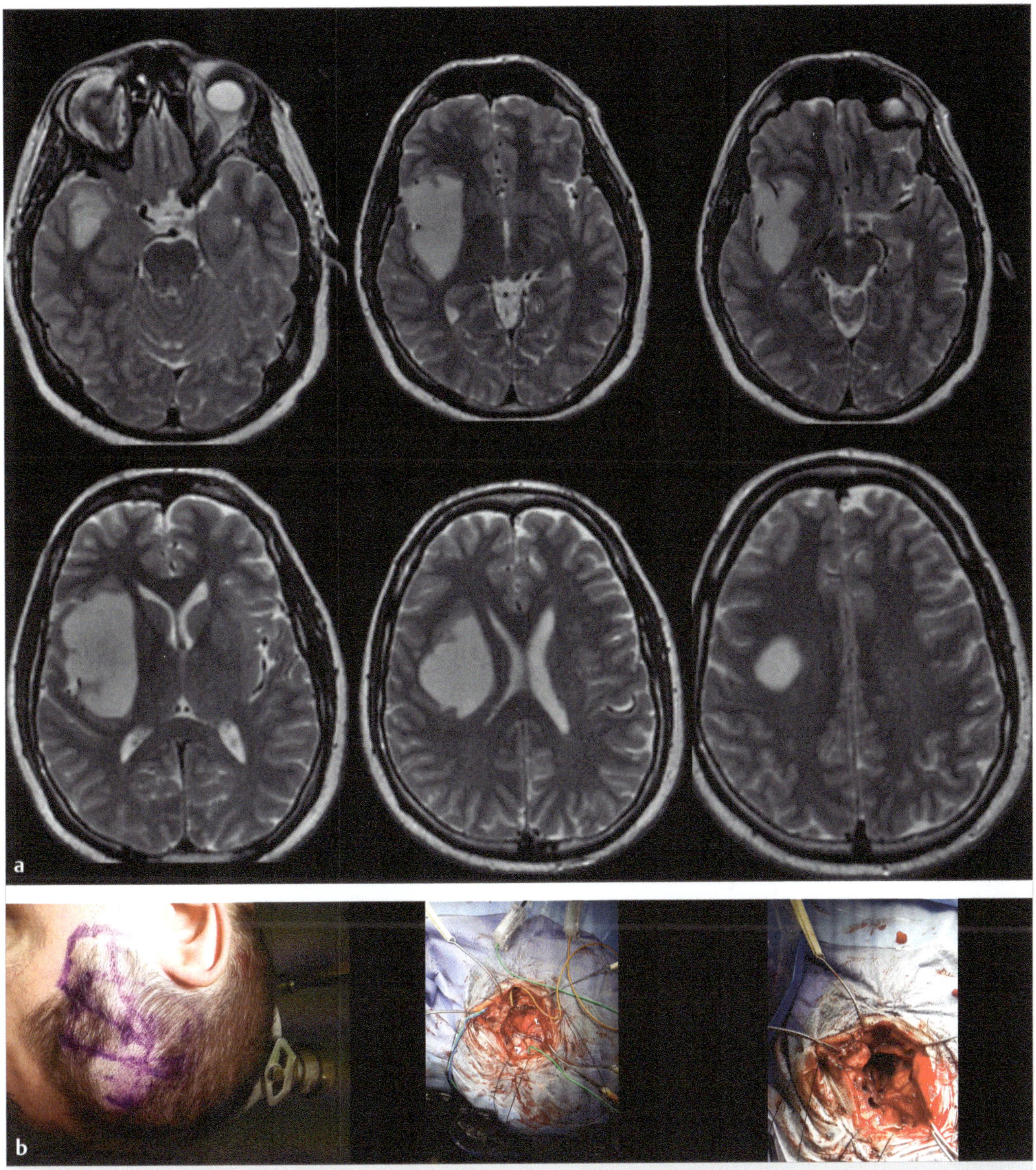

Fig. 12.20 A sizeable insular glioma resected via a combined above and below approach; (**a**) preoperative images, (**b**) images of the approach. (*Continued*)

due to the challenge of reaching high enough under the central core when the head is not tipped downward. Note that despite this, a fair bit of tumor was removed under the operculum and neglect was still avoided. However, at some point, you can only mobilize an unresected operculum so far, and you do not want to be blindly sweeping for tumor in a corner near a key tract. All things considered, we removed a good piece of this large tumor, but obviously not a complete resection as with other cases.

▶ Fig. 12.21 demonstrates a massive right insular glioma which had a history of open biopsy, radiation without success. After resecting the tumor up to the basal ganglia, we put patient on temozolamide to treat the residual disease and had excellent success.

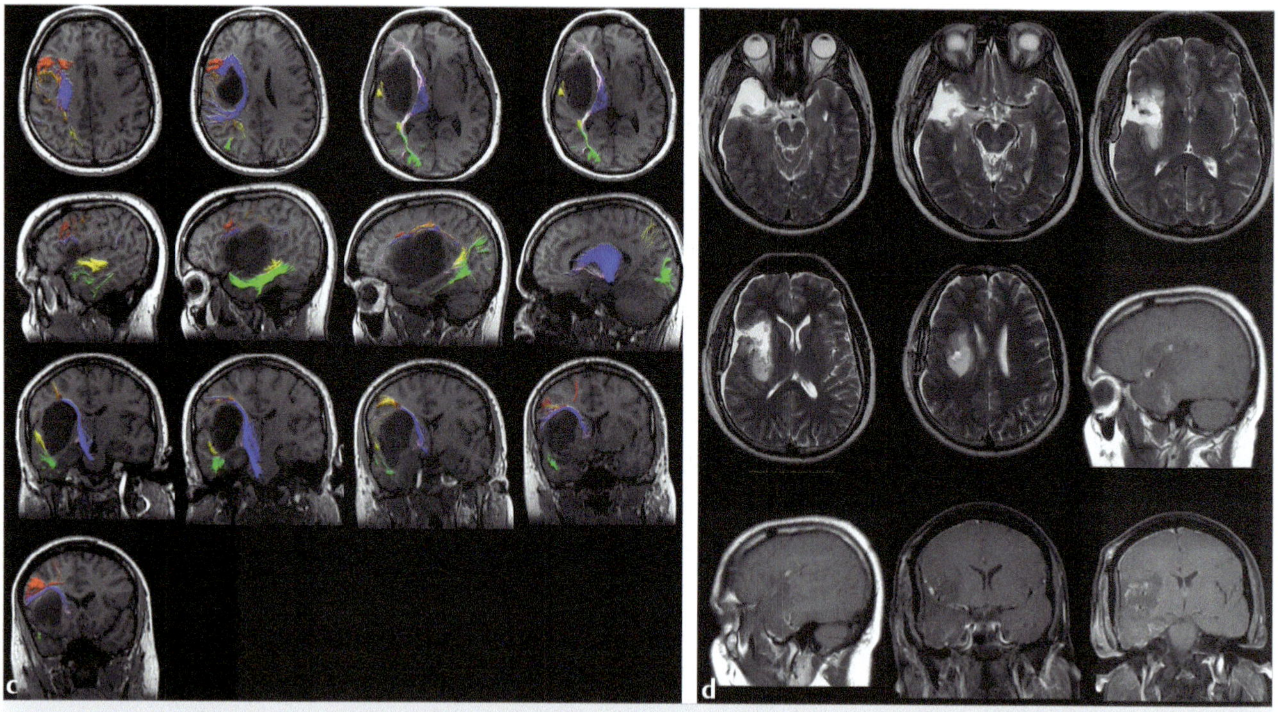

Fig 12.20 (*Continued*) (**c**) DTI tractography (**d**) postoperative images.

a) This tumor was operated on at a high profile academic hospital, radiated, and allowed to progress under surveillance for years until reaching this stage, which is the full blown appearance of an advanced insular glioma. It densely involves the temporal lobe (and was causing 10 or more complex partial seizures a day), the insula is massively enlarged, and the tumor extends upward into the premotor areas and forward following the uncinate. The putamen may be pushed or invaded (it's hard for me to tell), but the lenticulostriates are in the tumor and have been radiated in all likelihood. Regardless, our goal is similar to the earlier case: remove the temporal lobe and insula, debulk as much frontal tumor as possible, and isolate the deeper tumor for later adjuvant therapy.
b) We were forced to use the previous incision given the need for frontal and temporal access. The before and after resection images highlight that resecting a glioma like this requires removing a large piece of what appears to be normal brain.
c) The right IFOF is running through the middle of this tumor, and it is unlikely we can meaningfully save this and deal with this massive tumor. We elected to take it in this case. The descending motor fibers are also running through the superior and posterior part of the tumor on the coronal images. We will not be able to completely come over the top of this tumor without destroying the motor network (look at FAT as well). The SLF is in a favorable location.
d) The majority of this residual tumor is located in the subthalamic region and the premotor areas. The safe portions have been aggressively resected.
e) This long term follow-up image 9 months after finishing a course of temozolamide demonstrates while some T2 changes remain, most of the T2 change in the subthalamic region and he has responded well to this combination of cytoreduction and adjuvant therapy. He might have seen shrinkage of these areas with therapy alone, but presently has the smallest amount of tumor burden we can obtain for him. Also note that the insular vessels are now up against the dura after the brain has shifted in the long term. This is an important consideration when performing repeat surgery following an aggressive anatomic resection. This issue is discussed in Chapter 15.

▶ Fig. 12.22 demonstrates a challenging case of a large, recurrent, radiated anterior left insular grade 3 oligodendroglioma.

a) Review of the images reveals that much of the tumor is actually in the orbitofrontal cortex, and that the insula is pushed significantly posteriorly. The presence of tumor in the temporal lobe tells us that this spread is through the uncinate. The previous resection cavity is very far anterior, likely with the goal of avoiding dealing with the insula and speech networks; however, this has not been very effective at dealing with the problem. It is critical to recognize that this cavity has shifted the insula towards this cavity. The face of the insula now is oriented in the coronal not the sagittal plane, which is a set-up for disorientation if you are not aware of the effects of previous surgery on tumor anatomy. Most of this tumor is not located in the putamen, but it is likely that some tumor is in there as the tumor seems to reach the internal capsule.

The attack strategy I had for this tumor is as follows: 1) Remove the STG to define the insula location and make room to work, 2) perform a lateral frontal disconnection to isolate the anterior insula, 3) extend that disconnection anteriorly above the involved orbitofrontal cortex paralleling this in the axial plane towards the midline, 4) remove the orbitofrontal cortex until

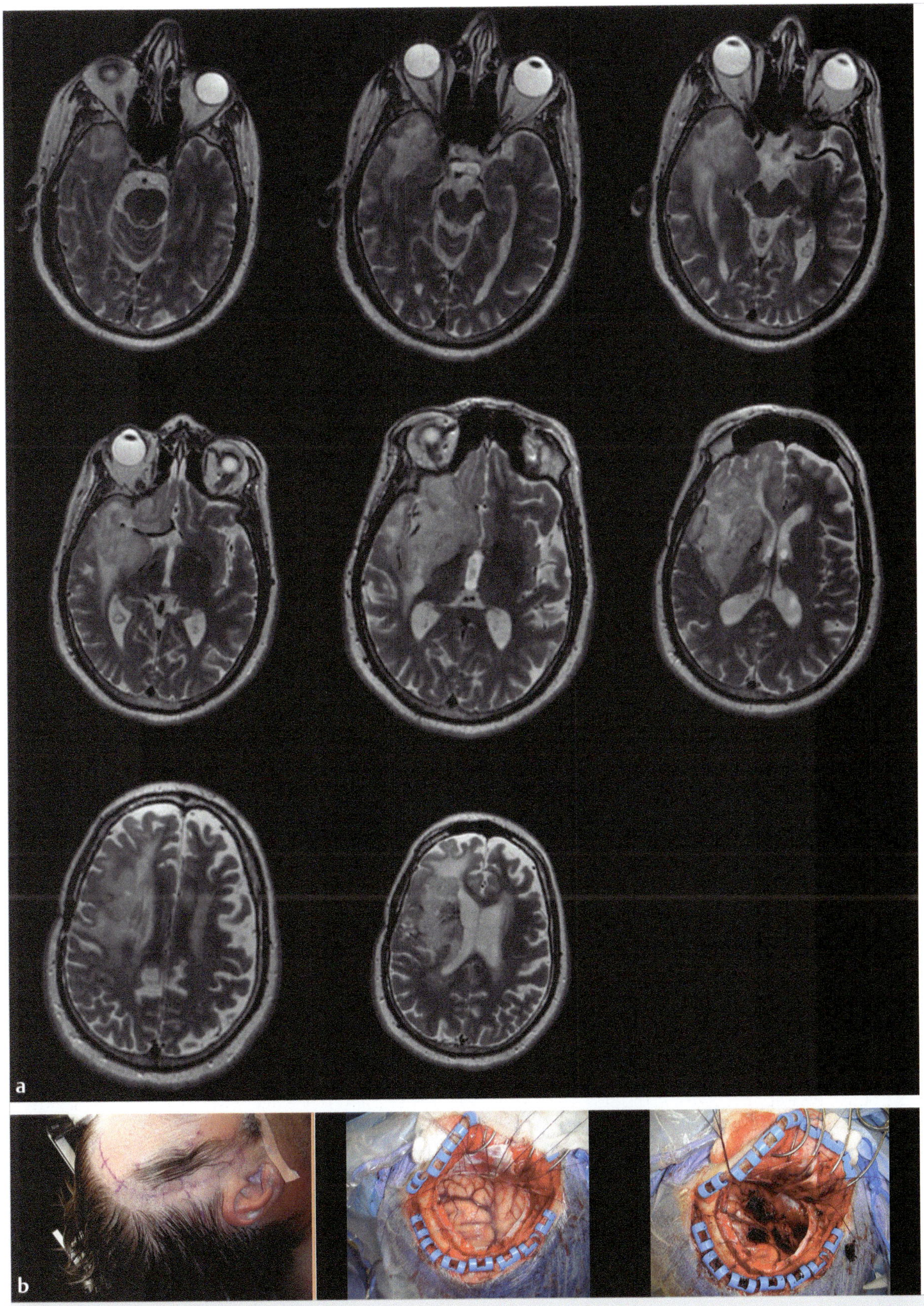

Fig. 12.21 A massive right insular glioma which had a history of open biopsy and radiation without success; (**a**) preoperative images, (**b**) images of the approach. (*Continued*)

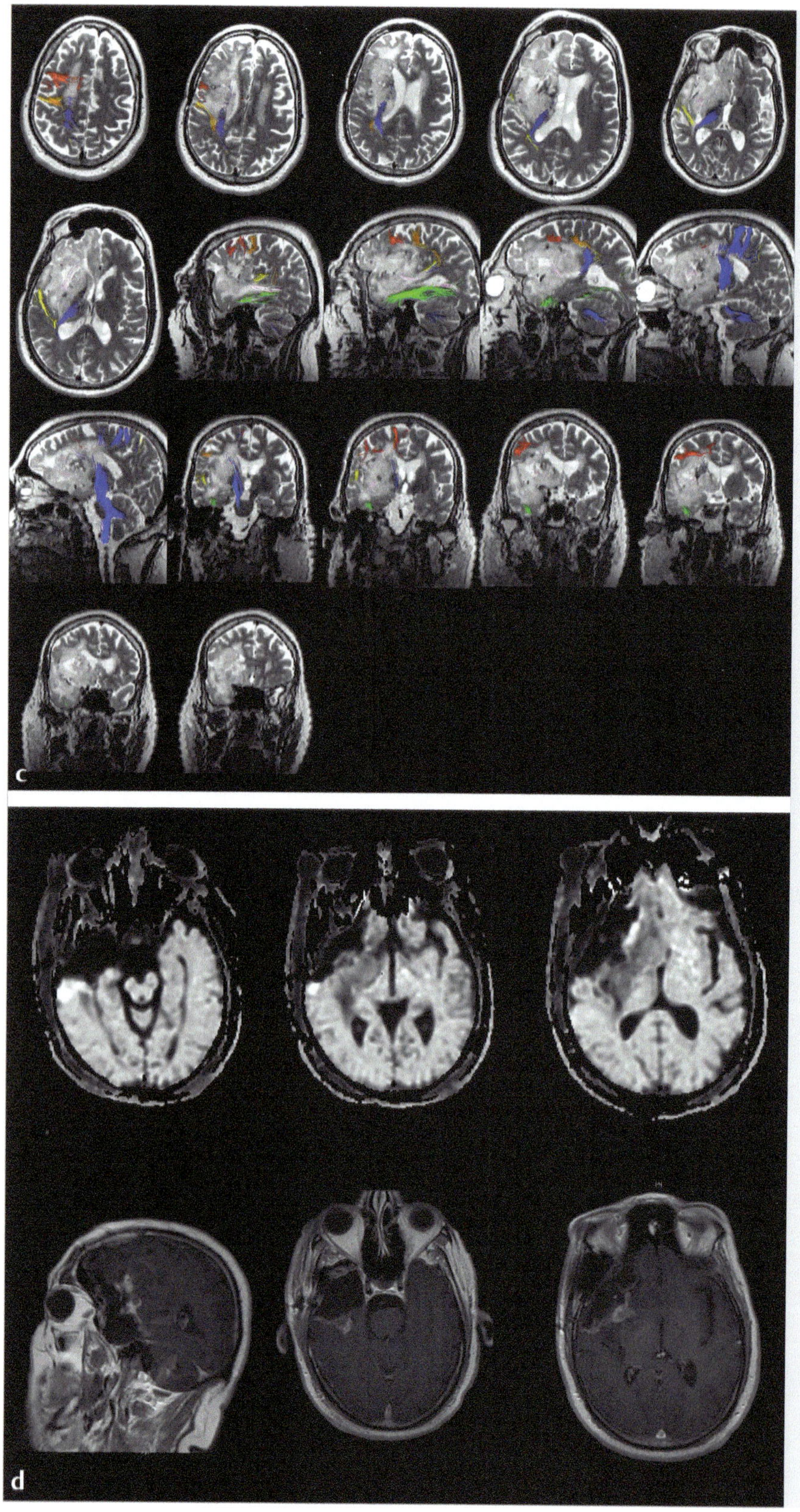

Fig 12.21 (*Continued*) (**c**) DTI tractography, (**d**) postoperative images.

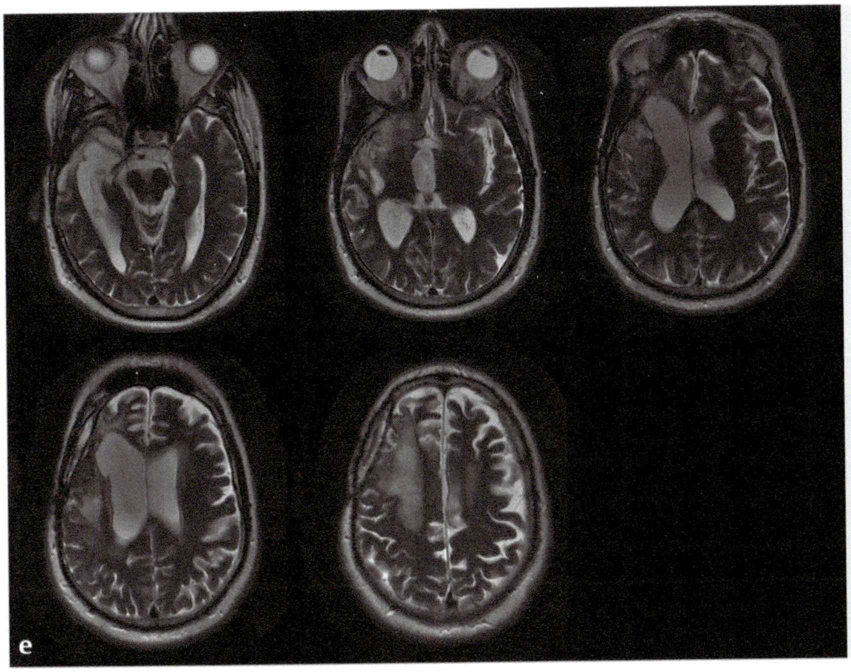

Fig 12.21 (*Continued*) (**e**) Long-term follow-up images.

flush with the M1, 5) identify and remove the insula as much as tolerated by IFOF, 6) completion temporal lobectomy.

a) None.

b) The frontal rami of the SLF are shifted very anteriorly due to the previous surgery (and this is real as it lined up with the mapping exactly). The IFOF could not be located on tractography, but given that the patient had normal preoperative speech, this is likely not really gone but simply cannot be imaged in this T2 bright tumor. The speech aspects of this case made the working room quite challenging and limited.

c) Overall, I was happy with this resection, and the patient did very well. There are places it could have been better worth discussing, however. The tumor in the basal forebrain was expected, and some of the insular tumor left likely contains the IFOF as naming problems limited us posteriorly. The purpose of identifying the M1 early and staying in front of it in cases where orbitofrontal involvement and basal forebrain involvement or basal ganglia might be running together in a massive tumor, is that staying in front of the MCA basically always tells you were these structures are, and keeps you from injuring the lenticulostriate. I do, however, wish I had pushed the resection into the gyrus rectus up to its medial pial boundary to ensure a better resection of this disconnected gyrus.

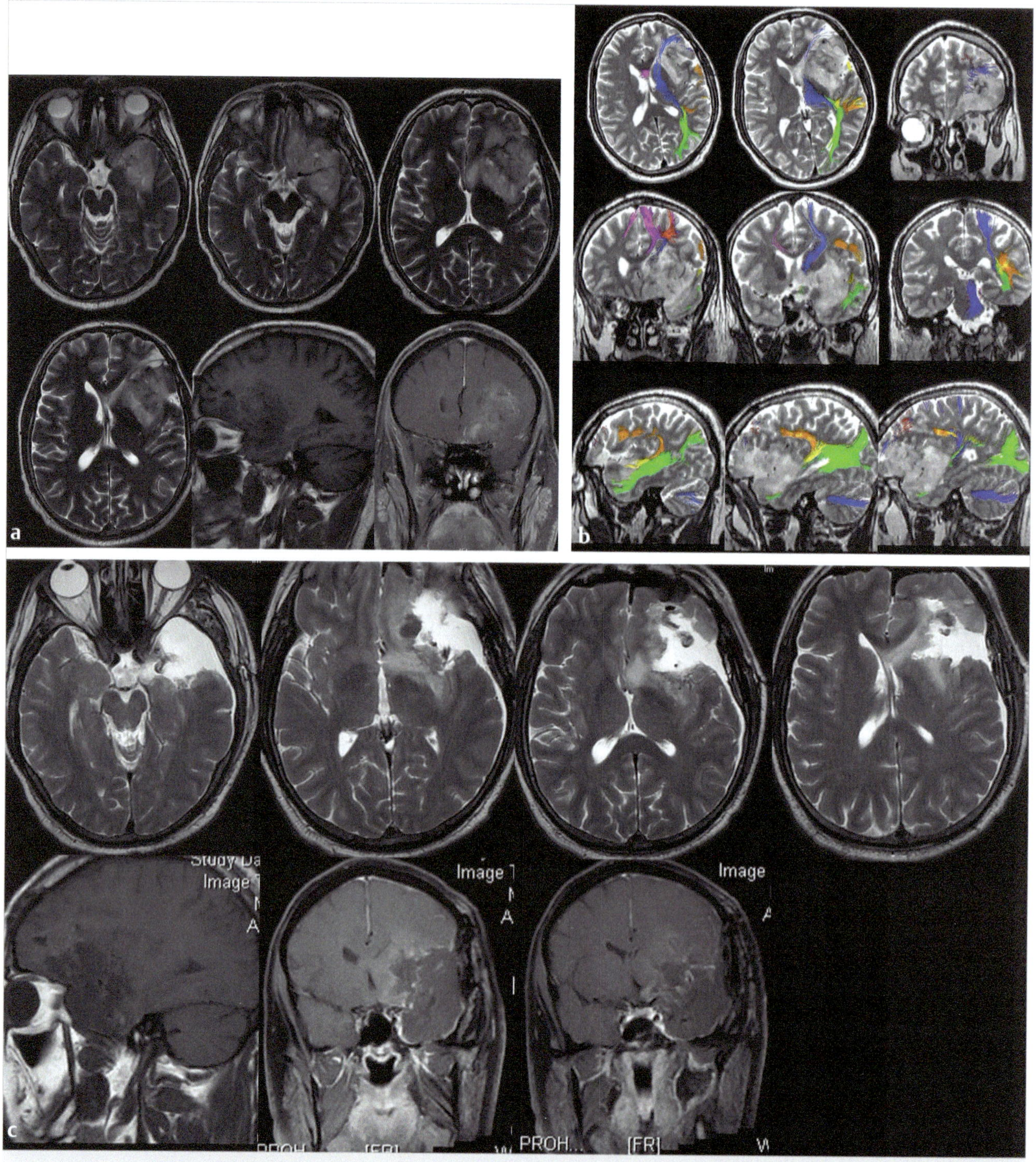

Fig. 12.22 A challenging case of a large, recurrent, radiated anterior left insular grade 3 oligodendroglioma: (**a**) preoperative images, (**b**) DTI tractography.

13 Parietal and Occipital Gliomas

13.1 Introduction

In the section on AVMs in his classic text, Yasargil spoke of parietal AVMs with a great deal of respect, noting that in his more experienced years, he had become more cautious with offering surgery for these lesions. When I read that during my training, I was somewhat surprised, as I had never considered the parietal lobe to be as treacherous as the motor strip, the brainstem, or the thalamus. However, experience has taught me that he is probably right on this, as it is quite simple to profoundly affect someone's quality of life with misadventures in the parietal lobe. The gross anatomy of the parietal lobe is simple, but the microanatomy is exceptionally complex.

I have combined parietal and occipital gliomas into the same chapter, as in many ways the issues with these cases do not substantially differ between the two lobes. Many times these tumors cross the arbitrary boundaries we have made to define these lobes, making such distinctions irrelevant. More importantly, these tumors threaten the same systems and thus the cuts used to remove them follow similar principles. Fundamentally, surgery in the parietal and occipital lobes is surgery around the visual processing system, flanked by the two pathway systems (SLF/IFOF) (speech/praxis or neglect) laterally, and the sensorimotor system anteriorly.

Despite being anatomically simpler than, say, surgery in the insula, parietoccipital lobe surgery involved highly functionally complex brain areas, which integrate fairly abstract aspects of sensation, attention, and cognition. The obvious result of this is that the majority of these cases are mapping cases aimed at identifying and preserving function, with a significantly less demanding anatomic resection than other areas, such as removing the corpus callosum. In other words, this area can only be meaningfully defined in terms of functional anatomy.

13.2 Specific Demands of Parieto-occipital Surgery (▶ Fig. 13.1)

The best friend of a surgeon doing surgery in the parieto-occipital region is the bilateral nature of much of the visual system. While there are neuropsychological syndromes which result from injury to parietal or occipital regions, a large percentage of them require bilateral injury to occur, making them harder to cause. This redundancy results from the richly bilateral networks which doubly represent much of the visual system. Most of these are homotypic connections and connect analogous medially positioned cortices; however, some heterotypic connections exist and also maintain the bilaterally of visual processing and its use.

While this feature gives some parts of the parietal lobe a forgiving nature, it also points out the need to take bilateral connections into your consideration for maintaining the flow of visual information with relevant association areas, such as the semantic networks. For example, a left occipital lobectomy does not on its own cause anomia or alexia; however, damage to the heterotypic connections between the right visual system and the left-sided semantic networks in addition to an occipital lobectomy will. This raises the interesting idea that in the context of an occipital lobectomy, that the corpus callosum becomes eloquent brain tissue worthy of stimulation mapping to preserve the speech network.

It is also critical to have a firm grasp of what parts of the parietal and occipital lobes are not sufficiently expendable and cannot be compensated from the other side. The most obvious lateralized networks are the sensorimotor networks, which are the determinants of the anterior cuts in many of these cases. The SLF connects parts of the parietal lobes involved in visuospatial information to frontal lobe premotor areas which are often critical for useful hand functioning, but equally critically it joins the semantic areas to (SMG, STG, MTG, etc.) to the frontal premotor areas, a critical aspect of the speech, praxis, and neglect networks. These networks are well established to be highly lateralized, and generally less tolerant to unilateral disruption as they generally lack strong homotypic connections from their partner gyri on the other side.

The visual system obviously can be disrupted unilaterally, causing a typical homonymous hemianopia picture or other similar variations on that theme. This is well known to be due to entering the optic radiations. Notably, this may result not only from disruption of the primary fiber from the LGN to the calcarine fissure and its banks, but such injuries likely disrupt communications with the pulvinar and superior colliculus necessary for higher visual processing. What is interesting is that interruptions of later parts of the pathways (dorsal or ventral), can often be compensated for. For example, transecting the left IFOF in the occipital lobe often does not cause a semantic speech loss provided visual information can reach these areas from the other side; however, the subinsular IFOF is not a bilateral tract and cannot be compensated for if cut.

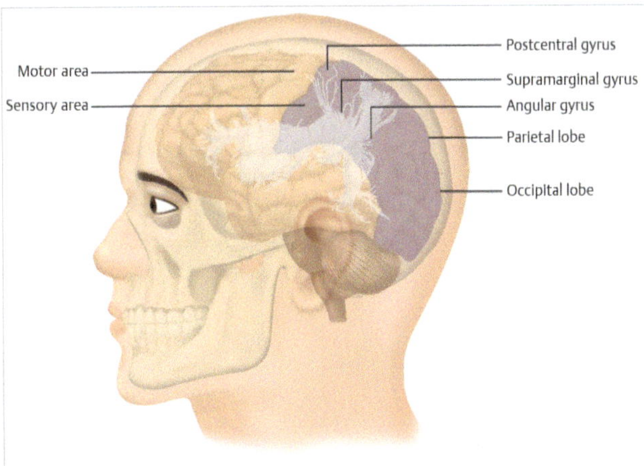

Fig. 13.1 This schematic demonstrates the key connections driving parieto-occipital glioma surgery.

13.3 The "Define" Phase (▶ Fig. 13.2)

The diversity of parieto-occipital tumors that I describe below overestimates their differences. The key questions one needs to ask prior to cutting are always the same, and the classification system thus are different views of the same fundamental problems.

Question 1: Can I save the ipsilateral visual system?

It's always best, if possible, to try to avoid a field cut, as a hemianopia prevents one from safely driving, among other problems. Sometimes this is not possible. For example, a patient who presents with glioblastoma invading the lateral wall of the atrium is unlikely to avoid a hemianopia in the long term, even if they don't initially present with one. In a low grade glioma, it may be possible to save the fibers without compromising the oncologic plan. DTIs can be very helpful in this decision making.

Question 2: If the visual system is unilaterally compromised (or will be), how will visual input be transmitted from the other side?

Visual input is a critical component of semantic function. The absence of visual information from one hemisphere mandates that the other side visual information reach there from the other side, which means that fibers crossing in the corpus callosum (specifically the splenium and posterior body) need to be worked into the operative plan. Extension into the splenium can make the goal to save these fibers very challenging.

Question 3: What is the relationship of this tumor to the SLF?

With the exception of tumors in the medial bank of the polar occipital lobe, almost all tumors in the parieto-occipital region have some association with the SLF complex. Performing glioma surgery on these tumors involves dividing the tumor from the SLF on the tract's posterior or medial border. With tumors in the TPO junction (STG, SMG or angular gyri) the SLF can be involved along a substantial length of the tract.

Question 4: What is the involvement of the motor system?

For some tumors, such as the anterior occipital tumors, the motor system is generally uninvolved. Most parietal tumors have components of the motor system in their anterior aspect, at least parietal association and sensory contributions to the motor network. At the other extreme, TPO Junction tumors can extend into the internal capsule at their deep border.

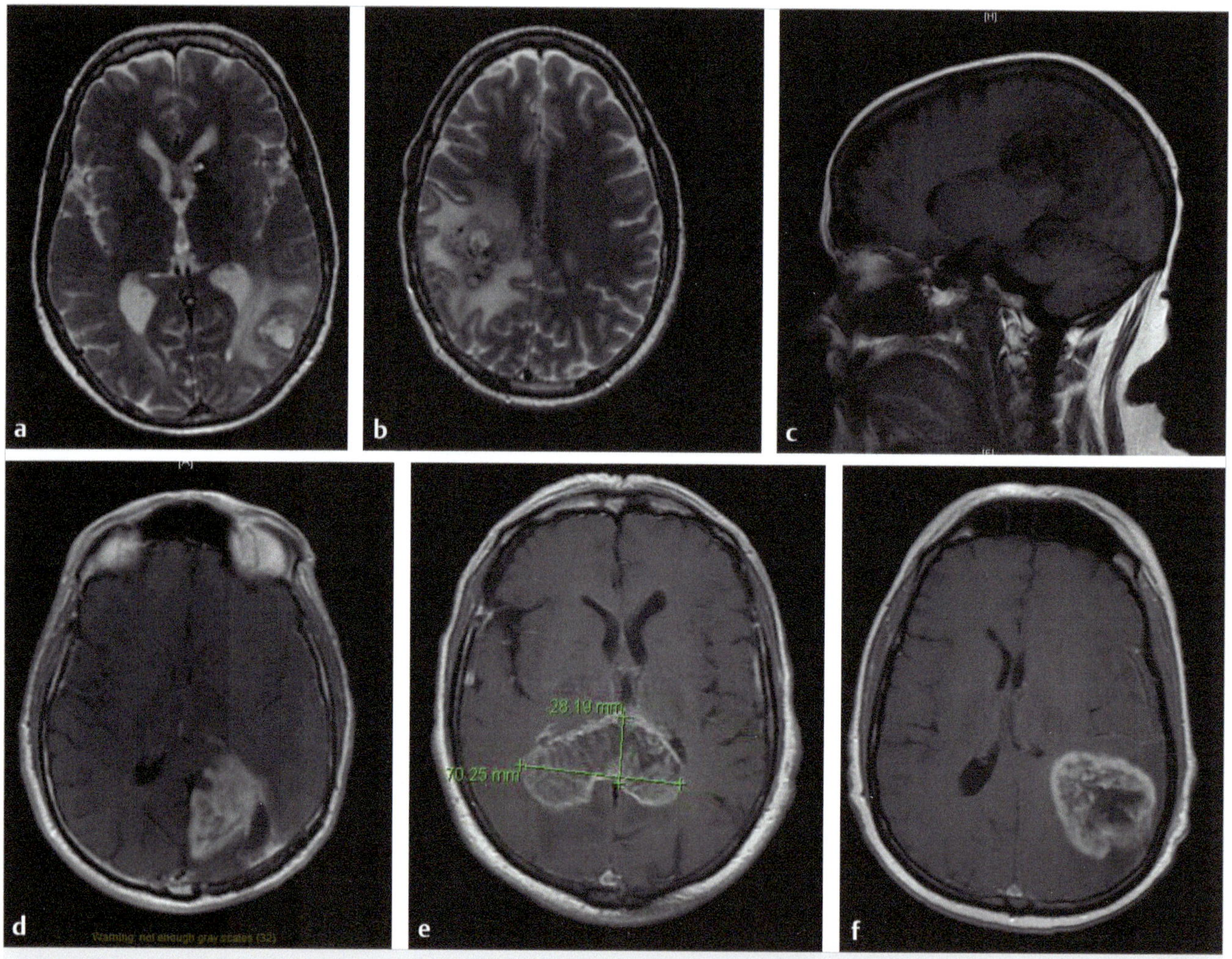

Fig. 13.2 Images depicting the basic types of parieto-occipital gliomas: (**a**) anterior occipital, (**b**) medial parietal, (**c**) posterior cingulate, (**d**) occipital pole, (**e**) splenial butterfly, (**f**) temporal-parietal-occipital junction tumors.

Question 5: Are the posterior cingulate gyrus or parahippocampal gyri involved?

The presence of tumor in the cingulum network changes the case significantly as it raises issues of risk to the default mode network, and the memory consolidation circuits. Tumor in these gyri can cause functional reorganization of these networks to an extent. They can also require one to follow the cingulate sulcus under the motor strip or down into the medial temporal lobe.

Based on these distinctions, I subclassify parieto-occipital tumors into the following basic groups (▶ Fig. 13.2).

1. Anterior occipital tumors: These lie in the inferolateral occipital lobe and the principle cut is with the SLF anteriorly. They are principally tumors of the ventral visual stream, and one unique risk (other than the typical risk of causing a field cut and/or speech/neglect problems) is to reading which is uniquely in this part of the brain on the left.
2. Medial parietal tumors: These tumors lie in the space between the motor system anteriorly, the SLF laterally, and the visual fibers and IFOF inferiorly and posteriorly.
3. Posterior cingulate tumors: These are often part of a medial parietal tumor case, but can arise independently, in which case I plan the case as a transcortical surgery similar to a medial parietal tumor. They pose specific risks to memory and alertness, and defining the cingulate sulcus and its boundaries is critical for safety, especially when the tumor extends below the motor and sensory areas.
4. Occipital pole tumors: These tumors involve many of the same basic cuts as a medial parietal tumor, but generally are far less risky. The visual system is ipsilaterally at risk, and in many cases this cannot be saved, but with attention to the contralateral visual contributions, the overall cognitive benefits of maintaining connections between vision and other systems will persist.
5. Splenial butterfly gliomas: Pure butterfly gliomas are discussed in Chapter 14 with anterior butterfly tumors. It is important to note that many occipital region tumors invade the splenium secondarily and this is a serious threat to overall vision, and it is important to address this when it occurs.
6. TPO (temporo-parieto-occipital) junction tumors: these are among the most difficult tumors in the cerebrum to remove given that they can involve multiple networks at once and primarily arise in the semantic networks of the brain, in other words compromising those functions that most makes us human, which are centered in the inferior parietal lobule and its connections to the frontal lobe. Being surrounded on all sides, starting with neurologic deficits, working in distorted anatomy, and being forced into limited goals are par for the course in these cases.

These TPO junction cases are discussed in the next chapter on difficult gliomas.

13.3.1 Cortical Mapping

Cortical mapping aims to define the motor network, the attention networks, and the termination points of the SLF. We usually test numerous functional domains up front in these cases, as the redundancy between tests can often double check these tests. For example, testing neglect system function with target cancelation tasks rechecks motor planning.

I check motor planning, speech, and neglect tasks in every case. This is not because I necessarily plan on always finding positive sites for these functions (neglect is usually a right-sided function and speech is usually on the left), but because I always assume the SLF networks might be partially bilateral, and they may need the side I'm operating on.

13.4 The "Divide" Phase

Conceptually, there are really only two basic cuts in these cases: the anterior occipital cut and the medial parietal cut. This does not mean than we always take a resection of a tumor at the occipital pole up to the sensorimotor cortices; however, the more limited resection we perform in these cases is based around the principles based around these cuts.

Both cuts aim to preserve the SLF, and to maintain at least some visual input to the semantic system from either the ventral stream ipsilateral or the contralateral visual system. The principle differences between these disconnections lie in the relationship between the cut and the optic radiations, and the relationship with the sensorimotor network.

13.4.1 Anterior Occipital Disconnection (▶ Fig. 13.3)

This cut principally aims to separate the tumor from the temporal rami of the SLF complex. Similar to a posterior temporal disconnection, once the lateral white matter system is separated from the tumor, the medial temporal lobe can be removed working medial to the ventricle and SLF. Obviously, the optic radiations are at risk, and you are by definition operating within the ventral visual stream; however, the IFOF is usually identifiable and salvageable, maintaining visual connection to the semantic networks. On the left, reading is clearly at risk.

13.4.2 Medial Parietal Cut (▶ Fig. 13.4)

This is a challenging cut. It is L-shaped based anteriorly and laterally and requires a deep cut which will seem aggressive until you have experience doing it. The posterior and medial boundaries are with the core of the visual system (the posterior cut parallels the ventral stream and optic radiations and you are inherently sacrificing at least part of the ipsilateral dorsal stream which can be compensated for), and the falx, respectively.

The lateral cut is with the SLF, and this puts several systems at risk, notably speech and praxis on the left and neglect and the dorsal attention network on the right. I do this cut first almost always because problems with the motor network can make higher testing impossible, even if they are temporary. The cut essentially extends to the roof of the atrium and aims to follow the SLF down to the atrium remaining medial to the tract which similarly protects the optic radiations. Note that the roof of the atrium can have corpus callosum fibers, which include the semantic crossing loop, a small tract linking the bilateral semantic networks.

The anterior cut is a coronal cut which parallels the sensorimotor system anteriorly. It is essential to note that this network can be variably extensive, and you will often note coordination problems when working behind the sensory strip. This is due to

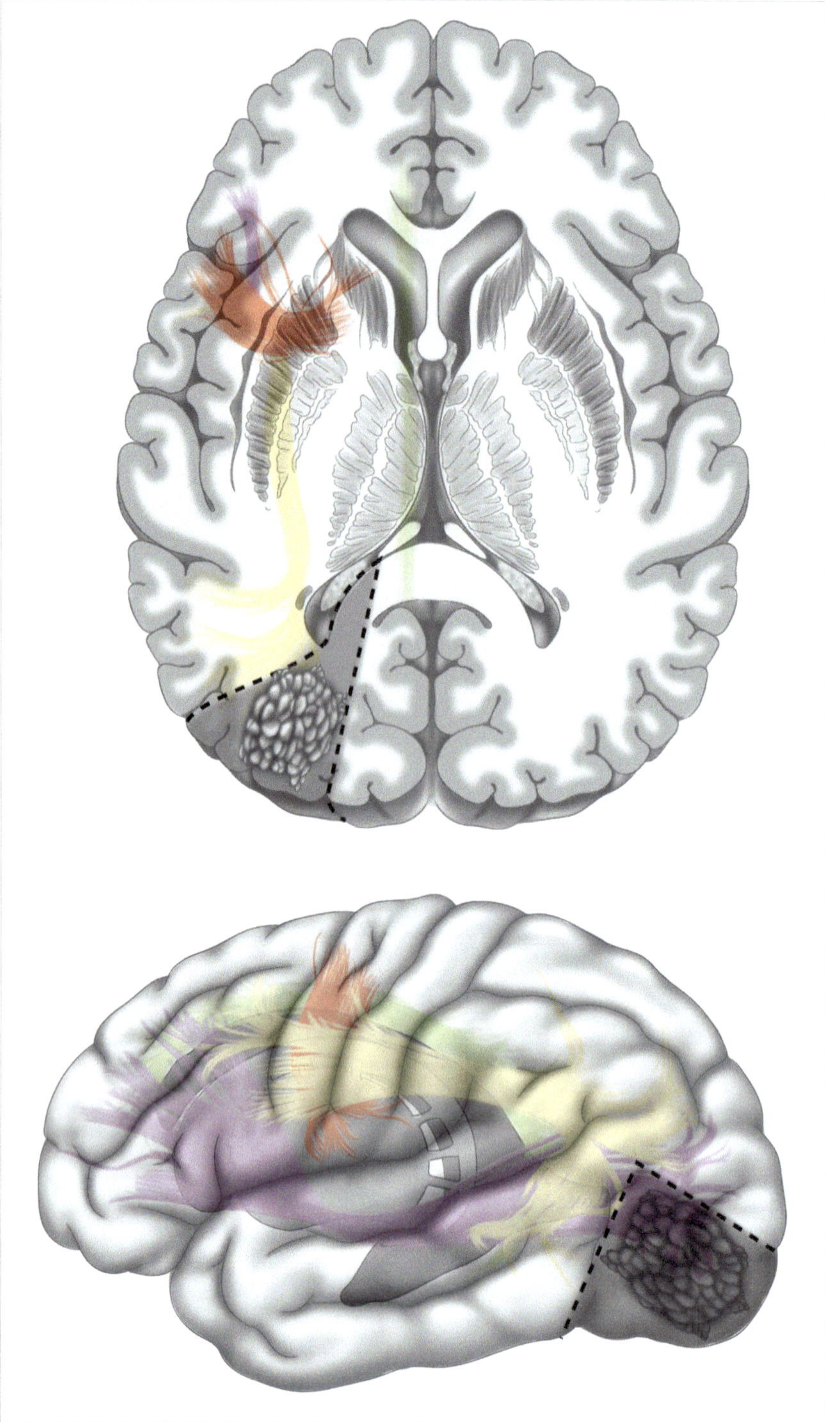

Fig. 13.3 The steps of the anterior occipital disconnection. This cut principally aims to divide the tumor from the SLF anteriorly and is primarily a linear cut behind the temporal ramus of the SLF. This angles internally towards the ventricle, landing as far anterior as permitted by the mapping, and as far superior as allowed by the IFOF and MdLF in the depth of the cut. Whether to enter the atrium depends on the goals of surgery and the tumor anatomy, as this risks a complete hemianopsia.

manipulation of the parietal contributions to visuomotor coordination, which should be figured into your calculation.

One additional aspect of this cut involves the cingulate gyrus and the corpus callosum. While tumors can invade the posterior cingulate gyrus from the parietal lobe, as with frontal tumors, they often don't as these white matter systems are quite distinct. If uninvolved, you should try to save the cingulum, using stimulation mapping for concentration tasks, and the cingulate sulcus to define the boundaries and stay out of the cingulum and DMN. This is especially true if you plan on entering the splenium. These should be planned for ahead based on tumor anatomy, the preoperative function and your goals of treatment.

13.5 The "Destroy" Phase

Most of a parieto-occipital case is usually consumed with the division and the mapping, with the anatomic resection comprising a lesser component. As noted above, the gross anatomy is usually simple compared to other parts of the brain. In many cases, once the cuts are complete, I finish the case in about 10–15 minutes.

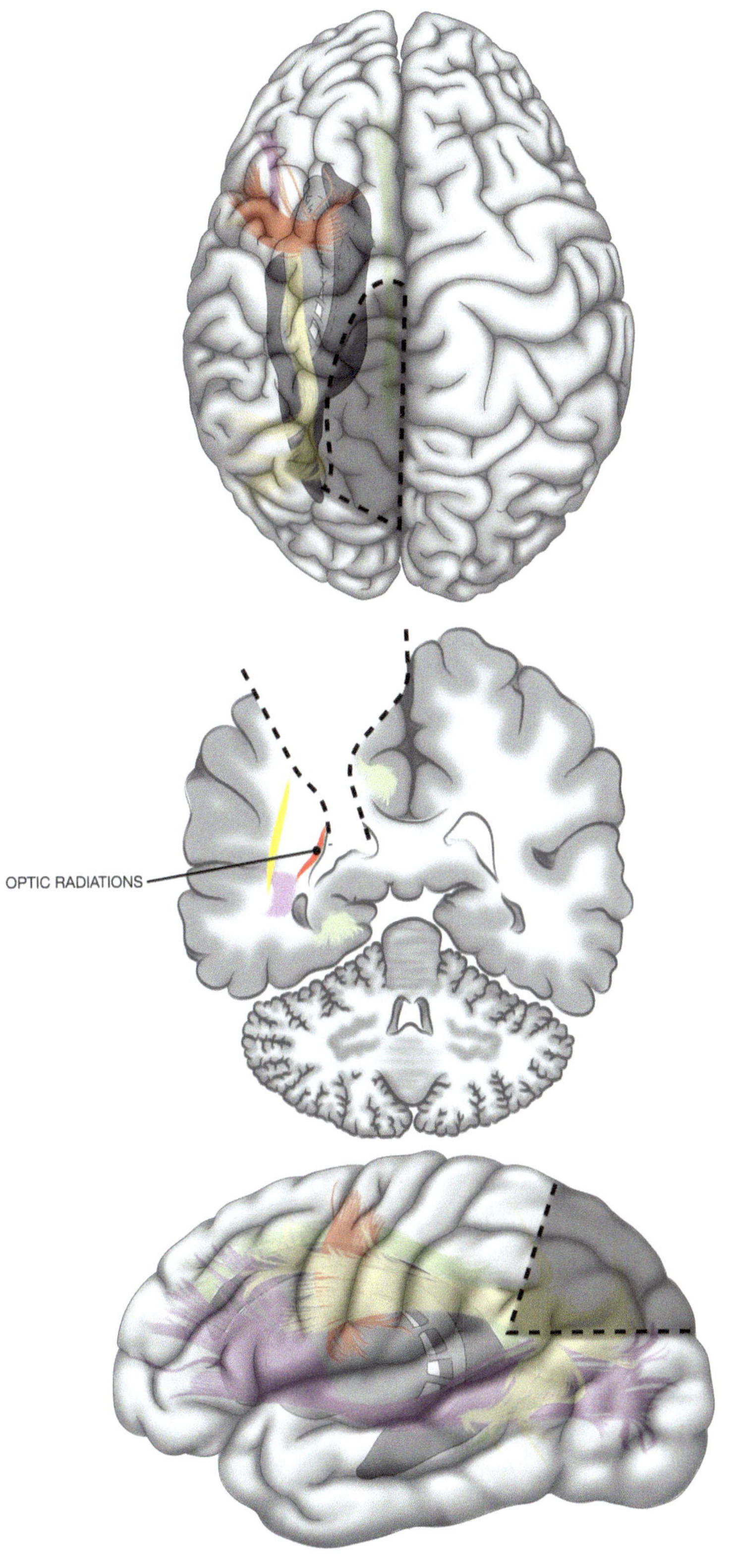

Fig. 13.4 The medial parietal disconnection. This division is L-shaped, separating the tumor from the sensorimotor system anteriorly, and the SLF laterally. Both cuts should continue until they enter the superior wall of the atrium, taking the sematic limb from the other side into consideration as necessary.

There are many reasons for this. First, unlike most other gliomas, the arteries are not en passage vessels, they almost always are going to the part of the brain you are removing as they are distal ACA and MCA vessels. Further, once you have finished the separation, you are behind the thalamus and central core, making the risk of significant disorientation much less. Finally, depending on the tumor, you either have committed to removing the occipital pole or you haven't, making the endpoint of the "destroy" phase either limited (i.e., you don't have much work to do posteriorly) or with a simple obvious endpoint (you go until the occipital pole is out) (▶ Fig. 13.5).

A few additional steps can be used to tailor the resection to specific situations, as discussed in the following sections.

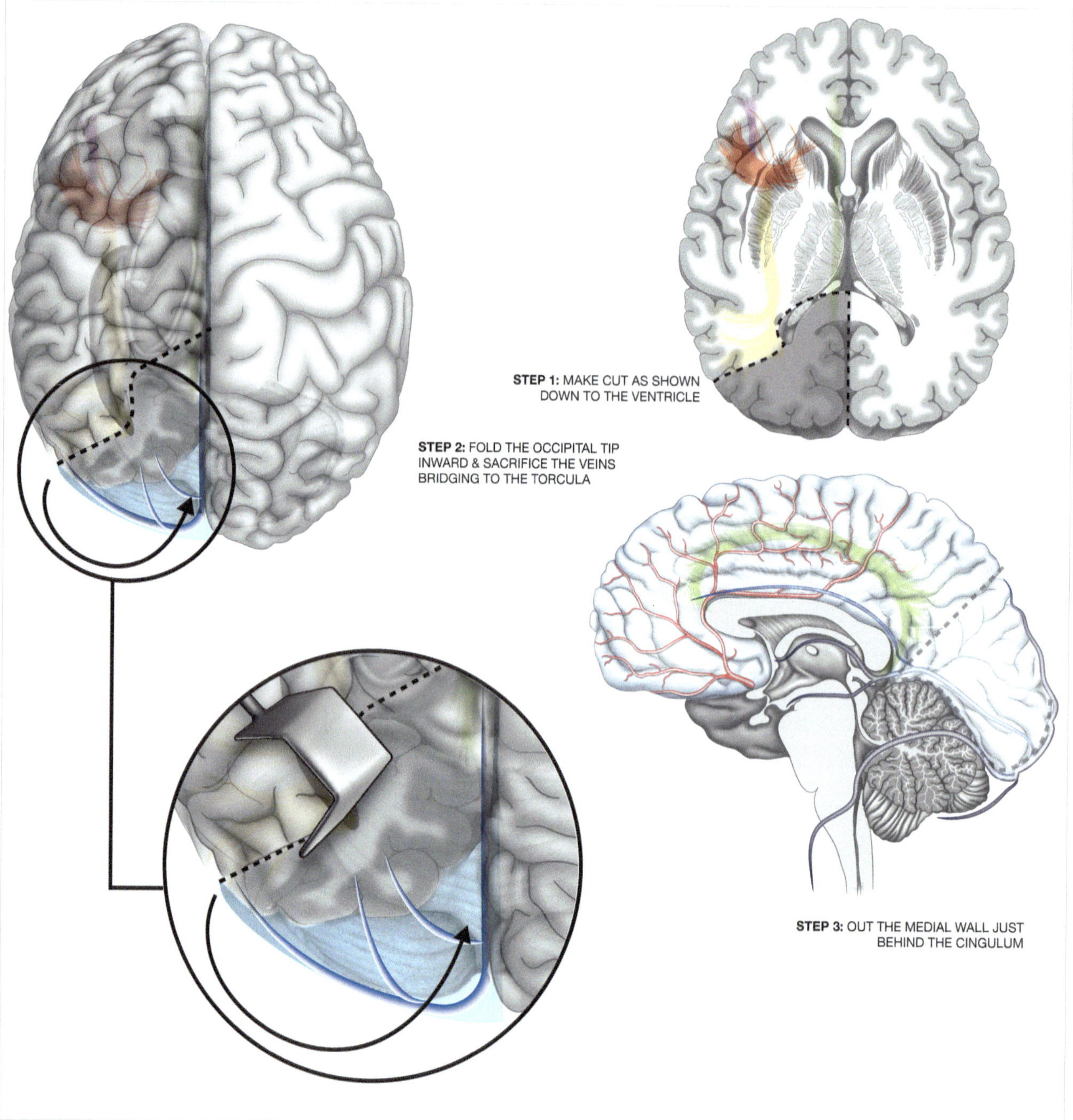

Fig. 13.5 This diagram demonstrates the steps of an occipital lobectomy. A complete lobectomy, involves at least some form of an anterior occipital and/or medial parietal disconnection (in smaller tumors, these can be very conservative cuts, far away from the tracts, but the tract position should always be taken into consideration. Once both of these cuts have been taken into the atrium, then the PCA branches (not en passage in this case) and the bridging veins should be divided and the lobe folded inward. As with frontal and temporal lobectomies, it is unnecessary to extend the bone flap to the pole of a lobe which is coming out.

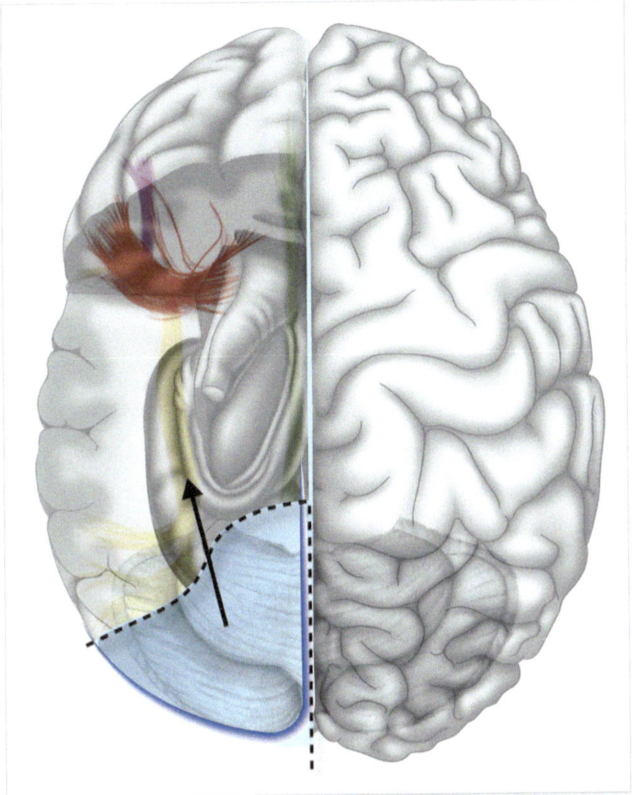

Fig. 13.6 Accessing the medial temporal structures from the occipital side: Note that the principle barrier to safely accessing the medial temporal structures, is the lateral white matter system. While occipital tumors do not commonly enter the medial temporal lobes, they can gain access to them via the lingula-PHG connections, or via the cingulate to PHG connections of the cingulum. Once a lobectomy or medial parietal disconnection is complete, the SLF and lateral system is out of the way, and tumor extension into the medial temporal structures is simple, as shown in this diagram.

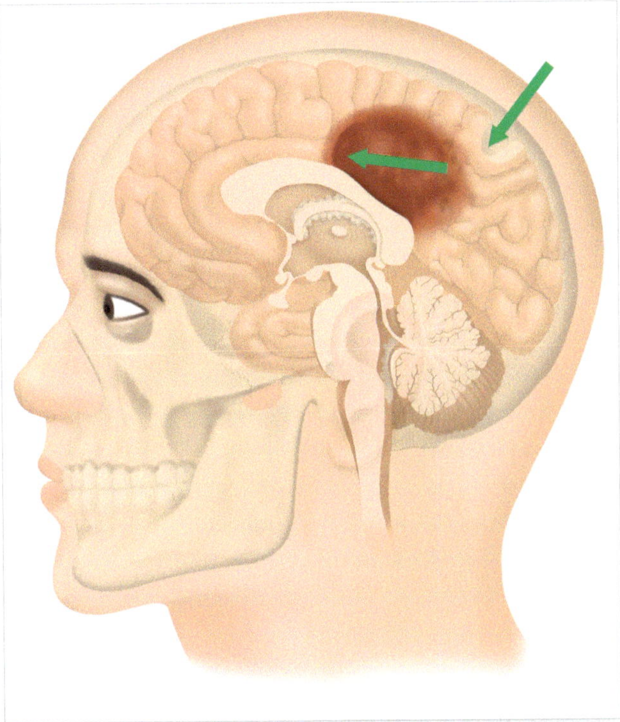

Fig. 13.7 Tumor involvement of the posterior cingulate first involves entering the cingulate from a medial parietal approach, and separating its lateral boundaries from the parietal lobe. The correct way to think about removing the posterior cingulate is to envision yourself clearing out a tunnel. The walls of that tunnel are the sensorimotor system, and the floor is the corpus callosum. Once you have identified the relevant sulcal boundaries, you should use monitoring to confirm that the cingulate tissue being removed is not necessary,

13.5.1 Resection of the Medial Temporal Structures (▶ Fig. 13.6)

Occipital and parietal tumors typically enter the inferior and/or medial temporal lobe by either following the ILF into the fusiform gyrus or by following the cingulum into the parahippocampal gyrus and/or hippocampus. This can be removed from the parietooccipital side by remaining inferiorly and medial to the atrium and temporal horn and following this from posterior to anterior. Extreme caution must be taken to avoid disorientation which can take you into the thalamus, the internal capsule, or the SLF/IFOF/optic radiations laterally, which is easy to do when the head is rotated.

13.5.2 Removal of the Posterior Cingulate Gyrus (▶ Fig. 13.7)

When the cingulate gyrus is uninvolved, it is best to leave it alone as this is a critical path involved in the DMN and memory. However, if involved with tumor, it may be nonfunctioning and/or reorganized/compensated for.

From the parietal side, these tumors often extend below the sensorimotor cortices. Note that as with the cingulate everywhere, the gyrus is a tubular tunnel surrounded by other cortices and the corpus callosum. Thus, by staying below the cingulate gyrus and medial to the sagittal plane bounded by this sulcus, you can safely work below the motor and sensory cortices and follow the cingulate as far anteriorly as you like. It is important, I think, to orient your microscope such that you are looking down the long axis of the cingulate gyrus, and to check your angles repeatedly as exiting the gyrus can lead to disaster.

13.5.3 Removing the Splenium (▶ Fig. 13.8)

The principle for removing the splenium is similar to removing the genu and rostrum from the frontal approach: you proceed until you have a wide biventricular opening, and you utilize anatomic boundaries to guide what is callosum and what is not. There are some differences which are summarized below.

1. Removing the splenium involves entering the atrium. The posterior wall of the atrium is the splenium, and as with the frontal callosum, entering the ventricle allows you to get

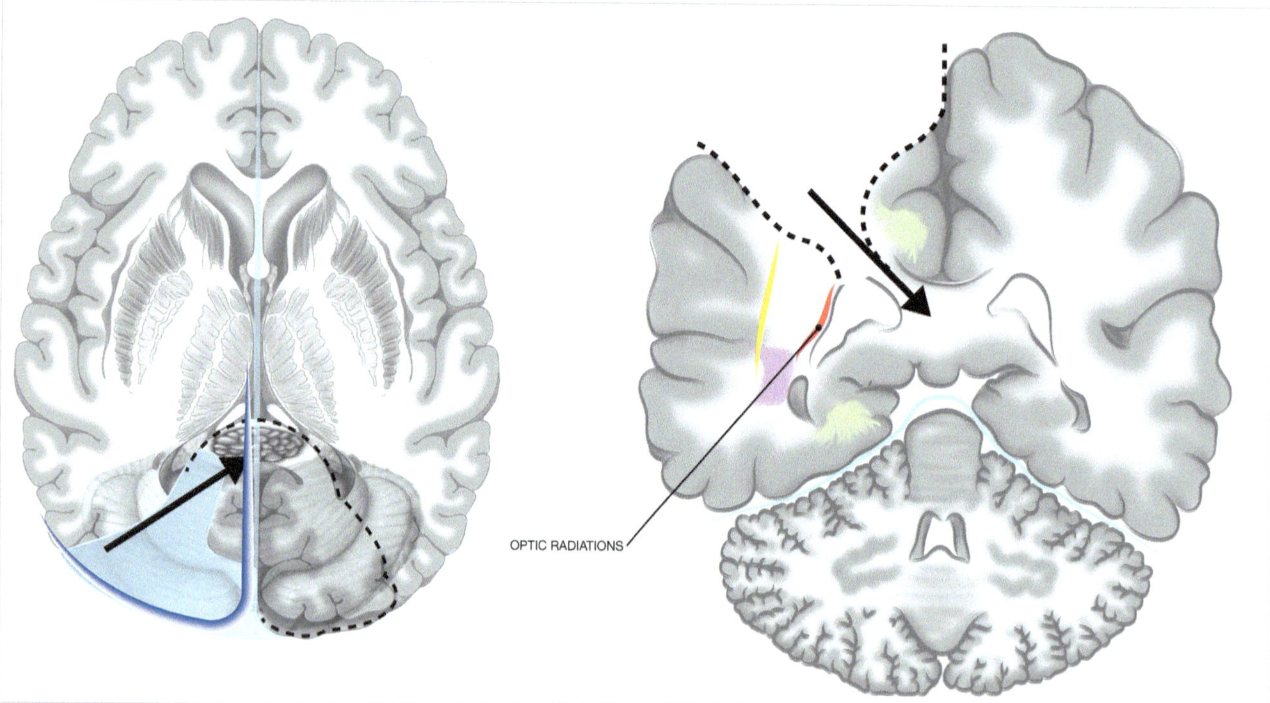

Fig. 13.8 This schematic demonstrates the steps of removing the splenium. First, you need to make a cut into the atrium lateral to the tumor and medial to the SLF and other fibers. By doing so, you can remove the splenium from the occipital lobe, and define its boundaries. The front wall of the splenium is the back wall of the atrium, the bottom surface abuts the vein of Galen, and the posterior surface is the lower edge of the falx and the posterior cingulate. The splenium is removed by resecting all tissue within those boundaries until you have widely entered the other side. The contralateral splenium is hidden behind the falx, which usually requires a 30 degree endoscope, and angled instruments to reach.

oriented and to separate the involved callosum from the ipsilateral brain so it limits the ability for this tumor to spread. Entering the atrium safely usually means a division with the SLF, done awake.

2. The posterior boundary of the splenium is the falx. Thus, by removing everything between the ventricle and the falx, you have removed the splenium. Of note, the internal cerebrals and vein of Galen delineate the inferior boundary.
3. The fornices and thalami are at risk anteriorly.
4. The superior aspect of the splenium fans out triangularly (▶ Fig. 13.9). Our white matter work suggests that the bihemispheric connections between the semantic areas run through this part and this should be worked into your considerations.
5. The posterior bend of the contralateral splenium is behind the falx. This typically requires an endoscope and angled instruments to follow this bend into the contralateral occipital lobe in most resections.

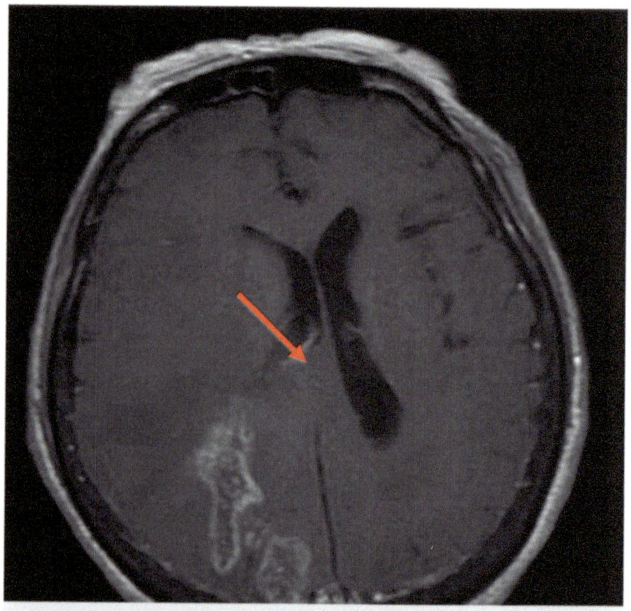

Fig. 13.9 This figure depicts the upper boundary of the splenium, which forms a triangular structure of fibers fanning out into the parietal lobe. Tumors occasionally extend that superiorly, but you should be aware of the semantic fibers passing through this part of the callosum to the other side.

13.6 Case Examples

13.6.1 Anterior Occipital Tumors

▶ Fig. 13.10 demonstrates an anterior occipital GBM. The cut is anterior with the SLF and the principle challenge with removing this tumor is the risk to the ability to read which we found two sites specifically for reading. We were able to remove the enhancing part of the tumor without causing alexia, but a larger anatomic resection was not possible.

a) At the time I did this case, I was somewhat surprised to find reading in this area, but I have since seen this many times.

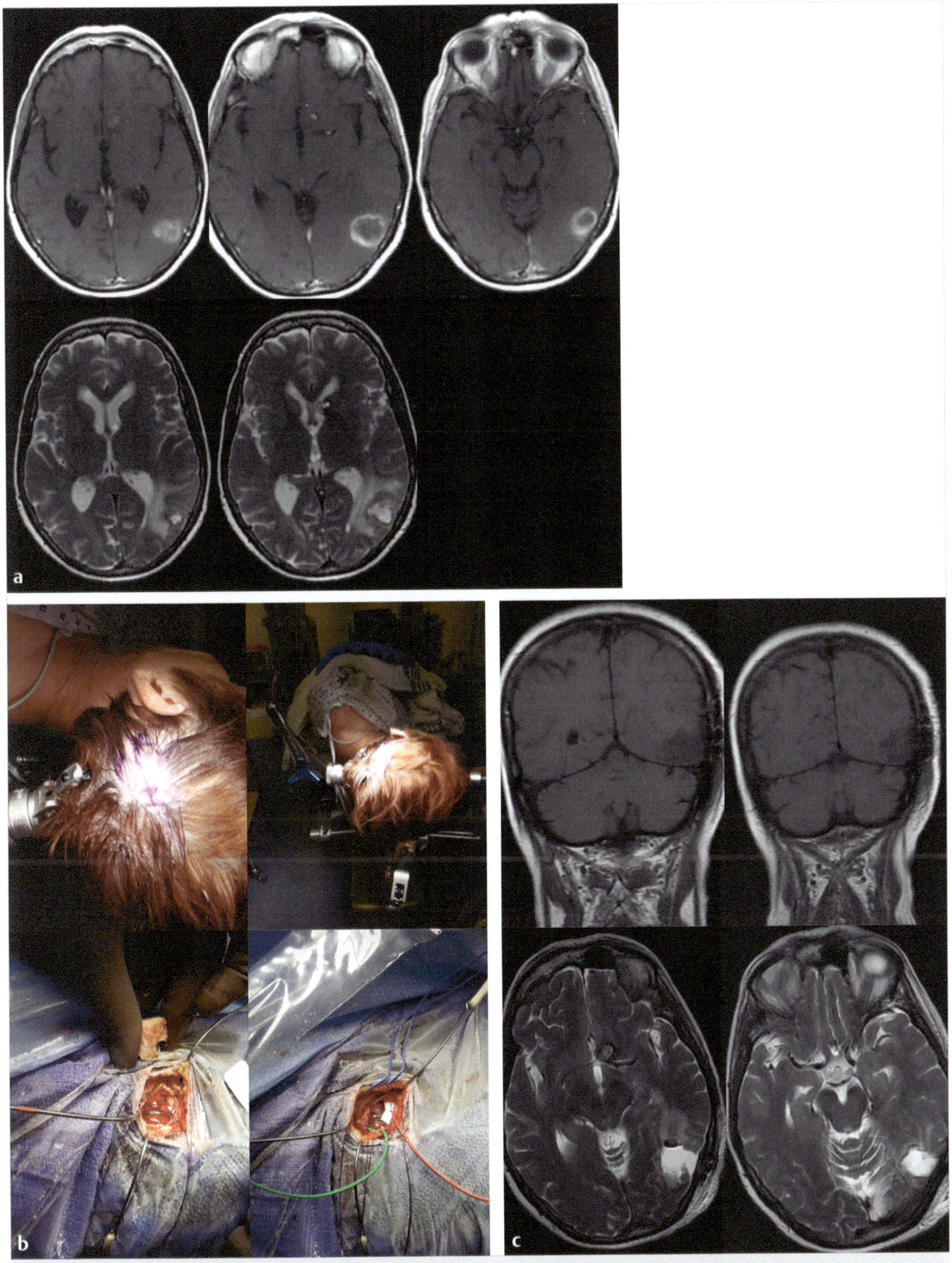

Fig. 13.10 An anterior occipital GBM; (**a**) preoperative images, (**b**) images of the approach, (**c**) postoperative images.

The maps in Chapter 6 make this obvious that this is a visual to speech case, and that reading is front and center.

b) This small craniotomy behind the ear took us down to the tentorium. As noted by the markers, which indicate alexia sites, speech areas were located in front of an over the top of this tumor, and we had to extend the bone flap with a kerrison to work behind this.

c) None.

d) Note on the postoperative scan that a low anterior occipital disconnection is used to avoid this network. This tumor took a lot more time to do than similar ones usually take me, as I had to stop many times due to alexia. I was eventually able to avoid this.

▶ Fig. 13.11 demonstrates a deeper anterior occipital tumor. The mapping found naming sites on the anterior border, and we cut just behind them to access the tumor which was mostly medial to the SLF. Note that it is possible to remove the amygdala and hippocampus from this angle. The patient had normal speech after surgery and for some time after except the reading was affected by this. In retrospect this makes sense, now that I understand macroconnectivity better.

a) When I did this case several years ago, I did not think this would be a complex speech case, and I did not consider reading as a major risk (most surgical maps I have seen have localized this to the parietal lobe, where I personally have not found it outside of other speech sites). I ultimately chose an anterior occipital approach after examining the DTI and seeing how close they were.

b) You can see from the anterior occipital approach, how close language areas were to the front edge of this tumor, exactly as the DTIs predicted.

c) The tractography clearly shows that the SLF is anterior to the front edge of this tumor and is very much at risk with this case. Note that the IFOF is pushed upward by the tumor and this tumor sitting anterior to the pre-occipital notch is threatening the ipsilateral ventral visual pathway. The ILF is likely involved as well given its position in this pathway. Thus, reading is clearly at risk in this case, which I know now.

d) The resection is good. The patient had good naming and speech function for over 2 years after this surgery, until it finally progressed within the SLF. He did have alexia, which did not entirely recover in the long term.

▶ Fig. 13.12 demonstrates a large lateral anterior occipital grade 3 glioma. The cut is made anteriorly with the extensive semantic network and we work underneath it to remove the tumor. A small amount of tumor had to be left anteriorly.

a) This tumor is located in the angular gyrus, and it should be obvious that it threatens both the SLF and IFOF as well as the semantic networks on its anterior edge. It appears to be following the apically exiting white matter fibers which leave this gyrus and head to the junctional white matter.

b) The intraoperative images demonstrate the extensive semantic network of sites threatened by this tumor as all of these markers indicate anomia sites. Note that some posterior sites lie in the clearly abnormal appearing gyrus at the front edge of this tumor. This required us to work posteriorly to avoid them. The first step in a case like this is to remove some tumor in the safest area you can find to relax the brain and make room.

c) The SLF clearly runs through the front of this tumor, consistent with our intraoperative finding that there were language areas in the anterior edge of this tumor. The IFOF also runs along the deep boundary of this tumor. While some of this may be compensable from the other side via the crossed semantic loop, it is probably best to go slow at the depth and to not plan to widely open into the atrium as your landing site for this disconnection.

d) There is a fair size piece of tumor along the anterior edge, as expected. One thing I have learned to do when looking at films like this is to compare them side by side in multiple planes. It is quite easy in a case like this to feel like you got out less than you really did, as the cavity collapses inward, edema spreads on the boundaries, and blood can confound the interpretation. It is important to remain honest with yourself about how you are doing, but post-operative scans can leave you over critical in some cases when they are not in context with the starting point.

13.6.2 Medial Parietal Tumors

▶ Fig. 13.13 demonstrates a recurrent medial parietal GBM, which is mostly non-enhancing in a patient with mild neglect due to tumor located in his SLF. We performed a medial parietal disconnection and resection taking care to preserve the SLF and motor network.

a) As with many recurrent GBM cases, it is critical to set a goal of what you are going to try to get out and this case is a key example. There is an area of enhancement in the middle of the tumor, near the SLF; however, the T2 change is extensive. You cannot realistically expect to get all of that out and leave a functional patient. At the same time, just removing the enhancement is usually not very helpful, and can make the edema intolerable. Finally, you don't want to do a giant anatomic resection of the T2 changes and leave the enhancing part for some reason (it's not all the tumor but it's the worst part). I approach this issue by creating a mental plan that first addresses the enhancement, and then plans an anatomic resection in as many directions as I think are reasonably possible and helpful. I do not perform a wide lobectomy type of operation if I believe a lesionectomy of the enhancement will be treacherous and difficult.

In this particular case, I chose to address the enhancement with a medial parietal type resection and to continue this resection as wide medially as possible. This would leave some T2 changes in the motor system and SLF, anteriorly and superiorly but would at least reduce problems on the posterior and medial boundaries of the enhancement.

a) None.

b) The patient initially presented with mild neglect and it's easy to see why as the tumor is densely involved with the parietal ramus of the SLF and the posterior components of the motor network. The disconnection should be tailored to address these two areas, which are the two main cuts of a medial parietal disconnection.

c) The postoperative film demonstrates a medial parietal disconnection and anatomic resection. There is some blood on

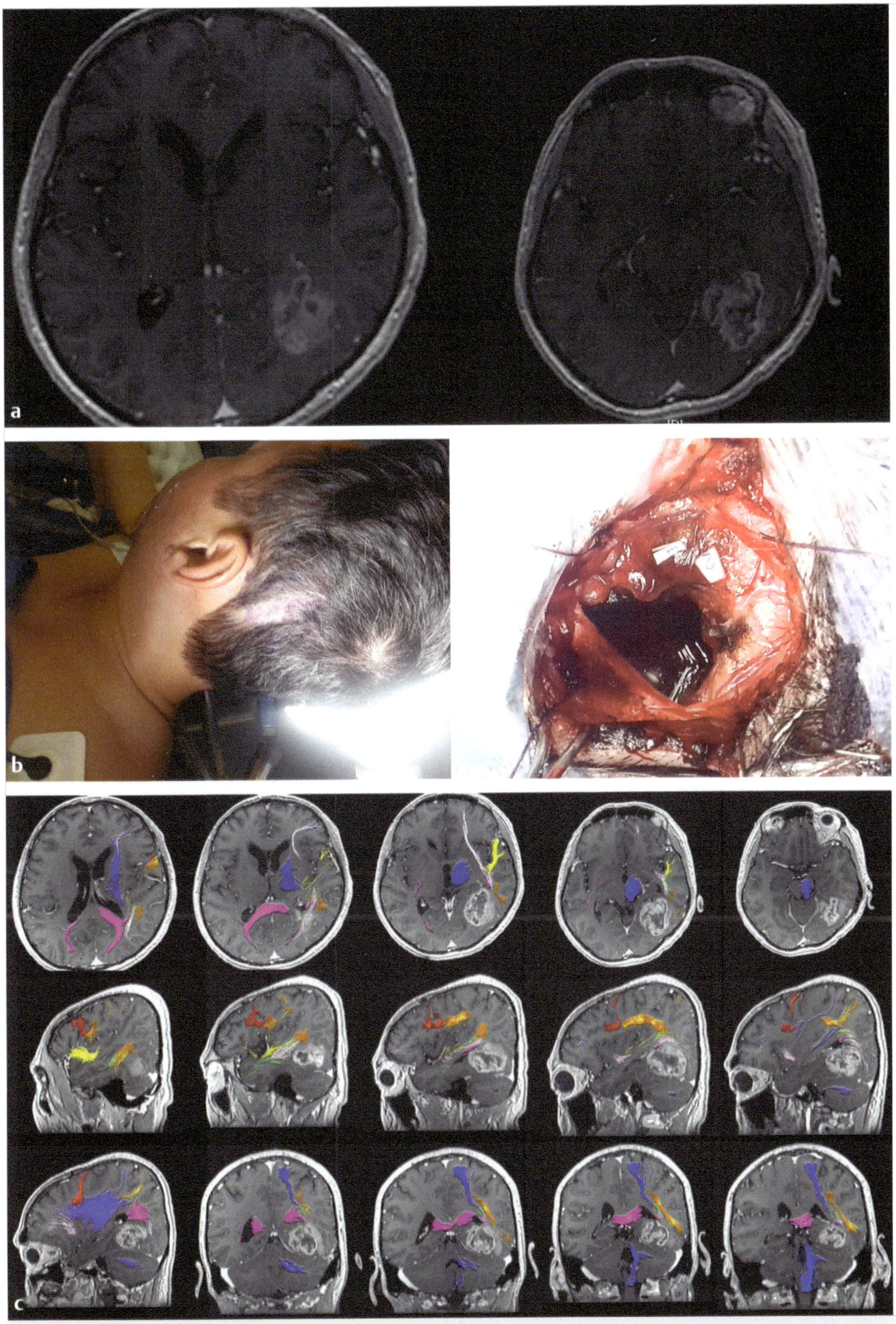

Fig. 13.11 A deeper anterior occipital tumor; (**a**) preoperative images, (**b**) images of the approach, (**c**) DTI tractography. (*Continued*)

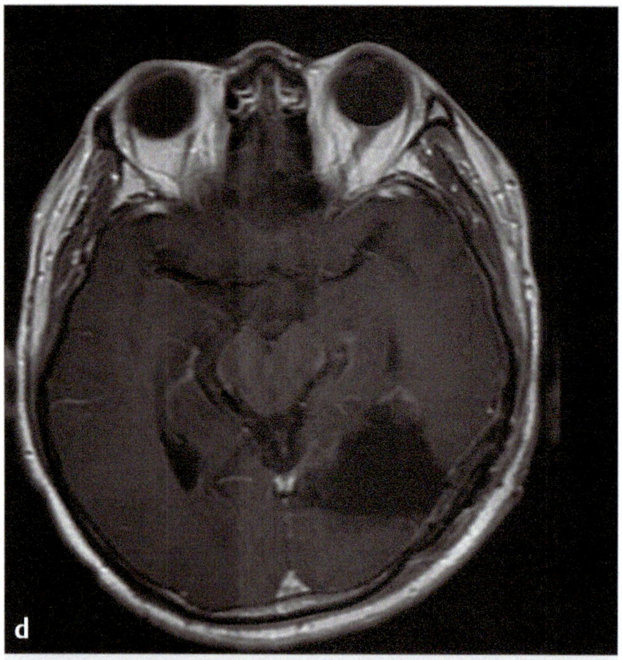

Fig 13.11 *(Continued)* **(d)** Postoperative images.

the pia of the postcentral gyrus which may contain some enhancing tumor. This patient tolerated this quite well and was doing well at 3 months when he died suddenly of a pulmonary embolus from a pre-existing DVT.

13.6.3 Occipital Pole Tumors

▶ Fig. 13.14 demonstrates a GBM in the occipital pole in a patient who has a dense homonymous hemianopsia.

a) The images reveal two key facts. One, the tumor is in the optic radiations, as they pass around the atrium, and thus the field cut is neither recoverable, nor worth trying to do so. Two, the tumor is beginning to enter the splenium. If you are doing an occipital lobectomy then there is no reason to avoid working in the splenium, other than what it takes to preserve the posterior cingulate which is not usually involved and which contains the DMN. We have not found any evidence to date that the splenium has any non-homologous connections outside of the occipital lobes, and the key thing is to avoid cutting the crossed semantic loop which will cause anomia in this left-sided tumor. This tract is a bit more anterior in the callosum and does not run in the splenium.
b) We are committing to an occipital lobectomy with this case, and so our principle goals are to avoid damaging the SLF and semantic networks laterally, and to avoid cutting too high in the parietal lobe. The operative images demonstrate a craniotomy centered around these cuts, and which is close enough to the torcula and sinuses so we can cheat under the bone flap to deliver the occipital tip. As always it is best to avoid exposing up the sinuses as it is unnecessary to be gentle with an occipital tip which is coming out.
c) None.
d) The post-op axial and sagittal images nicely show the cuts of a standard occipital lobectomy.

▶ Fig. 13.15 demonstrates a similar case of an occipital pole GBM treated with occipital lobectomy. The cuts are with the SLF and the parietal lobe, similar to a medial parietal tumor, but are obviously less aggressive.

a) This is a transformed, radiated low grade glioma operated previously elsewhere. Removing the enhancing part of this tumor will destroy the ipsilateral visual system, and thus there is little reason to preserve visual pathway intermediates as far as I can tell. They are full of tumor in this case
b) The torcula and sinuses are outlined, as is the planned craniotomy. Note that this is an older case which I did asleep, but today I would do this awake to preserve the crossed semantic loop. Notably, he did have some anomia postoperatively which partially improved, which I suspect comes from this issue.
c) None.
d) The postoperative images show a nice resection.

▶ Fig. 13.16 demonstrates a tumor in the occipital pole which is far more extensive.

a) A careful review of the images demonstrates that this tumor is following the visual fibers to the thalamus and pulvinar, as well as following ILF fibers into the inferior temporal lobe. Despite this complexity, these extensions are deep in the brain, thud the operation is grounded in the occipital lobectomy as shown in these images, and the initial cuts are similar. Taking the lateral cut into the atrium from posteriorly, allows you to define the extensions of this tumor, including clearing this from the thalamus, and following tumor into the temporal lobe and hippocampus, as needed. Note that this is easy to do, as you are working down the long axis of the temporal lobe at the depths of an occipital lobectomy; however, caution is advised as it is easy to become disoriented from this angle. Disorientation from this angle usually takes you into the internal capsule or central core.
b) The craniotomy is planned like a standard occipital lobectomy. The bed is rotated when we remove the medial temporal portions so that the lip of brain along the lateral cut does not fall into our way.
c) None.
d) Note that once you locate the atrium and the edge of the tentorium, you can follow the medial temporal structures as far anteriorly as you wish provided you stay below and medial to the temporal horn.

▶ Fig. 13.17 demonstrates a lateral occipital lobe GBM which was resected without a margin early in my series. This patient presented without a visual field cut.

a) This tumor is primarily localized to the lateral occipital cortex. The deep part of this tumor abuts the optic radiations, and this tumor is clearly in visual processing areas. You can discuss at length whether a marginal resection or a lesionectomy is better for this case: I performed a compromise between lobectomy and lesionectomy. This is obviously a very difficult decision, as we would wish to save the ipsilateral visual system if possible, in patients where it is functioning. A few arguments for aggressive resection based on anatomic boundaries: 1) the depth of this tumor is close to the optic radiations, making them hard to save and still remove the tumor, 2) as the maps in Chapter 6 demonstrate that visual

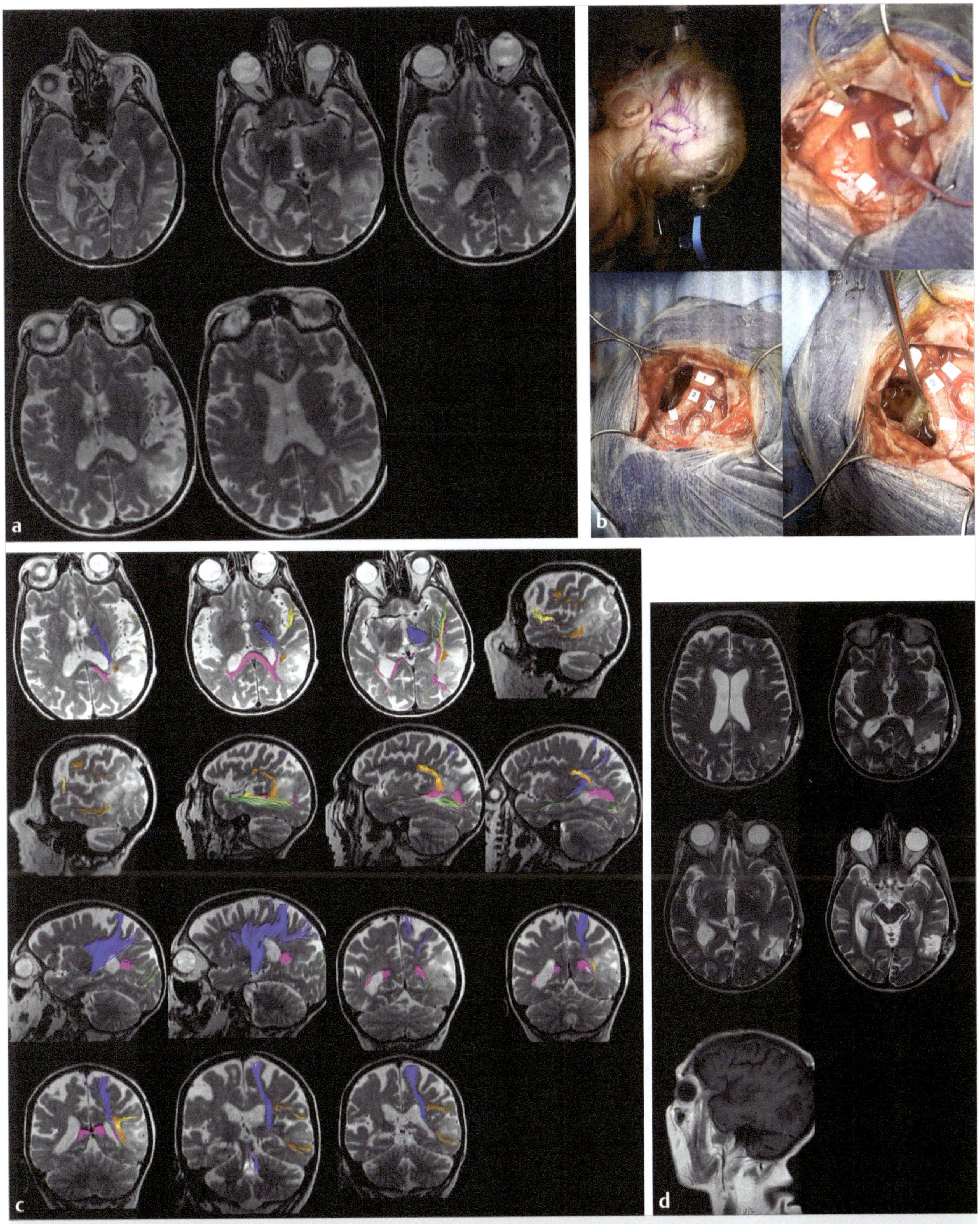

Fig. 13.12 A large lateral anterior occipital grade 3 glioma. They are case examples and the files are organized as follows: (**a**) preoperative images, (**b**) images of the approach, (**c**) DTI tractography, (**d**) postoperative images.

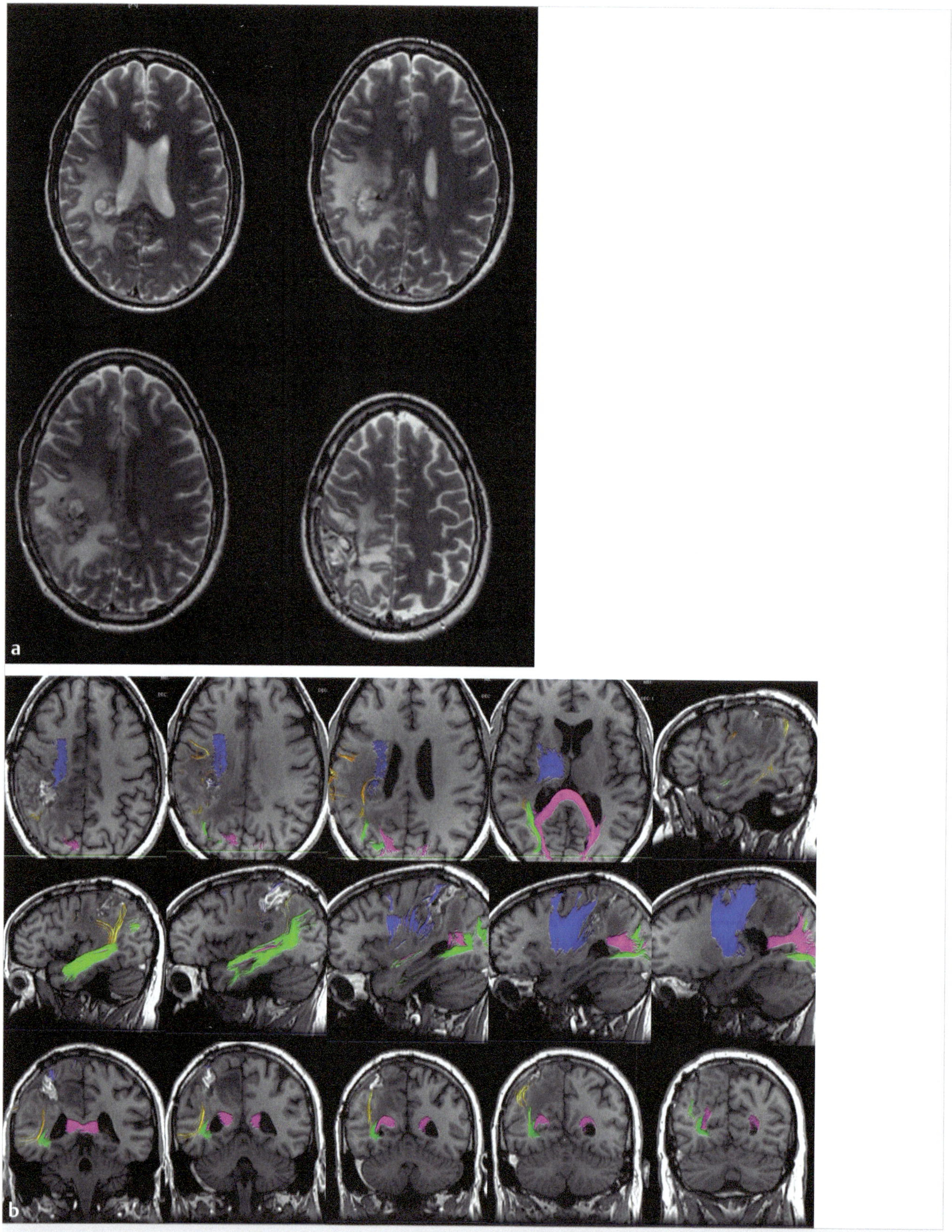

Fig. 13.13 A recurrent medial parietal GBM, which is mostly non-enhancing in a patient with mild neglect due to tumor located in his SLF. They are case examples and the files are organized as follows: (**a**) preoperative images, (**b**) DTI tractography.

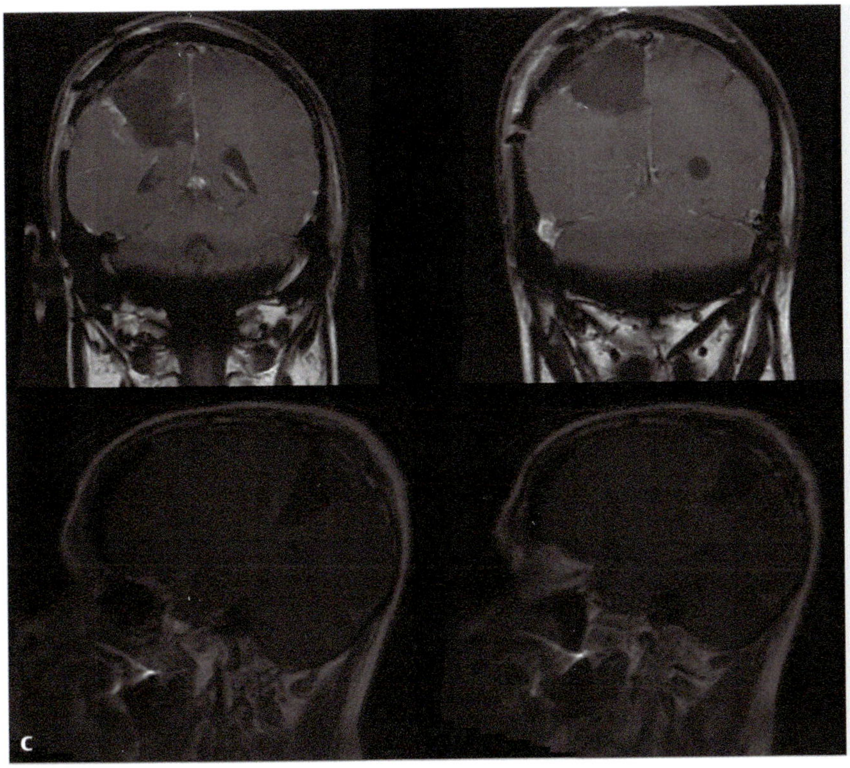

Fig 13.13 *(Continued)* (**c**) Postoperative images.

processing is a series of sites which process in sequential fashion and are connected via numerous small local connections and interconnections. They are also interconnected with the thalamus at multiple steps, and I feel that it is likely that cutting anywhere along the chain (especially early stages such as V2 or V3) would eliminate visual output in the same way as resecting V1. I am not certain that you can make cuts in this network without disrupting its function, as there isn't a main connection which defines it, and which preserving it saves the function in the same way the SLF defines speech or neglect. 3) It is unclear that you can save a visual system by leaving tumor in it in the long term, 4) unilateral visual loss causes a field cut which limits driving, but otherwise patients can have a meaningful life without assuming information can come from the other side, and finally 5) by trying to save the optic radiations in a case like this, we may get a lose-lose situation, where we neither save the ipsilateral optic function nor adequately address the tumor. Again, those willing to sacrifice tumor control for function often end up with neither, and we should always be aware of this in our tradeoffs. In short, I am not advocating for an occipital lobectomy for all tumors like this, especially for low grade gliomas without deficits, the risk benefit of increasing the resection by 1–2% by finishing off the optic radiations is far less overwhelming, and you realistically might be able to save the pathways, but instead I wanted to outline the conflict in my mind on this issue at present.

b) None.
c) None.
d) The resection is aggressive but I did try to spare at least some of the visual system (which admittedly I didn't understand at the time as well as I do now) and the optic radiations in the false hope of sparing at least part of his visual fields on this side (it didn't work).
e) This patient had an early recurrence, and at recurrence the tumor not only regrew in the surgical cavity, but also followed the connections with this area to the pulvinar, which is predictable based on the connectivity of this region.

Of course we cannot be certain if taking the radiations would have prevented this early recurrence, but certainly we didn't do him a favor by trying to save, especially in light of spread across the splenium and into the thalamus. The answers are never as clear in prospect as in retrospect, but in hindsight, I view this as a poorly thought out tradeoff on my part between function and tumor control that ultimately achieved neither for long.

▶ Fig. 13.18 demonstrates a lateral occipital GBM with an anteromedial extension into the TPO junction as it follows the fibers to the thalamus. An untrained eye might not appreciate the risk to speech such a case presents; however, an analysis of DTIs demonstrate that the tip of this tumor was tucked between the IFOF and the SLF and was quite challenging.

a) At first, glance, it is easy to view this as a lateral occipital tumor, which has its own set of issues as described in ▶ Fig. 13.19. But a closer look shows that this tumor is following the lateral occipital pathways into the deep white matter, and thus puts numerous pathways at risk. Blindly trying to fish out the tip of this tumor with an asleep patient, and no tractography might work out well, but don't be surprised if it doesn't and the patient has some speech problems afterwards.
b) None.
c) By this point in this book, a tractography set like this should concern you. The tip of this tumor is wedged between the

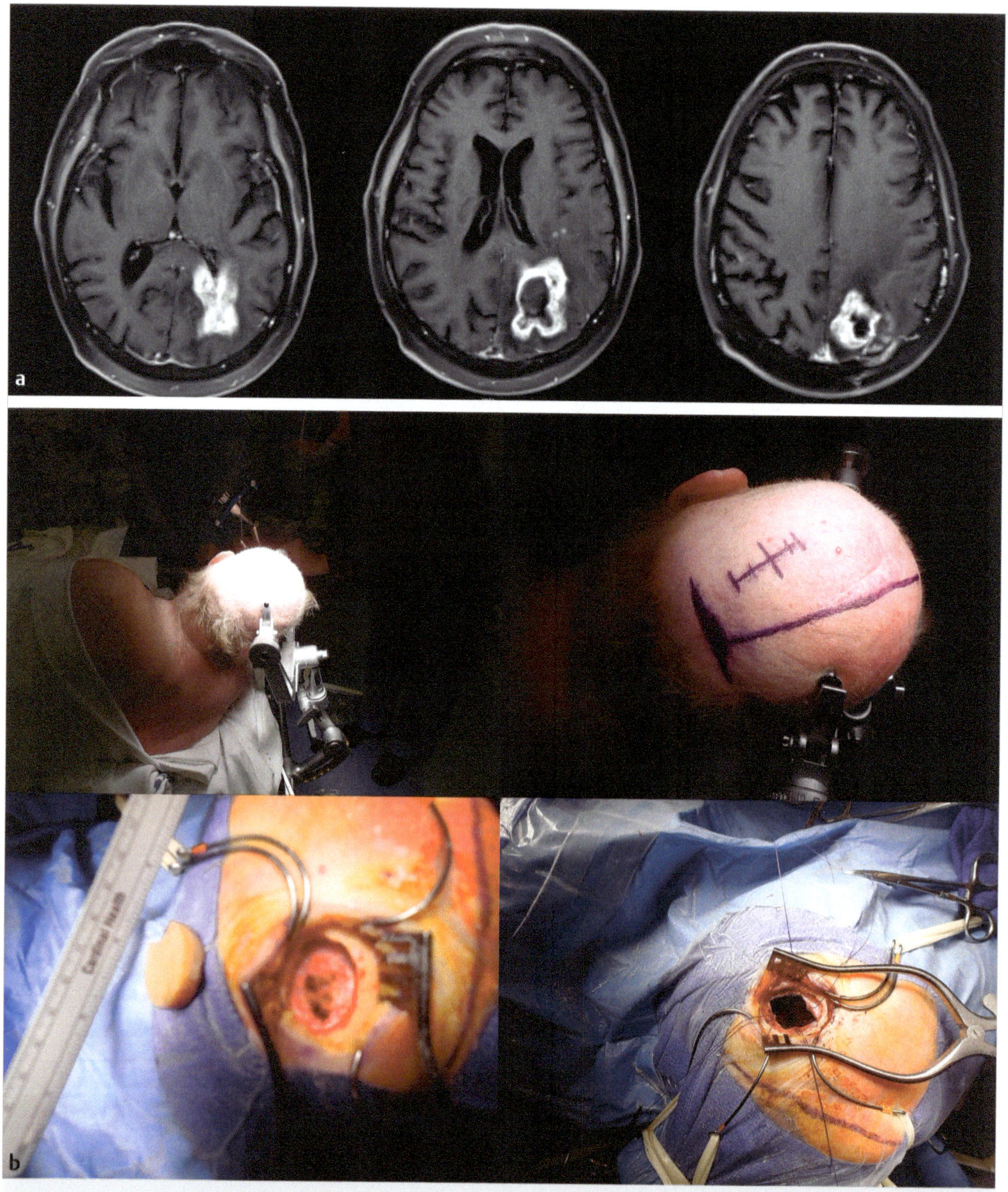

Fig. 13.14 A GBM in the occipital pole in a patient who has a dense homonymous hemianopsia. They are case examples and the files are organized as follows: (**a**) preoperative images, (**b**) DTI tractography.

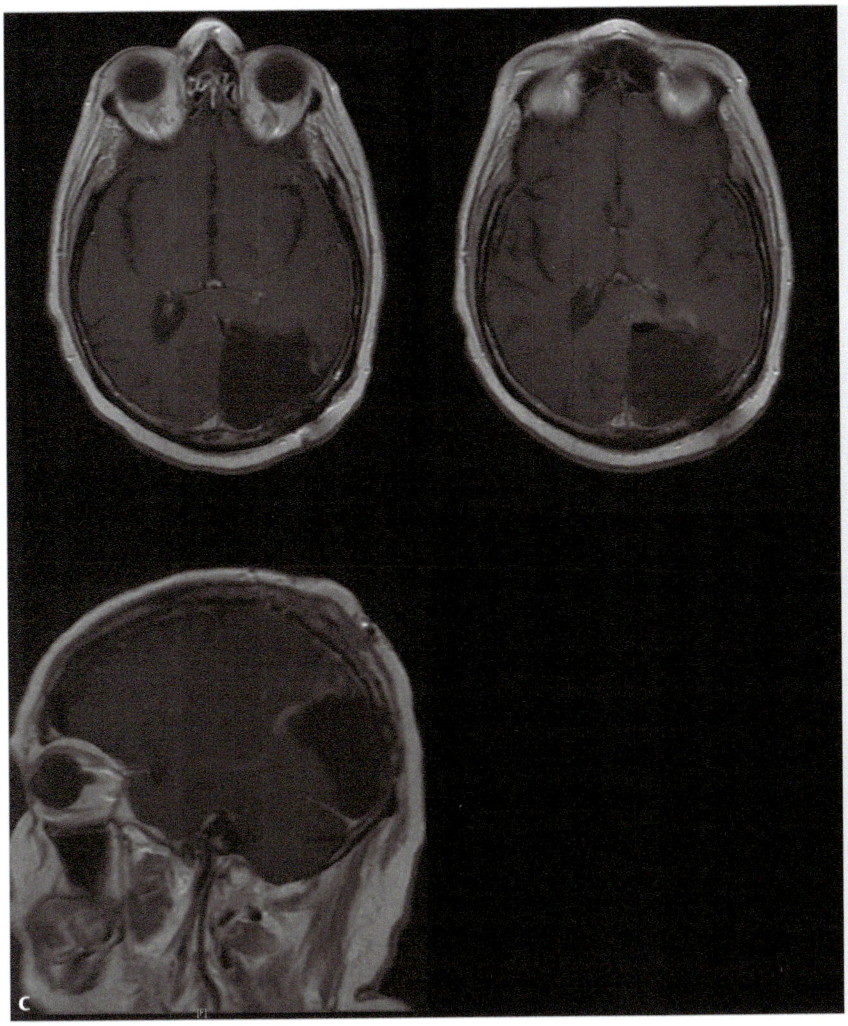

Fig 13.14 (*Continued*) (**c**) Postoperative images.

SLF and IFOF in the TPO junction. Further, the IFOF is at risk over a fair length (as we would expect with a tumor starting in the lateral occipital cortices and following its pathways, which roughly parallel IFOF). This is a very difficult tumor to completely remove and have normal speech.

d) I spent several hours in this case patiently teasing this tumor away from the deep white matter. Anatomic resection was not realistic here, so we based the resection on gross appearance and functional information. This involved numerous subcortical speech arrests, especially at the depths. I settled for the resection seen in these images, and was very happy I got out as much as I was able to without any speech problems.

13.6.4 Posterior Cingulate Tumor

▶ Fig. 13.13, ▶ Fig. 13.14, ▶ Fig. 13.15, ▶ Fig. 13.16, ▶ Fig. 13.17, ▶ Fig. 13.18, ▶ Fig. 13.19 demonstrates what at first glance looks like a recurrent medial parietal tumor; however, closer examination demonstrates that the majority of this tumor is mainly centered in the posterior cingulate. These tumors provide the challenging feature of extending below the sensorimotor cortex by following in the cingulate gyrus. The technique for removing them is similar to a medial parietal case (they often are in these parts of the parietal lobes given the interconnection with the cingulum and superior parietal lobule). After providing access to the posterior cingulate, I determine what aspects of the posterior cingulate can be removed, with concentration tasks, usually I find that it has reorganized and can be taken in most cingulate tumors. It is then critical to define the cingulate sulcus and stay between it and the callosum as you remove the cingulate under the sensory and motor strip. You need to be monitoring leg function as this is the area principally at risk.

a) When you first see one of these uncommon tumors, you generally will mistake it for a medial parietal tumor. The key is to examine sagittal images on all cases, which make it obvious. It is also critical to note that this is not only a posterior cingulate tumor, it is also in the medial parietal lobe and even threatens the SLF. Like an insular tumor, cingulate tumors involve a two-step process. The first step is a standard approach to access the difficult area. In insular tumors, this is an opercular resection, but in this case it is a medial parietal resection. Once this is complete, you have excellent access to the boundaries of the deeper structure, and can see what you are doing. You need to mentally separate these parts out, or it is quite easy to find yourself working in a deep hole not entirely clear where you are. You can get lost in the cingulate just like the insula and you need to identify and remain in the safe boundary landmarks.

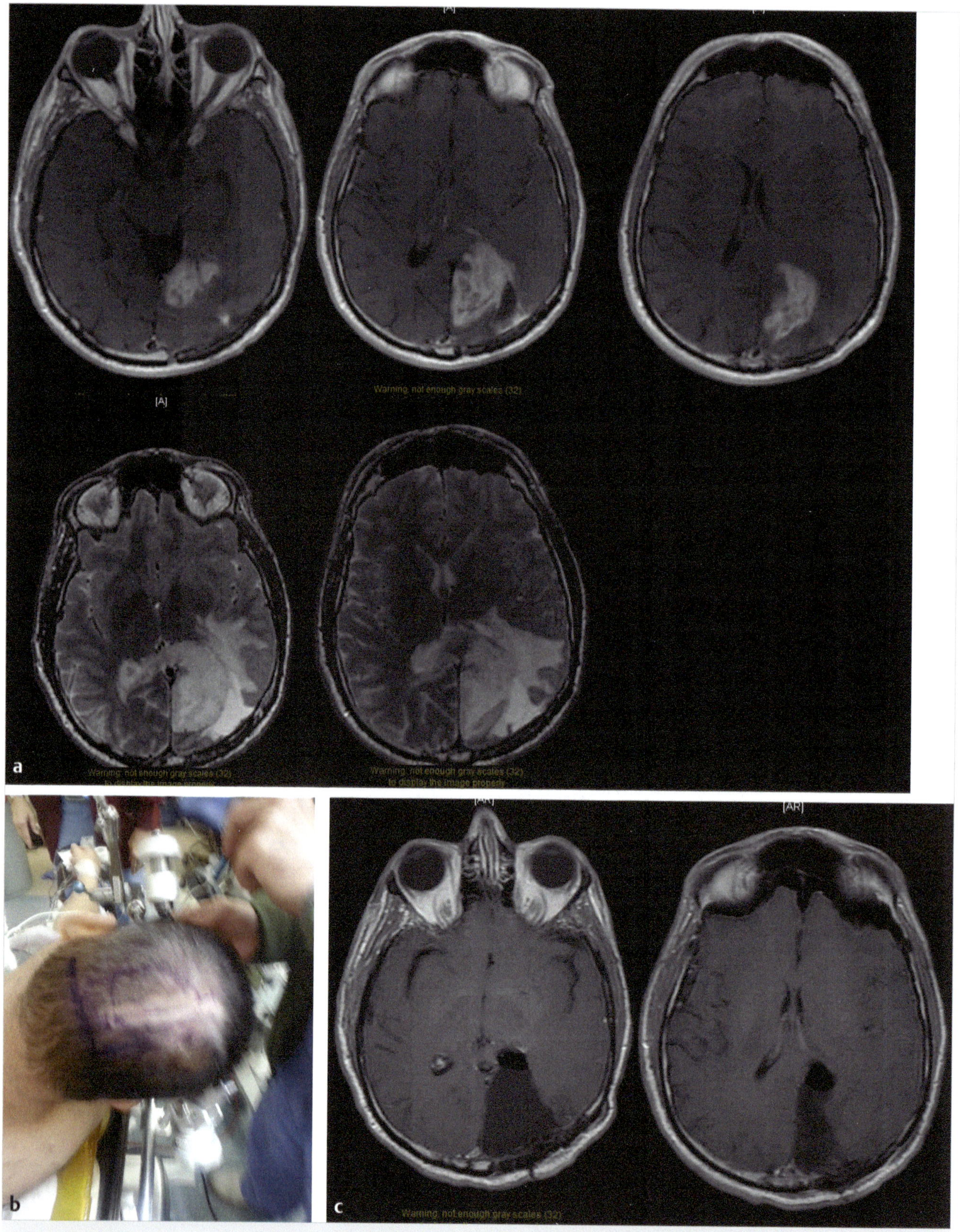

Fig. 13.15 A similar case of an occipital pole GBM treated with occipital lobectomy; (**a**) preoperative images, (**b**) images of the approach, (**c**) postoperative images.

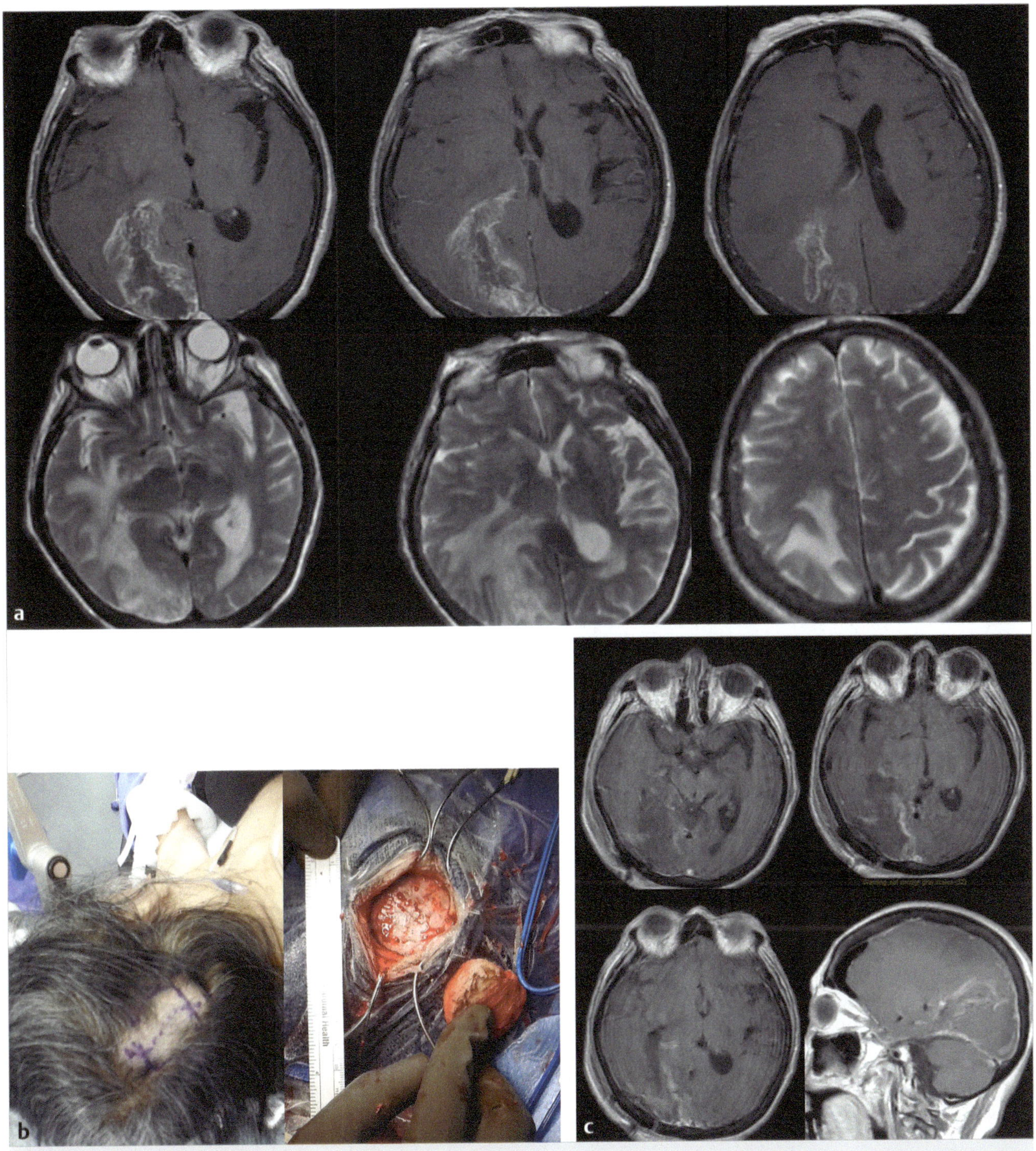

Fig. 13.16 A tumor in the occipital pole which is far more extensive; the files are organized as follows: (**a**) preoperative images, (**b**) images of the approach, (**c**) postoperative images.

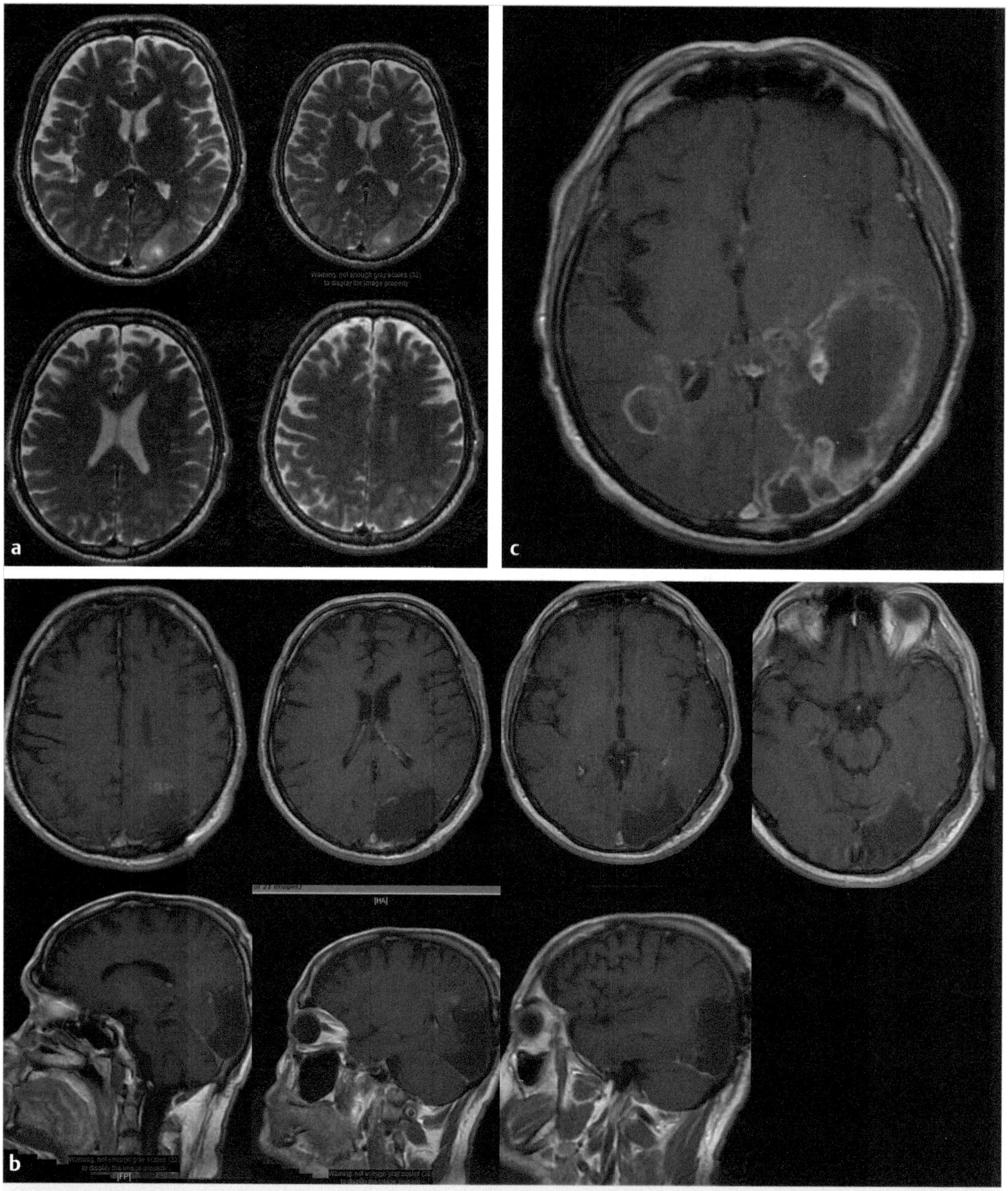

Fig. 13.17 A lateral occipital lobe GBM which was resected without a margin early in my series; (**a**) preoperative images, (**b**) postoperative images, (**c**) long-term follow-up images.

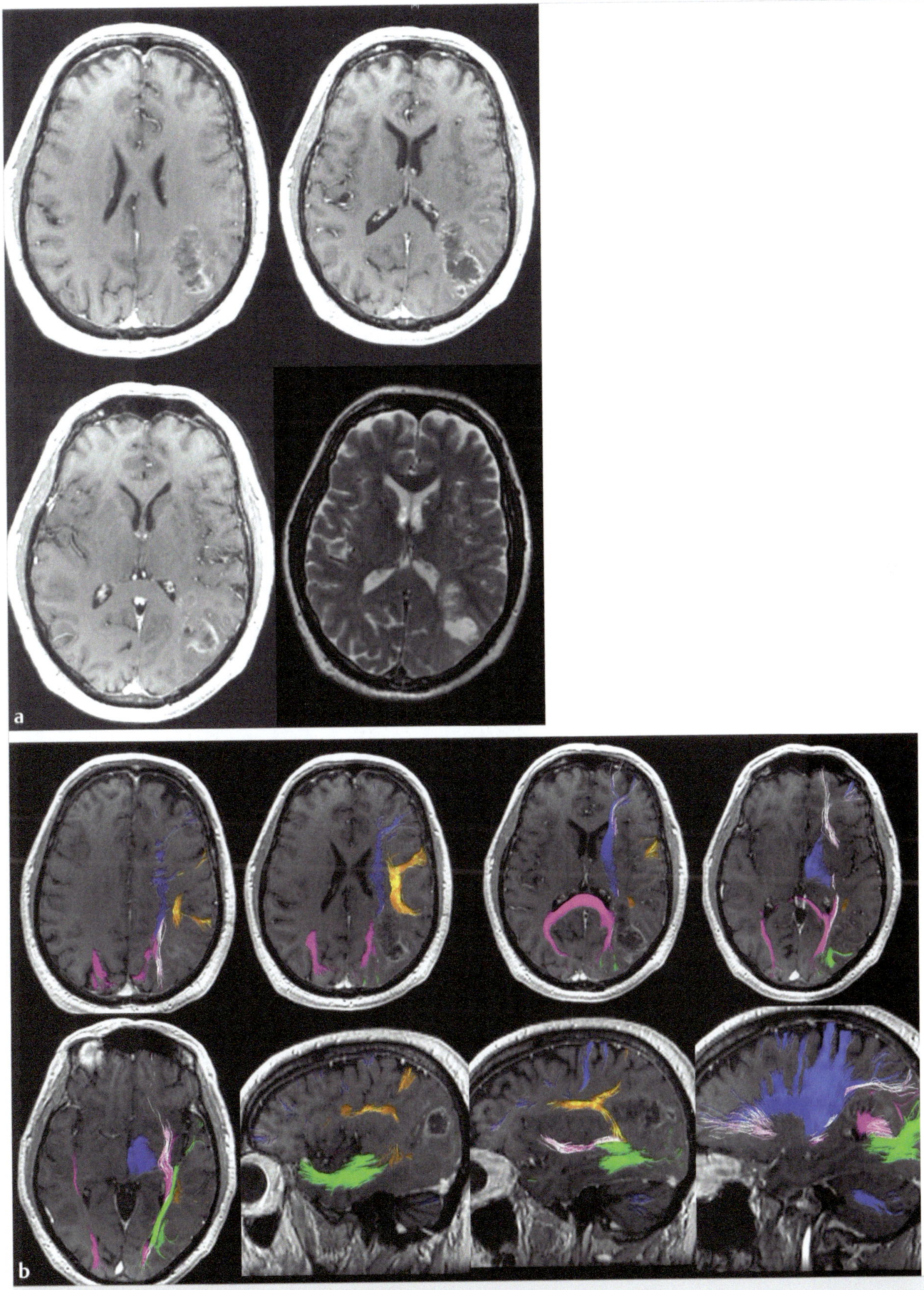

Fig. 13.18 A lateral occipital GBM with an anteromedial extension into the TPO junction as it follows the fibers to the thalamus; (**a**) preoperative images, (**b**) DTI tractography.

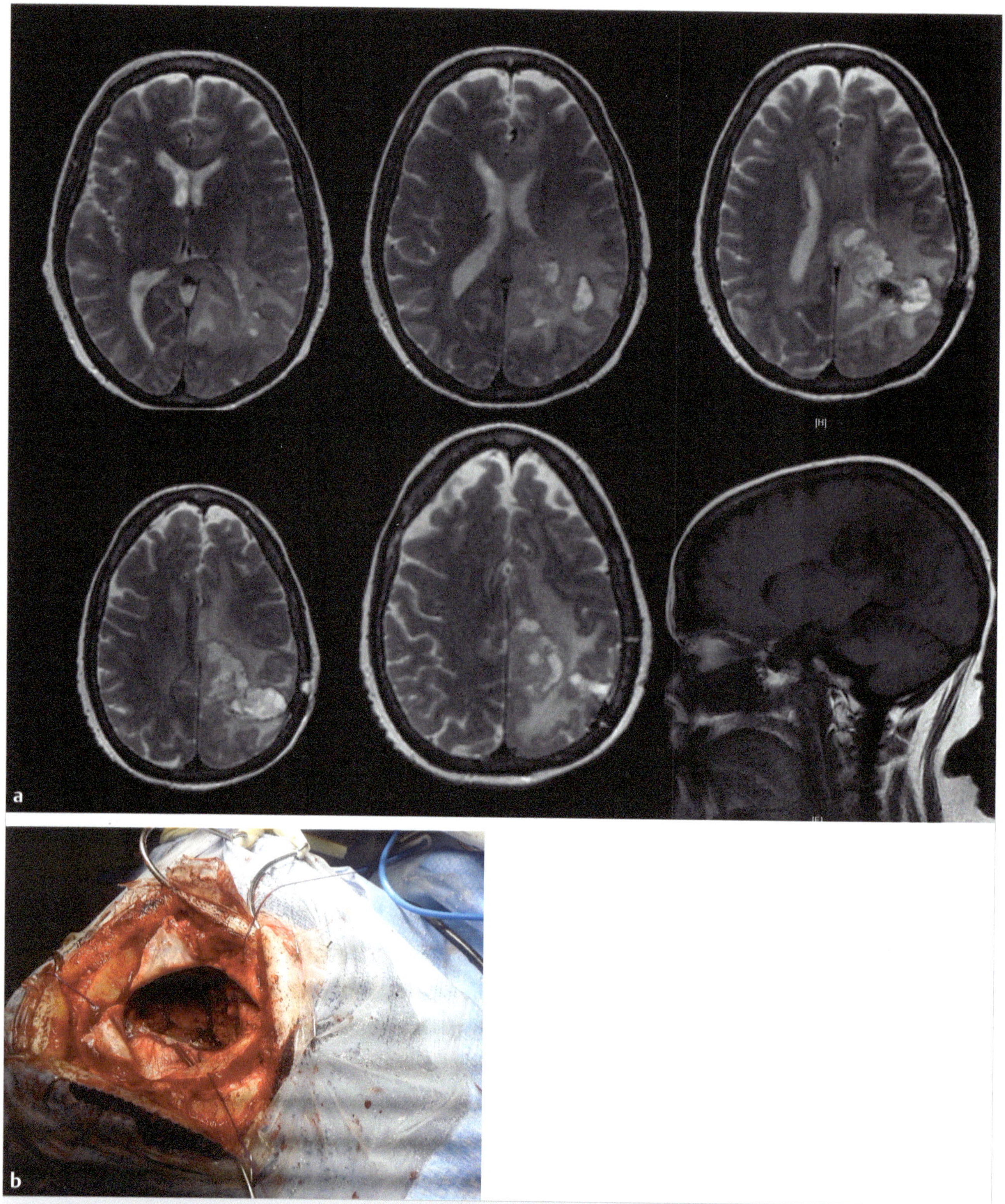

Fig. 13.19 A recurrent medial parietal GBM, which is mostly non-enhancing in a patient with mild neglect due to tumor located in his SLF. They are case examples and the files are organized as follows: (**a**) preoperative images, (**b**) intraoperative image.

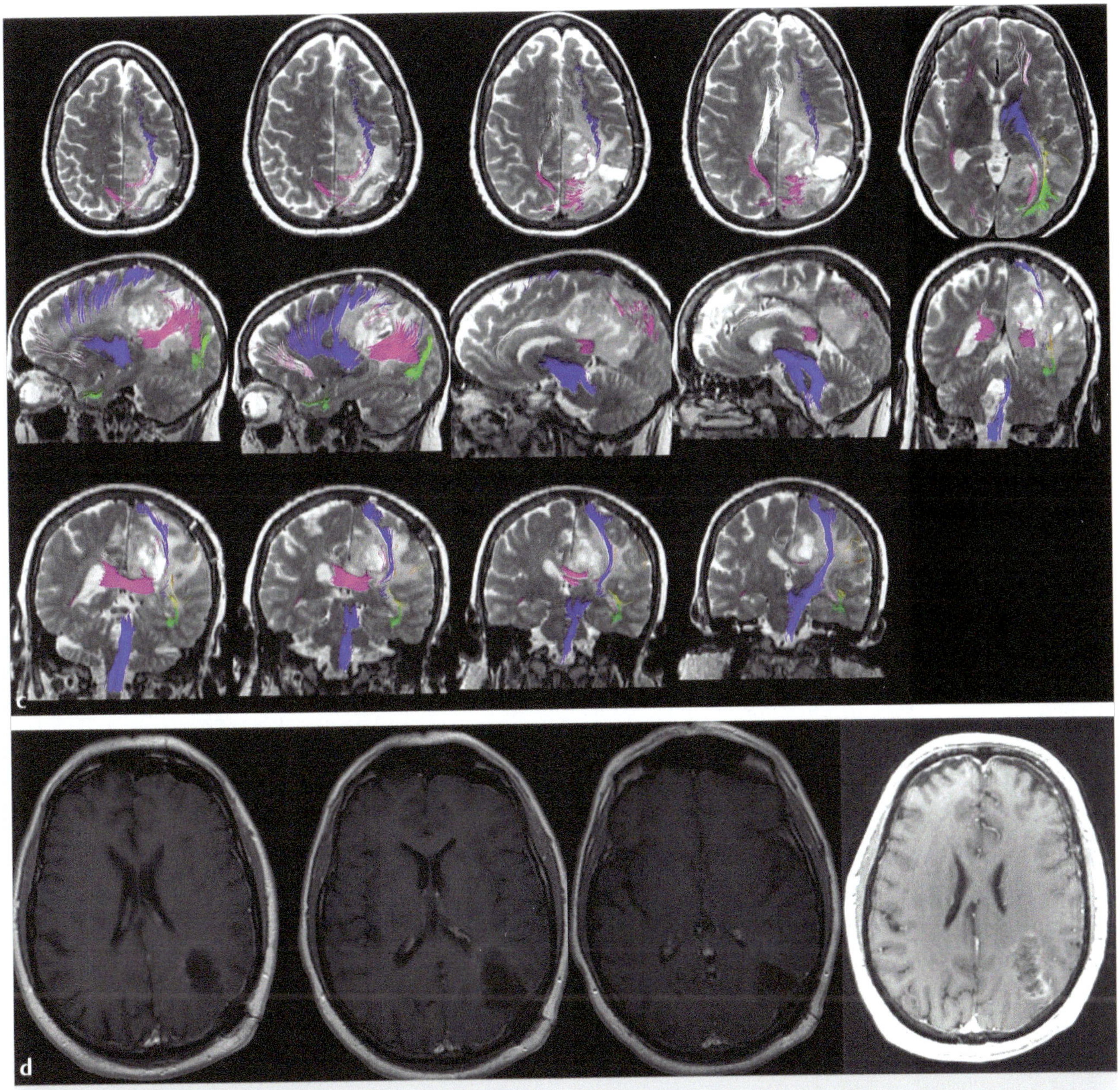

Fig 13.20 (*Continued*) (**c**) DTI tractography. (**d**) Postoperative images.

b) Note that in this case, with the left side upward, that the medial parietal cuts with the SLF (bottom) and motor areas have been performed. It is harder to appreciate the work under the anteromedial lip of the motor network cut (about at 2 o'clock in this field), which extends for several cm under the motor network within the cingulate boundaries.

c) If you closely observe the DTI sequences, and look at the motor fibers in blue on sequential images. This can be appreciated on all sequences, but especially on the sagittal, where the motor fibers create a tunnel where the cingulate tumor must pass through. The callosal fibers are colored in purple as well, and these also form a tunnel for the cingulate. Staying within this tunnel is critical for success.

d) While there are still T2 changes in the motor system, overall this is a good resection. Note that there are distinct aspects of this resection cavity which reflect a medial parietal resection followed by cingulate removal.

14 Difficult Gliomas

14.1 Introduction

This chapter is about taking on the bad boys. These are tumors which are obviously high risk, and ones which many, often good tumor surgeons deem "inoperable." They are in diverse areas of the cerebrum, and many of the anatomic aspects of these tumors are diverse, yet I will make the following observations which will make clear why I put these tumors in a common chapter towards the end of the book.

1. The tumor resection in these cases is almost always a lesionectomy: anatomic wedge type resection like lobectomies are rarely part of the operation as they are inadvisable in these parts of the brain.
2. The tumors are often surrounded on all sides with critical brain. There is no "destroy" phase of the surgery as you are frequently dealing with essential functional areas on all sides. Thus, the end of the mapping is usually the end of the case.
3. The 3-dimensional anatomy of these tumors is unfamiliar and complicated. Most of us can visualize the temporal tip because we have seen it in its entirety, but operating in the forceps major exiting the splenium and extending into the occipital white matter, or in the thalamus demands a great deal of thought to visualize what you are doing. Many of these resections require you to work based on a mental reconstructions of anatomy from conceptual knowledge, more than they are based on actual visual knowledge of the structure. Getting lost is easy to do with tragic consequences.
4. The patients are often sicker. Many of these types of tumors are high grade gliomas, and edema in these parts of the brain have major functional consequences. The patients are harder to map, and harder to achieve results you are excited about. Worse, many times, these patients have undergone a biopsy (after being deemed "inoperable"), radiochemotherapy, and a long run of steroids and physical deterioration prior to an attempt to resect the tumor, making it even harder. Your goals need to be realistic and brave. Remember that the only thing worse than being paralyzed or aphasic from a GBM is being paralyzed or aphasic from a GBM which is still there killing you.
5. Often, the fibers of interest are small and unpredictable. For example, it doesn't take a major transgression of the ascending alertness fibers from the midbrain during a thalamic tumor to lead to disaster. Nor does it take a major misstep to disconnect the motor network, or to veer into the SLF at the TPO junction.

14.2 Common Pieces of Advice for Tumors Like These

1. Go slow. The margin for error is small and the risk of disorientation is high. There is often not a great volume of tumor to remove, and the cases are rarely very long (none of these cases takes anywhere near as long as a frontal lobe resection or an insular glioma), but it is important to force yourself to slow down, stimulate more often than usual, change tasks as often as needed, and reorient yourself frequently. There is no prize for cutting 30 minutes off the resection.
2. Do not neglect the deep boundary. If you are doing these cases in the manner described in this book, you know well that you often depend on a clear anatomic boundary to signify when you are complete. Reaching the ventricle, the falx, or a well-defined sulcus, provides you reassurance that your cut is all the way past the fibers at risk. In contrast, one common feature of these cases is you really never get this kind of event to reassure you that you are done with the cut as the deep boundary is usually a white matter tract or a critical element. Failing to spend time addressing the deep boundary ends in either transgression of the tract at the bottom of the cavity (many times this is the SLF) or the critical structure at the bottom. On the other hand, if you are not aggressive with the deep margin, then you can expect to be disappointed with your extent of resection.

In short, these cases involve a cut into the white matter on the deep surface, which is usually based on functional considerations, and loosely guided by anatomic estimations (like comparing your depth to neighboring sulci, etc). I never stop the mapping until I am certain all of the boundaries are clear, especially the deep one. Conversely, once the mapping stops, I force myself to stop addressing the deep margin. It's tempting to keep going and trying to get more tumor; however, either functional preservation is important or it's not, and you cannot guarantee that the tumor doesn't possess relevant brain tissue if the patient is asleep.

3. The visual appearance of tumor tissue counts a lot in these surgeries. In most gliomas, a good anatomic resection of an area functionally disconnected brain is the best way to ensure an oncologically satisfactory resection. In other words, there is no residual tumor in the center of a hole. This avoids the issue of fingers of infiltrative and unclear tumor mixing in making it hard to know when to stop.

However, resecting to anatomic boundaries is not advisable in tumors like these. In many cases, the areas we are operating in areas that if transgressed in normal patients, would have devastating consequences. In some cases, surgery is made possible by cortical reorganization. For many of these tumors, especially the deeper ones, the more likely situation is that the resectable part of the tumor is that which is densely full of cells, pushing function out of the way, and the infilitrative portions of the tumor on the boundaries are unresectable. The visual features of glioma are described in Chapter 2 and they are critical in these cases as often this is all you can safely resect (i.e., it is the dense, noninfiltrative part).

4. Use the concepts and techniques helpful in other more straightforward gliomas as building blocks for simplifying these tumors. Many times a disconnection used in other settings can be helpful for part of these cases. The anatomy of the insula, and of major white matter tracts can also be helpful in defining boundaries for more complicated tumors, or

approaches to deeper tumors. There is a reason I waited till the last section to tackle these tumors, as you need solid fundamentals before setting out to tackle these monsters.

5. Deal with the tumor everywhere else also. It is easy to fixate on tumor in a dangerous area and to neglect a fair bit of tumor somewhere else. Doing a bunch of work in a dangerous area and not addressing the tumor elsewhere in a less dangerous area is easy to do and oncologically inadequate. There is no reason to do a risky part of the case like a butterfly glioma and neglect tumor in the frontal lobe. Again, the goal is always to leave as little disease as possible, and this is not accomplished by getting excited about the unusual part and not maximizing the mundane parts of the case.
6. Study the T2 images closely. It is critical to have a detailed understanding of where the tumor is exactly. This is always true but here it is essential for success. The T2 can tell you the position of the internal capsule, basal ganglia, thalamus relative to the mass (they are usually not in their normal positions) which is essential for picking an entry point into the tumor. It can define the exact gyri involved, and where the vessels are. The difference between a motor strip tumor, and a tumor in the parietal lobe which has pushed its way to the area where the motor strip usually is, is enormous.
7. Use anatomy wherever you can. You are not going to get a lot of anatomic clues during these cases as they often involve taking something amorphous out of the middle of an amorphous mass in the center of the brain. Defining sulcal and/or ventricular landmarks is ideal prior to making any irreversible moves.
8. Check your angles often. Many of these approaches involve deep targets and some are done in a non-neutral head position. Both of these make it quite possible to lose Anterior-posterior orientation and to veer into something terrible. Image guidance is no substitute for a good understanding of anatomy, but it is peerless in reorienting in a deep hole with few landmarks.

14.3 Methods for Resecting Specific Tumors

This chapter deviates from the organization of the rest of the book as these tumors do not fit the system very well. The "division" is a "surrounded on all sides" cut, there is no "destroy" phase, and the mapping never stops until the tumor is out as the most dangerous cut is on the blind side. Instead, what follows is a run through of the steps I use to remove these tumors.

14.3.1 Sensorimotor Region Tumors

It is unpleasant to remove gliomas from the motor strip, and sometimes this can be unrewarding in the short term. However, two points which will bring the goals of these surgeries into light:

1. The only thing worse than being paralyzed by a motor strip GBM is being paralyzed by a motor strip GBM that is still in there.
2. The motor strip is the tip of a very deep iceberg. Note that deep to the motor and sensory strips, is the entire SLF complex, inferomedial to it are the cingulum and the corpus callosum crossing from the other side, and at the end of its fibers are the basal ganglia, thalamus, and brainstem. You don't think it can get worse than hemiplegia? Try letting the tumor find its way into those structures.

Ultimately, as with many situations with gliomas, there is no peace without war, and there is no functional preservation without tumor control. Thus, while we all pat ourselves on the back when a patient walks out of the hospital perfectly normal, this is not about our pride, it's about putting a patient in the best possible situation based on the starting point and likely trajectories after different treatment strategies. In this area, it means trying to save the motor function if this is possible, but also to prevent the tumor from accessing anything else in the neighborhood for as long as we are able to do so, and it minimizing the edema that spreads into the neighboring brain regions by controlling the tumor. It has been my experience that this is usually only possible by removing the tumor.

14.3.2 Planning these Cases

As the anatomy of previous chapters should make clear, the sensorimotor system is a vertically oriented system (▶ Fig. 14.1), which is unlike the orientation of most non-thalamic projections in most networks. It is best considered as looking like a bouquet of flowers: somewhat conical and widening near the top of the branching. Most of our cuts in previous chapters addressed protecting this system by cutting parallel to these fibers with cuts in the coronal plane paralleling the precentral or postcentral sulci, which maintain the cortical motor networks, and their connections with the cerebellum, basal ganglia, thalamus and spinal cord.

It is important when planning a case for a tumor which is actually clearly in the sensorimotor system, that we consider this region as a network, and plan a way to disconnect as few parts of it as possible. This starts with a clear definition of involved gyri. For example, it is critical that if the tumor is invading the motor cortex from posteriorly, that you do not approach mistakenly from the anterior side, as you will be adding SMA syndrome or a dysfunctioning PMA system to the problem list. Similarly, a posterior approach to an anterior tumor, not only destroys the sensory and visual input to motor planning, but also probably crosses the descending motor fibers in the process (▶ Fig. 14.2).

DTI tractography is critical. As stated many times in discussions of thinking in terms of networks, there is no benefit to sparing the motor cortex if you cut the fibers. These can be pushed or infiltrated, and it is not always possible to resolve them in some cases when they are densely involved with the tumor. Equally critical is the fact that the SLF is running underneath the sensorimotor system, and this is the deep boundary of this resection. It is essential to note that you can add neglect or aphasia to a hemiplegic patient by neglecting the SLF in these cases (or by not removing the tumor and letting it destroy these fibers).

Finally, goals matter here and they should drive the surgical decision making. Sometimes patients can regain some function with careful resection, but this is not always the case. While we do not wish to be nihilistic, we should also be realistic, and try to put everyone in the best situation we can, even if that situation is still bad.

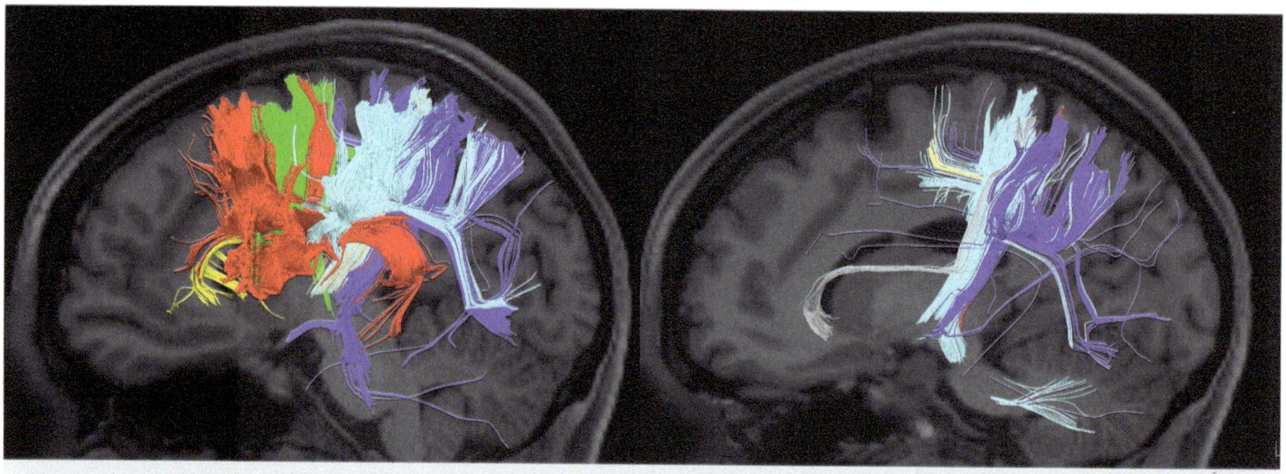

Fig. 14.1 These maps of the lateral and medial motor system are presented to emphasize the rostro-caudal nature of the motor networks. The cortical aspects of this network are box like and together the networks form a bouquet at the top of the stem, which are the descending and ascending fibers. Operating around this network means to work in the coronal plane first and foremost to respect this plane of organization.

14.3.3 Executing the Case

Lower Sensorimotor Gliomas

It is at first, important to note that sensorimotor cases of the inferior (opercular) third are substantially simpler than removing tumors from the other parts of the motor and sensory cortices. Not only are the face and mouth bilaterally innervated and compensable, but they do not directly overlie the descending corticospinal fibers the way the hand motor cortex does. Further, the insular cortex gives you a key depth gauge (▶ Fig. 14.3), as it tells you the approximate depth of the SLF, and of the stem of the descending motor fibers (they are just medial to the SLF). Cortical mapping can define the key players in the network, but I tend to be aggressive in these cases, on the assumption that the mouth/face motor and sensory function can be taken unilaterally if absolutely needed, and that speech will be preserved in the long term if the SLF remains intact in the depth (▶ Fig. 14.4).

Lower sensorimotor tumor cases begin with cortical mapping. It is usually best to look for spontaneous movement and sensation, as this is easy to find and useful for interpreting premotor sites. It is important to also look for SLF functions, such as speech or neglect, as they can have contributory sites throughout the area worth noting. Motor planning tasks can also be used to define the network before making a cut.

Once we have made an overall plan, resection of these tumors starts by subpial resection of the involved gyrus. The first goal is to find and preserve all en passage arteries exiting the Sylvian fissure (they are very likely going somewhere important). By resecting the brain around them, you provide slack and allow them to move out of the way. The goal eventually is to remove the opercular tissues to find the Sylvian cleft and follow it until the insula is visible, as this is the key landmark in these cases.

Once the insula and its orientation is clear, I direct my attention to the superior cut, which is the key step in the operation. This is made across the gyrus in the sagittal plane as you are disconnecting the tumor from the rest of the sensory and/or motor strip. It is important to make this cut aggressive and square with the initial axial trajectory (in other words, to not try to shortcut towards the insula too quickly); however, you must realize that this is the dangerous cut which risks injury to the SLF and motor fibers, and thus functional considerations will often push you off your geometrically ideal path.

At this point, I skeletonize the anterior and posterior pial boundaries of the involved gyri (it is rarely more than one or two gyri in this region), and join all of the cuts along the deep boundary of the tumor just lateral to the sagittal plane of the insula. By removing this piece, I can get a clear view of the deep margin without opercular brain in the way. I then slowly advance the deep boundary in all directions as far as motor and/or SLF functions will allow me to do. It is important that if the tasks don't overlap (i.e., a hand task to test neglect on the right overlaps both major tracts whereas speech and hand function are less overlapping) that you rotate tasks often so you are not missing something. The insula serves as a critical landmark to remain aware of the SLF and its position.

14.4 Case Examples

▶ Fig. 14.5 demonstrates a simple lower motor cortex low grade glioma, and this was removed without deficit as the mapping demonstrated reorganization of the face motor function superiorly in the motor strip.

a) By tracing out the right angle (superior frontal sulcus and precentral sulcus) and using the "hand knob:" as land mark, we can follow this tumor down to see that this tumor is mainly located in the face/tongue motor cortex. The critical thing to note here is on the coronal images which show the tumor following U-fibers into the superior insula at the circular sulcus. We need to take the cut into the motor strip as far superiorly as possible based on mapping to address the top of these U-fibers, and to see the circular sulcus clearly. The insula will serve as the depth gauge as well, so we need to know where it is.

b) None.

c) None.

d) The face motor was at the top of this cut (best seen on coronal images). This cut has drifted down inferiorly and underestimates its height. We did not feel we needed to sacrifice ipsilateral face motor in this case to get a good resection

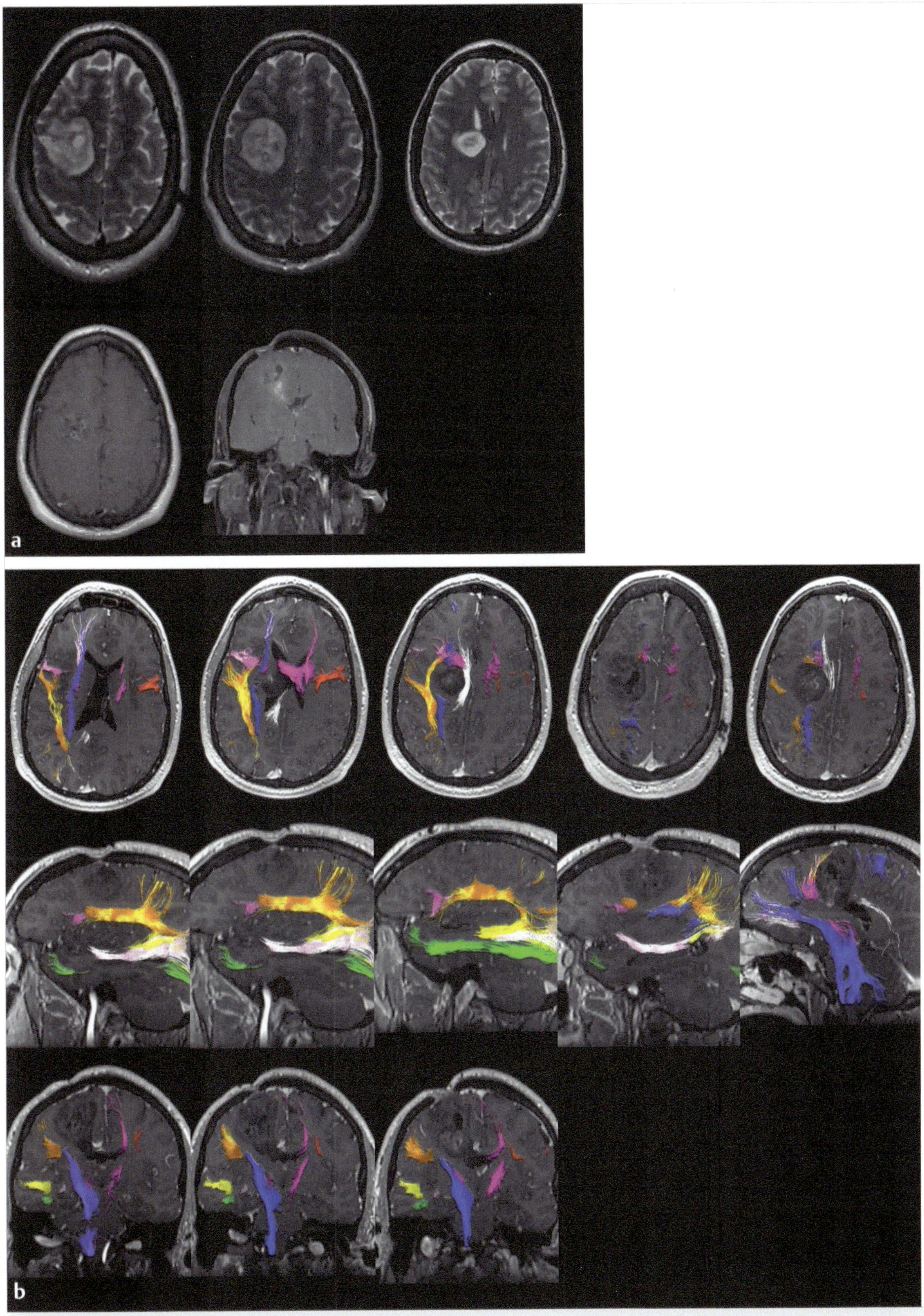

Fig. 14.2 This case depicts the importance of approaching a sensorimotor glioma from the correct side. This is a remarkable glioma which splits the SMA and motor cortex. As seen from the images, the tumor was able to be completely removed without neurologic deficit by respecting the networks, but this is in large part due to carefully studying the network organization prior to surgery; (**a**) preoperative images, (**b**) DTI tractography. (*Continued*)

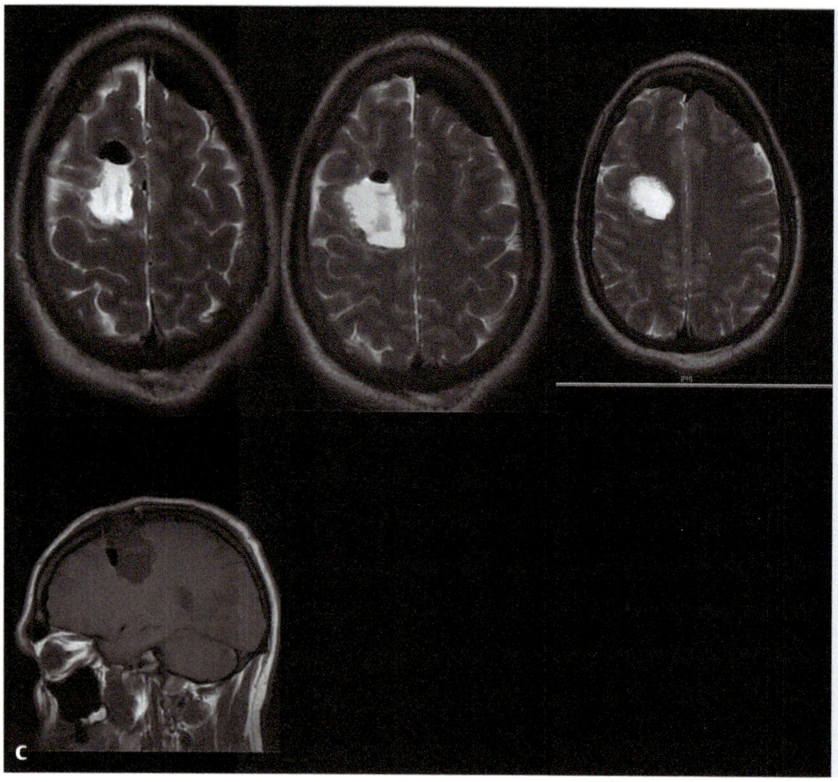

Fig 14.2 (*Continued*) (**c**) Postoperative images.

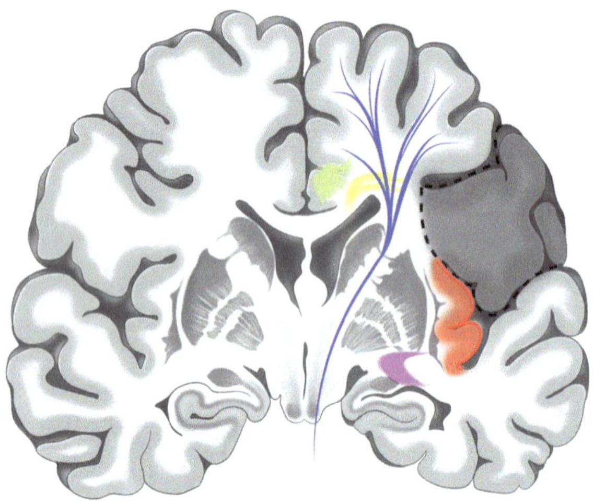

Fig. 14.3 The insula provides a helpful guide as to the depth of critical brain structures such as the descending motor network, and the SLF. In many lower sensorimotor gliomas (and TPO junction tumors discussed later), knowing the position of the insula can help keep you oriented in an otherwise featureless brain area.

▸ Fig. 14.6 demonstrates a lower sensory strip GBM.

a) At a glance, this may seem like a motor area tumor, but careful evaluation of the T2 suggests that it is in the sensory strip, and is pushing the motor strip slightly anteriorly. This enhancing part of this tumor was able to be completely removed.

b) The pre- and post-resection images demonstrate the depth of this resection, and how distorted sulci can be shortly after opening. A low lying biopsy site can be visualized and this was made after motor mapping, under the microscope to ensure that the opercular arteries were not injured.

c) As is typical for these tumors, the SLF and motor fibers are running along the deep border of these tumors. Looking at the coronal image, will reinforce the need to use the insula as a depth gauge in lateral sensorimotor tumors, the SLF and motor fibers really are never lateral to the insular surface.

d) There is some T2 change left in the more superior sensorimotor cortex, but in a case like this, this is a satisfying result, especially given that the patient was intact afterwards.

▸ Fig. 14.7 is the remarkable case of an extensive low grade glioma filling the lower third of the motor and sensory strips, and the posterior IFG. Surprisingly, the entire cortical surface had no function in it, and we were able to resect the tumor until encountering the SLF running deep to the cortical surface which we left tumor in. The patient had no neurologic problems with this surgery despite an aggressive resection of the tumor.

a) This is a very extensive tumor in the motor and sensory regions as well as threatening the speech networks. The greatest risk is the depth of this tumor, which extends nearly to the ventricle. Note that this tumor seems to have a denser area (which is reasonable to expect might be noninfiltrative), and a less dense area (more likely to be infiltrative). We should be very concerned about the lateral part given its proximity to critical tracts.

b) None.

c) Not surprisingly, the SLF and motor are plastered on the deep surface of this tumor. Simply put, they have nowhere else to go. What is encouraging is that the frontal, parietal, and

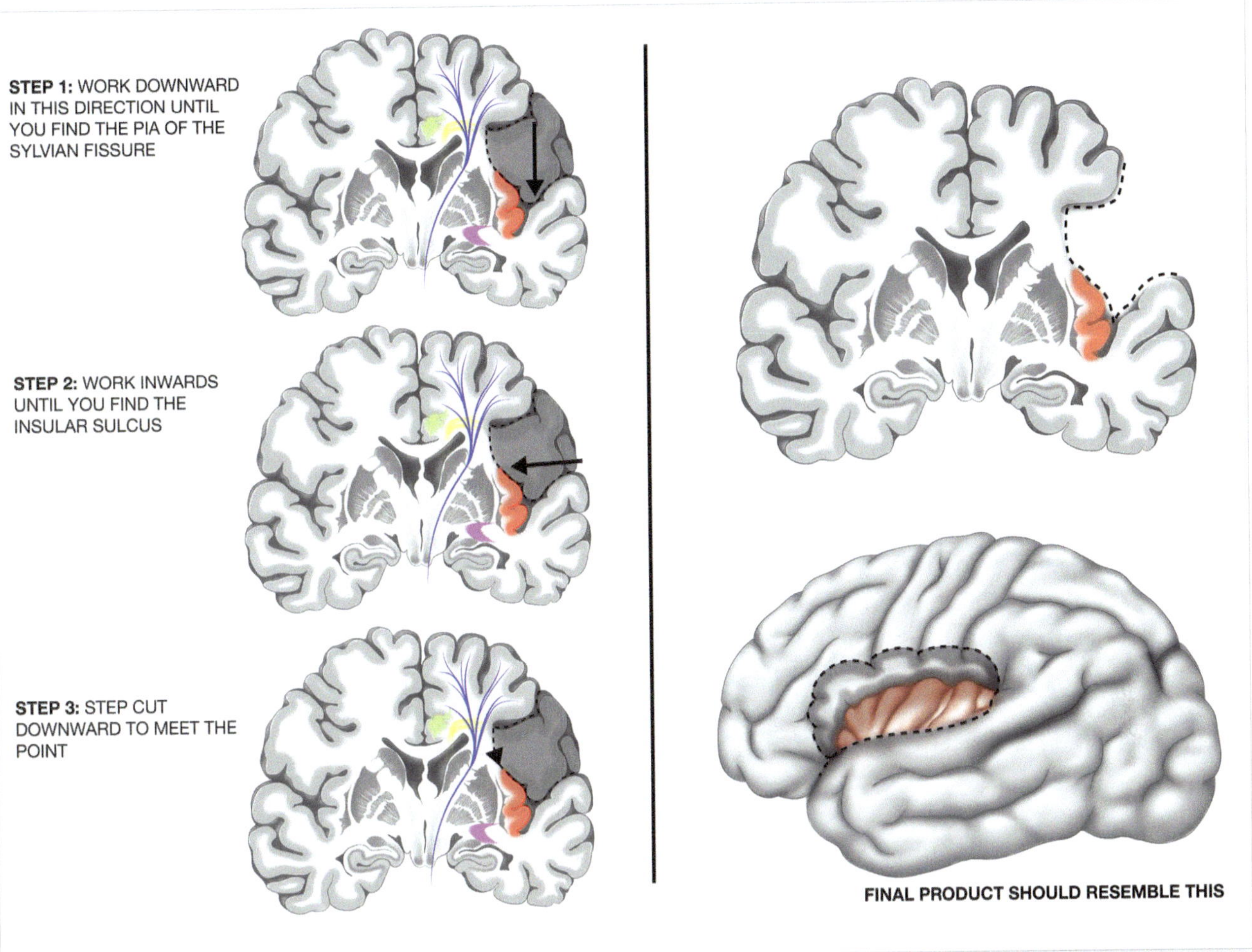

Fig. 14.4 These images demonstrate the technique of resecting a lower sensorimotor glioma. After mapping the cortex, the first step is to subpially remove the opercular cortex down to the Sylvian fissure. This helps you find the insula. The final, key step is to make the dangerous superior cut, continuing as aggressively as possible based on the mapping. Once this reaches the depth of the insula, it curves inferiorly to join the insula, which minimizes the chance of entering the SLF or the descending motor fibers.

temporal SLF ramus, and the FAT do not seem to run through it, but rather around it. Remember that we cannot assume that there are no areas in this tumor which feed to it, DTIs are not that accurate presently and you shouldn't follow it off a cliff. Tractography shows you bus routes, not all the stops. But it is promising, and should be studied with the possibility that this tumor can be aggressively removed.

d) The amount of reorganization in this case was remarkable, and an aggressive resection was possible with no neurologic sequelae. In this case, we left a rind of tumor in the SLF but otherwise the involved brain was nonfunctional.

14.4.1 Middle and Medial Sensorimotor Gliomas (▶ Fig. 14.8, ▶ Fig. 14.9, ▶ Fig. 14.10)

These are a much bigger problem. They clearly overlie the descending motor fibers, and the SLF is underneath these areas throughout their length. Further, hand and leg function is rarely compensable from the other side with motor cortex injuries. Interestingly, these features render the resection schematically simple: it is a box or circular resection, involving whatever is possible based on the map, with the SLF at the deep margin. You should assume you are surrounded on all sides even if the initial cortical map suggests otherwise. A few points follow:

1. Often, both leg and arm functions are at risk (▶ Fig. 14.8). You should switch often during the resection to make sure you are monitoring both. If you do both at the same time, you are probably not going to get the patient to double task and name at the same time which reduces the sensitivity (it doesn't stress both systems).
2. Cortical mapping and DTIs can often give you an idea if the tracts are still anatomically connected, and if so where they lie. They may not work, especially if the SMA or premotor areas are destroyed, but it gives you some idea which direction (anterior or posterior) is the best to approach from.
3. If it is unclear which side to approach from, the parietal side is usually better if possible, as it maintains the motor planning areas and their connection to the motor strip, providing some hope of recovery, especially if resection can be achieved from the superior parietal lobule. Sometimes a longer path in which parallels the SLF is better than going

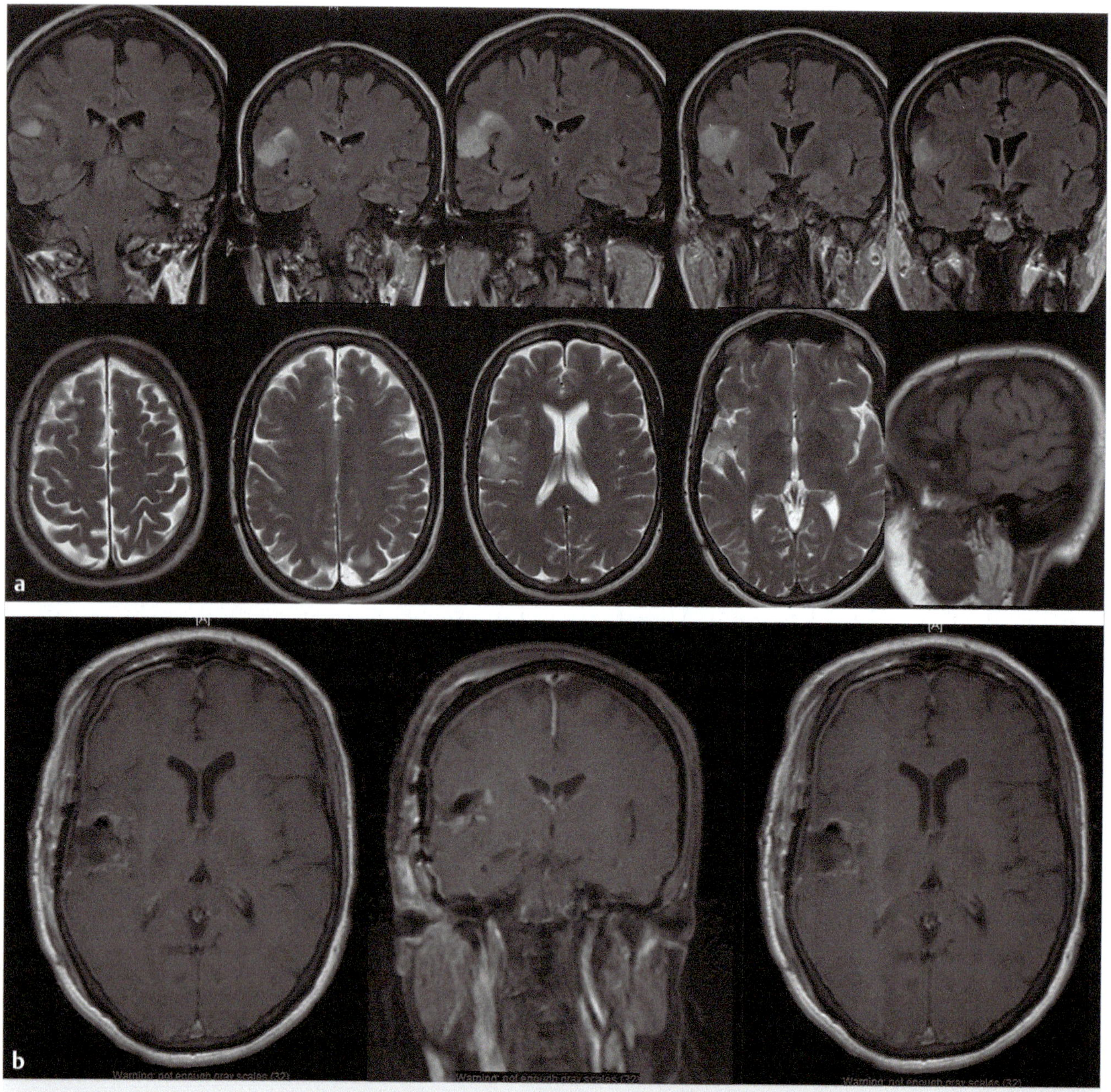

Fig. 14.5 Demonstrates a simple lower motor cortex low grade glioma, and this was removed without deficit as the mapping demonstrated reorganization of the face motor function superiorly in the motor strip; (**a**) preoperative images; (**b**) postoperative images.

directly through the motor cortex. Sometimes a small path into the motor cortex is the right way.

4. While it may be flashy to use a transsulcal approach to access these tumors, remember that these are not metastatic tumors or cavernomas, and not only are some of these approaches awkward, but they are incorrect for minimizing damage to the motor system. The central and intraparietal sulci are not aneural fissures, but instead are cortex and white matter which are parts of eloquent networks of brain function. As I have repeatedly expressed, gliomas are a unique disease, and often a smart route through the brain is better than a slick route which avoids transgressing the brain but provides poor or disorienting angles, or bad functional preservation options.
5. Remember that the SLF is running in the deep margin of this resection.
6. Do not follow tumors in the motor areas into the corpus callosum. They will probably need as much information from the other side as possible.
7. If you can preserve the FAT and motor planning networks you provide the hope for some return of function, especially for tumors limited to a modest part of the motor cortex.

14.5 Case Examples

▶ Fig. 14.11 shows a prototypic anterior approach to a medial premotor glioma. The degree of enhancement underestimates

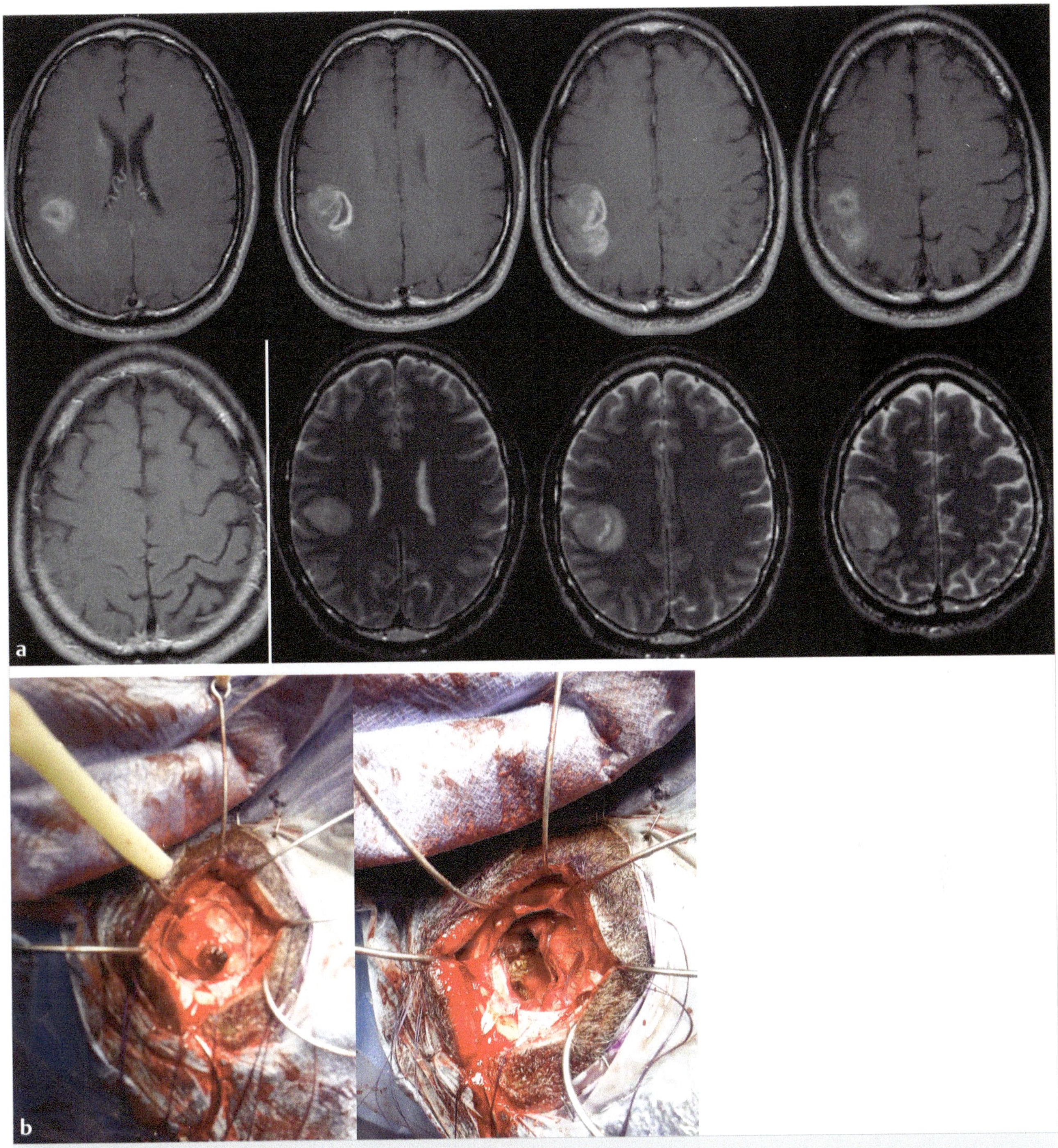

Fig. 14.6 Demonstrates a lower sensory strip GBM; (**a**) preoperative images, (**b**) images of the approach.

this avastin treated tumor. Note that the cut proceeds vertical and parallels the direction of the sensorimotor system as allowed by the mapping.

a) The preoperative image, as usual in these cases, is complex, and defining goals is critical in a case like this. The enhancement begins in the SMA, and appears to follow the descending motor fibers towards the basal ganglia. This is unfortunately not the only time I have seen this ominous pattern of spread. The T2 changes are extensive and fill much of the premotor and SMA regions. The goal was to make a posterior frontal type disconnection as best possible given the functional anatomy, and to perform a large anatomic resection of as much of the T2 change as possible. Of note, the patient had significant preoperative weakness from this tumor, but was not hemiplegic, being weaker in the leg than the arm. Our goal is to try to save whatever function we can in this case, recognizing that without an aggressive turn of events, his motor prognosis is poor.

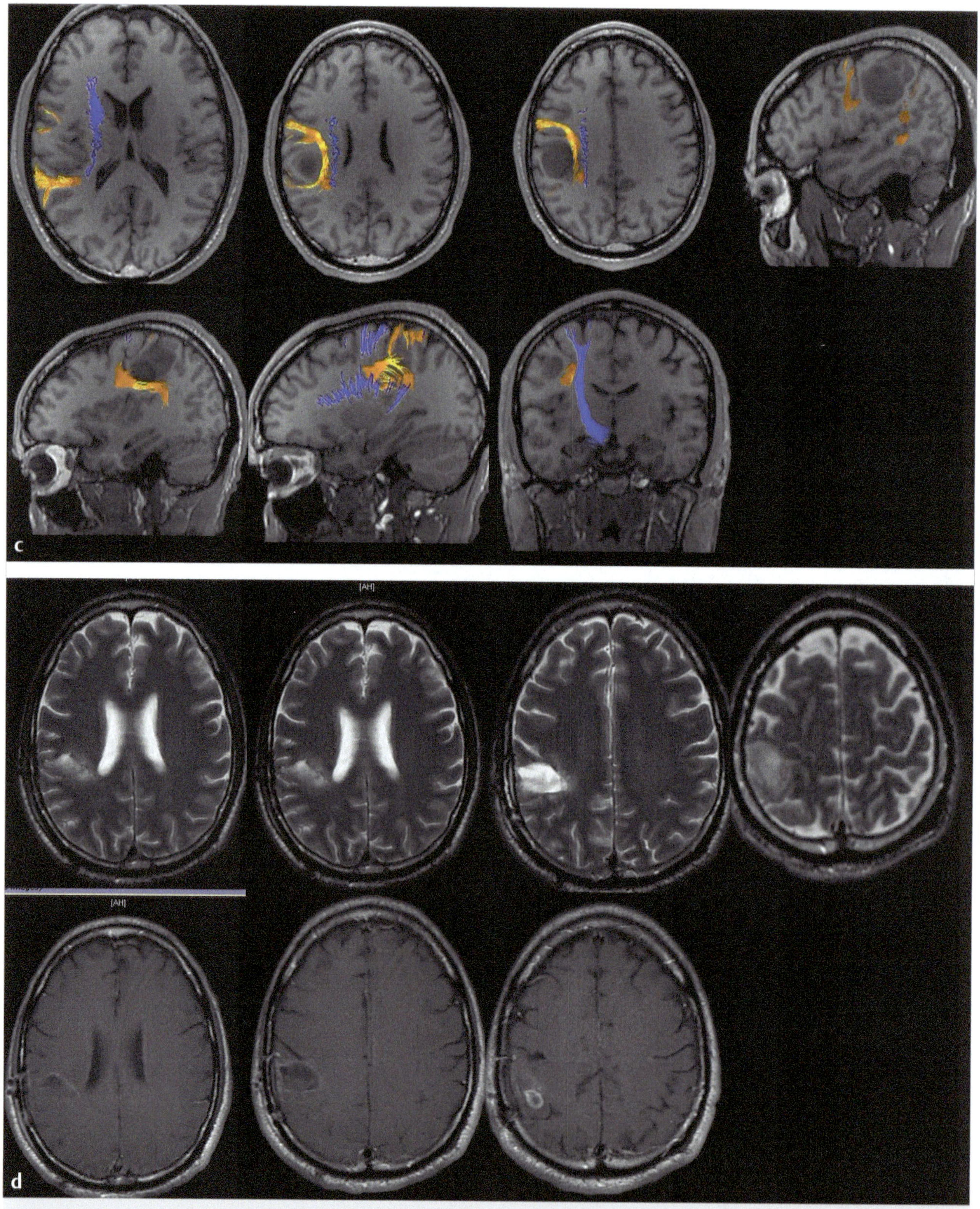

Fig 14.6 (*Continued*) (**c**) DTI tractography, (**d**) postoperative images.

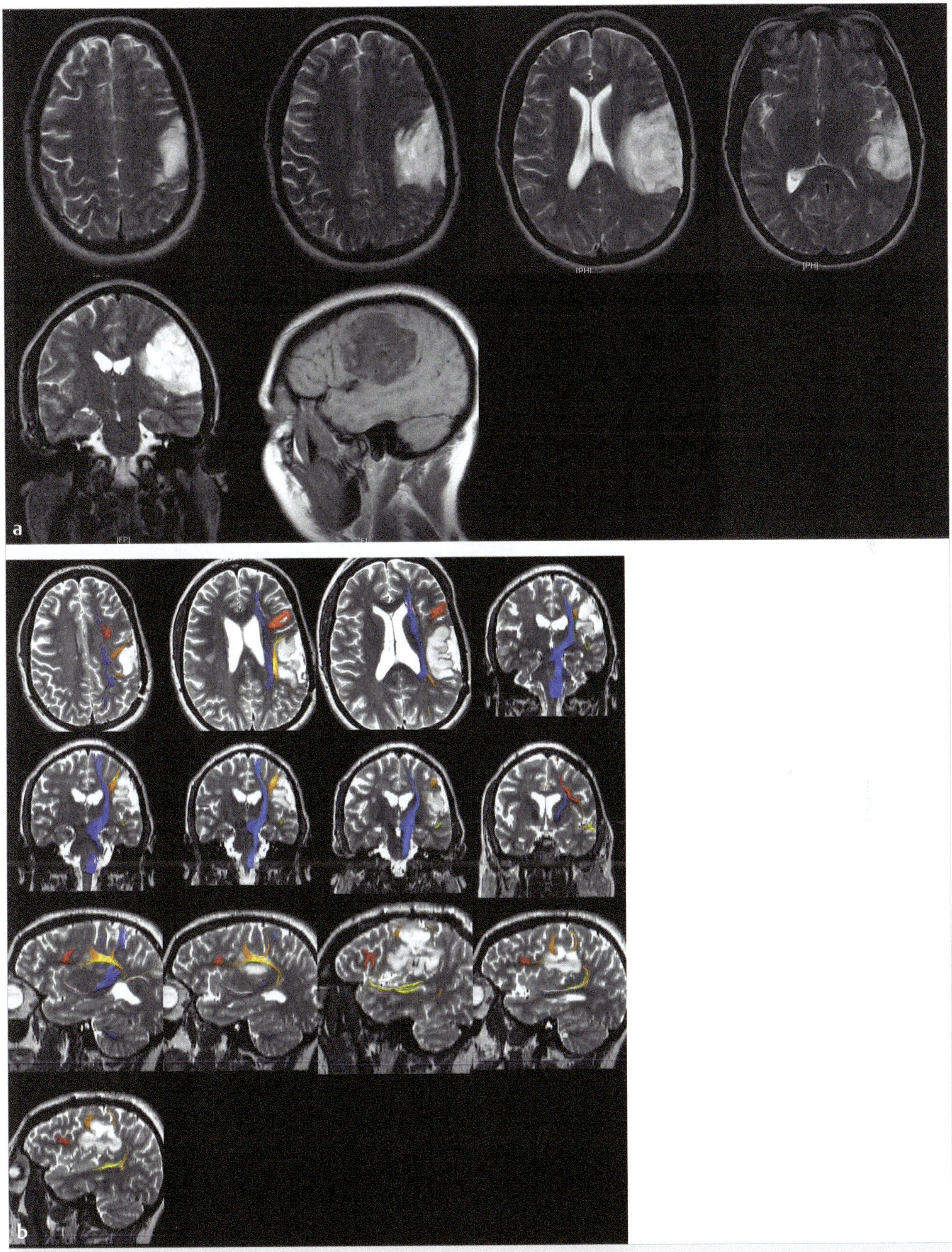

Fig. 14.7 Extensive low-grade glioma filling the lower third of the motor and sensory strips, and the posterior IFG; (**a**) preoperative images, (**b**) DTI tractography. (*Continued*)

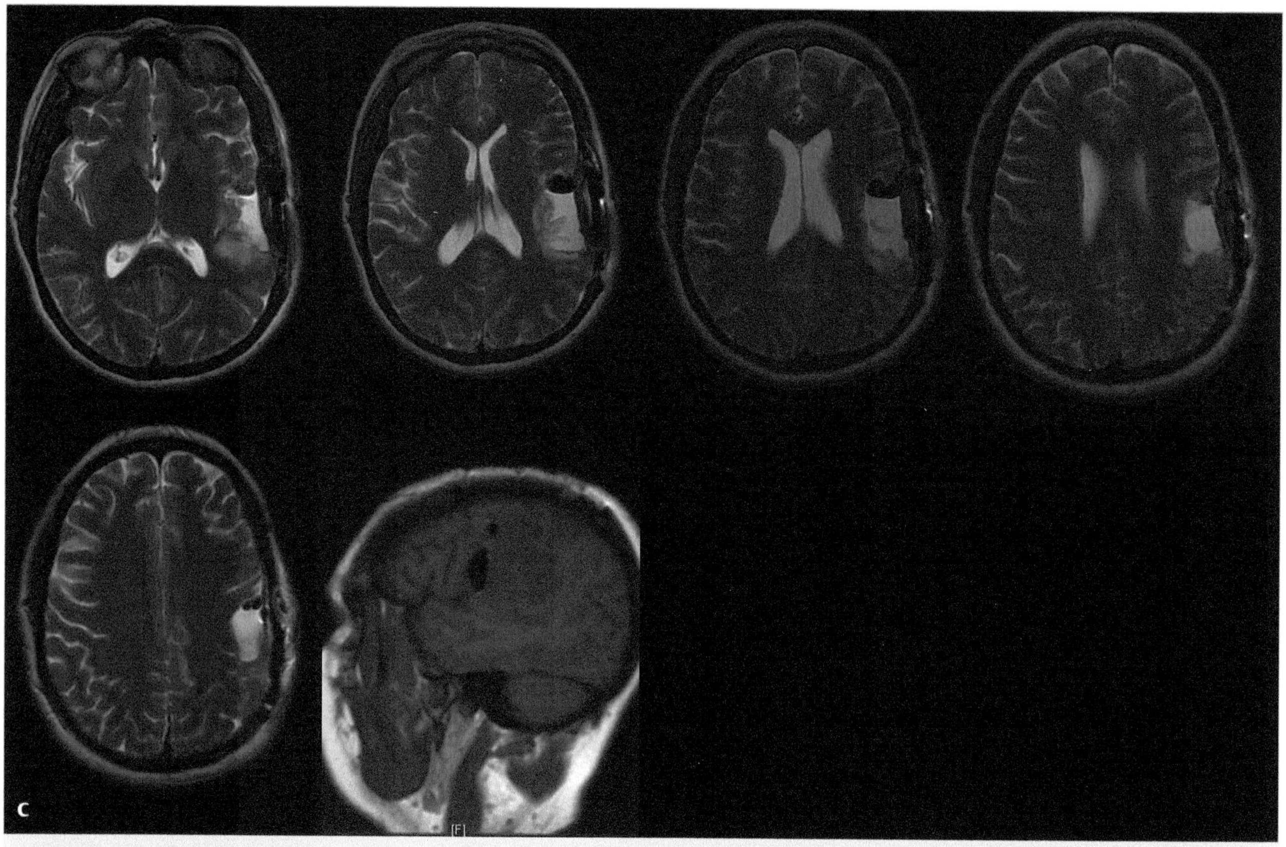

Fig 14.7 *(Continued)* (**c**) Postoperative images.

b) The incision follows a previous open biopsy incision and parallels the cuts. Note in the post-resection images that this cut is quite irregular and complex, and this is due to the need to define appropriate safe paths to cut parallel to the motor planning system, which can be quite complex in the coronal plane. Slow detailed subcortical dissection is critical in these cases.
c) The DTIs quickly reveal the nature of his motor problems. The FAT no longer enters the SMA and this has likely been disrupted by the tumor or the biopsy, or at least it is hard to visualize on the tractography. The motor system is splayed outward around the tumor and contibutions to the corticospinal tract are pushed quite far anteriorly. There are almost certainly connections that we do not see in this tumor due to edema. An additional noteworthy feature is the fact that at first glance it seems to be crossing the midline, but in fact this is simply an enlargement of the midline frontal lobe herniating under the falx. The coronal images demonstrate that the callosum is largely uninvolved but is merely pushed by the tumor bulk.

This patient on presentation has a kind of zoned-out affect, which I have seen many later staged GBM patients look like (this man came to us for a second opinion 6 months after completing radiotherapy elsewhere, when he was quite a bit worse than initial presentation). By this I mean he is responsive, conversant, able to follow commands, etc., but he is not driving the conversation mainly, he is passive. I think this happens for a lot of reasons, including fatigue, but in his case I suspect much of it stems from compromise of the DMN and cingulate seen in this image.

a) The resection is aggressive, and we did not make him any worse; however, he had a marginal recurrence in about 3 months and by this point his poor functional status made all of us decide not to treat him further. One thing this case highlights the need to get these tumors under control if at all possible, as early as possible. It is much easier to manage a patient through subsequent treatments when they haven't been accumulating edema and steroid toxicity for many months prior to starting an aggressive strategy. I try to aggressively treat all with gliomas that seek my help and understand the risks, but it is beyond question that it is much more fulfilling when we get to them early and treat them aggressively from the start.

▶ Fig. 14.12 demonstrates a case of a patient who presented hemiplegic from this GBM straddling the motor strip and SMA. Despite his inability to participate with motor tasks, we used direct stimulation to identify and preserve motor cortices and descending motor fibers, while resecting the enhancing portion of the tumor. His function improved to 4/5 the following day, but we could only preserve motor function in him for about 6 months before the tumor destroyed it.
a) As usual, the enhancing part of the tumor underestimates the T2 changes, and much of the T2 change is in the motor strip and not worth going after. The degree of T2 change is less than the previous case though, and given the more posterior location, we decided that a lesionectomy was all we should try, as an anterior resection would be in the SMA and not really be in the T2 areas.

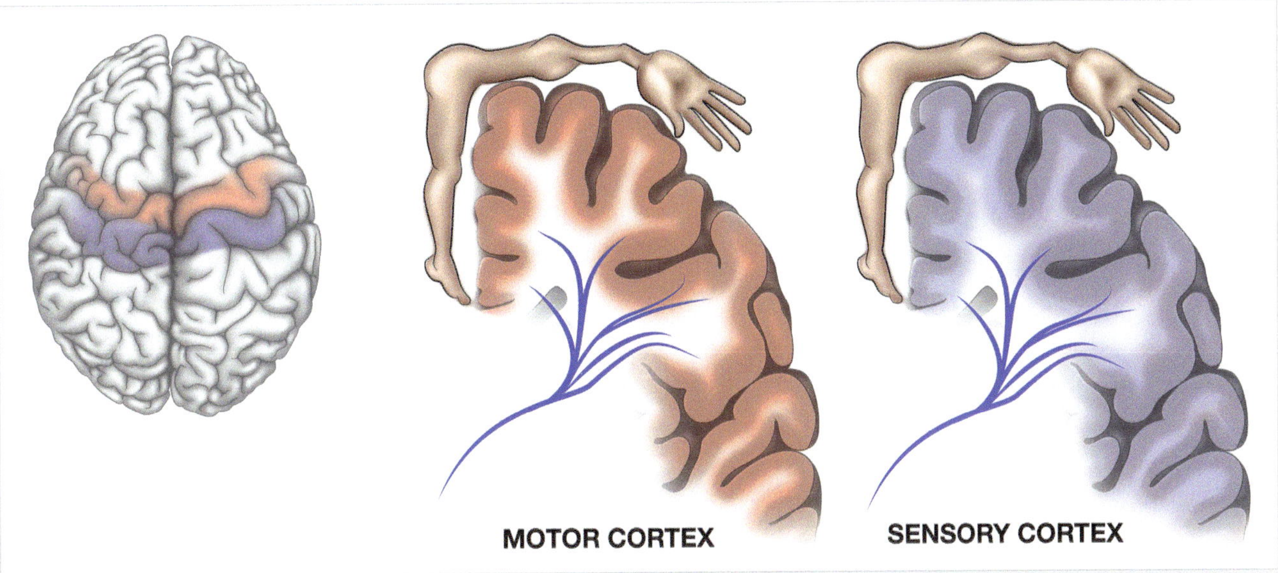

Fig. 14.8 This diagram demonstrates that in many medial or middle sensorimotor gliomas, both arm and leg can be at risk, and you need to change frequently between these two tasks during the mapping.

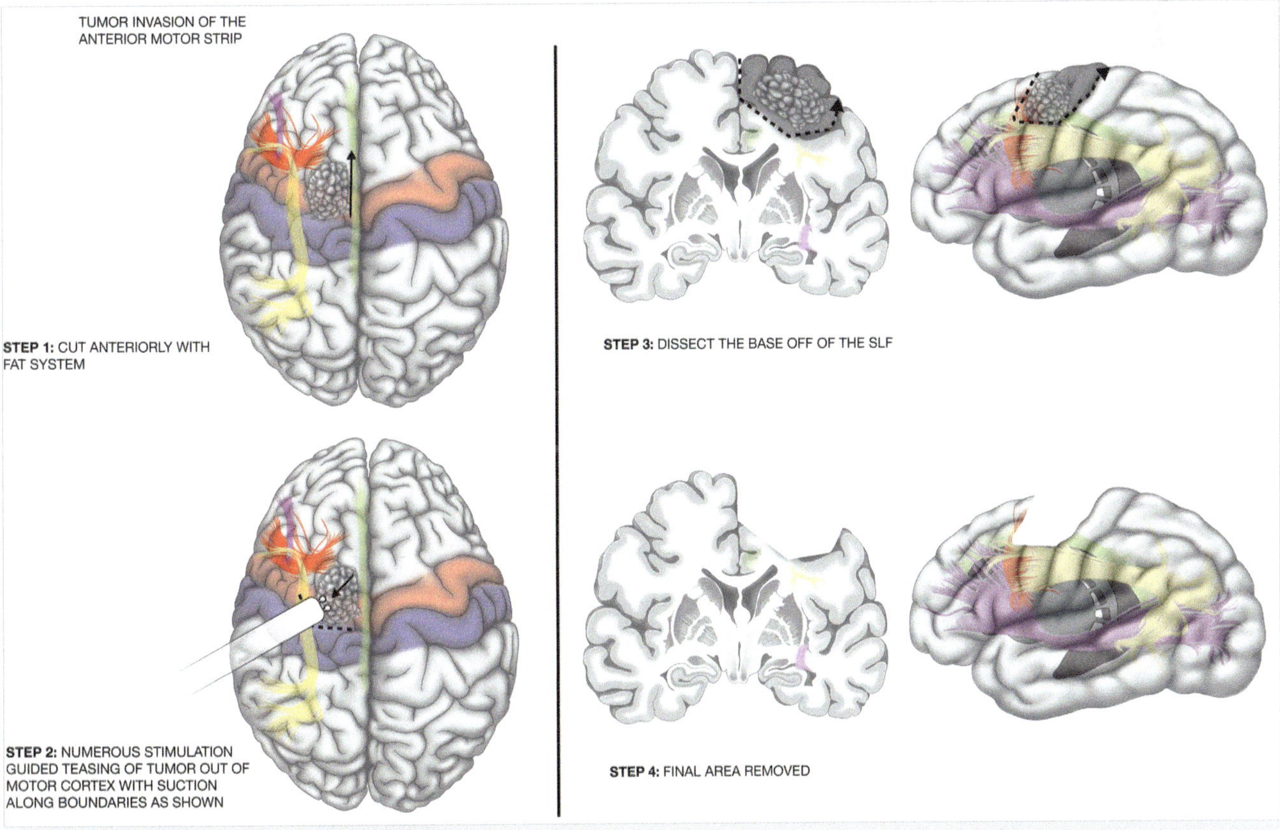

Fig. 14.9 This diagram demonstrates the steps of resecting a middle/medial sensorimotor glioma from an anterior approach. The key steps are to identify the motor planning areas and motor regions, and to work slowly to approach them and teach tumor from them. Once this back cut is complete, the inferior cut is with the SLF to scoop this tumor from its deep border.

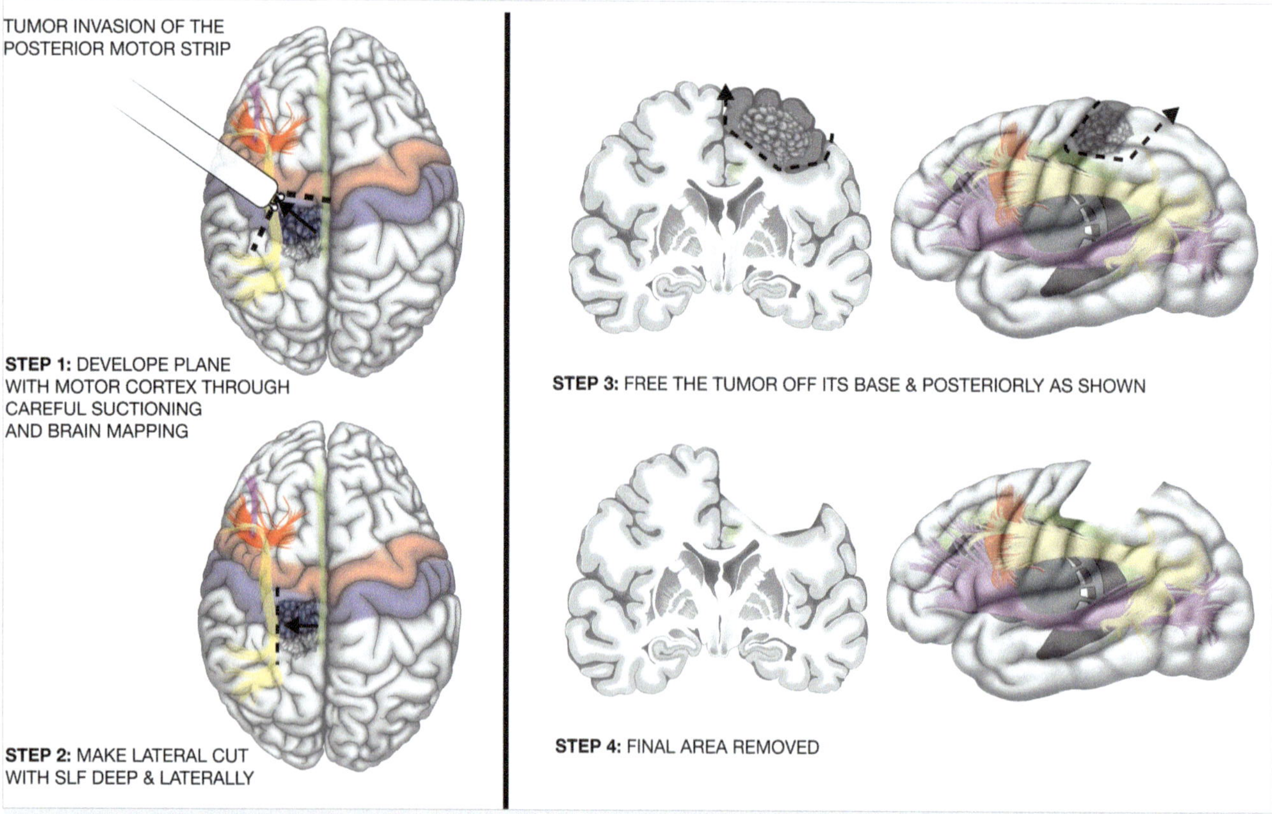

Fig. 14.10 This diagram demonstrates removing a medial/middle sensorimotor glioma from a posterior approach. The key consideration in this area is sensory input to the extremities, and this should be monitored as you work anteriorly.

b) The incision looks similar to the previous case as it had been similarly resected. The tumor was clearly visible upon opening the dura, and the markers demonstrate areas where we were able to stimulate motor responses with a cortical stimulator. We used this technique to define boundaries and primarily resected abnormally appearing areas.
c) The DTI shows an interesting pattern: the tumor lies between the SMA and FAT complex, and the motor strip. The fact that he regained his function following a lesionectomy argues that the key communications between the motor strip and SMA are not through the U-fibers.
d) The resection is limited to the enhancing region but with that as the goal this scan looks good.

▸ Fig. 14.13 demonstrates the case of a premotor glioblastoma operated at another facility who suffered hemiplegia immediately after the resection which only improved to 0/5 in the arm and 3/5 in the leg. Examination of the DTIs demonstrated that although the entry point selected was anterior, the resection drifted in the subcortical white matter entering the descending motor tracts. We were able to preserve his remaining function at the repeat surgery with our standard techniques.
a) There are a number of points to be made with these images. First, note that the enhancement is mainly in the premotor areas with extension into the deep white matter. I speculated that the tumor may be following the premotor communication with the basal ganglia (see Fig. 6.4 for an example of this). The main epicenter is in the inferior frontal gyrus and operculum. Second, there is the common issue with defining what is tumor and what is treatment effect in these cases. As always, I try to work a margin around the tumor as much as I can under the assumption that there almost always are tumor cells in this T2 change around the tumor, and by taking it out, if functionally possible, I am reducing tumor burden to its lowest reasonable amount.

Finally, the cortical entry path for the previous resection starts relatively premotor, and in a traditional view of the brain where cortex comes first, this should be good enough to avoid motor problems. But careful examination clearly demonstrates that the resection continues medial and inferior into the motor network and even into the basal ganglia, which were plausibly mistaken for tumor (the tissue looks so similar that if you are not relatively certain where you are and that you might be near it, your mind will not connect the fact that you are in the basal ganglia). This is easy to do if the patient is asleep for the subcortical portion, or if your subcortical angles are off. The surprising part wasn't that there were motor problems in a case with a "safe" anterior entry point, it was that it improved at all.
a) In the left panel, the cortical mapping has been completed. In this picture, the right Sylvian fissure is at 12 o'clock in the image and is a bit under the bone flap. The gyri are clearly enlarged and distorted. The two small anterior sites indicate premotor sites, where we found negative motor events (i.e., freezing) which in this setting represent probable motor planning areas. The more posterior marker indicates positive motor sites for the face found in the anatomic location of the motor strip. Following this, we performed a complex version

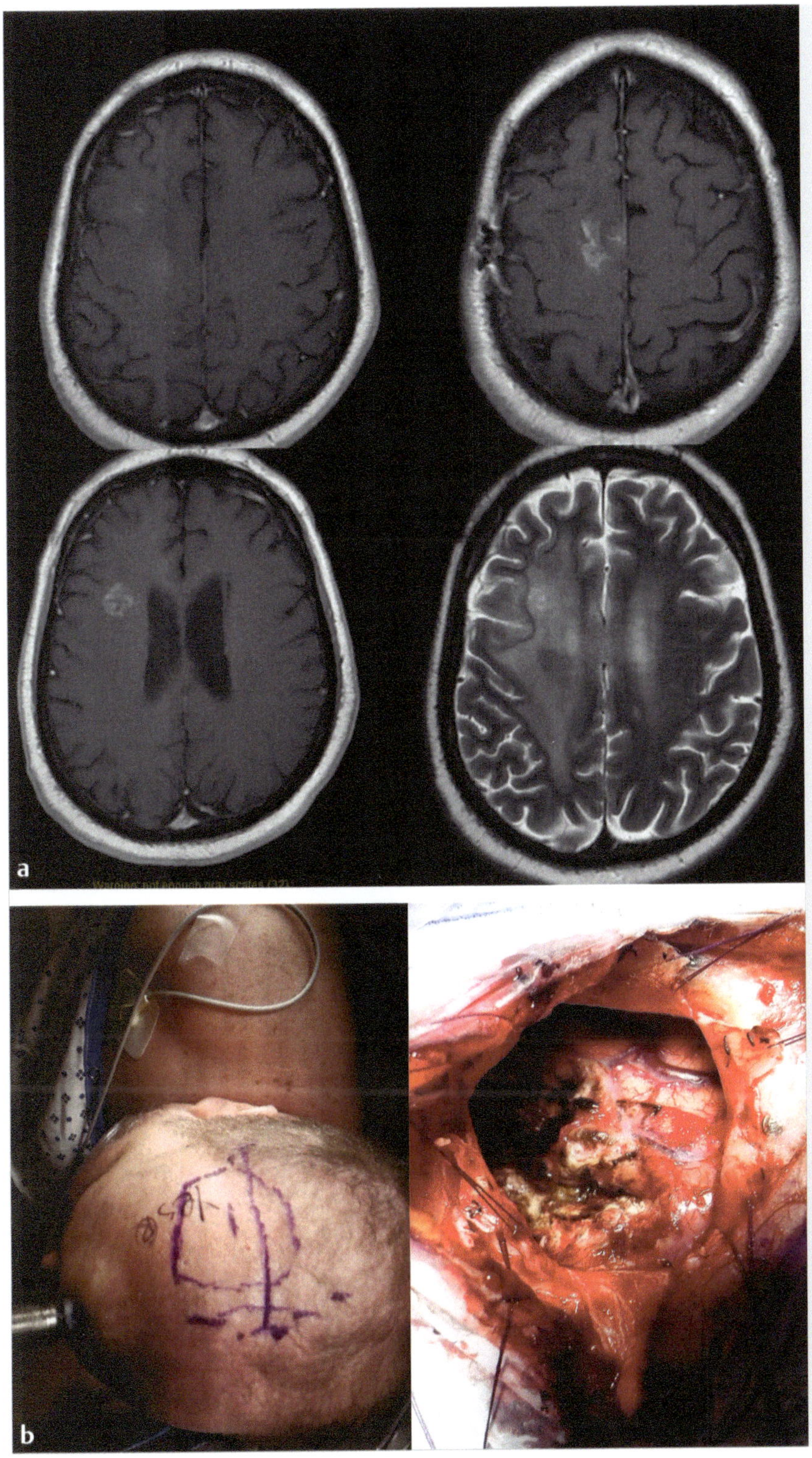

Fig. 14.11 Prototypic anterior approach to a medial premotor glioma; (**a**) preoperative images, (**b**) images of the approach. (*Continued*)

of a lateral frontal disconnection. This had to account for the fact that the FAT is running on the medial (i.e., deep to us) surface of the tumor, and may or may not be participating in this patient's motor function. It has to parallel these sites in the coronal plane to respect the coronal orientation of the motor system. It has to extend deep to the insular level, but should preserve the IFOF. Regardless, the steps are ultimately the same: subpialize the operculum and find the insula for orientation, protect the arteries, make the cut with the premotor areas ensuring that the cut remains oriented roughly parallel with the sulcal orientation, make the superior cut and then disconnect the deep boundary to free up and remove the tumor.

b) The DTIs make clear that the SLF and motor fibers have been entered at the previous surgery, especially on the axial images. The FAT has also likely been transected partially as well,

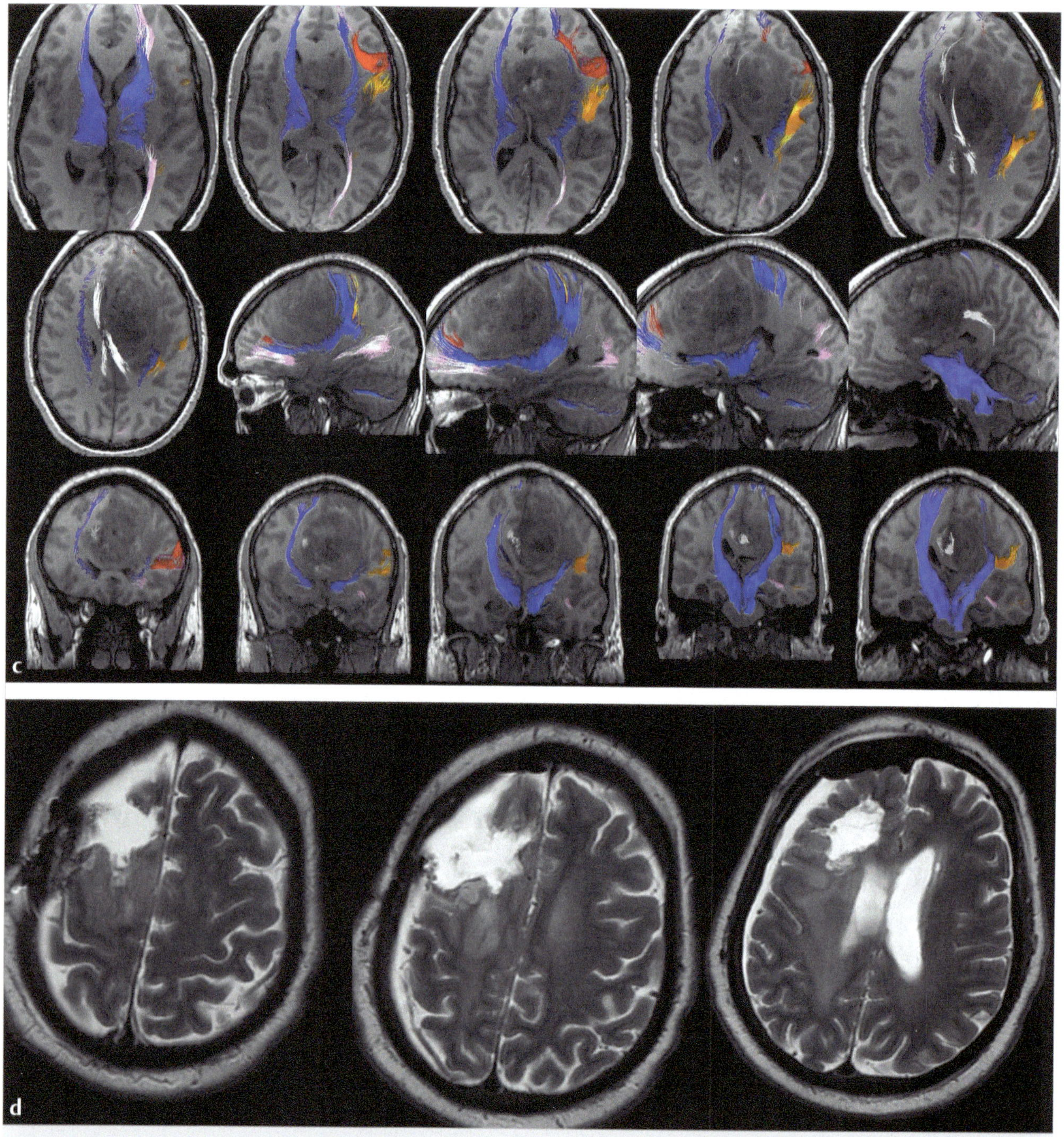

Fig 14.11 (*Continued*) (**c**) DTI tractography, (**d**) postoperative images.

as only a small number of fibers connect the SMA to the premotor areas and the coronal images suggest that the previous resection tract enters them as well. It is always difficult for me to interpret networks of previously injured brains, as it is unclear how they recover, but my working assumption in this case was that the recovery this patient saw resulted from recovering from an SMA type syndrome, and the permanent deficit resulted from the partial transection of the descending motor fibers. I think in this case, working on that assumption, that it is probably wise to try to save whatever FAT and SLF is still remaining, as they may contain some crossed FAT fibers or other mechanism for rewiring this area to allow him to recover spontaneous motor function. I think this may account for the more prominent premotor mapping in this case: in the setting of this injury, more of it may be essential then normal.

c) The resection is aggressive, but it is important to compare the postoperative coronal to the DTI to note how the deep cut tries to conform to the residual FAT. This patient did not lose any additional motor function as a result of this resection.

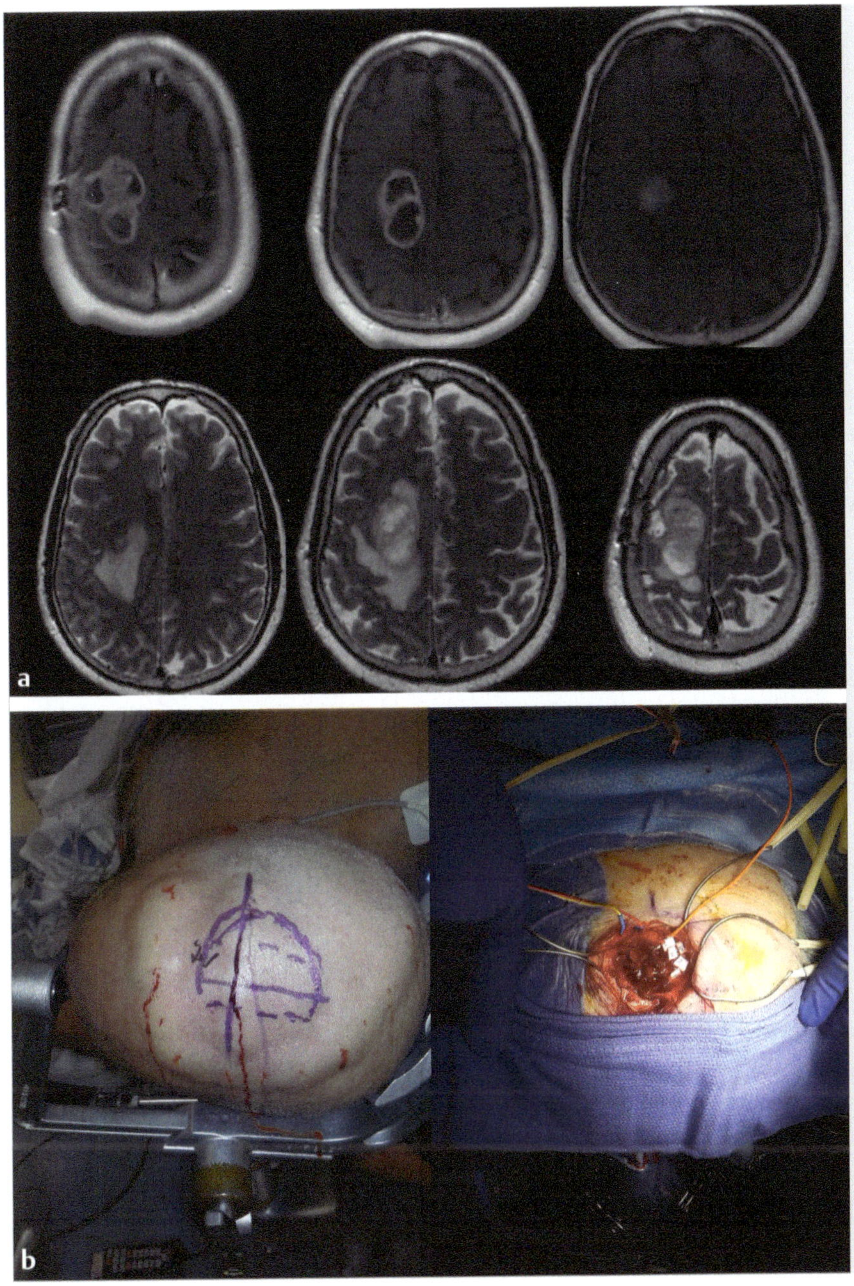

Fig. 14.12 Case of a patient who presented hemiplegic from this GBM straddling the motor strip and SMA; (**a**) preoperative images; (**b**) images of the approach. *(Continued)*

▶ Fig. 14.14 demonstrates a left-sided premotor tumor. Tumors like this add the additional problem of protecting speech, as well as the FAT/crossed FAT, needed to initiate speech.

a) This tumor has undergone a lesionectomy at another facility as seen, and has recurred within 3 months of completing chemoradiation. We are returning to complete the resection and obtain a better margin including the T2 changes in hopes of improving his chance of responding to a new agent.
b) None.
c) The DTIs highlight the complexity of a case like this. First, like previous cases, the tumor splits the SMA/FAT complex and the motor strip, putting both aspects of this system at risk. The SLF is at risk on the deep and lateral parts of this resection. Even the DMN is potentially in play in this case. This will require a lot of work for a small amount of tumor removal.
d) This postoperative scan demonstrates the aggressive resection we achieved. He has some issues initiating speech, but otherwise is high functioning, working full time, and recurrence free at 2 years after this surgery.

14.6 TPO Junction Gliomas

These tumors force you to operate in a part of the brain that makes us uniquely human. Not only are the gyri eloquent (SMG, STG, MTG, angular), but they are complex anatomically. The SMG and angular gyri are c-shaped and fold in a conical fashion with their white matter descending in a spiral hydra like fashion to enter the SLF and IFOF. The relationship with the insula is complex: while these gyri are opercula, the Sylvian fissure is quite shallow at this posterior section, and the untrained eye

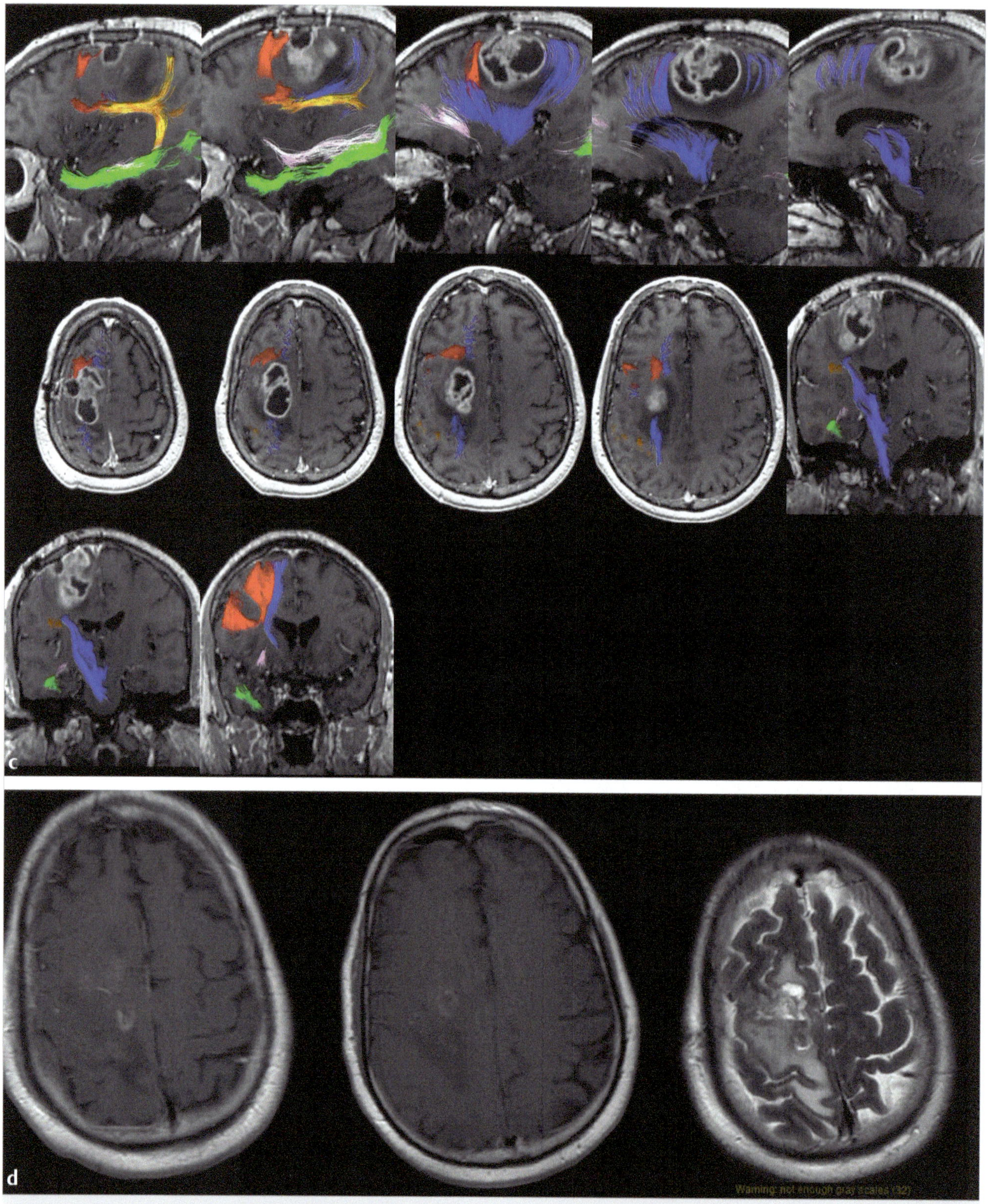

Fig 14.12 (*Continued*) (**c**) DTI tractography, (**d**) postoperative images.

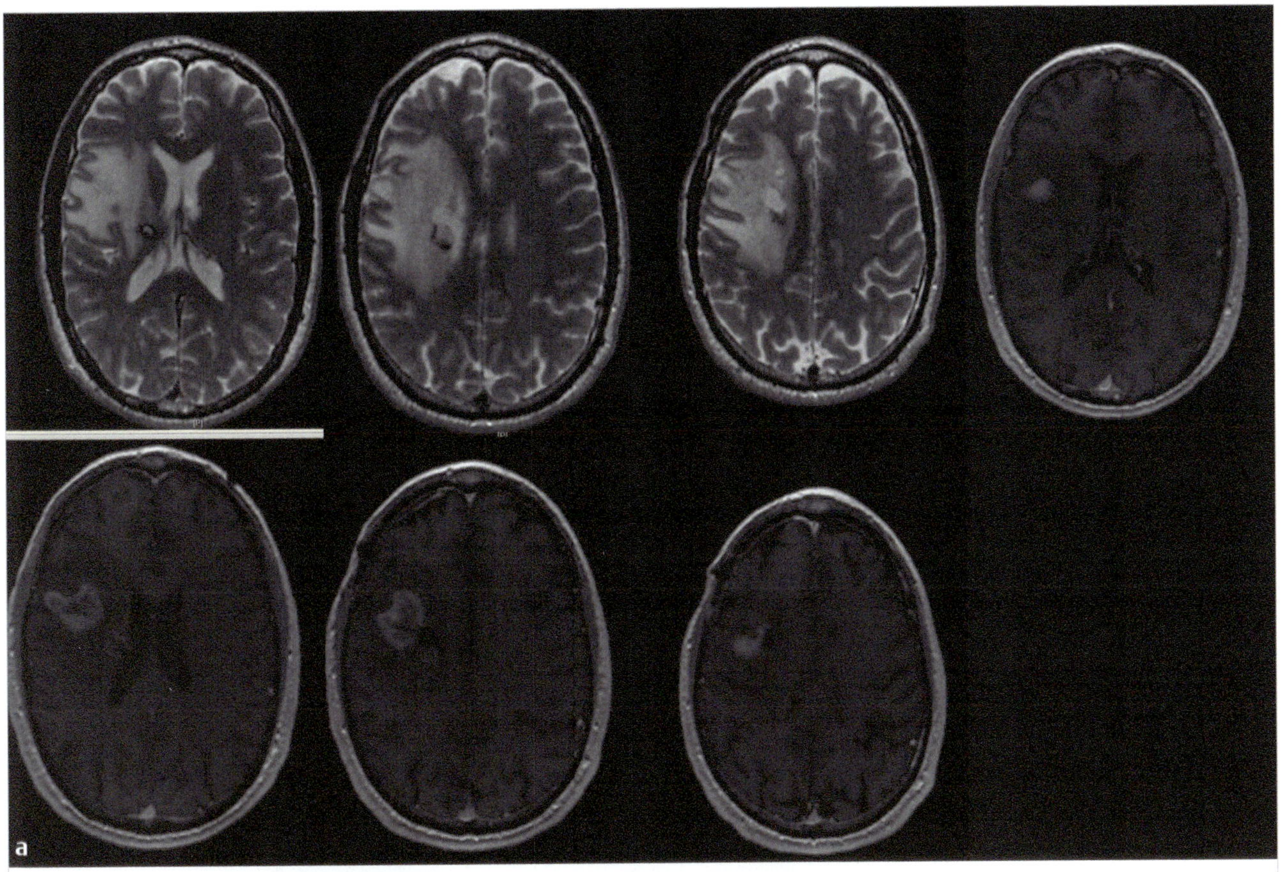

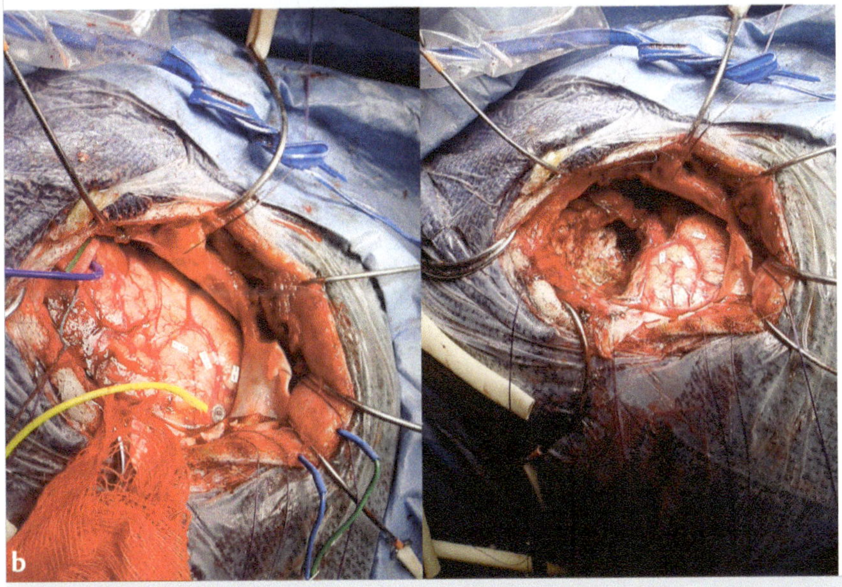

Fig. 14.13 Premotor glioblastoma of a patient operated on at another facility who suffered hemiplegia immediately after the resection which only improved to 0/5 in the arm and 3/5 in the leg; (**a**) preoperative images, (**b**) images of the approach. (*Continued*)

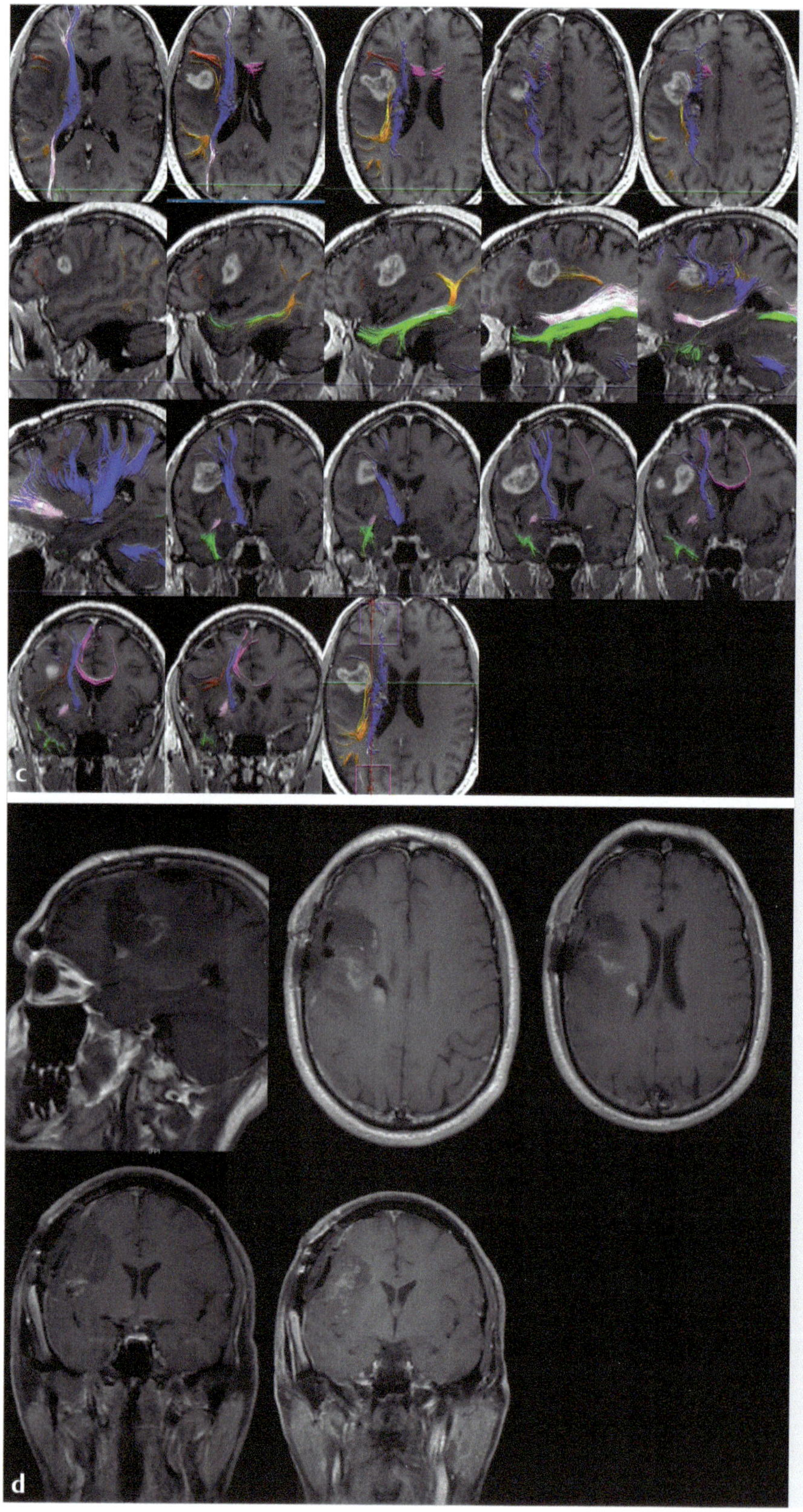

Fig 14.13 (*Continued*) (**c**) DTI tractography, (**d**) postoperative images.

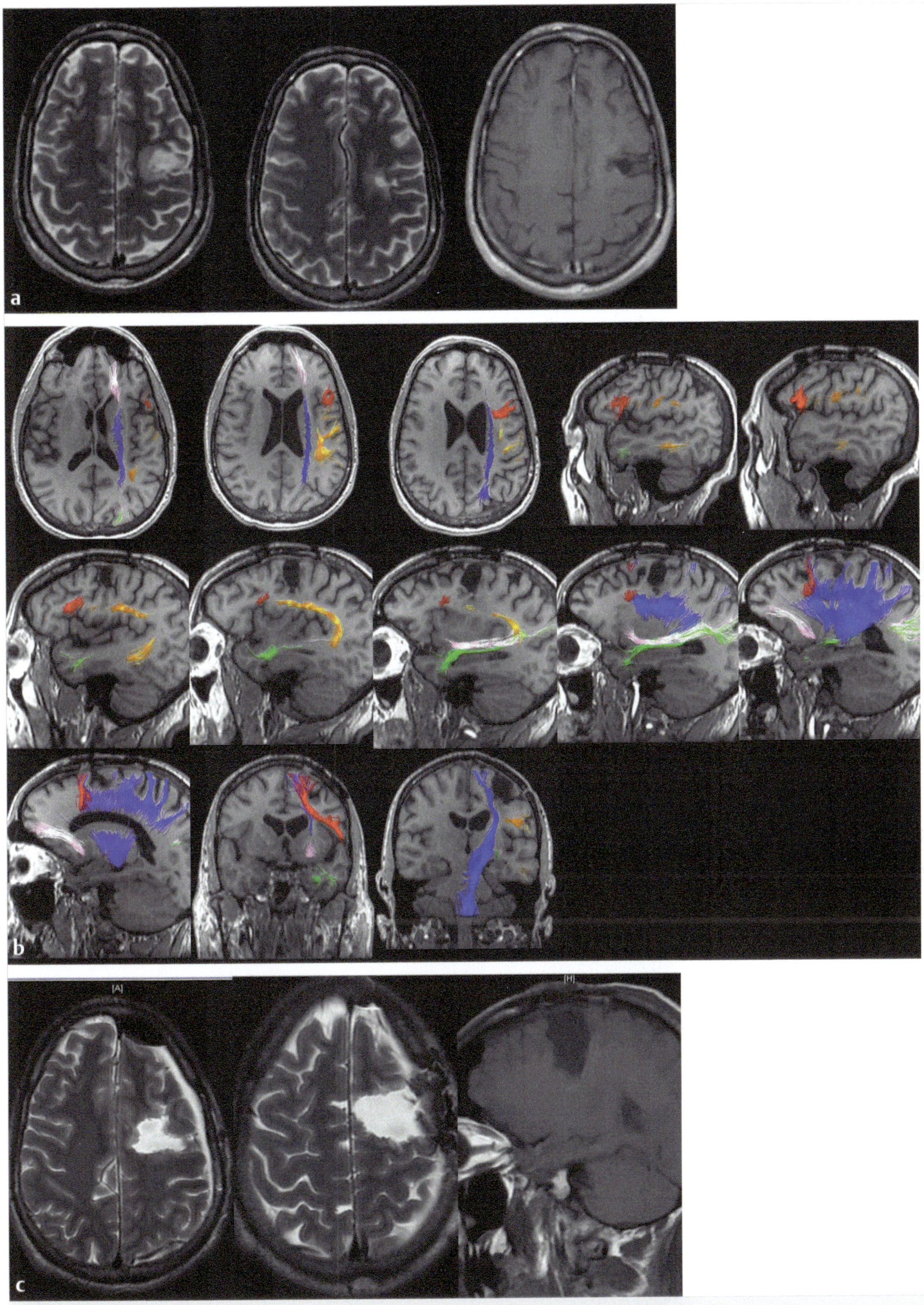

Fig. 14.14 A left-sided premotor tumor; (**a**) preoperative images, (**b**) DTI tractography, (**c**) postoperative images.

can easily miss the boundary between insula and opercula. Finally, nearly every major association fiber tract of the lateral system (SLF, IFOF, optic radiations, MdLF, posterior thalamic peduncle, not to mention the basal ganglia and the leg portion of the internal capsule) passes under this area, making it easy to destroy numerous functional systems in a small area of work. This is not to mention the fact that most of the arteries in this region are en passage to one critical brain area or another, including the artery of death.

These tumors are never easy, and you are generally happy with a lesionectomy that doesn't cause too much damage, but a few tips follow (▶ Fig. 14.15):

1. Minimize contact with the artery of death, this is the blood supply to the semantic network and the ventral visual stream.
2. Assume that the SLF and IFOF in these regions are bus routes and that any site in these areas could be a stop on that route. In other words, any part of these cortices (even in a sulcus) can have a small contribution to a two pathway network (SLF or IFOF) which is not obvious on DTI (which does not show small tracts extending to the surface very well) In other words, nowhere is definitively safe until it has stimulated negative multiple times.
3. The first order of business is to remove any opercula of the junctional area that stimulate negative. This defines the insula, finds the arteries early, and makes the deep tumor into a surface problem. If you are working in a deep hole without good visualization or landmarks, then remember you are working blindly near the SLF, and IFOF, with the goal of safely removing a tumor which has an anatomic propensity to follow them.
4. Once you have disassembled the junction, you need to determine the position of the SLF which can be anterior, posterior, deep, or surrounding the tumor. Careful thought is needed to determine what type of cut is possible with the SLF based on extrapolation from other more common cuts. Often only a lesionectomy is possible.
5. The optic radiations are often invaded and you will need to make a decision on them. Obviously, it's best to save them if possible. If not realistic, entering the atrium is quite helpful at defining the location of deep and dangerous anatomy, and should be undertaken early if the optic radiations are gone.
6. The TPO junctional fibers have an anterior bend which takes them into the deep junctional white matter at the back of the insula and posterior temporal stem. Not only is this an easy place to meet critical white matter, but loss of sagittal plane orientation is an easy way to enter the thalamus or internal capsule.

14.6.1 Case Examples

▶ Fig. 14.16 demonstrates a mostly nonenhancing GBM of the TPO junction. The tumor involved the SLF anteriorly, but we were able to resect the majority of this tumor without difficulty.

a) The cyst and nodule appearance of this tumor might fool you into considering that this is a pilocytic tumor, or some other benign tumor. The extensive and thick T2 changes along the cyst wall tell you this unfortunately likely untrue. So does the fact that this is a supratentorial tumor in a 52 year old. Either way, if you do awake surgery routinely, then you will never be caught doing a left TPO junction glioma in an asleep patient if there is minimal threshold for doing a surgery awake. There is no way in which an asleep surgery improves the safety or efficacy of a case like this. At worst, you have done a very safe lesionectomy, and added a few minutes of extra time.

Evaluating this tumor like a glioma, you will note that while the enhancing part of the tumor is superficial, the T2 changes involve the junctional white matter, the motor strip and most of the SMG. Completely removing this will be challenging and may not be possible. As stated in other cases, at minimum, we should try to ensure that the enhancement is dealt with first and foremost, and try to address as much of the T2 change as possible.

In Chapter 10, I discussed a similar case of a cystic glioma. It is noteworthy, that draining the cyst, and removing its lateral wall, only addresses part of the tumor, as the walls of the cyst likely are tumor involved brain. Sometimes, mapping these cases requires two stages of subcortical disconnection, one to disconnect and remove the lateral wall, and another to address tumor in the deep parts of the wall.

a) This craniotomy is small and centered over the cortical surface. The surface is clearly distorted. A speech site was found in the anterior aspect of the tumor, which the DTIs predicted. It is critical, in a case like this, that after deflating a cyst, that you hold open the lips of the cavity so they do not fall inward and cause you to lose your concept of where things are. I hold these open with telfa pads. The right image shows how much the brain can fall inward from simply draining a cyst.
b) The DTIs show that the SLF and its parietal ramus are running through the anterior boundary of the tumor, and much of the medial wall threatens the motor system. Obviously, this is not entirely favorable. A less obvious question worth asking in a case like this is how the visual information will reach the semantic areas. The likely options are from the ipsilateral side, possibly through IFOF or the ventral stream, or from the other side via the crossed semantic loop. If your resection cuts the semantic network from both sides, anomia is the result.
c) The resection completely removed the enhancement, but there are T2 changes remaining. The anterior portion of this was left to preserve the SLF, which was clearly involved in the anterior wall of the tumor based on DTI and mapping. Interestingly, we also got anomias when trying to resect the deeper part of wall, which I assume must have been due to loss of visual input to the semantic areas. Either way, it was left. This patient responded very well to adjuvant therapy and has not recurred for many years. Of course, this further clouds the question about whether the wall needs to be aggressively addressed in these cases, as we cannot know whether this resolved due to a good treatment response or because this was brain edema from the cyst and not tumor.

▶ Fig. 14.17 demonstrates a remarkable case of a TPO junction GBM which was resected at another facility where initially this was a small, enhancing tumor. He deteriorated on post-op day 4 and blew both pupils. This was found to be due to this recurrence which had transpired in the 4 days since the last surgery.

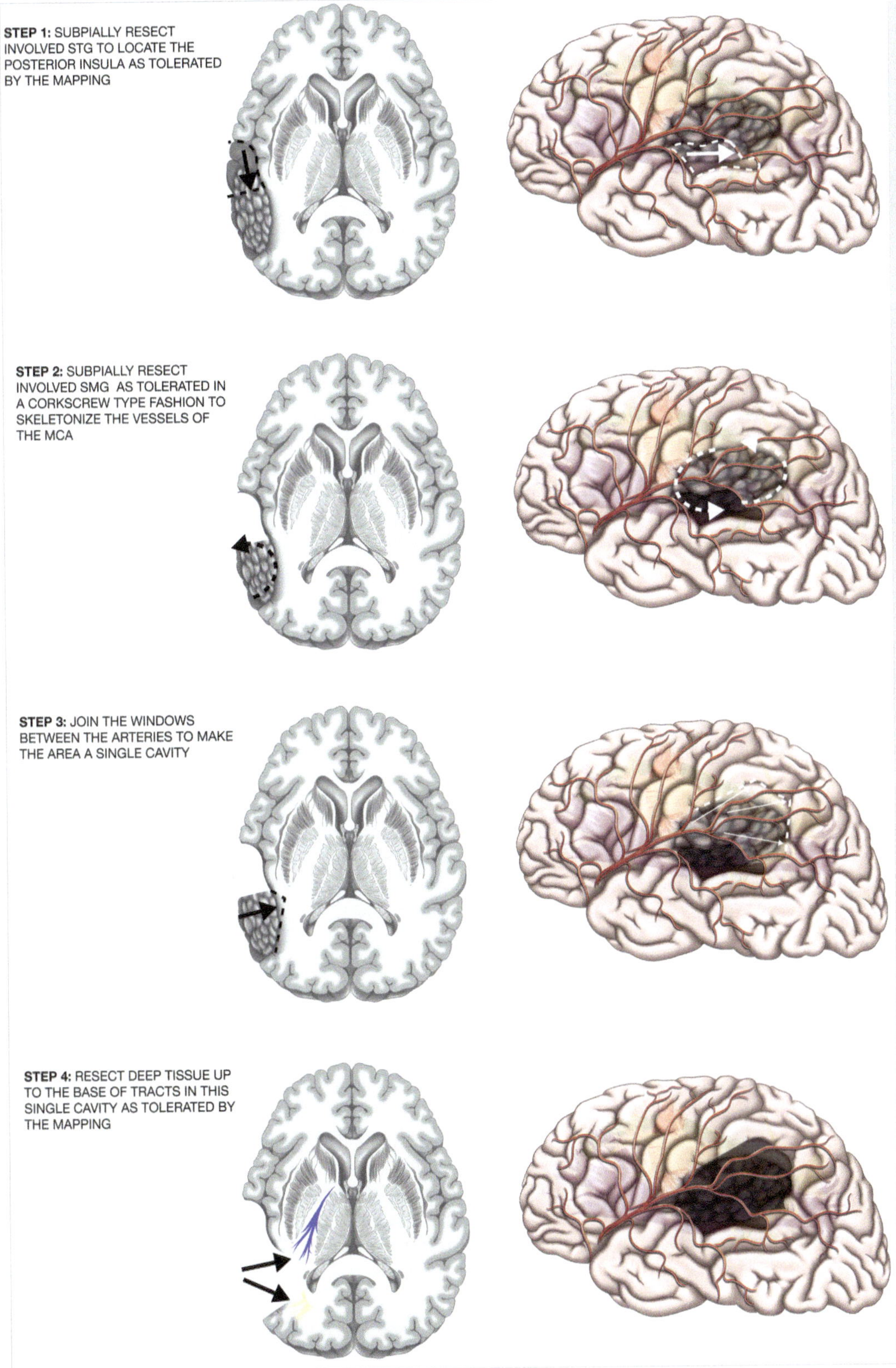

Fig. 14.15 This diagram demonstrates the steps of a TPO junction tumor. Obviously, these tumors have a high propensity to have eloquence inside of part of them, so these figures are idealized versions of the actual surgery. The first order of business is to remove all of the possible parts of SMG, and STG that your mapping allows. This simplifies this complex area, especially as you approach the critical issue of the deep white matter. Depending on what the functional anatomy allows, you can use a modified anterior occipital, medial parietal, or even posterior temporal disconnections to free the tumor from the lateral white matter system, or follow it into the deep junctional anatomy, if necessary. In many cases, a pure lesional resection is all that is possible.

When he recovered to alertness with mannitol, he was transferred to us where we continued to dry him out until he could participate with brain mapping.

a) This is a TPO junction tumor, so by definition, there are a lot of bad aspects of this case. A few good aspects worth noting: First, the T2 is limited, and nothing suggests there is tumor in the sensorimotor regions. Second, while there is tumor in the junctional white matter, this is not the tumor's epicenter (it is mostly in the angular gyrus). Finally, the tumor has filled the previous resection cavity, and is pushing to the dural surface, which limits our work to the edges of the tumor and not the need to resect overlying cortex.

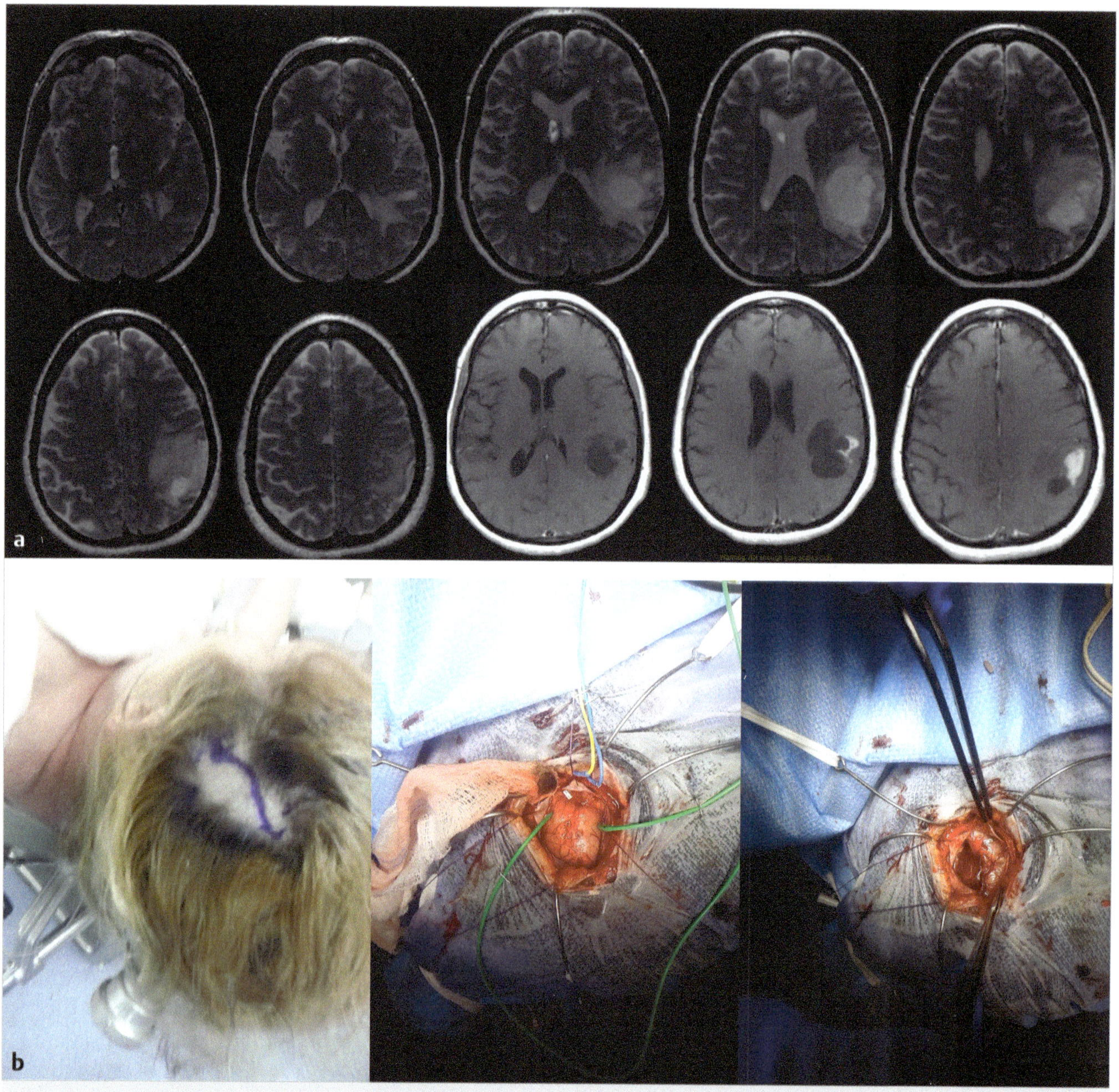

Fig. 14.16 A mostly non-enhancing GBM of the TPO junction; (a) preoperative images, (b) images of the approach.

b) We opened the previous linear incision and found obvious tumor presenting the to surface. Our initial mapping revealed that we were flanked with dyskinesias when we stimulated anteriorly and speech function inferiorly and to a lesser extent anteriorly.. The goal in this case was a lesionectomy of the enhancement as tolerated, staying within the obvious tumor tissue.
c) The DTIs show that the SLF is clearly cupping the tumor, but that the majority of these fibers are anterior and less inferior. This apparent discrepancy between the cortical location of speech function and the SLF location on the DTI can be explained by the observation that the semantic network is likely located on the anteroinferior border of this angular gyrus tumor, and the cortical mapping is locating the semantic network proper. The SLF can be found to be going to this area, especially if you closely examine the sagittal images, and it is likely that the intense edema in this region limits out ability to see all of these tracts. Indeed, we did begin to run into speech problems along the anterior border of the subcortical cut, which is what we would expect from this tract at this point in its path. Nevertheless, it highlights that while DTIs are a critical tool for understanding a network, they cannot supplant functional information during surgery.
d) With careful dissection, we were able to free the enhancing portion of this tumor completely and preserve most of his language function. After adjuvant therapy, he lived two years, demonstrating that it is possible to salvage even the worst recurrences. One way of thinking about this is that any tumor which recurs this quickly is likely dominated by rapidly dividing cells, which one would expect to be more radiation and chemotherapy sensitive.

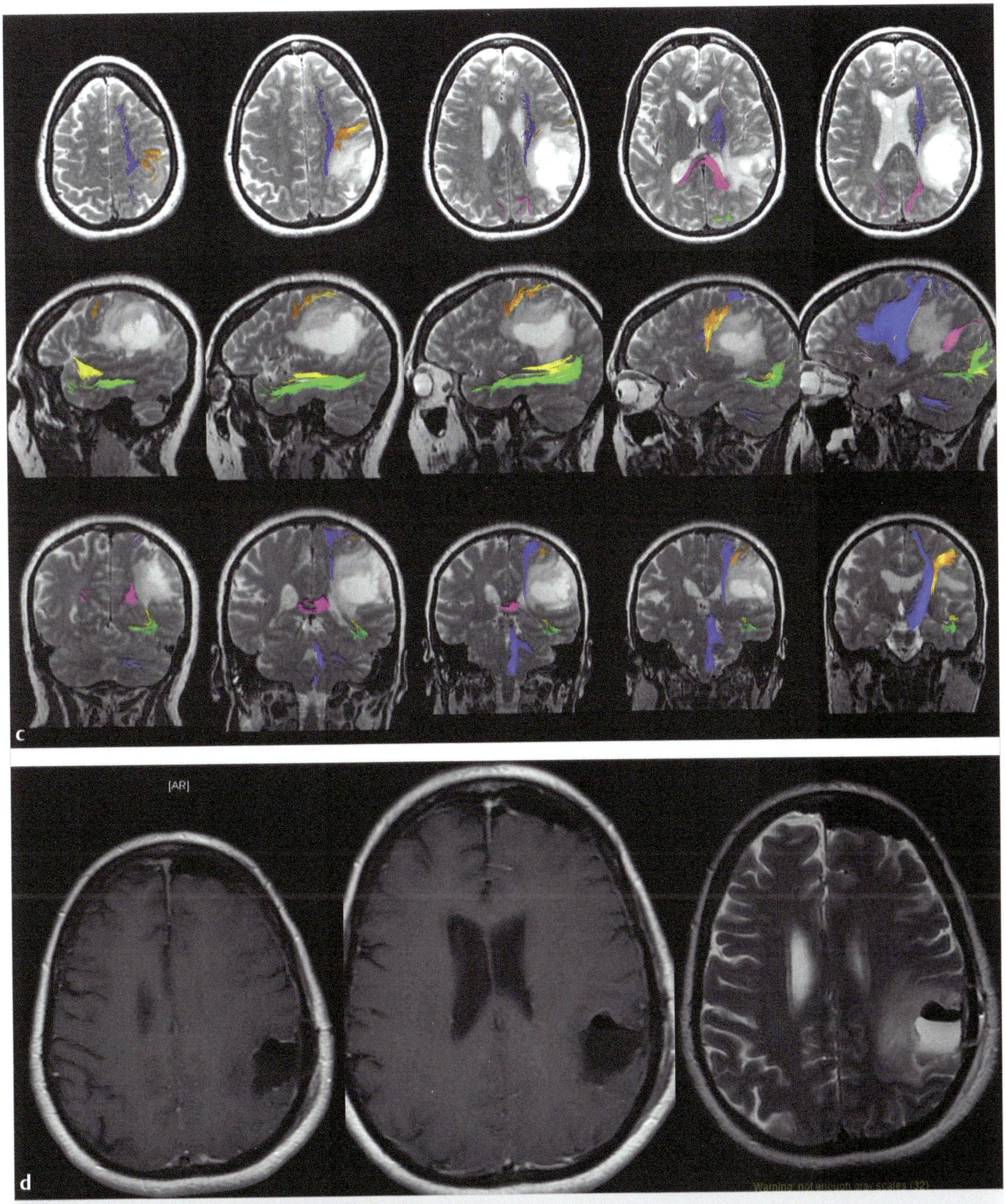

Fig 14.16 (*Continued*) (**c**) DTI tractography, (**d**) postoperative images.

▶ Fig. 14.18 demonstrates a TPO junction done asleep at another facility with dense post-operative aphasia. DTIs suggested that the SLF had been transected posterosuperiorly. We were able to remove the tumor and preserve what speech function he had left using counting as the only task he could successfully do. We remained conservative anteriorly given our inability to get much mapping function from him, and our desire to preserve what he had left.

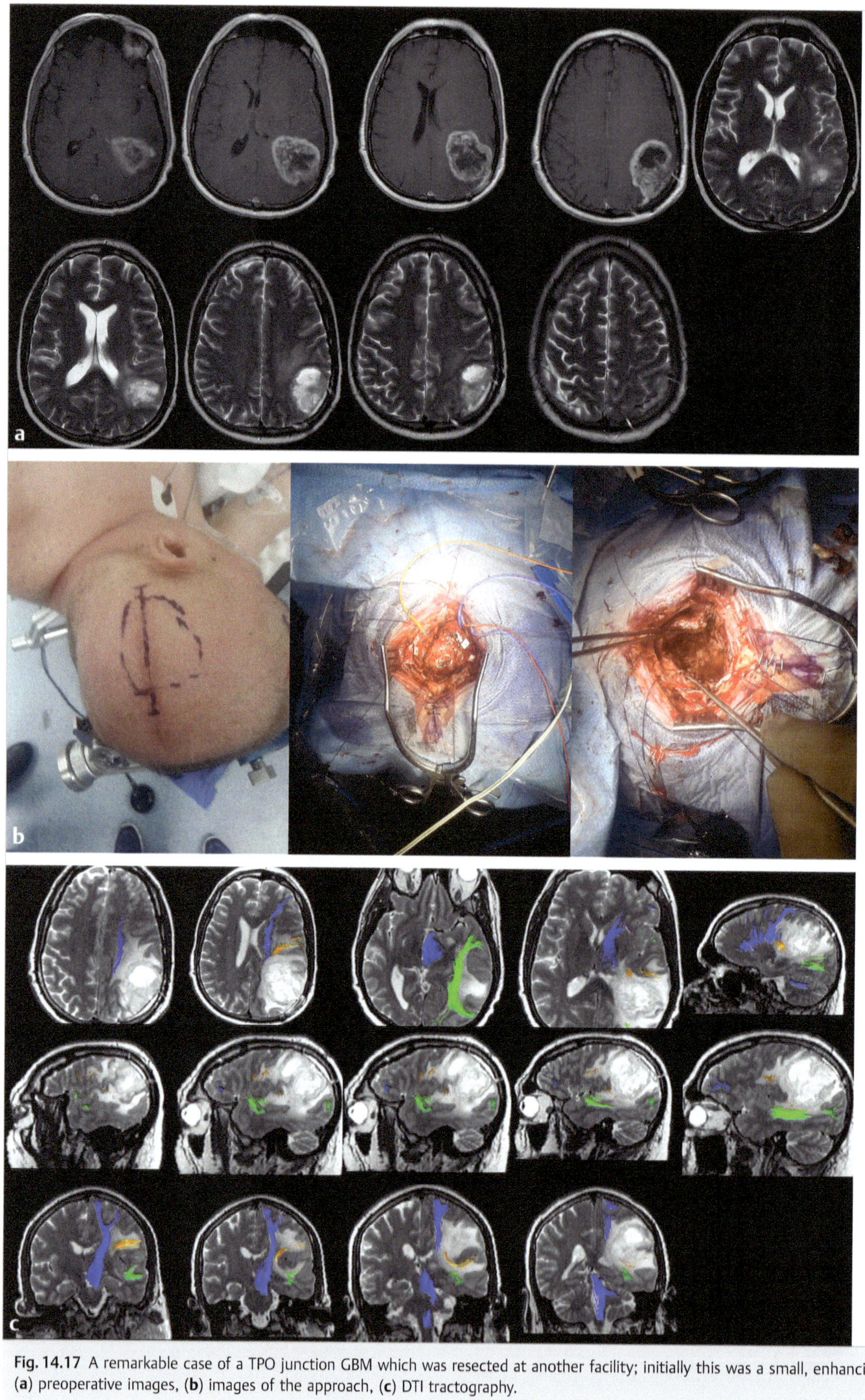

Fig. 14.17 A remarkable case of a TPO junction GBM which was resected at another facility; initially this was a small, enhancing tumor; (**a**) preoperative images, (**b**) images of the approach, (**c**) DTI tractography.

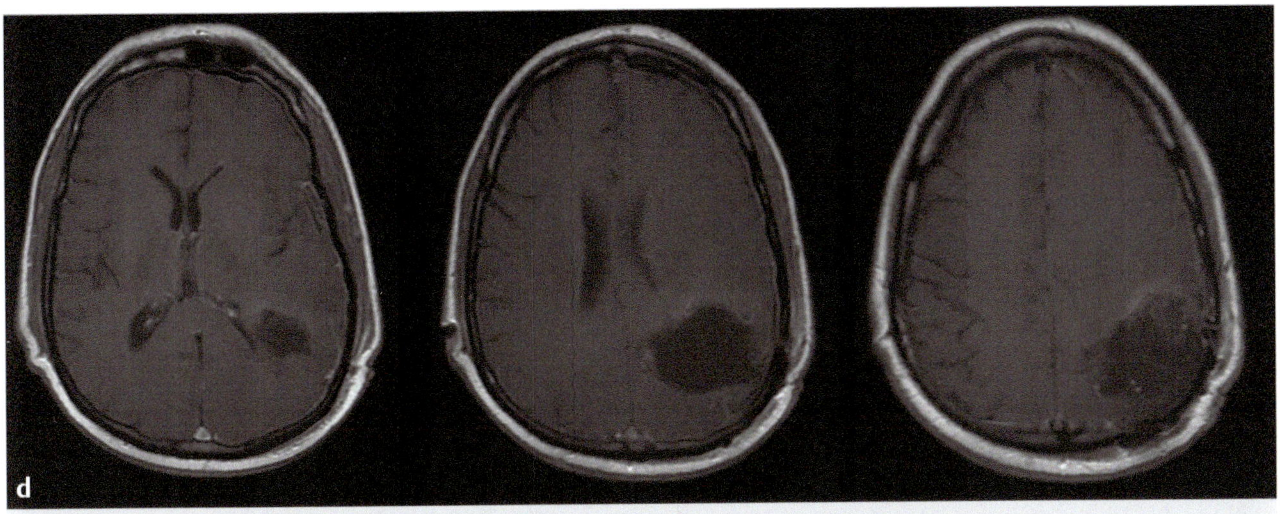

Fig 14.17 (*Continued*) (**d**) Postoperative images.

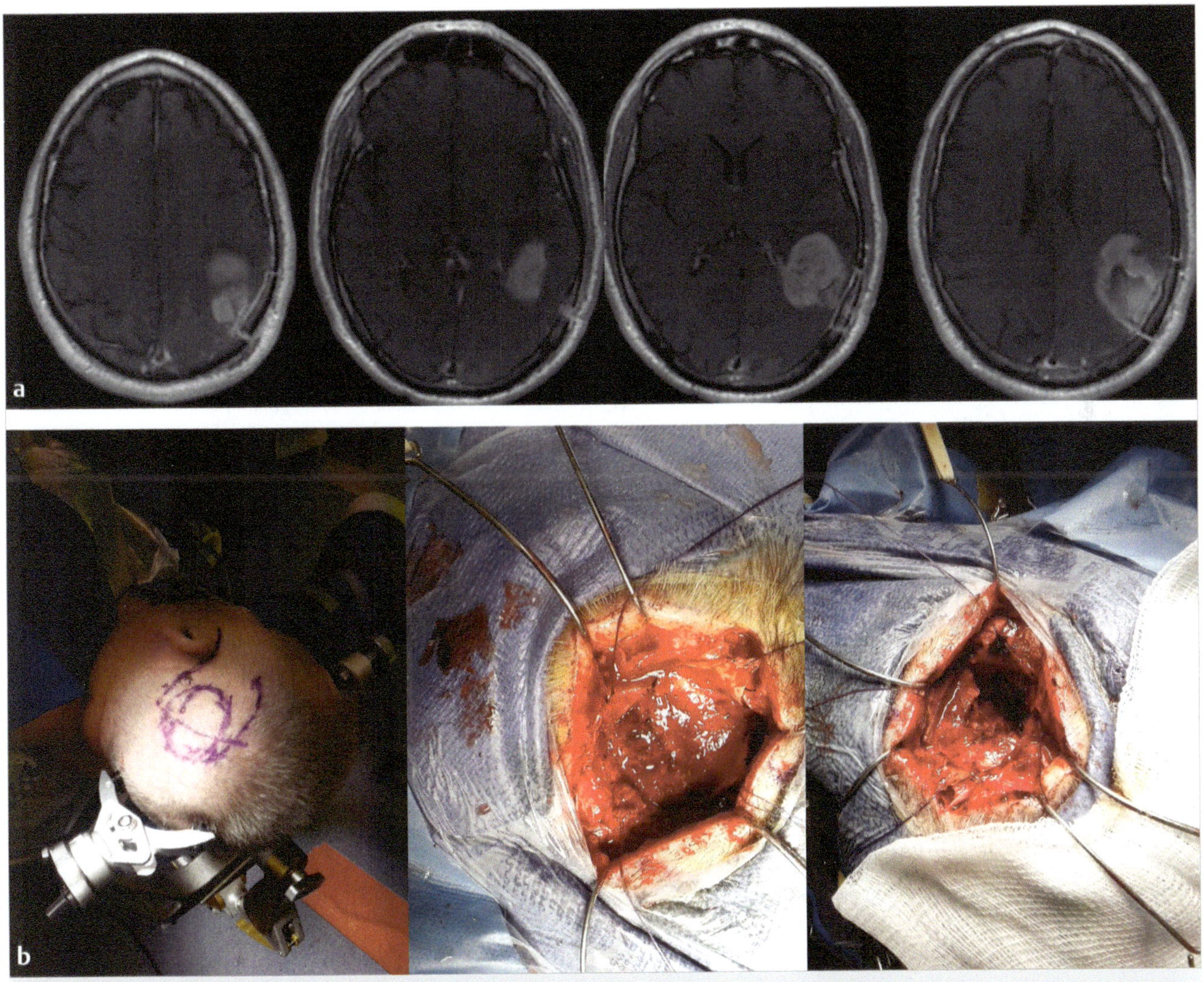

Fig. 14.18 A TPO junction done asleep at another facility with dense post-operative aphasia. They are case examples and the files are organized as follows; (**a**) preoperative images, (**b**) images of the approach. (*Continued*)

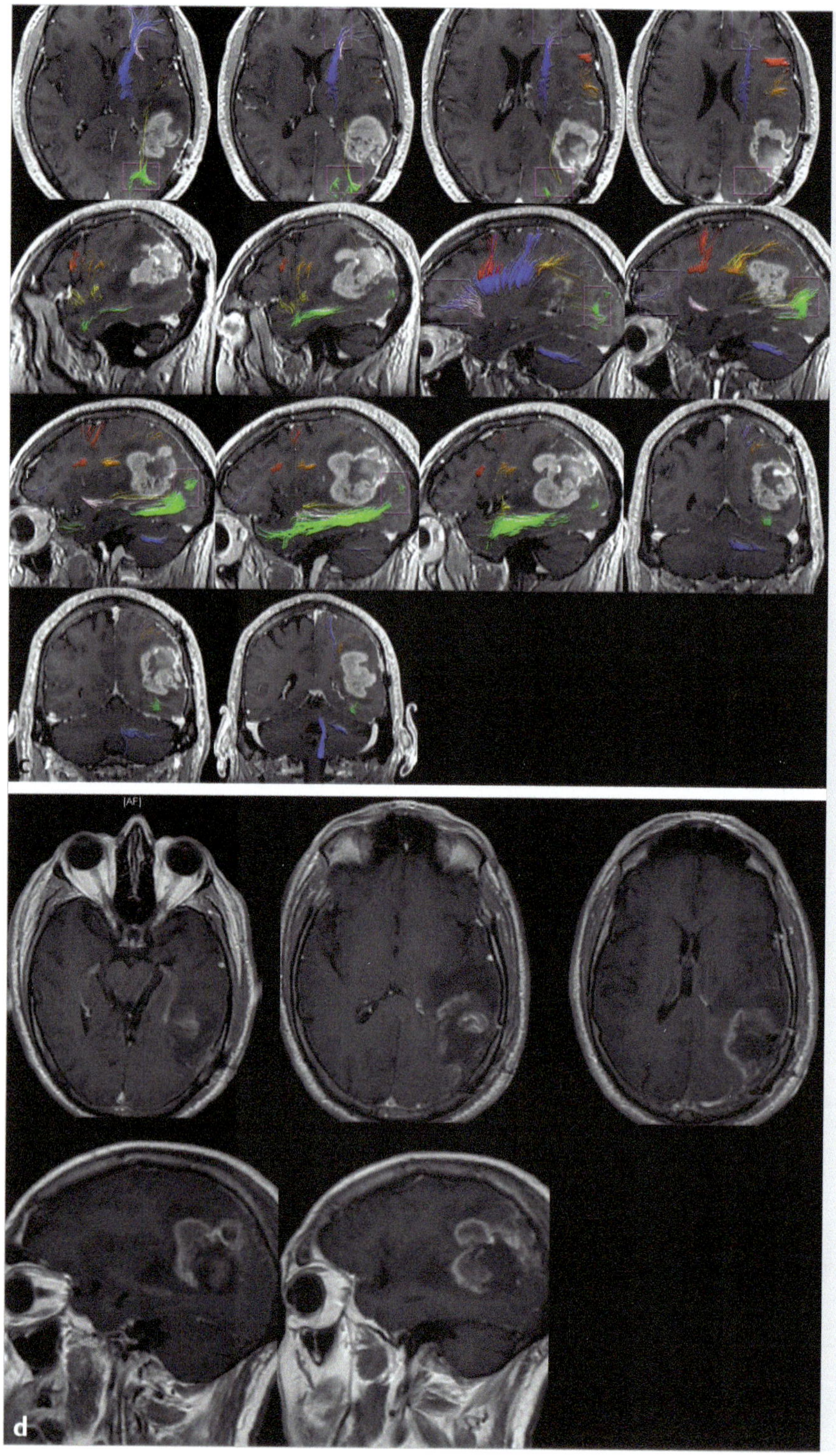

Fig 14.18 *(Continued)* (**c**) DTI tractography, (**d**) postoperative images.

a) When observing a tumor in this position, it is a reasonable guess that it is likely deeply intertwined with the SLF at minimum.
b) The location of the Sylvian fissure, the tentorium, and the tumor surface are indicated by the marks. The tumor dominated the surface visualized after opening the dura. Our goal was to preserve the SLF and thus we started the subcortical work relatively early, and attempted the best lesionectomy possible.
c) The SLF terminates in the tumor cavity. While it is conceivable that the tumor caused this transection, the chronology of events suggests that this was iatrogenic. Interestingly, there does not appear to be any temporal fibers on the other side of this cut, which we would expect. Again, this result is the consequence of choosing entry points based on a presumed concept of functional organization based around cortical anatomy and not white matter connectivity.

d) This is a difficult case due to the patient's poor speech function, which only worsens during surgery in almost everyone. We focused on the posterior and inferior aspects of this tumor, and tried to preserve the remaining SLF and IFOF pathways. Ultimately, we could only do so much to maximize the oncofunctional outcome in a case like this.

▶ Fig. 14.19 demonstrates a case that to the untrained eye might look like it involves the thalamus or basal ganglia. This is in fact a large TPO junction GBM which presented with neglect.

a) This at first glance looks like it might be in the deep core structures, but as I repeatedly stress, this is not a common pattern of spread in gliomas and you should skeptically evaluated this careful examination of the T2 scans demonstrates that this is not true as those structures are pushed forward, and that the tumor is mainly in the angular gyrus and following its deeper connections towards the temporal lobe as well as the optic radiations.
b) None.
c) The SLF is entirely unable to be resolved on tractography which likely explains the neglect. Whether it has been transected or is just not resolvable due to edema is not clear; however, it is fascinating that the entire tract's water movement is affected by this focal insult. Also of note is that the IFOF is running below this tumor, and should be saved if possible.
d) We were aggressive with this case given the lack of SLF function. We obtained a complete resection of the enhancement. Post-operative images demonstrate that the basal ganglia and thalamus were not involved in this tumor and have shifted back into position.
e) This is a 2-year post-surgery scan showing an excellent result. Of note, the neglect is mildly improved, but clearly present.

14.7 Butterfly Gliomas

I was taught as a resident at UCSF that butterfly gliomas were inoperable brain tumors. I was told when I asked why (for example the corpus callosum can be cut without life altering morbidity, so why resecting it when it was densely filled with tumor would cause this kind or morbidity didn't make sense to me) that the risk was too high of devastating the patient, and that the tumors were too aggressive to meaningfully change the clinical course. I was unable to find where anyone published data supporting this, but assume that people had tried to remove these with unsatisfactory results at some point.

My experience was that the idea that leaving these tumors in the patient was a reasonable strategy for preserving their quality of life was a myth. These patients generally did terribly with adjuvant therapy alone, and were often as bad as we would fear surgery would make them in a short time period. I wasn't convinced that these tumors were inherently more aggressive than any other glioma, only that they happen to start near the corpus callosum fibers. So I decided that I was going to figure out how to remove them.

As one could imagine, my initial results were mixed, conventional wisdom is often based on some truth, and some patients were clearly worse off for having surgery. What surprised me was how often they did quite well. Also, I found that the ones who did well often lived about as long as anyone else with GBM, which while not a cure, is a substantially better picture than the current one.

As I began to try to figure out why some patients did better than others, I had a case which broke the mystery open. While abulia occurring when operating in the medial frontal lobe to remove the anterior corpus callosum is not a notable problem and did not lead me to any new thoughts other than the medial frontal lobe has something to do with motivation (not a new idea), in this case the patient suffered a significant abulia (which eventually recovered) after removal of a butterfly glioma in the splenium, and careful study raise d the idea in my head that something in the cingulate gyrus was likely to blame. As I have done these cases awake, I have found that the eloquent areas which are needed to maintain task attention conform quite nicely to the DMN and cingulum. Since developing a practice of preserving this network, I have yet to have this problem since in over 30 cases. I currently believe that DMN problems are the cause of abulia in untreated patients, and the reason that unguided asleep resections which do not take this into consideration have had mixed results, is that if a tumor has not reorganized this network, then it is hard for a patient to compensate for its loss.

14.7.1 Key Anatomic and Clinical Considerations (▶ Fig. 14.20)

1. Having said that, it is essential to note that the corpus callosum and its fibers wrap around the cingulate gyrus and can surround it on all sides. Protecting it is paramount and this can be achieved by defining the cingulate and callosal sulci as early as possible, and to stay lateral to their deepest extent. Awake mapping looking for attention to complex tasks can also guide you to stay out of the cingulum, which you can drift into from the lateral side as there is not a pial bank to protect you as there is on other surfaces.
2. The cingulum and corpus callosum can be separated in the lab, and this is often possible in patients with careful patient dissection. There is a video which demonstrates this.
3. With as much notoriety as tumor in the corpus callosum generates, you should always remain aware that these tumors are mainly in the frontal lobe. If you spend your time fixating on the corpus callosum because it is unique to this case, you are leaving at least 60% of the tumor in the frontal lobe, and you will not be happy with your results. For this reason, the correct paradigm is to think of the case as a frontal lobe tumor that you enter the corpus callosum after clearing the caudate head and cingulate gyrus/DMN. If you really want to address these tumors, you need to go through the brain to do it, not the interhemispheric fissure. This is the long axis of these tumors.
4. While preserving the cingulate and DMN is a key part of these cases, it is essential to note that many of the cuts necessary to clear the tumor out of the cerebrum can bring you close to critical networks or structures on other sides. For example, frontal butterflies can requiring cutting near the FAT and motor networks posteriorly, the SLF posterolaterally, and the caudate head (and sometimes IFOF) posteroinferiorly. Splenial tumors need to be separated from the SLF laterally,

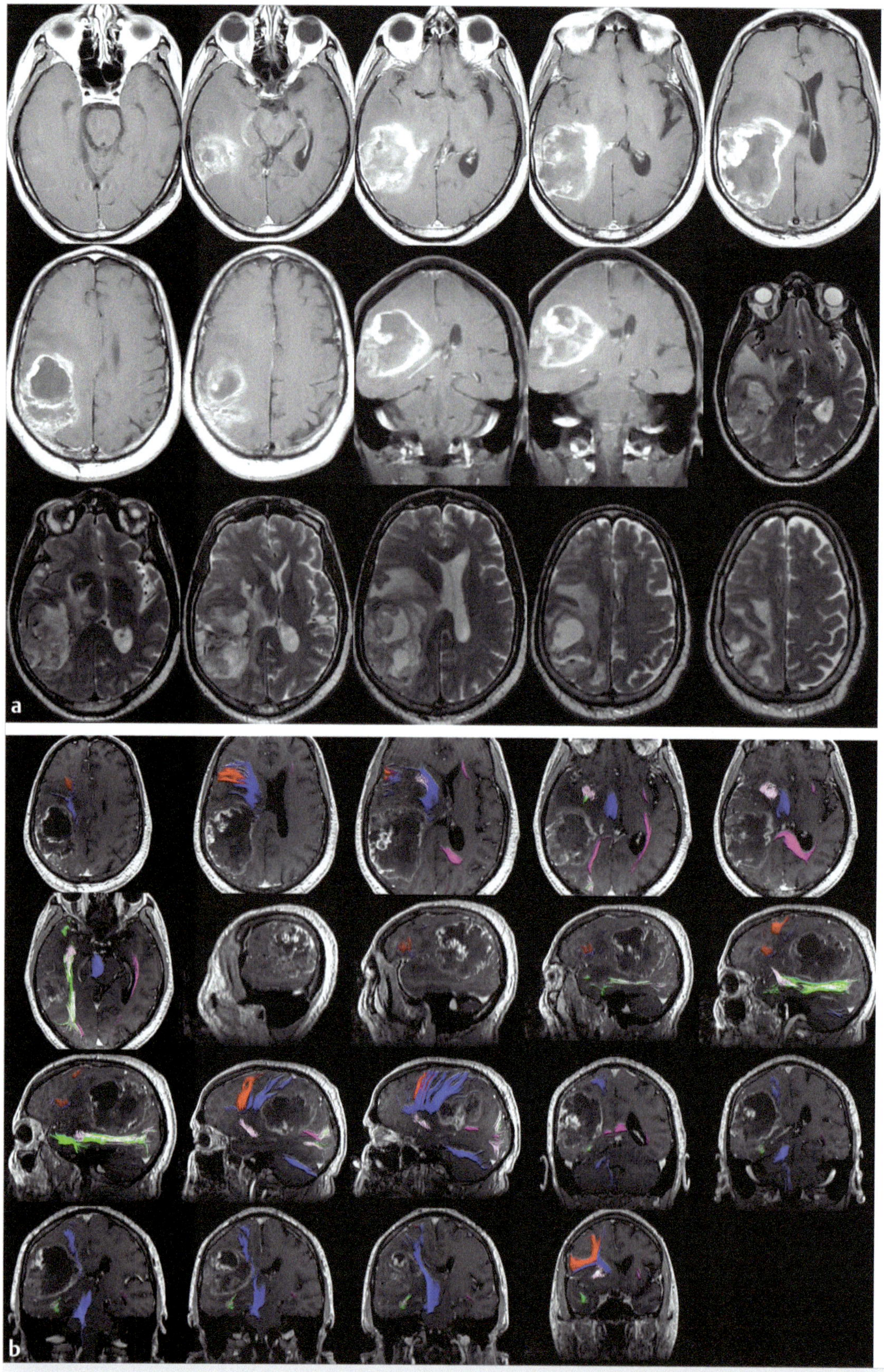

Fig. 14.19 A case that to the untrained eye might look like it involves the thalamus or basal ganglia. This is in fact a large TPO junction GBM which presented with neglect; (a) preoperative images, (b) DTI tractography.

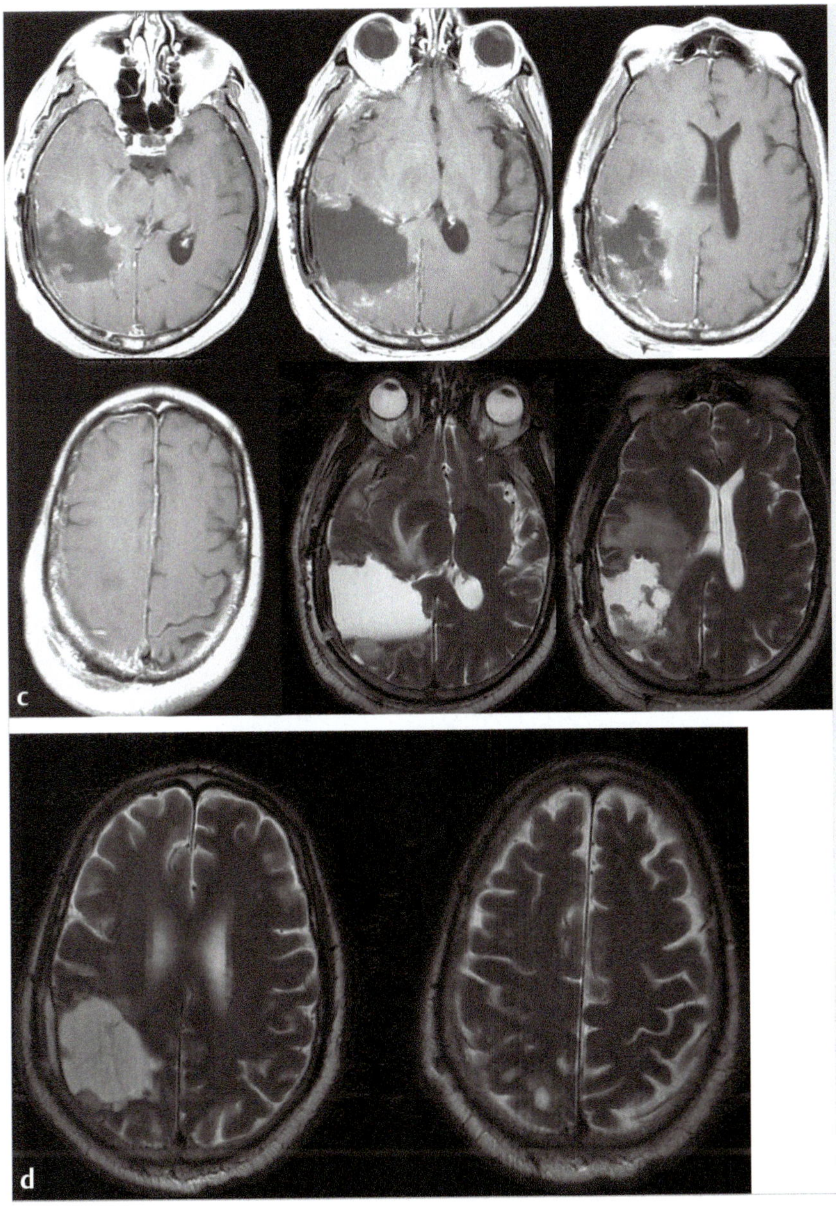

Fig 14.19 (*Continued*) (**c**) Postoperative images, (**d**) long-term follow-up images.

in addition to the cingulum. These tumors are described in a late chapter because they require you to build upon techniques and ideas learned from doing other gliomas, not merely because they are hard.

5. Removing a butterfly glioma means opening biventricularly. There is no way to avoid this and it would be unwise to try to do so (it is your best landmark). Shunts are often unavoidable.
6. You need to consider bihemispheric contributions to function and recovery in your decisions. For example, mid-callosal butterfly gliomas invade both SMA's or motor networks, as well as the connection needed for the other side to compensate for them. When you realize that the tumor is a bifrontal tumor more than a corpus callosum tumor, it is obvious that going for broke on a case like this is probably a recipe for disaster (trust me it is).

Similarly, cutting into the splenium or posterior callosum can interrupt bi-hemispheric transfer of processed visual information, and this should be considered in your calculations (though this sometimes does not cause problems and sometimes can't be avoided or the problem is present at initial presentation).

14.7.2 Technique

Anterior Butterfly Gliomas (▶ Fig. 14.21)

Butterfly gliomas are deep targets so the craniotomy needs to overly the planned trajectory but does not need to be excessively large. The trajectory you need is dictated by a balance between your desire to have a lateral trajectory which looks down the long axis of the callosum fibers, and the reality that the SLF and FAT may force you to deviate more medially. Usually, entry through the middle frontal gyrus is adequate.

You should spend as much time as necessary removing the tumor from the frontal lobe white matter. The cuts are as follows:

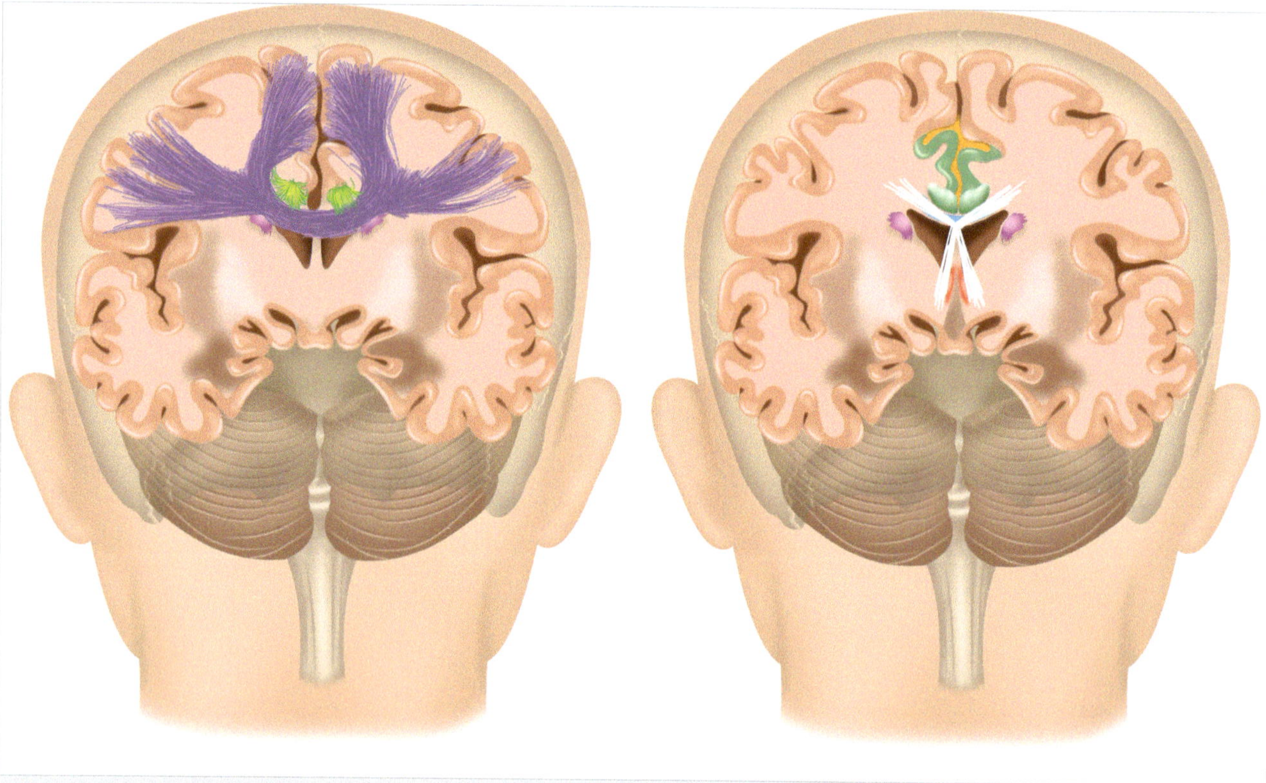

Fig. 14.20 Key relationships of the anterior corpus callosum: This diagram demonstrates the relationship between the fibers of the callosum with the cingulum, the SFG, the caudate and the septal nuclei. Because most of the callosum is not visible as a single extrinsic structure, it cannot be seen and has to be conceptually understood to perform safe surgery in it.

Medial: You separate the tumor from the cingulum along its entire anterior to posterior length. This is done with attention tasks.

Posterolateral: A cut to separate the tumor from the frontal bends of the SLF should be done under monitoring of SLF relevant tasks. It is essential that this cut be made sufficiently lateral and should follow the plane of the inferior frontal sulcus (i.e., parallel to the floor), forcing the cut as lateral and deep as the mapping will allow. Remember that with the patient in the lateral position, your natural angle is to work down towards the floor, which is towards the midline, not towards the patient's feet (i.e., a true sagittal cut).

Posterior: If the tumor is threatening the motor system or FAT, this cut should be tackled late in the game as an SMA syndrome can end meaningful mapping elsewhere. This is the standard coronal cut which typifies a medial frontal disconnection from the motor networks.

Inferoposterior: These tumors usually are running along the anterior face of the caudate head (look at the anatomy of the tracts). As stated elsewhere, the caudate parenchyma looks like glioblastoma with subtle differences. Entering the ventricle is critical for finding the boundary and staying out of it; however, manipulation of the caudate will often cause difficulty with multiple mapping tasks. Of note, the IFOF can also be encountered in this area.

Taking out the corpus callosum: At the angle you approach the tumor, removing the corpus callosum generally involves working down the long axis of the corpus callosum until you have widely removed the front wall of both frontal horns. The callosal sulcus and the ACA complex are key landmarks for remaining out of the cingulum and basal forebrain.

Here are a few points for remaining safe but effective while doing this. First, when working in the rostrum and genu, remember that the forceps minor has a superior and inferior radiation into the frontal lobe. You are generally approaching the tumor via the ipsilateral superior radiation, but you should be sure the mentally follow this as you approach the other side, and if needed, you should define the contralateral caudate head and work anterior to this. Also note that the inferior radiations form a pyramid as they exit the rostrum and enter the bilateral inferior frontal lobes. If you transgress these pyramids and head inferiorly, you have entered the subcallosal cingulate structures and/or the septal nuclei/basal forebrain. This can cause profound problems and should be avoided.

Additionally, the posterior portions of the callosum need to be separated from the septum pellucidum, raising the theoretical risk of damaging the fornices in more posteriorly extending tumors.

Finally, callosum resection is an anatomic resection, and thus everything between the ACA/ callosal sulcus and the ventricle needs to be resected. Subpialization is often the way to work but ACA injury must be avoided.

In short, the steps of this surgery are as follows:

1. Separate the tumor from the cingulum medially, the SLF laterally, and the motor system posteriorly.
2. Enter the ventricle and identify the boundaries of the caudate head. Clear the tumor from the anterior border of the

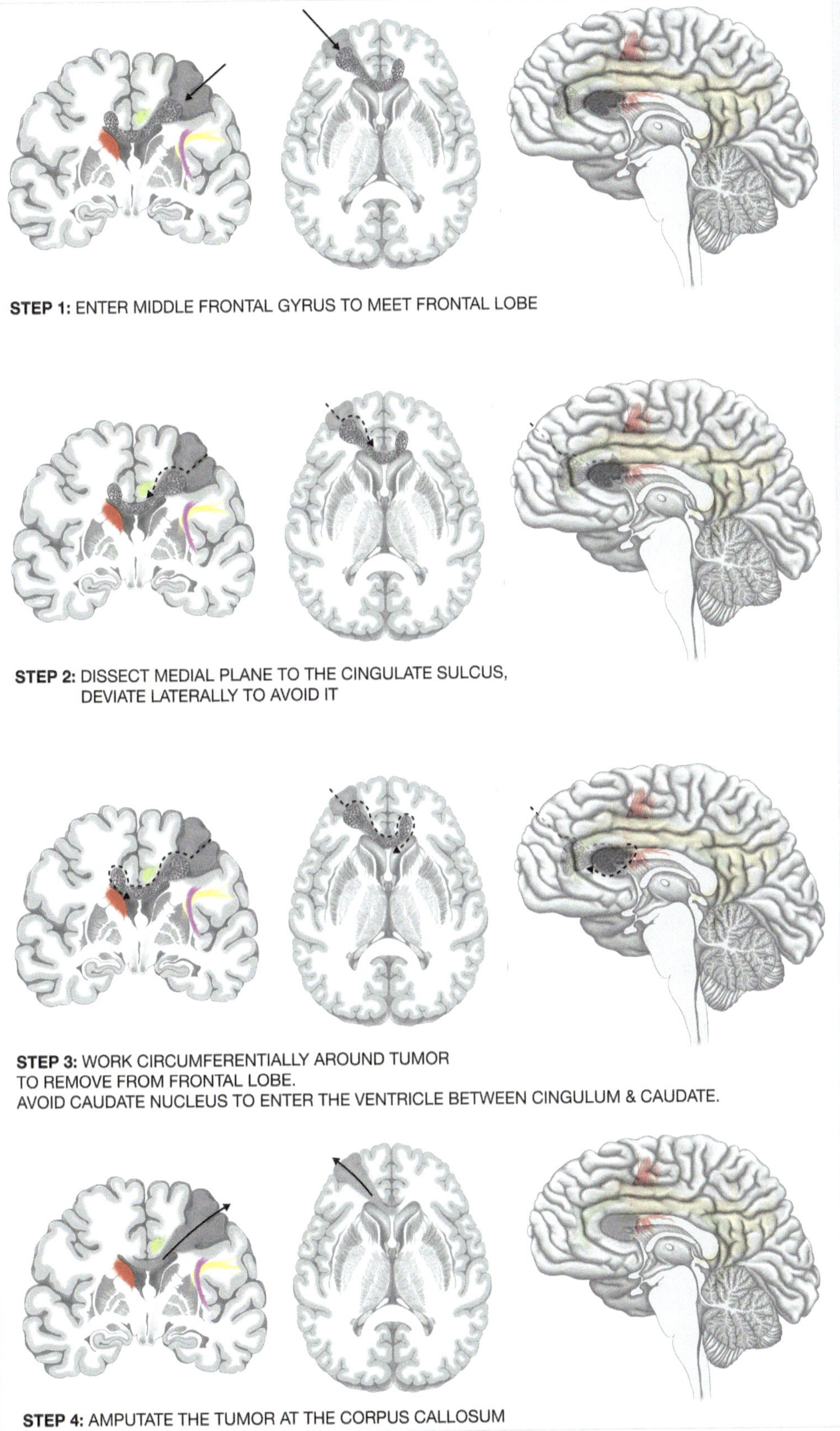

Fig. 14.21 This figure demonstrates the steps of removing an anterior butterfly glioma. The first step is to work circumferentially around the tumor to separate it from the frontal lobe. This involves separating it from the SLF and IFOF laterally, the FAT and caudate head posteriorly, and the ACA and cingulum/DMN medially. These cuts are complete when the cingulum is free from the tumor from the posterior tumor edge until the beginning of the callosal rostrum, and from the cingulate to the callosal sulcus. The ipsilateral frontal horn should be widely open, and the tumor free of the caudate. The ipsilateral tumor is truncated and removed.
The corpus callosum is then removed between the callosal sulcus and the frontal horns, until reaching the contralateral ventricle and widely opening it. The extension onto the other side can be followed by working in front of the other caudate head. Finally, it is critical to not extend the resection below the callosal rostrum, as this is the location of the septal nuclei.

caudate based on the landmarks in the ventricular wall and based on the gross appearance of the caudate tissue.
3. Remove the frontal lobe tumor on the ipsilateral side.
4. Identify the callosal sulcus and or ACA and orient yourself to the ventricular anatomy and ventricular walls. This shows you where the corpus callosum is.
5. Define the parts of the corpus callosum which needs to be removed. Follow this to the body and the rostrum to get a game plan.
6. Remove the corpus callosum until you have widely opened into both ventricles. Separate the tumor from the septium pellicidum.
7. Follow the forceps minor until you have cleared the other side, or functional considerations force you to stop. Take care to stay above the pyramid overlying the septal nuclei and subcallosal areas.

14.8 Case Examples

▶ Fig. 14.22 demonstrates a mostly unilateral butterfly glioma which was aggressively removed using awake mapping techniques.

a) This patient presented with mild abulia and this is likely due to the proximity of these tumors to the cingulate gyrus. Note that the tumor almost exclusively follows the corpus callosum fibers as shown in several figures in this book, and only has minor association with the cingulate.
b) Note that the craniotomy is small and the focus of this case is clearing tumor from the ipsilateral frontal lobe. You must resist the urge to fixate on the corpus callosum and make sure you deal with the bulk of the tumor in the frontal lobe. The craniotomy is intentionally not taken to the midline to encourage a more lateral to medial trajectory down the tumor's long axis. Note that most of the treacherous aspects of these causes involve structures near the midline (DMN, SMA, ACA, etc.).
c) The approach to taking these tumors out involves following the tumor into the window between the FAT and the cingulum. The cingulum is not well visualized in this case on either side, likely due to edema, and this requires that we preserve the anatomic structure of the cingulate gyrus, using anatomic landmarks, and functional mapping.
d) The tumor is mostly removed, though admittedly it is hard to tell in many of these cases what is blood and what is a small bit of residual tumor (a perfectly dry field without hemostatic material is rarely possible in this area. At minimum, it is quite hard to get the caudate head to stop bleeding without packing it off. The cingulate gyrus is mostly anatomically preserved, but thin in places. He recovered well from this surgery.

▶ Fig. 14.23 demonstrates the removal of a much larger butterfly glioma involving difficult clearance of tumor from the caudate head, and continued mapping on the other side to remove tumor from in front of the caudate head on the left side.

a) This tumor is bilateral and extends anterior to the caudate head both sides. Protecting the cingulate and FAT on the way in, and safely clearing the tumor from the caudate heads are important challenges.
b) The craniotomy does not need to be large, this is a deep tumor by definition and it merely needs to be centered down the long axis of the tumor and within the FAT-cingulum window.
c) The cingulum is surrounded by the tumor, but is structurally intact and salvageable.
d) This aggressive resection is possible provided you follow the tumor to the other side, remaining anterior to the contralateral caudate, and that you do not head inferior to the callosal rostrum where the septal nuclei are located.

▶ Fig. 14.24 demonstrates probably the most extensive butterfly glioma I have ever seen, which fills much of both SFG and cingulate gyri. I had limited goals for this case, as I did not think I could safely remove both cingulate gyri without devastating this patient and instead focused on a unilateral clearing of tumor with plans for adjuvant therapy for the other side. I think this is the best I could do for this extreme case.

a) It should be obvious that complete resection including resection of both cingulate gyri, is unlikely to end in a good outcome. Our goal is to try to make this unilateral, and to minimize neurologic morbidity while providing her with the least amount of tumor possible. This is an unusual case as it does not obey the typical anatomy of butterfly gliomas, and instead preferentially invades both cingulate gyri and the callosum extensively, while sparing the SFG almost completely.
b) None.
c) None.
d) This postoperative film demonstrates a fair bit of residual disease, but comparison with the preoperative films shows that a fair bit has been removed. It is important to point out the rationales for what was left behind and why: the contralateral cingulate was left to preserve at least one DMN/cingulate network, and the more posterior callosal involvement was left to maintain bilateral communication between the SMA's. The latter is a small amount of tumor left behind to avoid a potentially bad problem, which is a good trade off. This patient had significant abulia for about 3 weeks which eventually resolved to normal. She went on to receive adjuvant therapy and thus far has done well.

14.8.1 Splenial Butterfly Gliomas (▶ Fig. 14.25)

In many ways, splenial tumor surgeries are conceptually similar to anterior butterfly tumors. It is a transcortical resection of a parietal lobe tumor working down the long axis between the interval between the SLF and cingulum, which is followed into the ventricle, allowing you to identify the callosal boundaries, and to remove the corpus callosum down its long axis until you have a wide biventricular opening and have subpially resected the posterior boundaries of the splenium. So while the angles and views are slightly different, the overall concept of the surgery is the same.

A few specific points (▶ Fig. 14.26):

1. The SLF is at risk over a much longer length than with anterior corpus callosum tumors. In fact, the lateral mapping primarily aims to enter the top of the atrium just medial to the tract (if you don't get lateral enough you are leaving tumor in the splenium fibers, which is headed towards some less than desirable parts of the brain.
2. The optic radiations are running in the lateral wall of the atrium. Your approach from the posterior parts of the superior parietal lobule roughly parallels these fibers along their

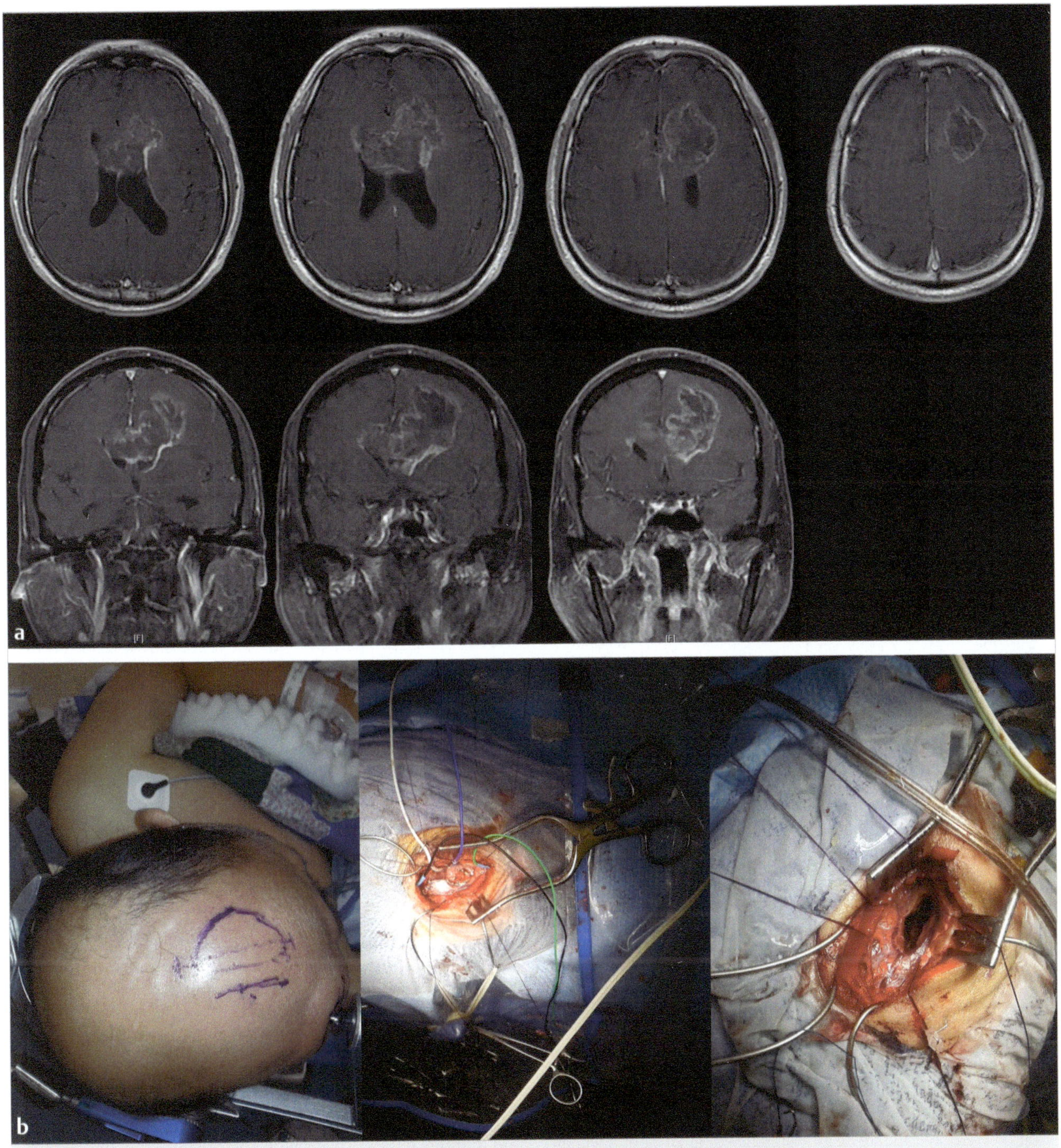

Fig. 14.22 A mostly unilateral butterfly glioma which was aggressively removed using awake mapping techniques. They are case examples and the files are organized as follows: (**a**) preoperative images, (**b**) images of the approach. *(Continued)*

anterior to posterior course, but it is easy to cut them by entering the lateral wall of the atrium.

3. The safest working angle in this corridor is to be as posterior and medial as possible as this parallels the visual radiations and ventral visual stream and is well behind the sensorimotor network and attention networks. This angle of attack is comforting, but wrong. You need to be more lateral and anterior to this or the falcotentorial junction will block your access to the opposite side, and will direct your angle anteriorly towards dangerous areas like the thalamus. You need to force your starting angle into the splenium forward and lateral so you are looking down the long axis of the splenium, of course limited by functional concerns.
4. After entering the ipsilateral atrium and clearing the tumor from the SLF, you need to circumferentially dissect the tumor out of the surrounding brain and the cingulum and truncate it across the base of the splenium. This is necessary to see the splenium running under the falx.
5. The boundaries of the splenium from the lateral approach are the two atriums anteriorly, the falx posteriorly, and the

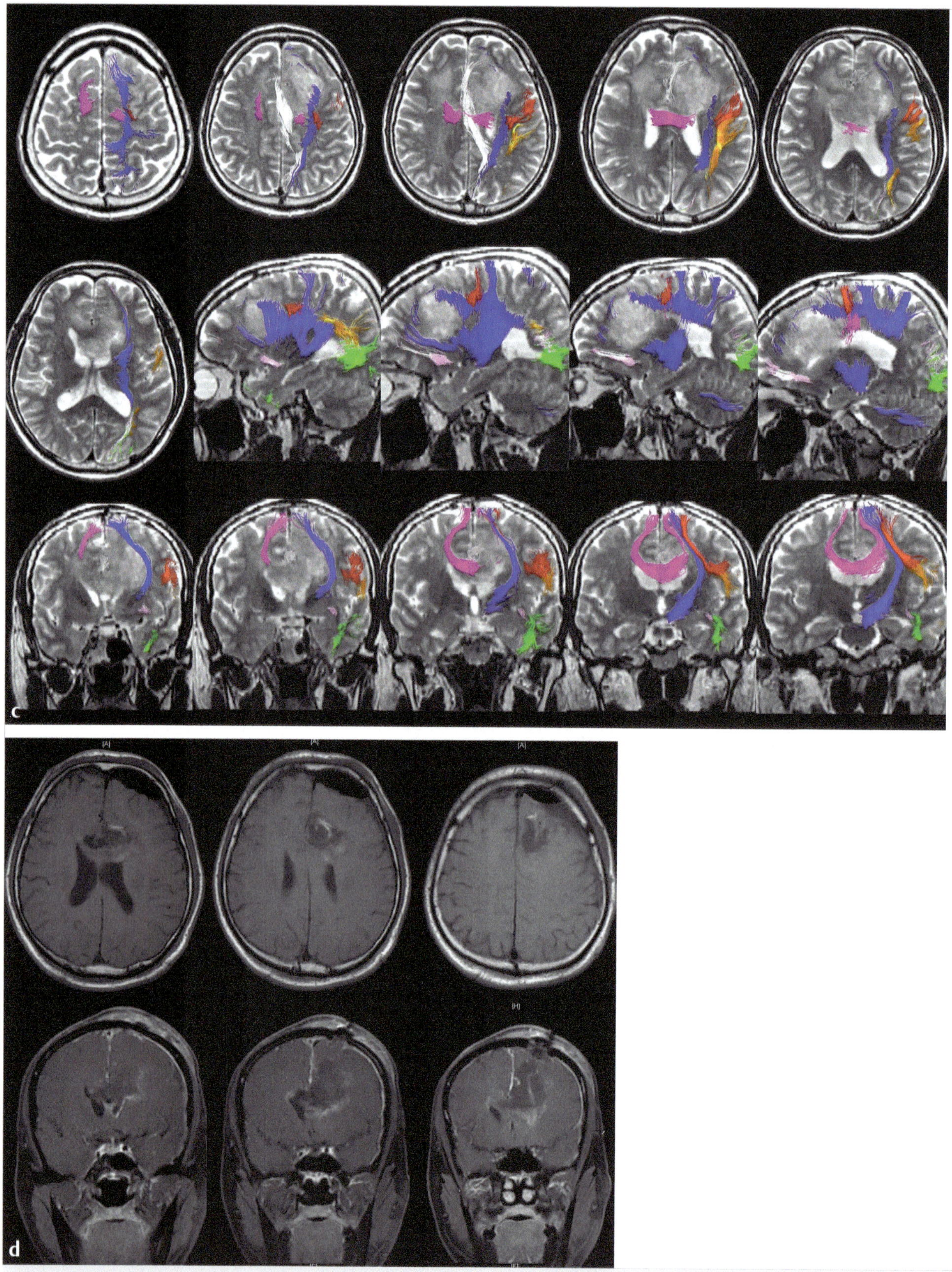

Fig 14.22 (*Continued*) (**c**) DTI tractography, (**d**) postoperative images.

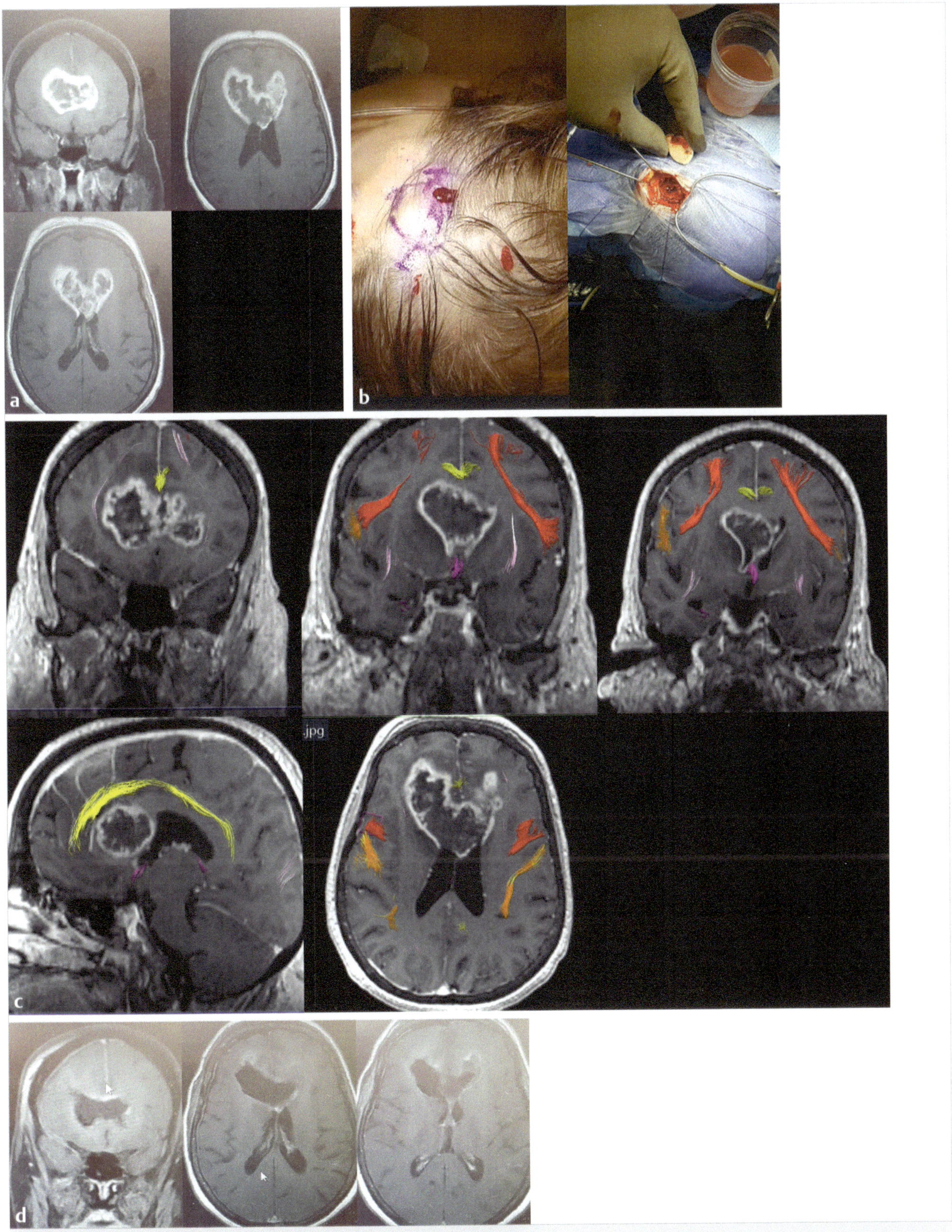

Fig. 14.23 The removal of a much larger butterfly glioma involving difficult clearance of tumor from the caudate head, and continued mapping on the other side to remove tumor from in front of the caudate head on the left side; (**a**) preoperative images, (**b**) images of the approach, (**c**) DTI tractography, (**d**) postoperative images.

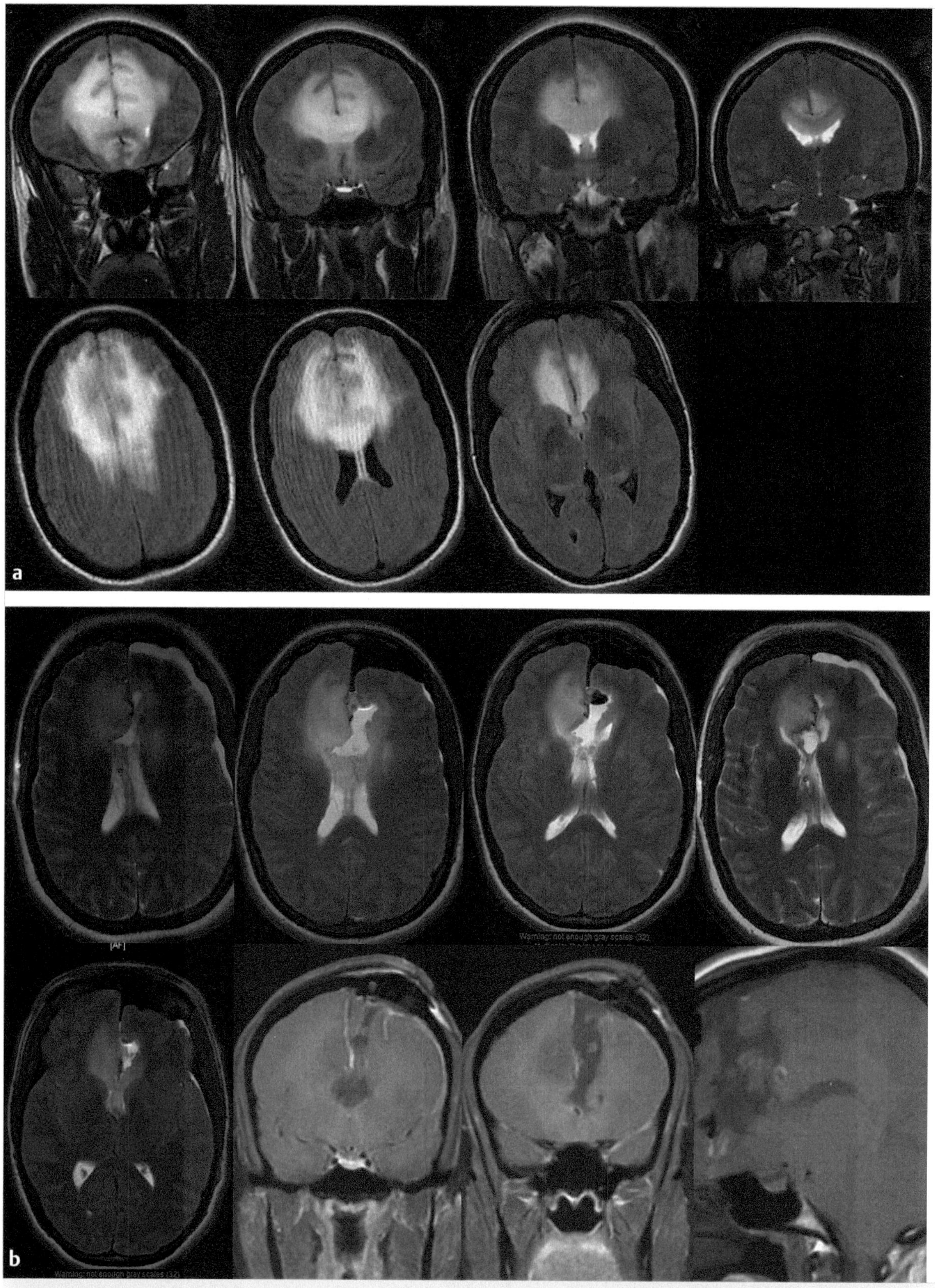

Fig. 14.24 The most extensive butterfly glioma I have ever seen, filling much of both SFG and cingulate gyri; (**a**) preoperative images, (**b**) postoperative images.

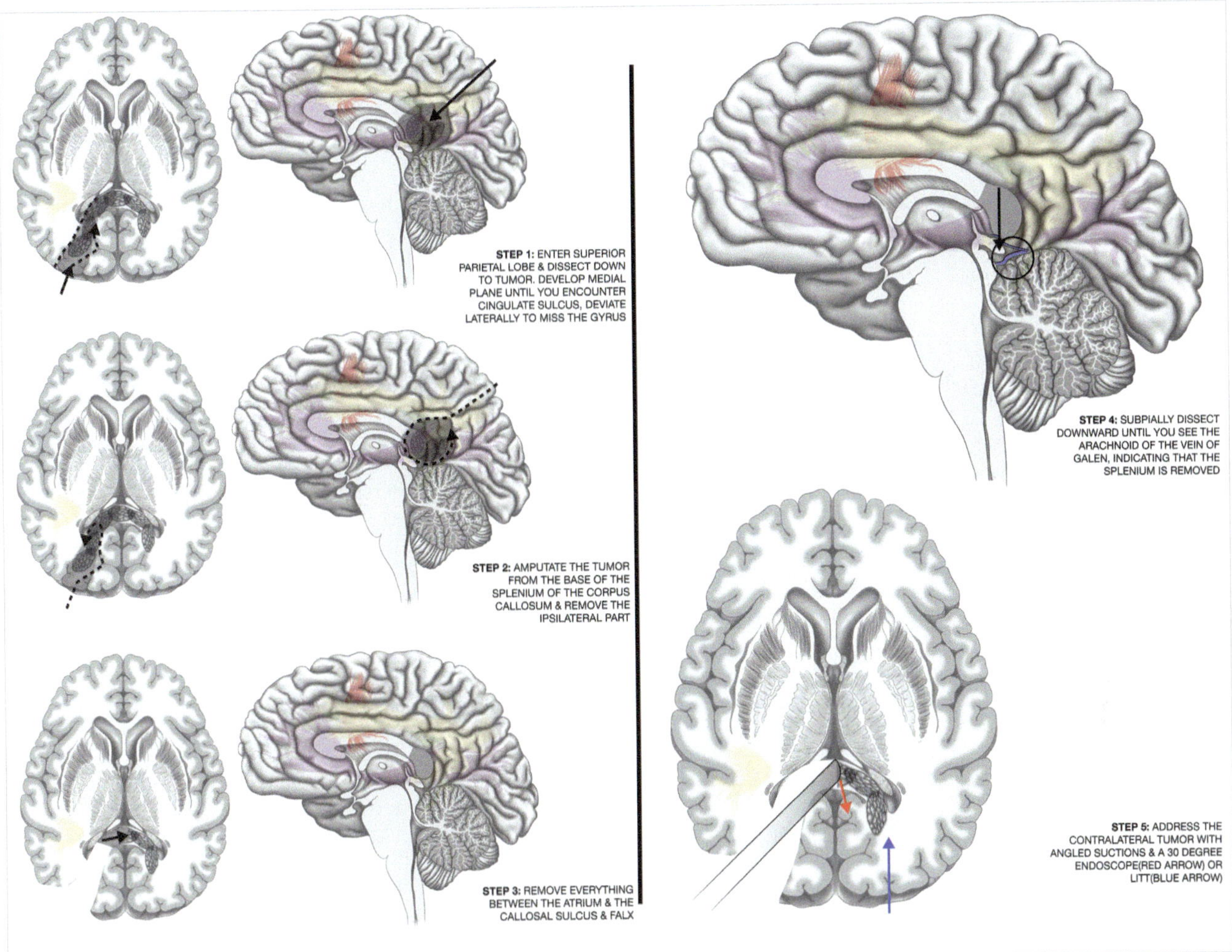

Fig. 14.25 These figures demonstrate the technique for resecting a pure splenial butterfly glioma. The angle of approach, unlike cases where the splenial resection is part of a larger parieto-occipital resection, is posterior through the back of the superior parietal lobule/precuneus, and as lateral as the SLF will allow. Once encountering the tumor, the first goal is to separate it from the SLF and optic radiations en route to entering the atrium. The cut is then continued superiorly over the top of the tumor. Attention is then turned to freeing the tumor from the isthmus of the cingulate gyrus which sits near the edge of the falx. Once this medial cut has identified the callosal sulcus, you have defined all of the splenium boundaries, and you can truncate the tumor. As described in Chapter 13, the splenium can be identified as the tissue between the callosal sulcus, the ventricle and the vein of Galen. It should be removed until biventricular exposure has been achieved, and the Galenic circulation is skeletonized. It is important to take this resection as high as desired, and to recognize the triangular superior portion (also mentioned in Chapter 13), and address it to the extent necessary. The contralateral side requires an angled endoscope, and may benefit from LITT therapy if it is significantly contralateral.

vein of Galen and internal cerebral veins inferiorly. Until you have subpially skeletonized this, you haven't finished removing the splenium.

6. A 30 degree endoscope and angled bipolars and suctions are usually necessary to remove tumor in the contralateral splenium which hooks strongly posteriorly behind the falx. If there is a very large amount or very posteriorly located piece of contralateral tumor, we utilize LITT therapy to treat this as bilateral approaches strongly risks visuospatial processing.
7. The superior body of the corpus callosum and its junction with the splenium are somewhat pyramidal shaped when resecting this from below. It is important to recognize this as you attempt to determine the top of your splenium resection; however, note that the semantic crossing loop, and its semantic information from the other side is running though this part of the callosum, and if you injure this, then you risk cutting off visual to semantic transfer in this patient. On the left side, this means anomia and alexia, usually.

14.9 Case Examples

▶ Fig. 14.27 demonstrates a large splenium butterfly glioma which we were able to get an aggressive resection on. Note that the blind spot of this approach is on the other side behind the falx posteriorly. If necessary, LITT treatments are useful for dealing with this without entering both parietal lobes.

a) This tumor is a pure splenial butterfly tumor, and it's important to note that the posterior cingulate gyri are not involved on either side and should be left alone. The goal is anatomic resection of the splenium via a transparietal approach.

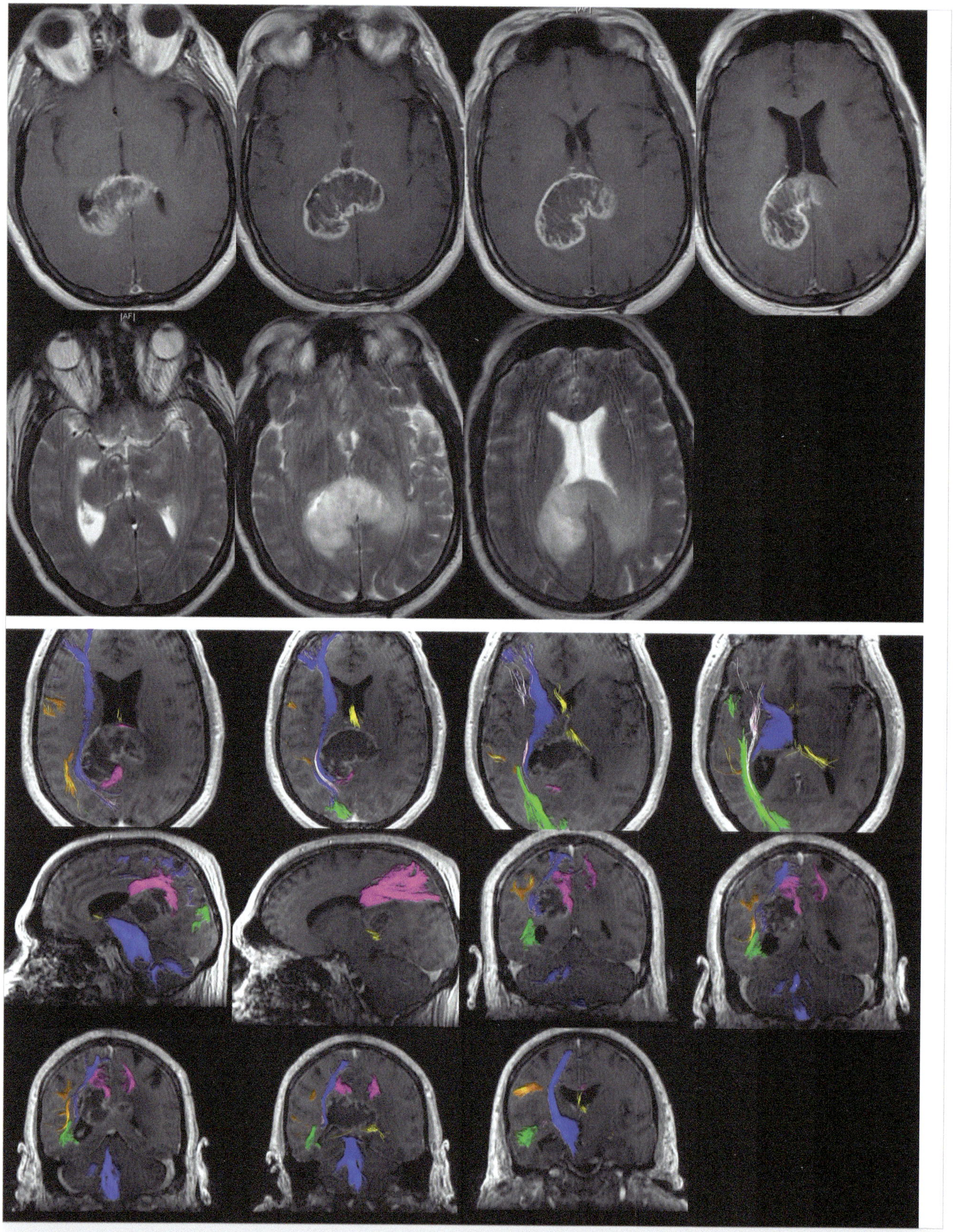

Fig. 14.26 Splenial butterfly glioma; (a) preoperative images, (b) DTI tractography.

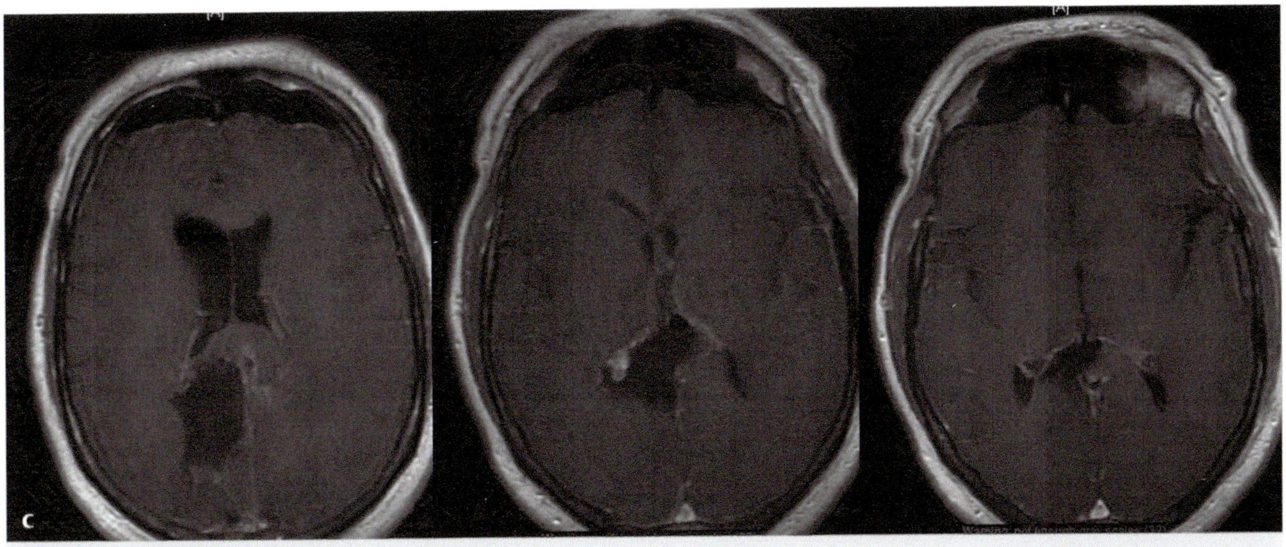

Fig 14.26 (*Continued*) (**c**) Postoperative images.

b) None.
c) The sagittal DTIs show some of the residual callosal fibers running over the top. The important thing in these cases is to avoid cutting the crossed semantic loop, especially if the ipsilateral visual system is compromised or at risk.
d) The resection is very good. Note that the endpoint of the resection involves removing the back wall of both atria with the choroid plexus exposed posterior as shown.

▸ Fig. 14.27 demonstrates a butterfly glioma following the cuneus fibers into the splenium.

a) The anatomy of this tumor perfectly highlights the splenium anatomy: it spares the cingulate and appears to be wrapping around to join the early visual cortices. As always, the key to butterfly gliomas is to address the tumor in the cerebrum thoroughly, and to not get too focused on the fact that this tumor is in the callosum.
b) None.
c) There is a lot of information provided on these images, which I will summarize. In short, you expect to disrupt part of the ipsilateral visual system with a tumor like this. Compensation from the other side is only possible by communication from contralateral later stage steps in visual processing, as the splenium is not there to provide earlier, unprocessed information. The goal here is primarily to focus on sparing as many later stage communicating tracts as possible, and to minimize injury to the posterior body of the callosum which provides bilateral communication between later stage visual processing areas. For example, the MdLF (in yellow) is threatened by the lateral boundary of this tumor, and if dorsal pathway information cannot reach the neglect areas on the right via either the crossed semantic loop, or the MdLF (which brings information from the later dorsal stream areas which in turn can use contralateral input passing through the posterior body as opposed to the splenium), then it is reasonable to conclude that visuospatial problems might occur. In this case, mapping helps to integrate the overall picture into your decision making. In other words, it doesn't matter exactly how the information gets there as long as it does.
d) We were able to get an excellent resection of this tumor and to save the cingulate without causing any neurologic deficits other than the expected hemianopsia. The important cuts to focus on here are the lateral cuts with the SLF, and the MdLF (both anterior and lateral), and the cut with the posterior body or the corpus callosum, where an over aggressive resection can cut off visual information from the other side. This means that the subcortical mapping does not stop until everything is cleared up to the falx.

14.9.1 Mid-callosal Butterfly Gliomas

Presently, I do not believe these can be resected using any technique I know of without considerable morbidity as I have tried to do so. Given that operating on these tumors involves entering an SMA region or motor region and following the tumor into the corpus callosum (where the crossed FAT is bringing information from the other side), I am not certain that this will be possible using conventional surgery. I am rarely pessimistic that something is actually inoperable, but these are bad tumors without question (in the context of the other tumors we take out in this chapter, this should obviously stand out), and I am not certain we can do much for these patients without a better understanding of the anatomy. Thankfully, these are pretty rare tumors.

14.10 Case Examples

▸ Fig. 14.28 demonstrates a mid callosum butterfly glioma which we attempted to resect awake.

a) This tumor is more posterior than the previous examples, and involves many of the bilateral communication between the motor networks. Thus, the usual strategy of focusing on addressing the tumor in the hemisphere first, risks injurying one SMA, and cutting off the ability to compensate from the other side.
b) The patient developed mutism nearly as soon as we entered the tumor, so we stopped the resection well short of our goal. The mutism did not improve.

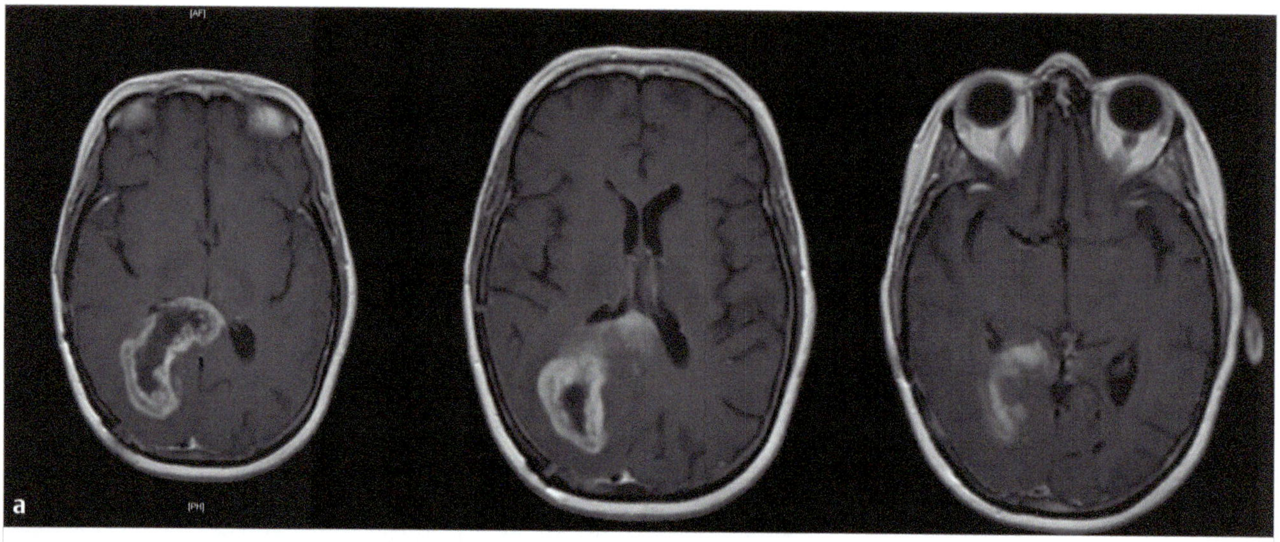

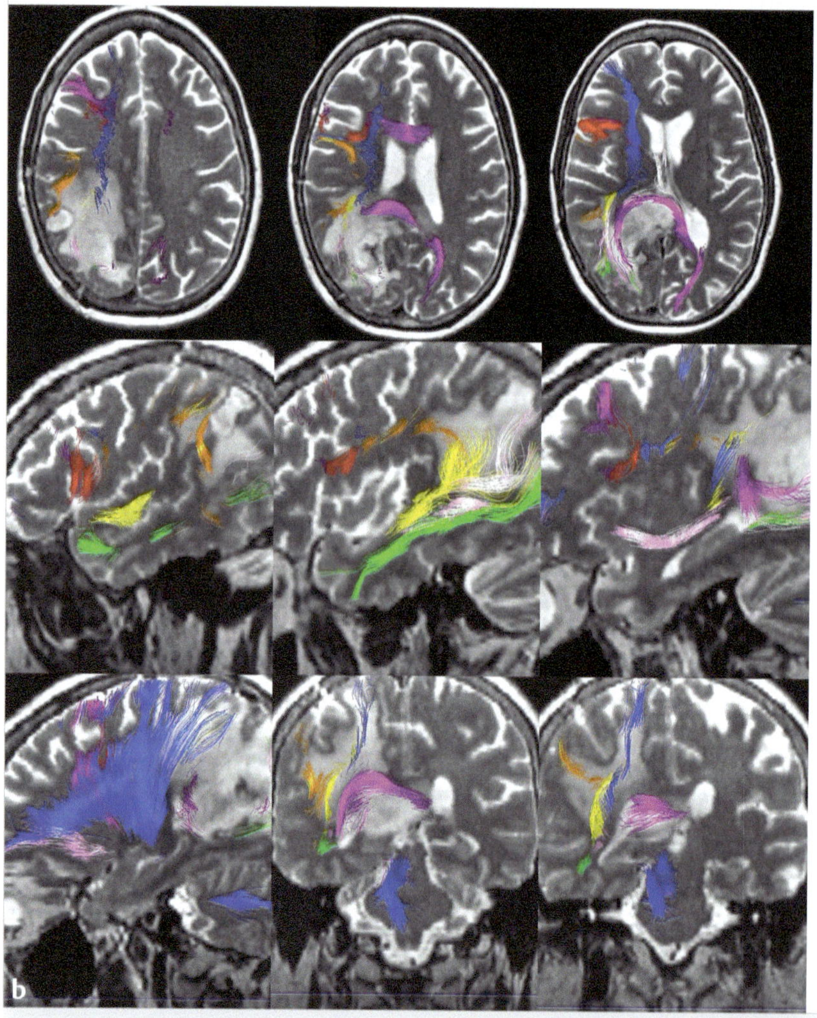

Fig. 14.27 A butterfly glioma following the cuneus fibers into the splenium; (**a**) preoperative images, (**b**) DTI tractography.

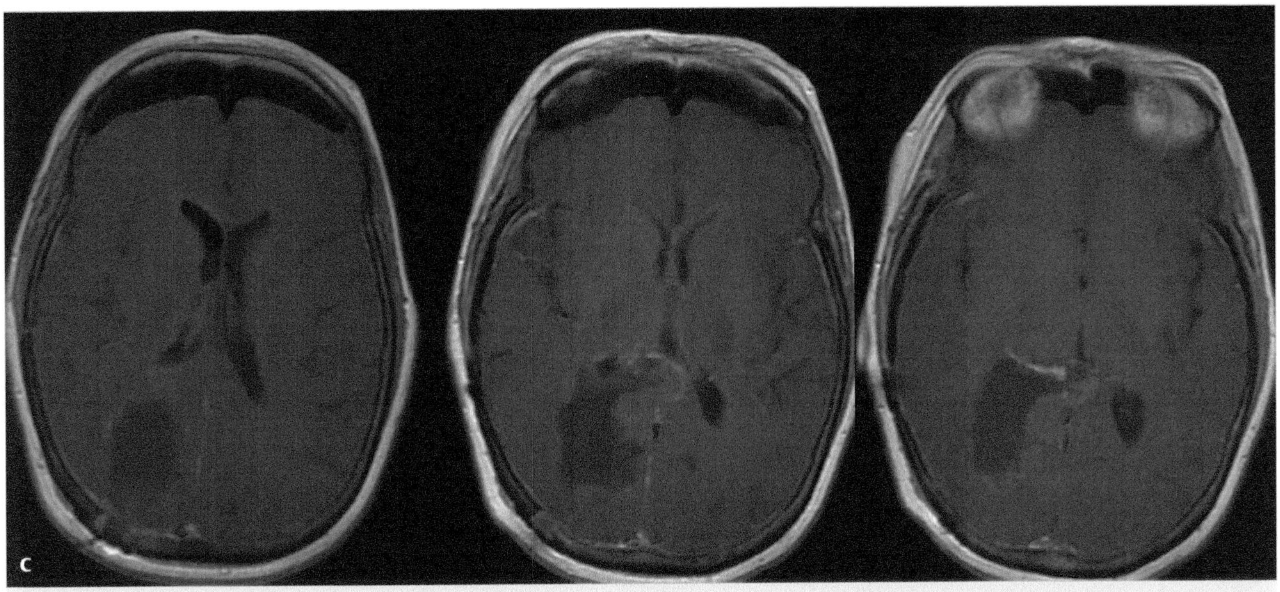

Fig 14.27 (*Continued*) (**c**) Long-term follow-up images.

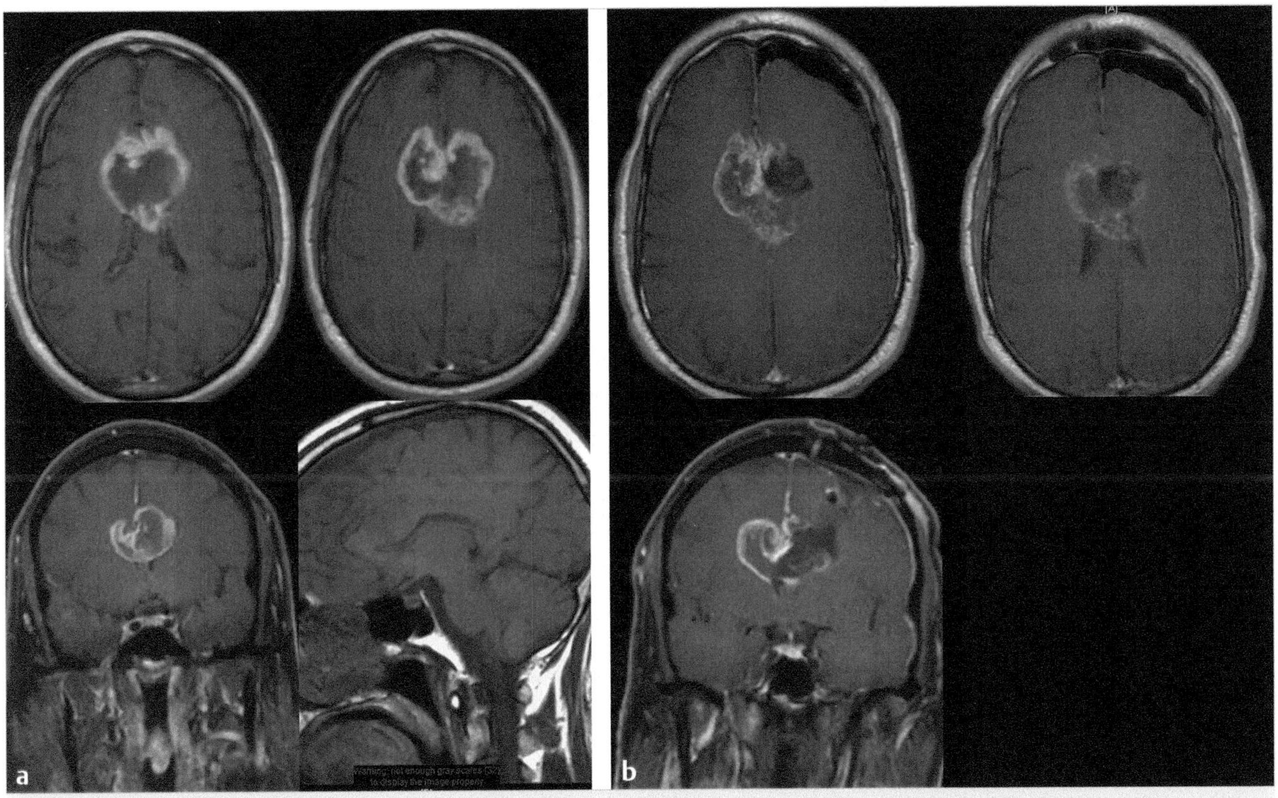

Fig. 14.28 A mid callosum butterfly glioma which we attempted to resect awake; (**a**) preoperative images, (**b**) postoperative images.

▶ Fig. 14.29 demonstrates a cingulate glioma which extends into the mid callosum.

While we entered and removed the middle callosum, as well as the involved cingulum, unlike the other case, this case was able to be resected without disturbing the SMA and motor network, meaning that the callosum was not needed to compensate for the ipsilateral motor network.

a) The preoperative images reveal a large number of challenges in this case. First, the SMA and corpus callosum are involved, as is most of the cingulate gyrus. The best explanation I had for this pattern of spread is that the cingulum gives off fibers into the SFG at places (such as its connection with the DMN cortices) and this tumor is following them, and thus is in both structures. Thankfully, this is uncommon; however, a

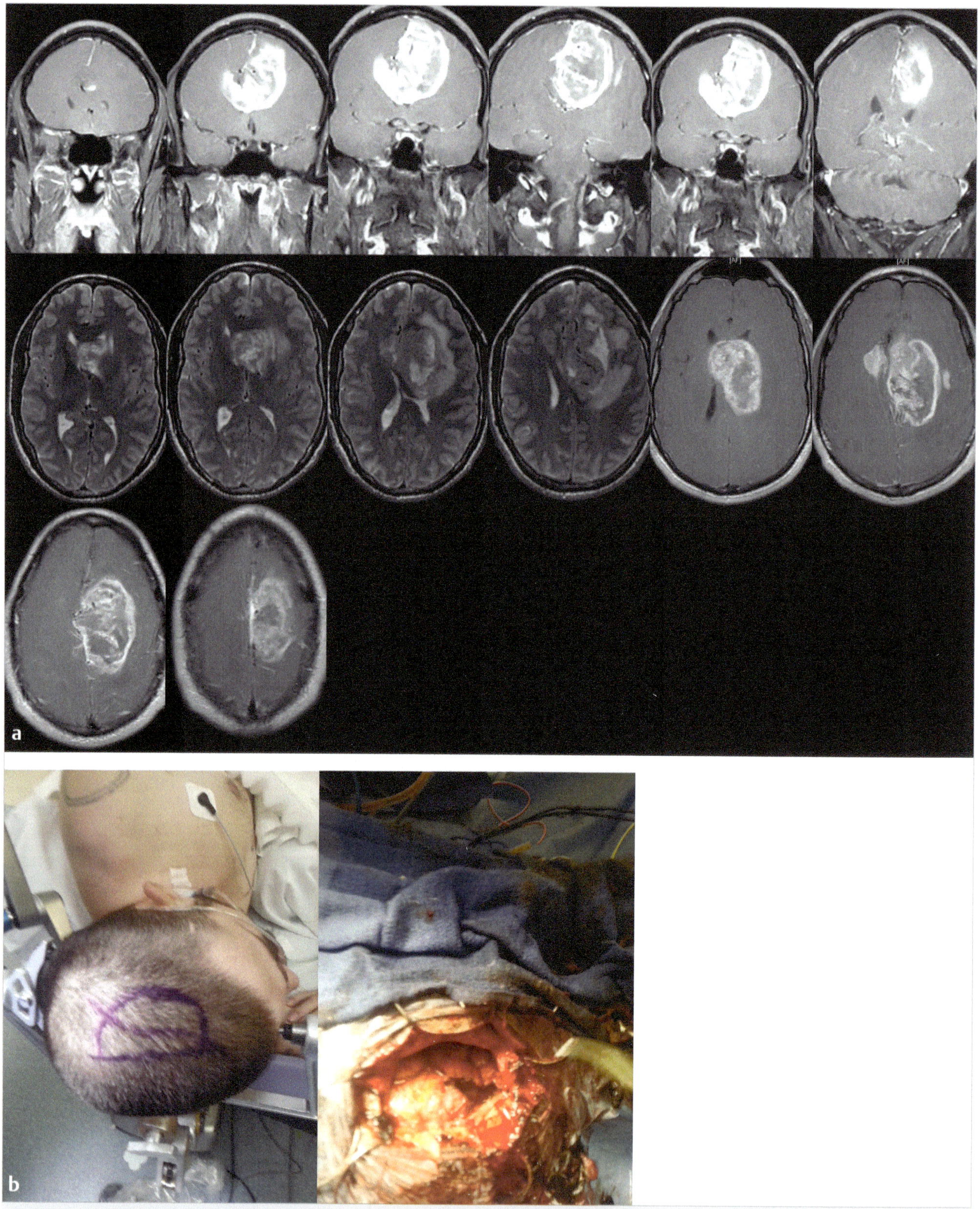

Fig. 14.29 A cingulate glioma which extends into the mid callosum; (**a**) preoperative images, (**b**) images of the approach.

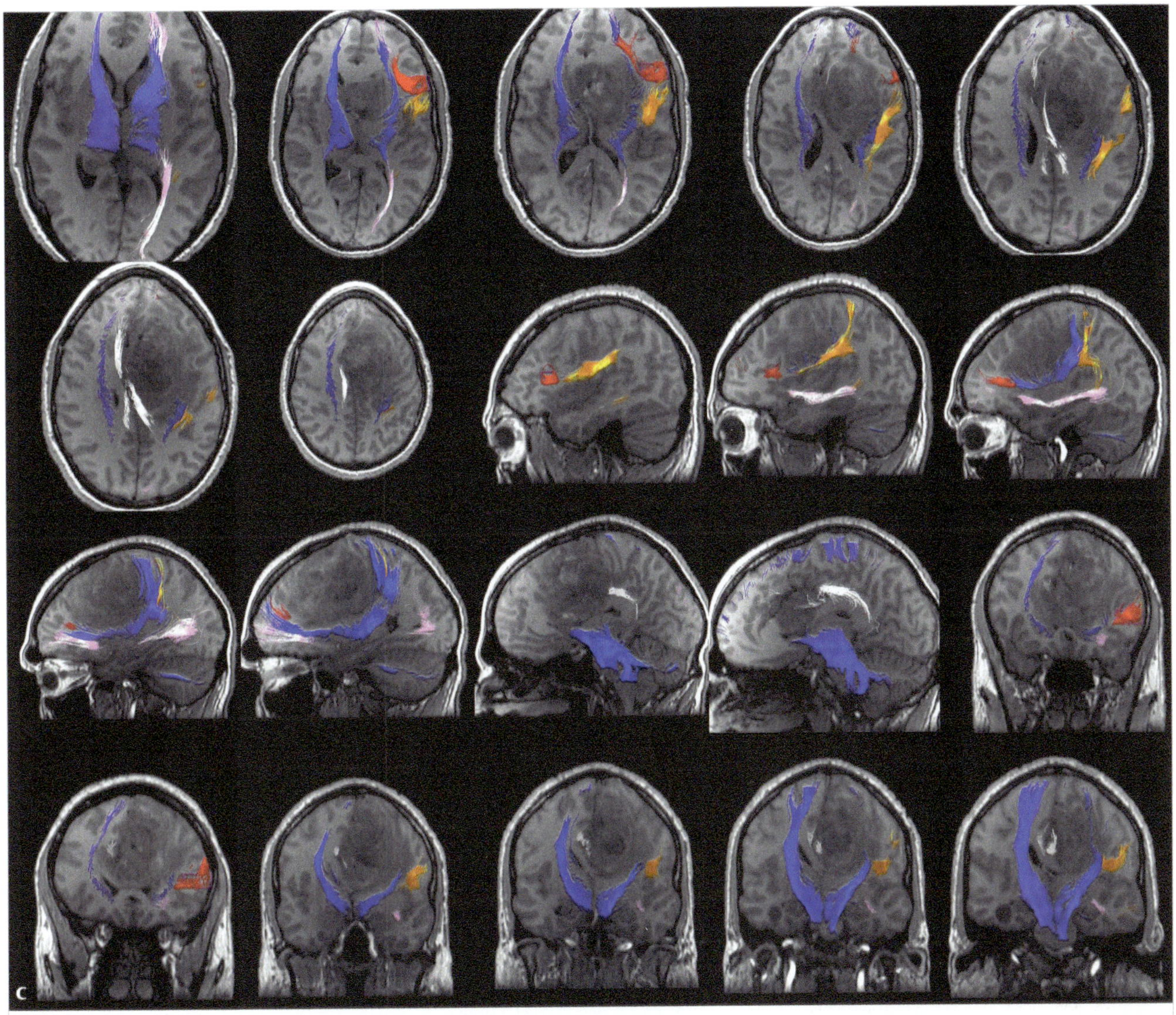

c

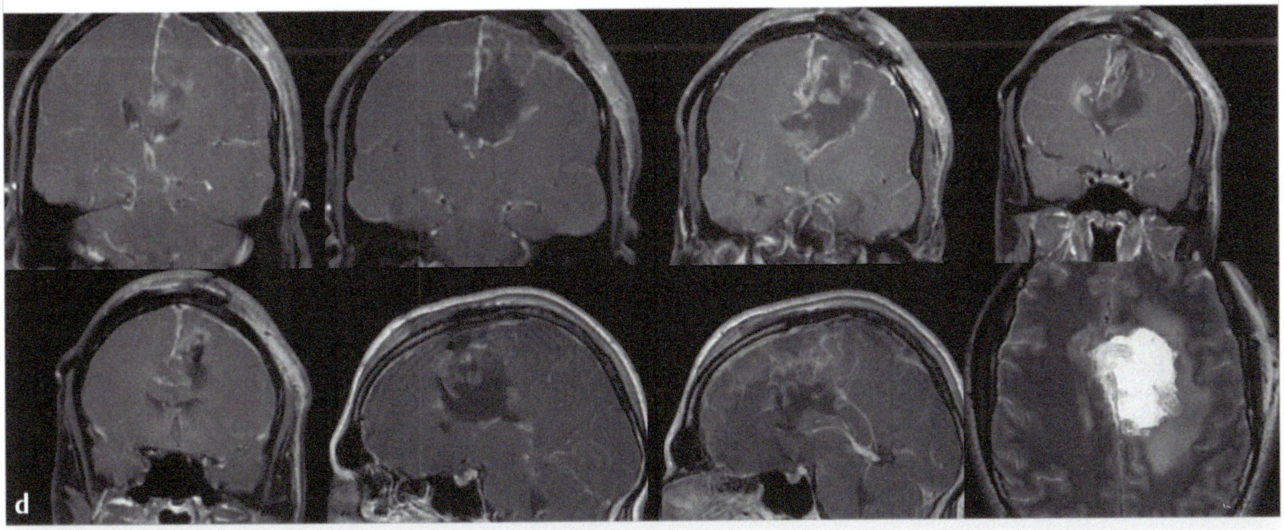

d

Fig 14.29 (*Continued*) (**c**) DTI tractography, (**d**) postoperative images.

case like this is a damage minimization mode, as there are a lot of ways you can wreck this patient's quality of life, and not many ways you can do this case right.

b) The case is approached as a two stage tumor, similar to the description of posterior cingulate tumors in Chapter 13. The first stage is performed similar to a medial/middle third sensorimotor tumor. This both addresses the SFG portion of the tumor, but also provides a good view of the involved cingulate. The second stage involves removing the cingulate gyrus under the sensorimotor area as tolerated. The tumor is separated from the callosum as much as is tolerated, understanding that this part of the callosum is probably quite eloquent after resecting the SFG like this case demands.

c) This tumor has many of the typical features of an SMA tumor. The FAT is pushed anteriorly and does not really go to the SMA at least on tractography. The anterior corticospinal contributions are splayed around the tumor. This is not surprising, but the possibility that some aspect of the FAT is still intact and runs through the tumor should be considered.

d) We were able to get an excellent resection on this tumor. The abulia the patient had preoperative, did not improve, but we did not make it worse. Again, these are very bad cases, and it is difficult to get perfect results.

14.10.1 Basal Ganglia Tumors

Obviously, these are challenging cases, and thankfully gliomas tend not to start in or invade the basal ganglia until they are quite advanced (often not even then). But they do occur, and they can surprisingly be removed with good outcomes if you approach them thoughtfully and apply techniques from other gliomas to these tumors. We have had many of these patients survive for several years even with aggressive tumors at presentation, though obviously we try to provide realistic goals for these patients.

It is without question essential to closely examine the T2 images to determine what structure this is actually located in, to confirm that this tumor is in fact in the basal ganglia and not in a neighboring structure (like the TPO junction, the fornix etc) that is not in the basal ganglia but has pushed itself into expected location of the basal ganglia (I see this mistake made very often), and to deduce the ideal angle to enter the tumor in that minimizes damage to the normal basal ganglia and equally important, minimizes disruption to the connections between basal ganglia structures and/or the thalamus. For example, passing through the anterior limb of the internal capsule is usually a bad idea, but sometimes the tumor has created that cleft, allowing some resection, in that interval. Tractography is equally critical to defining correct windows and planning your attack.

I consider basal ganglia gliomas in two basic types of cases which I approach from different directions:

1. Caudate head tumors: I approach these tumors from a transfrontal approach.
2. Putamen tumors: I approach these through a transopercular transinsular approach.

Thalamic tumors are distinct and discussed as a separate section. They are approached through the superior parietal lobule-transatrial approach.

14.10.2 Caudate Head Tumors

My preferred approach for removing a focal mass from the caudate head (like a cavernoma or a brain metastasis) is the contralateral interhemispheric transcallosal as it provides an excellent view of the caudate head looking straight at its face. This is not how I generally like to do gliomas in this area, as I generally go through the ipsilateral frontal lobe to do so, despite the fact that the angle of attack is somewhat inferior to the contralateral approach. This preference is based on the following observations:

1. A glioma is an area resection not a lesionectomy, and it is important to account for the common patterns of spread in your calculations of what to resect. The principle connections with the caudate head are with the anterior frontal lobe and I have found that this is almost always where the tumors recurred when I tried to remove them via a lesionectomy type approach.
2. An interhemispheric approach involves working past a large amount of dura to get to the target. If you have touched the dura in an awake patient, you know well that this patient is unlikely to cooperate for long in an approach where you are bumping the dura frequently. If there is anywhere I want to have an idea of how the patient is doing to guide my approach, it is in the basal ganglia, so I would rather give up a perfect angle
3. The IFOF and other structures are on the blind side of the contralateral approach, and it is generally disadvantageous to try to separate tumor from an eloquent tract on the blind undersurface of a tumor. I would rather it be on my lateral side of the surgery.

Key Observations (▶ Fig. 14.30)

1. This case begins as a medial transfrontal trajectory through the middle frontal gyrus, as far back as is needed to enter the tumor on the desired angle which minimizes disconnection of the caudate from the rest of the deep structures. The mapping and subcortical work are the same; however, we are generally not here to perform a lobectomy as the anatomic resection is focused on the superior and anterior shell of white matter around the caudate nucleus where the fibers are exiting. If you are concerned about cutting through this brain to get there, remember that these are the primary targets of the caudate head and you are essentially cutting them when you enter the middle frontal gyrus anyway.
2. Similar to butterfly gliomas, you need to widely open the frontal horn and orient yourself to the anatomy and the tumor location. Note that it is common to have a behavioral arrest when you drain the ventricle, so I give the patient a break when I am doing this.
3. Basal ganglia parenchyma looks like glioma. It is greyish red, it bleeds a lot, and it is soft and suckable compared to normal white matter and cortex. Often the only way to reliably tell the difference are the faint white spots of the basal ganglia, the texture of necrosis, and a general gestalt of where the tumor is relative to the parenchyma.
4. Point three and the fact that touching the caudate head often causes behavioral arrests should highlight the fact that these tumors require patience.

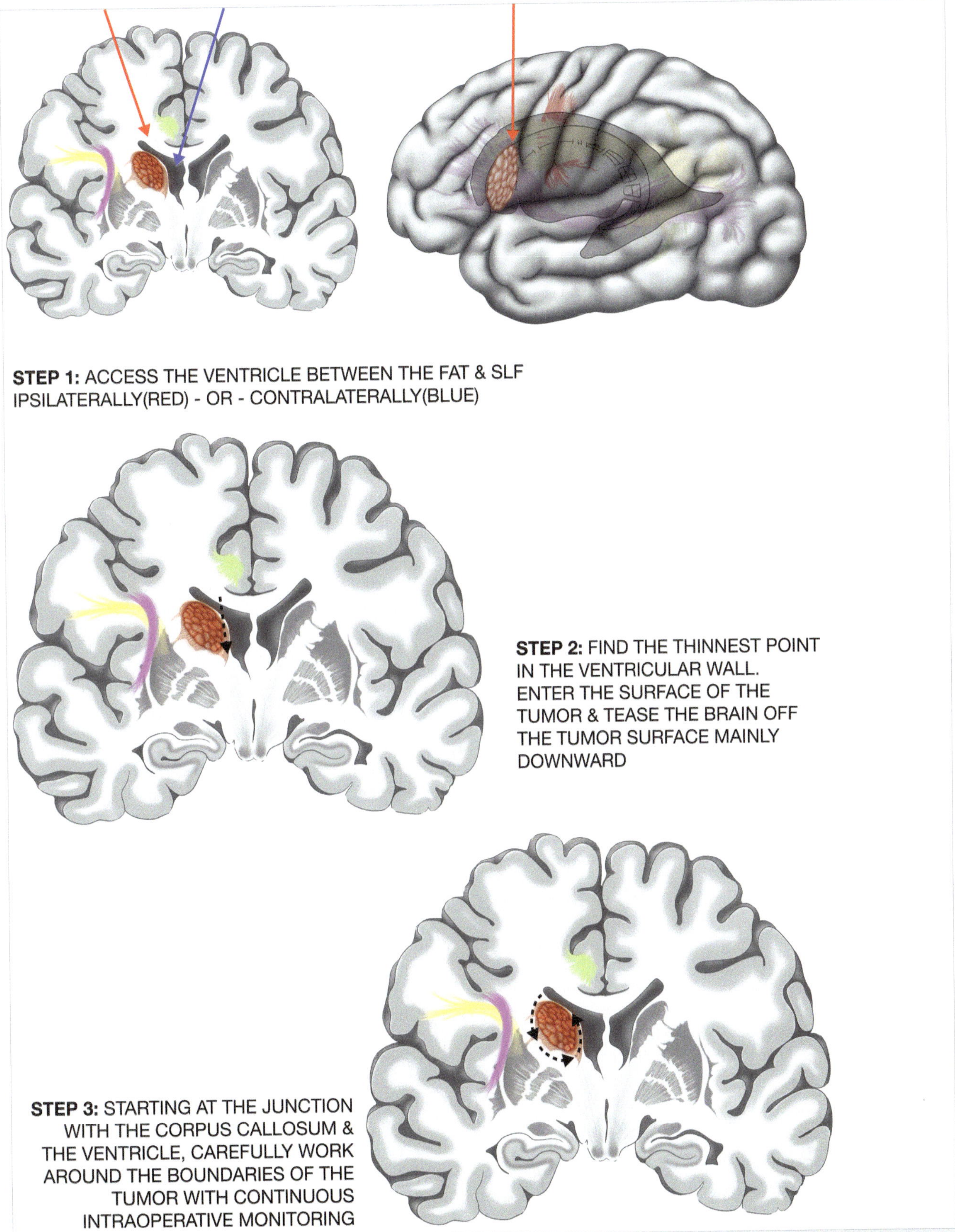

Fig. 14.30 This figure demonstrates the technique for removal of tumors from the head of the caudate. The approach is trans frontal, similar to a medial frontal surgery. Once you have entered the ventricle and identified the caudate head, you should carefully select an appropriate entry point and slowly and carefully remove caudate tumor.

5. Any medium-sized artery in this area should be assumed to be a lenticostriate and preserved. This often means leaving tumor and especially necrosis, but obviously increasing the extent of resection by 5% and causing a deep stroke is not a good trade off and these vessels are very sensitive to manipulation.
6. The task of choice is anything that requires attention, but our favorite is combining the peg board and naming in a high complexity double task. The mapping gives you courage to continue when it seems like you are doing something crazy, and also helps guide you to not do something crazy.

14.11 Case Examples

▶ Fig. 14.31 shows a caudate tumor I did asleep early in my series through a contralateral interhemispheric transcallosal approach.

This approach provides an excellent view and avoids the white matter en route; however, you cannot map the patient and this approach does not provide an easy way to address spread out of the caudate head. The resection and outcome were good, but I think a better resection can be done via a transfrontal approach.

a) In cases like these, it is essential to carefully examine the T2 images to find the least damaging approach into the tumor. While the shortest approach is usually the best, a slightly longer approach which avoids internal disconnections in the basal ganglia structures or transgression of the internal capsule is infinitely better tolerated than a short approach through these connections. In this specific case, the best route appears to be demonstrated by the provided T2 coronal image in this figure. The caudate head and putamen are largely pushed superolaterally and the tumor is accessible though a thinned part of the caudate inferiorly.
b) None.
c) None.
d) There is a thin rim of tumor around the edges of the cavity, but I was reasonably happy with how much we were able to get out.

▶ Fig. 14.32 demonstrates an awake transfrontal method of resecting a recurrent caudate GBM.

a) I had done the previous surgery asleep via a more lateral transfrontal approach about 18 months prior to this and had done a good resection (the films are less informative, so I have omitted them for space reasons); however, at this point, the tumor has exited the caudate into the frontal lobe entering the infraorbital cortex and with some extension towards the middle frontal gyrus. The plan is to utilize a medial frontal type resection to address the tumor radiating out from the caudate head into the frontal lobe, and then to follow the tumor into the caudate as tolerated, with plans to be cautious with these radiated lenticulostriates which are inside the tumor.
b) I performed an awake medial frontal lobe resection and followed this into the caudate. I removed tumor until I encountered the lenticulostriates and stopped after removing about 90% of the tumor.
c) The most informative DTI images is the coronal image second from the lower right. This demonstrates the "back wall" of the frontal lobe made up of the FAT and IFOF. This left IFOF, and the naming problems we encountered when we approached this, were the limiting aspects of the lateral cut in the orbitofrontal cortex.
d) Overall, the resection is good, while a thin rind of tumor was left as planned on the lenticulostriates, we have removed the majority of the enhancement and addressed the pathways of spread out of the caudate nucleus. This is the best state we can put this patient in given his starting point.
e) The patient was entered into an immunotherapy trial and responded well. At the time of this writing, he is alive three years after diagnosis. Thus, while basal ganglia gliomas are unquestionably a bad disease, good results are possible in these patients if we try.

14.11.1 Putamen Region Tumors

Basic Anatomic Considerations

Obviously, safely entering the putamen is a substantial challenge given the diffuse inputs and outputs passing between the putamen and the parts of the cortex, and the number of critical structures and pathways interposed between the surface and target. Careful study of tract anatomy will demonstrate that almost any attempt to enter the basal ganglia and deep core from the superolateral brain is highly likely to encounter at least some of the SLF complex, if not the core of the tracts. A very anteriorly originating frontal transcortical approach paralleling the SLF can access this, but this is a long approach in a deep hole, and without a clot to do some of the dissection, this involves a long path into treacherous ground. A temporal approach is not only mechanically disadvantaged (you have to work back on yourself) but also puts the IFOF at risk.

In most of these cases, the best route I have found into these cases has been through the insula. This is obviously challenging, but a review of tract anatomy demonstrates that this route provides a route which protects the SLF and IFOF, and minimizes injury to white matter connections to the putamen and other deep structures.

Key Points (▶ Fig. 14.33)

1. There is no role for skimping on exposure, which is at a premium in this part of the brain. If a part of the STG maps negative, it should go. You should tease the superior opercula upward to access the circular sulcus. Once you have identified windows into the insula, you should resect insular cortex to define the boundaries of the tumor. Failure to find anatomy in this case can equal disaster, as there is very little to guide you when operating this deep in the brain.
2. In an inverse of anatomic considerations for cases when approaching from the temporal side, the bottom of this tumor is the temporal horn (remember from the chapter on temporal lobe tumors that the roof of the temporal horn is the bottom of putamen, here we are exploiting this fact to know where the bottom of the putamen is).
3. Often these tumors abut the atrium, which can be used as a posterior boundary.
4. Obviously, this is a lesionectomy and care should be taken to tell tumor from basal ganglia tissue, as they can look similar.

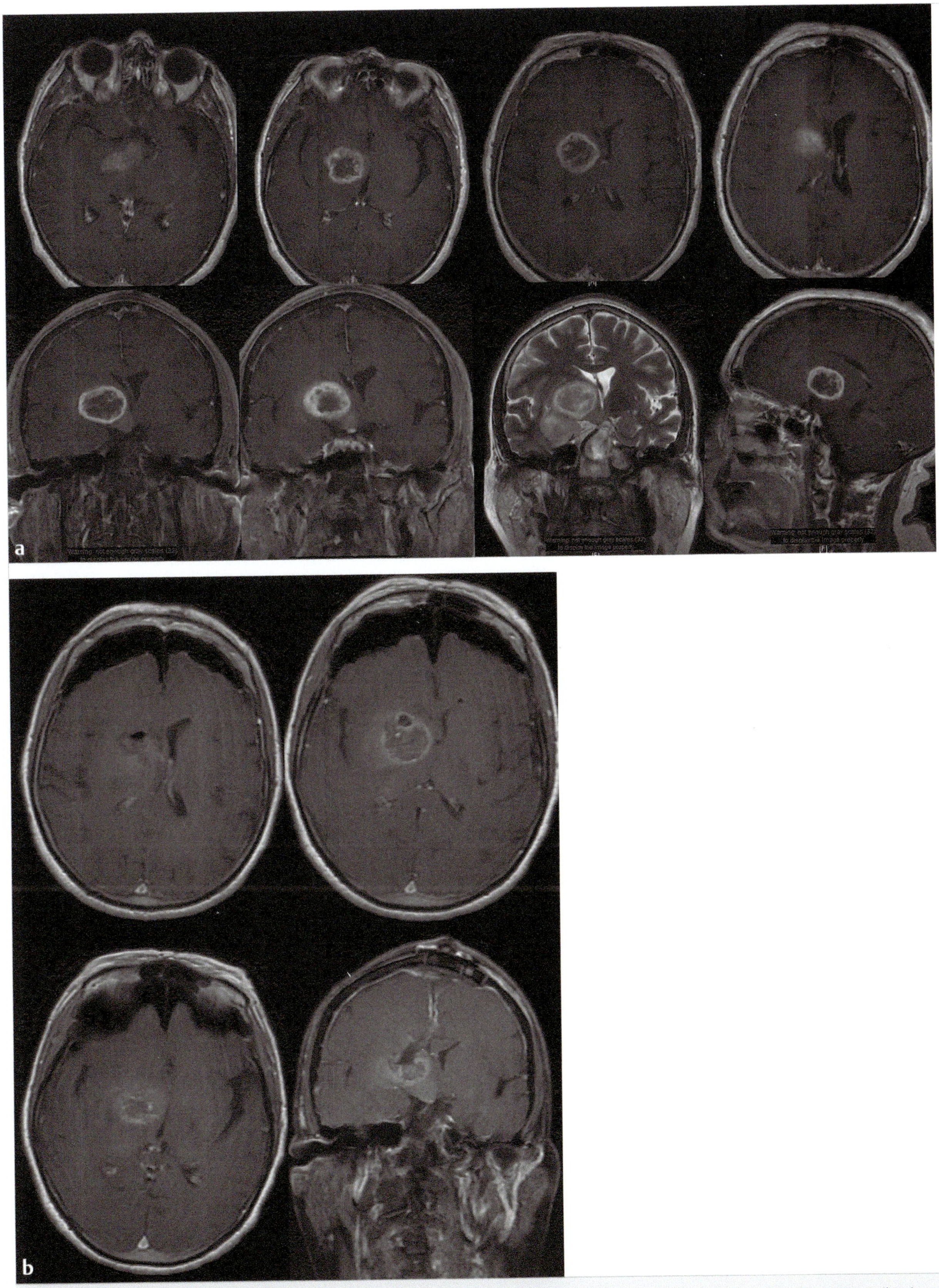

Fig. 14.31 A caudate tumor operated on while patient is asleep early in my series through a contralateral interhemispheric transcallosal approach; (**a**) preoperative images, (**b**) postoperative images.

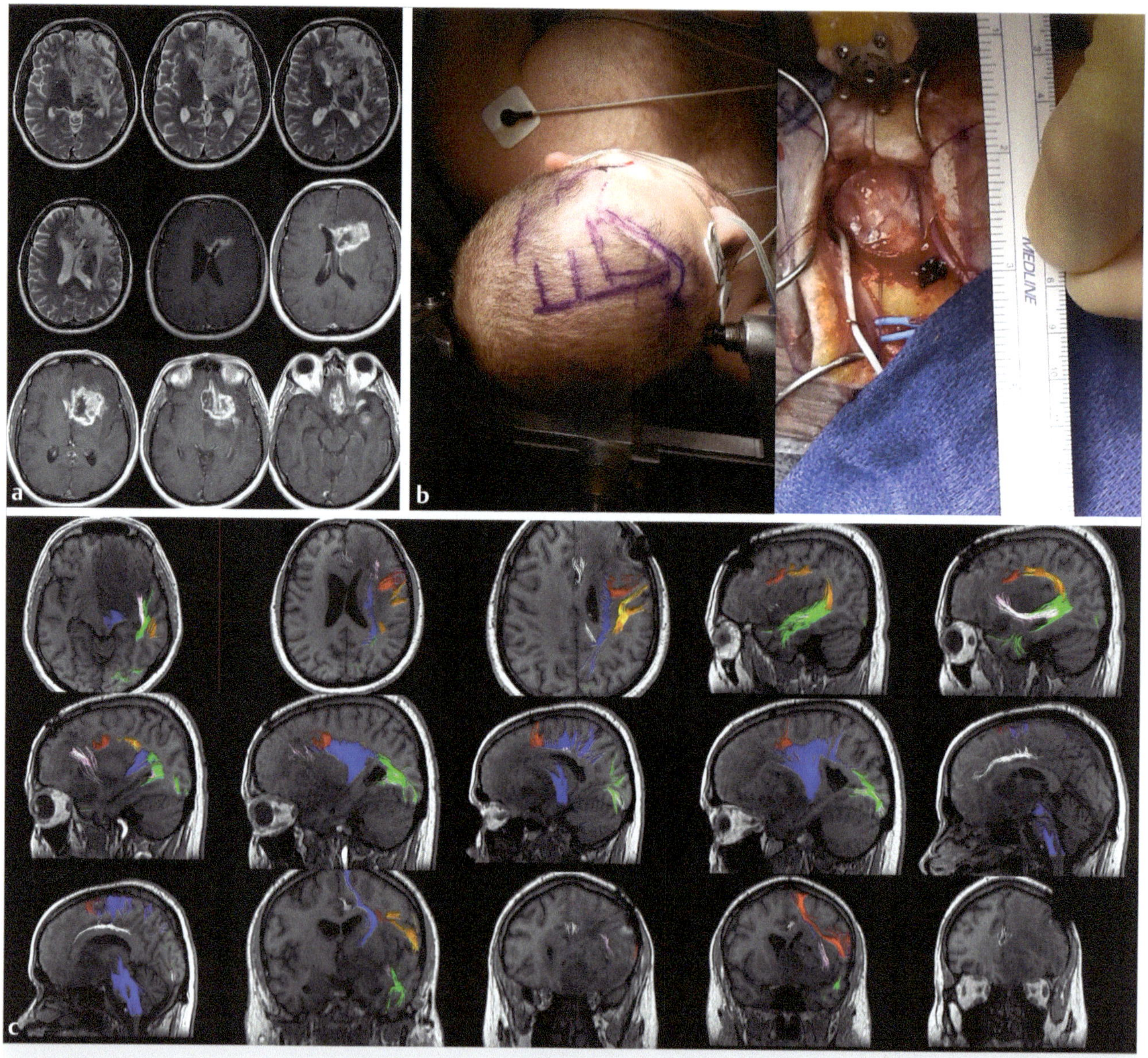

Fig. 14.32 An awake transfrontal method of resecting a recurrent caudate GBM; (a) preoperative images, (b) images of the approach, (c) DTI tractography.

5. As with caudate tumors, small vessels are highly likely to be lenticuliostriates and should be left alone.
6. The descending motor fibers are both medial and also superior to the tumor and this must be considered.

14.12 Case Examples

▸ Fig. 14.34 demonstrates a GBM in the putamen with a symptomatic cyst which someone has put an Omaya reservoir in without success. Shunting or serially draining tumor cysts are seldom as effective at controlling the cyst as is removing the tumor, which I did via a transopercular transinsular approach. There is some opercular subarachnoid hemorrhage from removing the Omaya.

a) This tumor has a small repeatedly symptomatic cyst on its deep surface which has an inserted omaya catheter which has failed to keep the symptoms from coming back. The likely origin of this cyst is the enhancing nodule on the lateral edge of the wall. It is clearly deep to the insula which has some T2 changes. The plan is to use the insula as a route into the tumor, which will be dissected free on all its borders ending in the cyst.
b) The exposure is planned by mapping out the location of the insula and planning which opercular resections will give us adequate access to the insula such that we can make a circumfrencial cut around the nodule and enter the cyst so that the enhancing nodule falls out. Due to speech considerations, we only removed a small portion of STG and because of this; we split the Sylvian fissure to maximize the exposure we could obtain. Unlike an insular glioma, we are using the insula resection as a route not the endpoint, so it's less essential that we identify all of the boundaries of the circular sulcus; however, this is a deep tumor, so you also need to make sure you resect enough of the insular cortex to see what you are

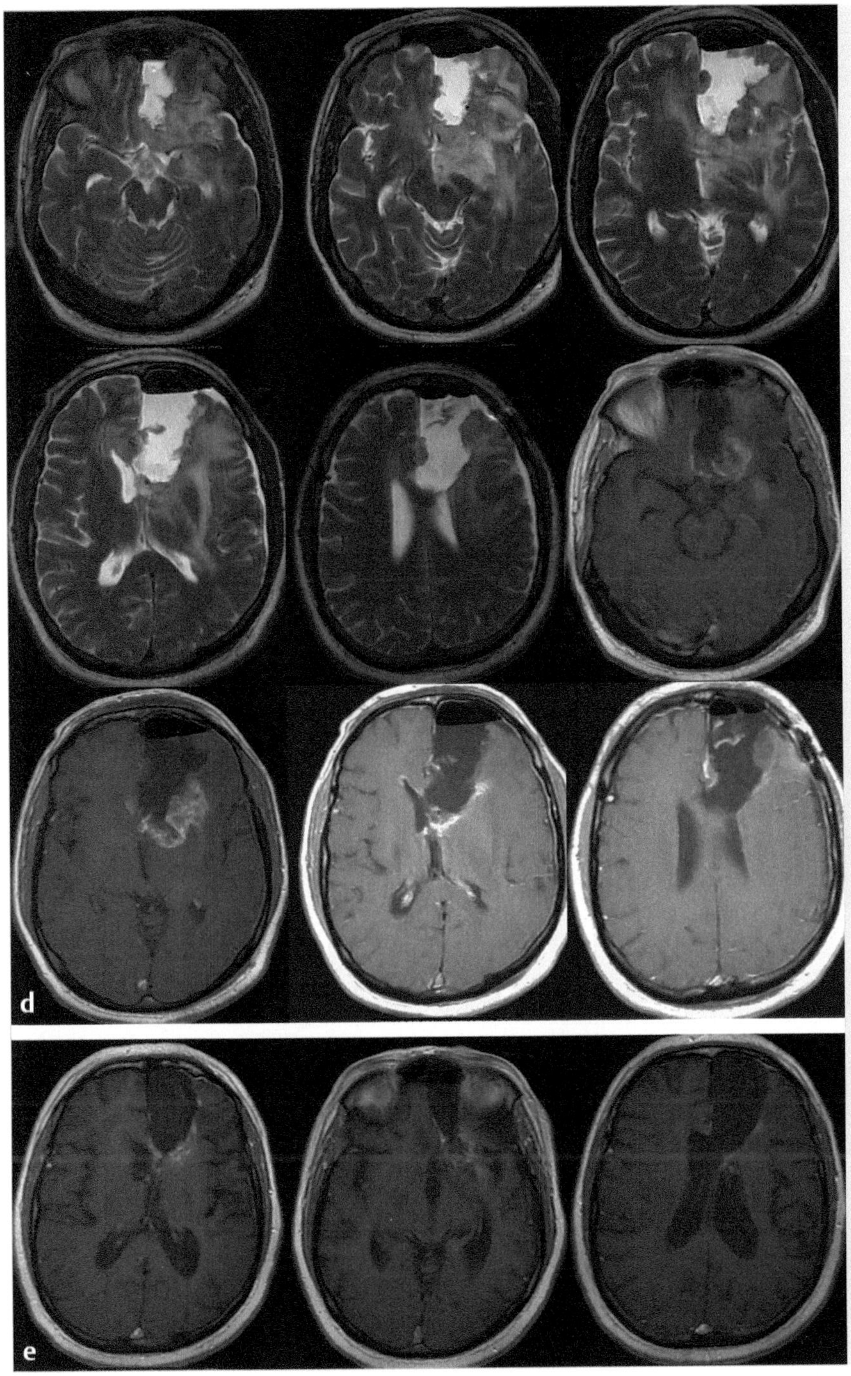

Fig 14.32 (*Continued*) (**d**) Postoperative images, (**e**) long-term follow-up images.

doing and to provide slack on the MCA branches to work comfortably between and around them.

c) None.

d) The resection of the nodule is reasonably good; however, there is a fair bit of blood in the cavity and this makes it more difficult to care for patients like this as it makes it hard to work out how much residual disease was left, and thus what is recurrence. This is especially true with insular tumors, where hemostasis can be very tedious and time consuming. It is very hard to asssess the extent of resection accurately in a bloody cavity in the insula. In general, even in these deep tumors, you should aspire to get the surgical cavities as dry as possible, for more than just safety reasons, but also it is helpful for the long term management of these patients.

▶ Fig. 14.35 demonstrates a GBM in the internal capsule. Remarkably, we were able to remove this without weakness, leaving only a small remnant in the descending motor fibers.

a) The single most critical question in a case like this—after you have determined that this is actually not in the insula or fornix, but instead really is as bad as you initially thought and is in the basal ganglia or capsule—is what is the least bad route into the tumor. In this case the transinsular route is somewhat complicated by the presence of a thin layer of putamen

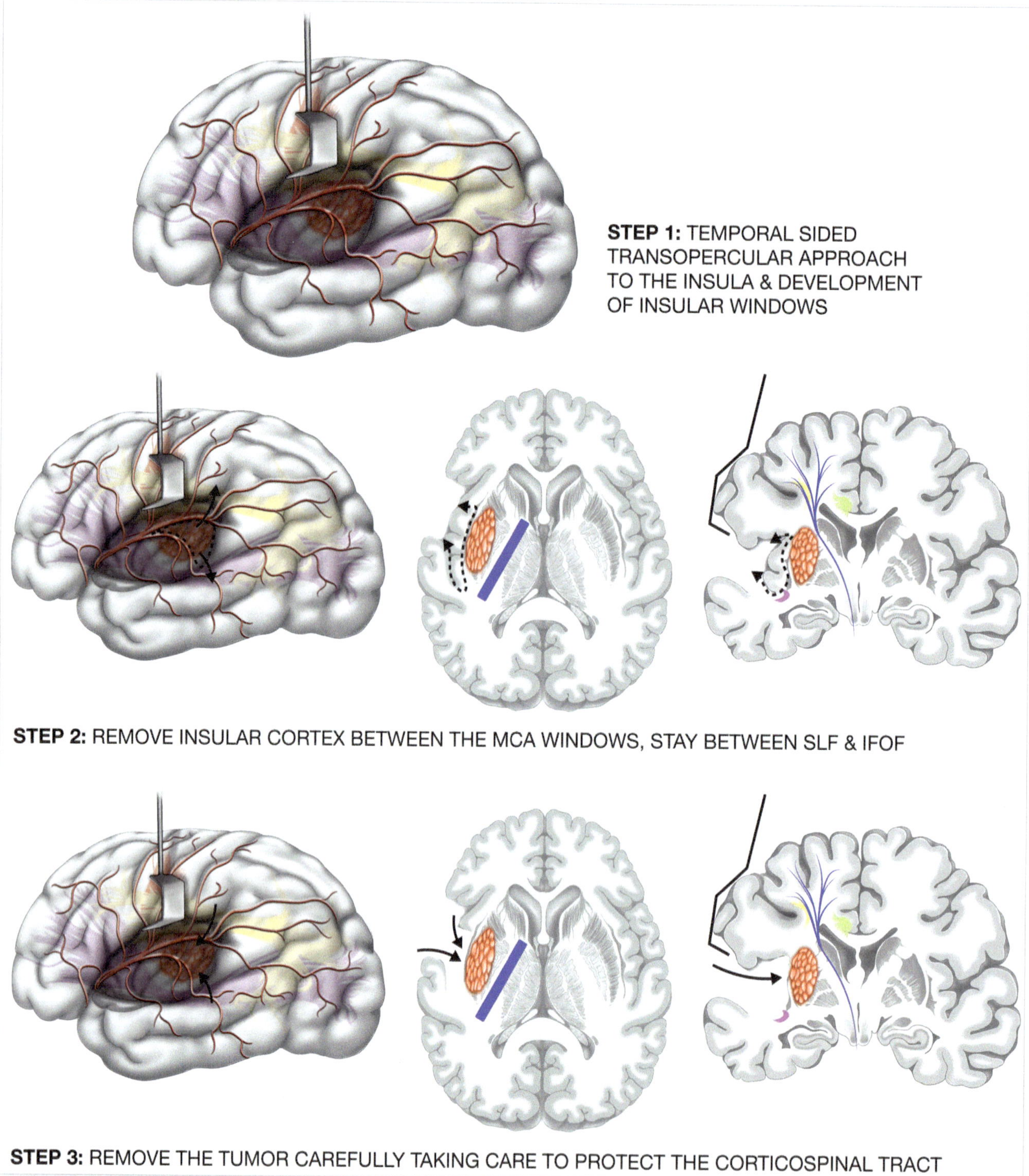

Fig. 14.33 This figure demonstrates the technique for removal of tumors from the head of the putamen. The approach begins with a transtemporal approach to the insula, which as described in Chapter 12, involves elevating frontoparietal opercula after removing as much of the the STG as possible. After defining and creating windows into the insula, you need to first work on the posterior and inferior border of the tumor until you find the temporal horn and atrium, which gives you landmarks in this deep area. The rest of the resection is a lesionectomy guided by mapping.

overlying the lateral surface of lesion, making the best angle a posterior to anterior one. This is a much more difficult angle which requires tangling with the junctional white matter and the SMG to an extent. While this involves adding a difficult approach to a difficult case, the only other option is to use a superior parietal lobule trans atrial approach, and entering the deep white matter lateral to the thalamus from angle while still staying medial to the SLF is likely not possible.

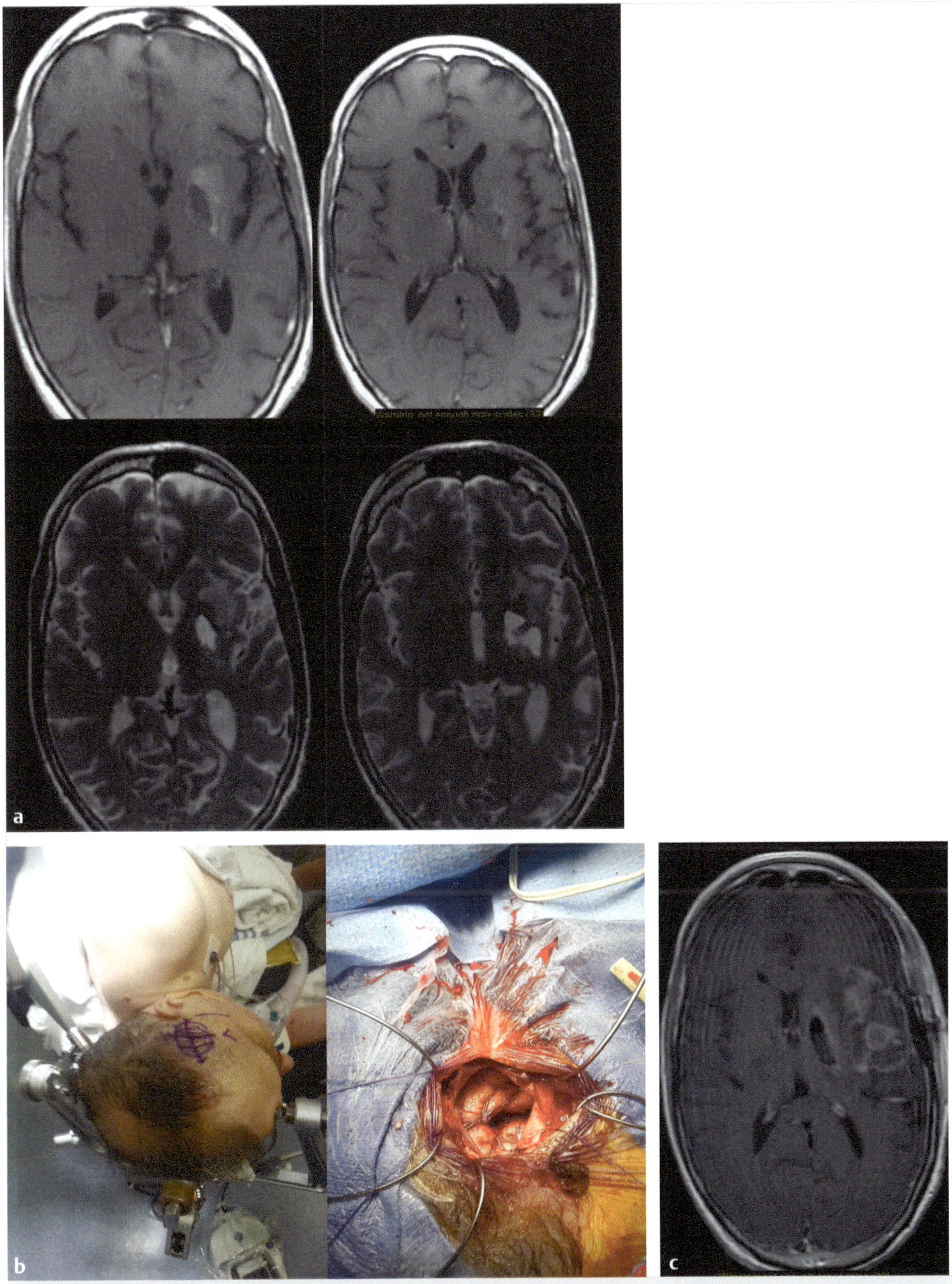

Fig. 14.34 A GBM in the putamen with a symptomatic cyst which someone has put an Omaya reservoir in without success; (a) preoperative images, (b) images of the approach, (c) postoperative images.

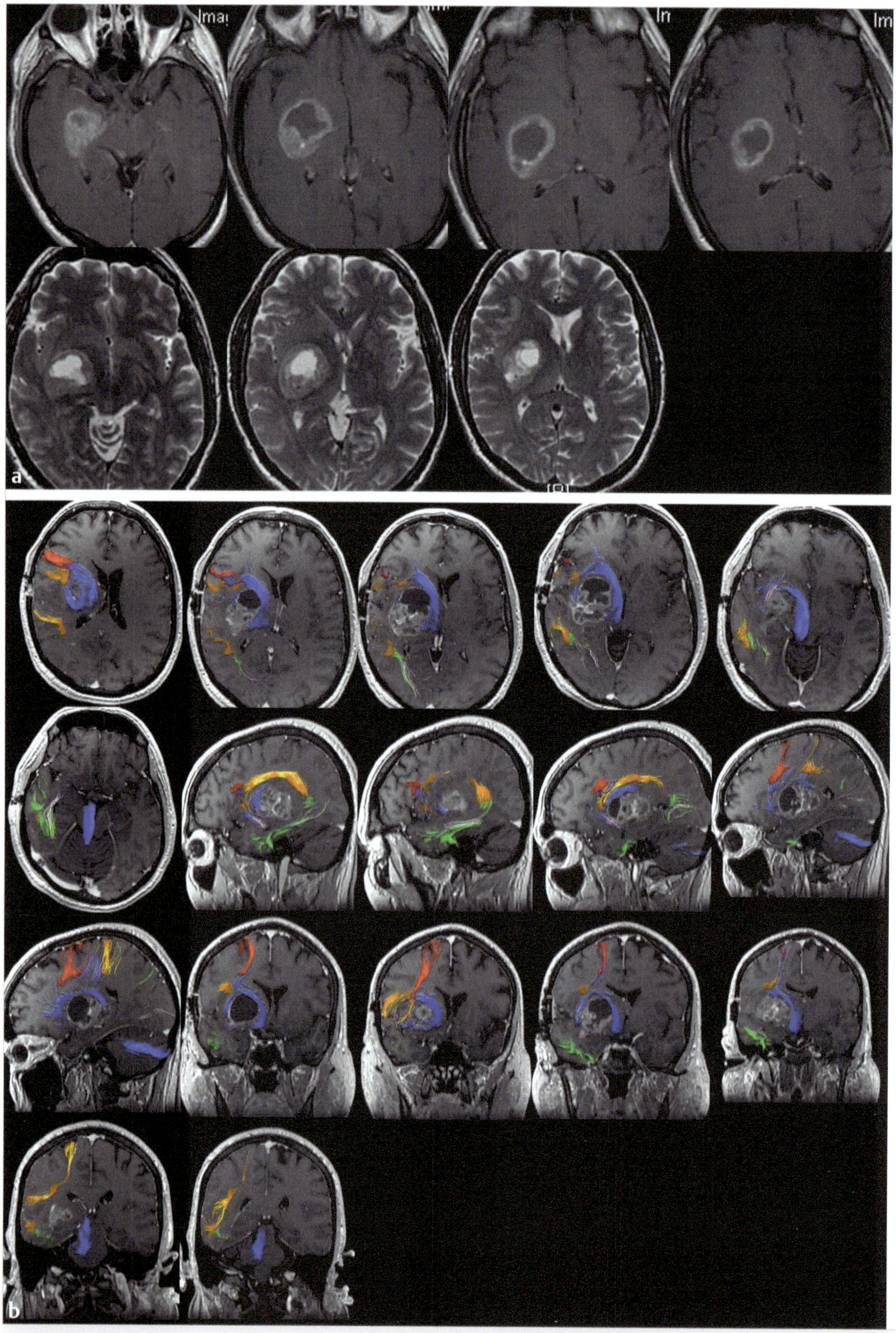

Fig. 14.35 A GBM in the internal capsule; (a) preoperative images, (b) DTI tractography.

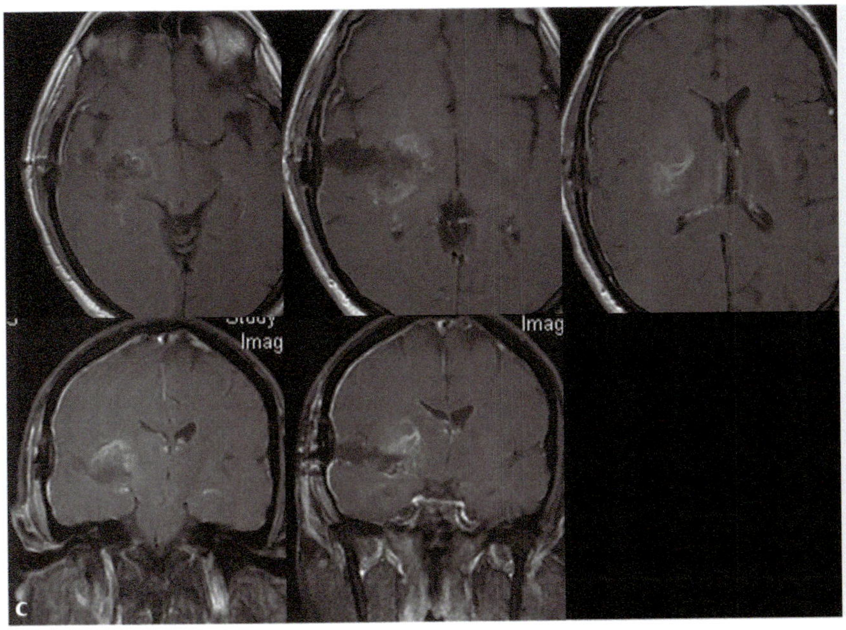

Fig 14.35 *(Continued)* (**c**) Postoperative images.

Thus, my plan was to remove the STG/SMG to create as big a window into the posterior insula as neglect mapping would allow, and to use this as a route into this tumor.

b) None.

c) The tractography shows that while the posterior window into this tumor is small, the SLF does not seem to go so far into the temporal lobe that this is impossible. The motor fibers are blanketed over the tumor, as is obvious from the coronal and sagittal images, which makes slow lesionectomy the only real option without paralysis. The IFOF seems to be low enough to give us some window into the tumor over the top. A field cut is probably certain entering this far back in the insula; however, the motor fibers seem more anterior than posterior.

d) This is about as good of a resection without paralyzing the patient (who walked out of the hospital the next day) as I could have realistically hoped for. There is some tumor anteriorly and superiorly which was left after stimulation suggested that fibers were running through those parts of the tumor. The key landmark in this cases is to continue until you enter the temporal horn and atrium from above and anteriorly, as this tells you have gone low enough.

14.12.1 Thalamic Gliomas

I will start this last section with a disclaimer that I do not have all the answers to thalamic tumors, as obviously this is a very bad place to have a glioma. I do think they are possible, and I have removed them with acceptable outcomes, though I am not sure a perfect outcome is possible for most of these cases. It is important to note that a lack of perfection does not imply that nothing can be done, and that it is best to leave the tumor growing in the thalamus as a way of avoiding a field cut: the natural history is abysmal for these patients. I admit, however, that these cases are a work in an earlier stage of evolution than say, butterfly tumors where I am more confident about what to do, and how to avoid problems. In part this is simply because they are less common. In a practice doing about 500 brain tumor surgeries a year, I presently average about 3–4 thalamic gliomas per year versus around 75–100 temporo-insular tumors, and 20 butterfly tumors per year. So it's a lot harder to refine technique on something you don't see very often.

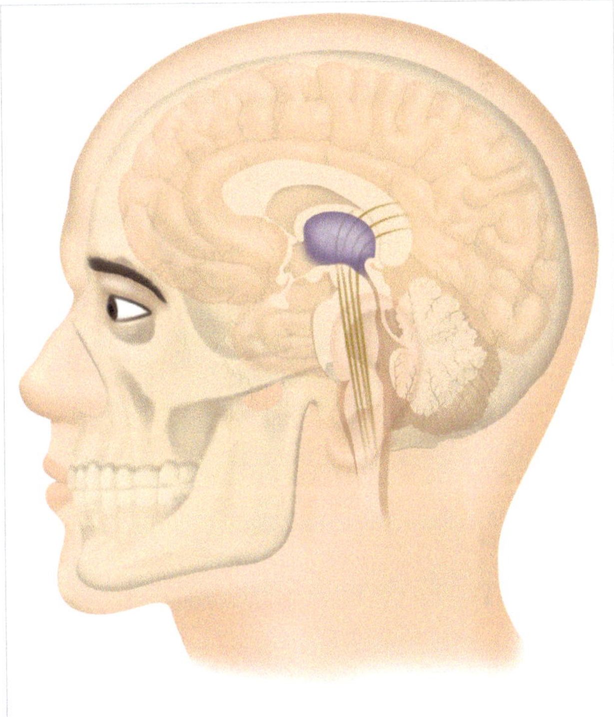

Fig. 14.36 White matter relations of the thalamus to surrounding structures.

What follows are observations on these tumors, with the hopes of stimulating further discussion.

Anatomic Considerations (▶ Fig. 14.36)

A quick glance at the thalamus suggests that there are three possible routes to physically enter the thalamus: lateral (i.e., transtemporal), posterior (transparietal-transatrial), and superomedial (transcallosai-transventricular). Knowledge of white matter anatomy suggests that the lateral route is generally a bad idea, unless the tumor has created this path for you somehow. Coming from the side to access the thalamus at minimum risks the SLF, the semantic areas, the IFOF, the optic radiations, the basal ganglia, and the back of the internal capsule. Further the angle is usually completely off the tumor's long axis.

The transcallosal route is anatomically acceptable as it does not transgress white matter pathways (other than the callosum) to get to the tumor. I personally do not use this as the large dural exposure and positioning of this approach makes mapping difficult or impossible, and I personally need the patient feedback to keep an eye on this very high risk case. Also, I find it difficult from this angle to judge how lateral I am in the inferolateral quadrant and temporal horn. As I explain below, failure to maintain patency of the temporal horn can take these cases from success to failure in a hurry. So I think it's a decent angle, I just don't think it's the best one.

I favor the transparietal transatrial approach to the thalamus. It is simple, fast and can be done in awake patients. The approach stays medial to the SLF, works in the interval between the SLF and cingulum, between the motor and visual systems, in an area which tends to be bilaterally compensated. Once familiar it is easy to stay oriented. It enters the thalamus in the pulvinar where these tumors often present to the surface (as opposed to the medial dorsal nucleus where they often do not approach the surface). Finally, and more subtly the angle is anterior to posterior, which makes it harder to drift inferiorly into the subthalamus and midbrain, which is more of a tendency with a superior to inferior angle acquired transcallosally.

What Are the Key Disasters in Thalamic Surgery?

If we are going to try to remove tumors from the thalamus, it is critical to not just say that operating in the thalamus is dangerous and stop there, but rather to specifically identify what is dangerous and why, and also to address things that are not really dangerous.

To my knowledge, I am the only person I know of who operates in the thalamus in awake patients (I apologize if someone else does but when I started doing this I looked in the literature for advice and found nothing). What was interesting when I first started doing awake surgery in the thalamus was that stimulating or manipulating thalamic tissue did not induce obvious problems with the patient's function, a finding I have repeatedly observed in every patient I have operated in. Importantly, despite its reputation as a seat of consciousness, disturbing the thalamus does not turn the lights out, paralyze someone, or wreck their attention or cognition (though if they do not have a field cut this may cause one.

I would suggest that the greater risk comes from damage to the ascending neurotransmitter systems (like locus ceruleus, etc), midbrain reticular activating system and subthalamic structures below the tumor. Damaging these structures can turn the lights out. Further, the lateral and superior borders contain the thalamic peduncle and the internal capsule. It is likely that one day we will understand the thalamus better that this, but at presently, my main goal is to prevent myself from drifting out of the thalamus, because the jungle is outside, not inside.

Thus, safety in the thalamus involves thinking of yourself working in a three-sided tunnel. The walls involve the internal capsule, the consciousness connections, and the densest thalamic outflow. The only safe areas are the medial wall to enter the third ventricle, and the temporal horn and its proximity.

The Unique Challenges

In my experience with these tumors, the events which happen outside the OR, before and after the surgery, often dictate success and failure more than the surgery. A few observations follow about events which I have experienced which are unique to this case.

1. These patients enter often with edema in the deep white matter and midbrain. If they are exposed to any anesthesia whatsoever, there is a real chance they will be overly sensitive to it, and will not map. I stress this to the anesthesiologist, as even low doses of medications may take hours to clear in these patients.
2. It is well known that glioma edema worsens temporarily after surgery. In the frontal lobe, this may cause abulia or speech problems which resolve. In the thalamus, the edema causes a very long time in the hospital, collecting complications and not getting radiotherapy. To prevent this, I argue that it is essential to dry these patients out for a few days prior to surgery to blunt the spike of edema before it happens. This is key to a faster recovery, and to lock in a victory with radiotherapy.
3. You must, must, must keep the temporal horn open in these cases. You should work to widely open the horn by removing tumor. It is also the only case where I leave a ventricular drain at the end to prevent even small amounts of blood from blocking the horn. A blocked horn can become the anchor which drags down the boat of a successful case.

Key Points (▶ Fig. 14.37)

1. The fornix is crossing your path from this angle. It is critical to keep the choroid plexus identifiable to keep yourself oriented to the plane of the fornix.
2. If you have not seen the third ventricle you have left a fair bit of tumor.
3. You need to map motor and or SLF functions as you extend laterally and/or superiorly.
4. The posteromedial boundary is defined by looking medially over the fornix and working until you see the pineal region and/or the Galenic vein
5. Do not stop in the inferoposterior quadrant until the temporal horn is widely clear.
6. Be careful and good luck.

14.13 Case Examples

▶ Fig. 14.38 demonstrates one of my earlier cases of a thalamic GBM done asleep.

a) A few observations. This tumor is quite big, but much of it is necrotic. It is unlikely that a lot of this tumor is at risk for eloquent fibers. This makes it likely that we will get a fair piece

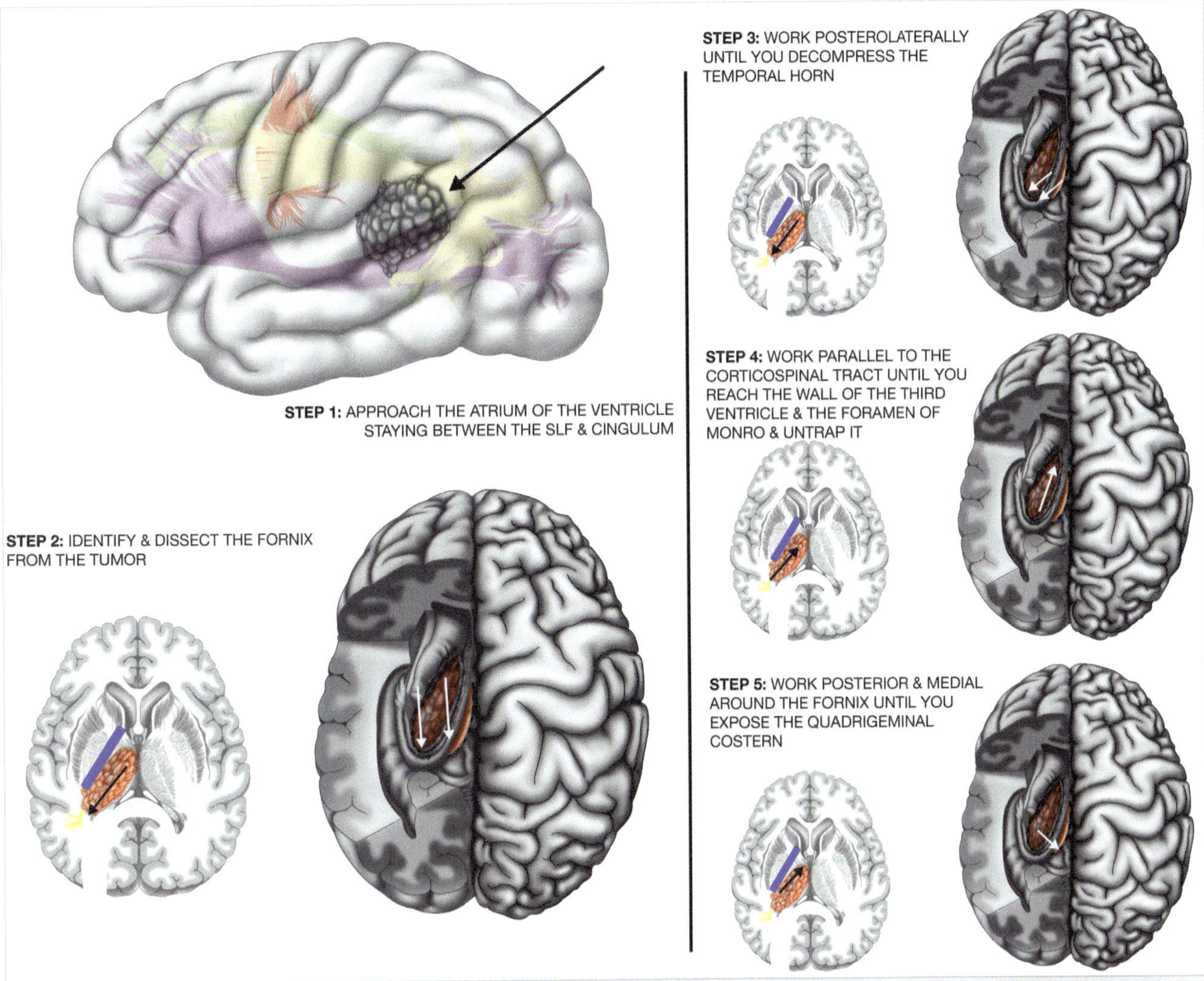

Fig. 14.37 Steps in the resection of a thalamic glioma. The approach passes through the superior parietal lobule and enters the atrium as lateral as possible based on the SLF. Once entering the atrium, the fornix is teased away from the thalamic tissue and as much normal anatomy as possible is identified. Thalamic resection begins inward and projects outward in three directions: first, laterally to find the temporal horn and ensure that this is widely open; second, superomedially to enter third ventricle to ensure you have cleared the tissue appropriately up to the body of the lateral ventricle; and finally, inferomedially to reach the quadrigeminal cistern. This last maneuver involves working over the top of the fornix.

of this out before risking danger. The basal ganglia and internal capsule are pushed anteriorly. Additionally, this tumor's long axis is lateral to medial. If approaching through the superior parietal lobule-transatrial approach, then it is absolutely essential that you work far more lateral and medial than you would expect otherwise you will leave a big piece of tumor out there.

b) The head in this approach is somewhat rotated to keep the parietal cortex from falling into your way. It is essential through to prevent over rotation as this really makes it substantially harder to maintain your orientation and that is a recipe for disaster. Further, awake patients cannot stay very rotated and also participate with testing, so you must balance these goals.
c) Two aspects of the tractography should be noted. First, the corridor into the atrium is a box which is behind the sensorimotor network, medial to SLF, anterior to the visual networks, and lateral to cingulum. This is actually much further posterior and medial that you would think, and longer, but it is the one that risks the long connections and networks the least.

Second, as concerning as operating in the thalamus is, note that the internal capsule is pushed anterior and lateral to you, and the midbrain reticular activating fibers are mostly below you. Keeping the fornix in its position can help to serve as a great orienting landmark keeping you away from both of these inadvisable deviations. It also highlights the value of coming from the back on many of these cases as opposed to the side.

a) The resection I felt was decent, and the patient's initial neurologic function was good; however, the long-term outcome was suboptimal, and in retrospect this was due to the following causes. First, by being asleep, I did not have the confidence to push superomedially until I entered the third ventricle and left a fair bit of tumor there. Second, I did not push inferolaterally and this set up the temporal horn to

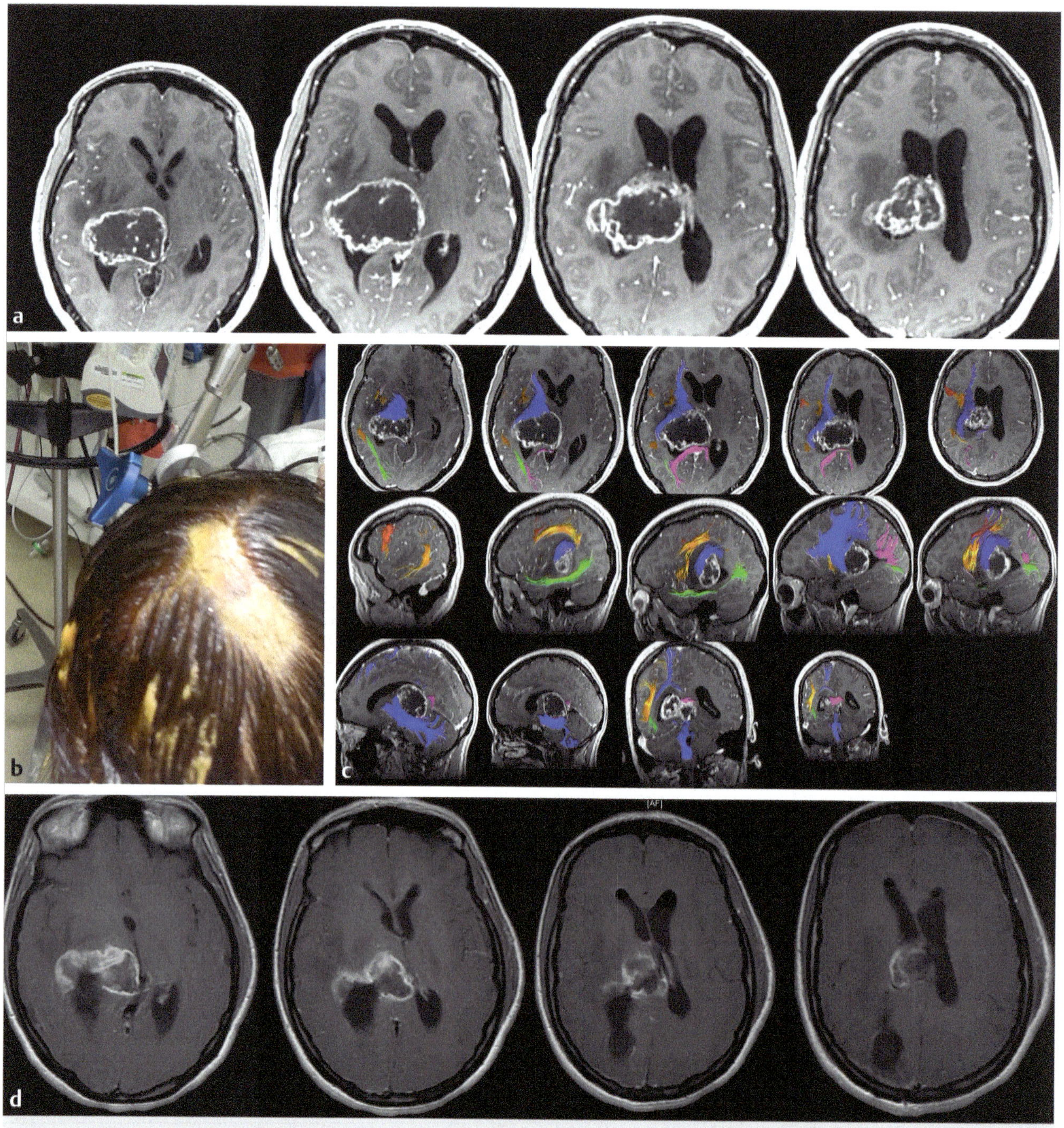

Fig. 14.38 One of my earlier cases of a thalamic GBM done while patient is asleep; (**a**) preoperative images, (**b**) images of the approach, (**c**) DTI tractography, (**d**) postoperative images.

become trapped. Finally, by leaving this much of the enhancing tumor, the brain swelling was far more substantial than with a GTR, and this is due to being asleep. Ultimately, the brain swelling and residual tumor near the horn lead to a series of a trapped temporal horn and complications stemming from that, which undid what could have been a good result.

▶ Fig. 14.39 is a case more typical of my usual approach. It is done awake, and I remain aggressive until I get an aggressive resection of I have to stop to save function. I have been surprised with cases like this, what can be accomplished if we try.

a) This tumor differs from the previous case in that it is somewhat higher (i.e., more superior) at its upper extent. It is critical as you are planning this case that you do not make

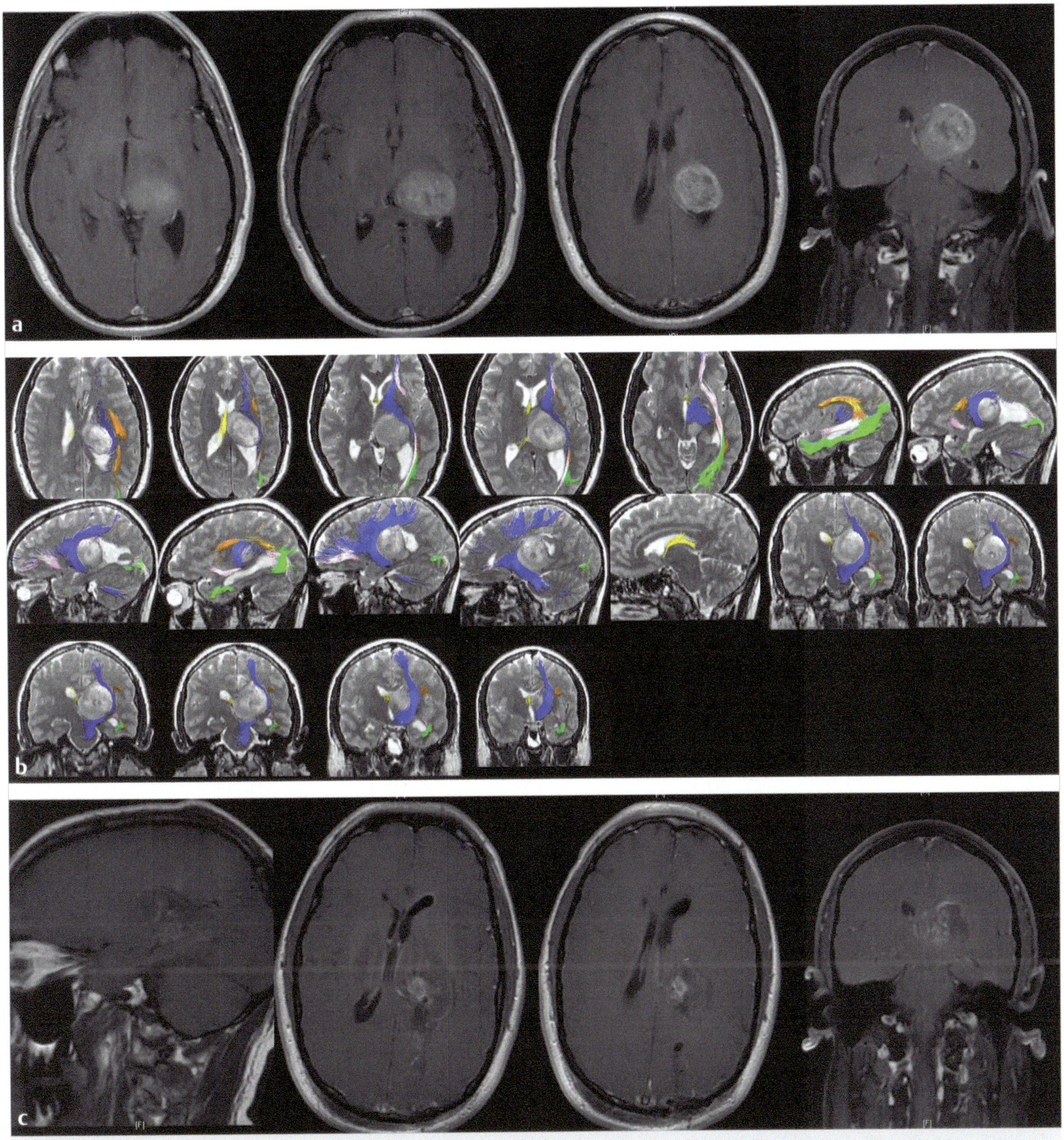

Fig. 14.39 A more typical case of my usual approach of a thalamic GBM; (**a**) preoperative images, (**b**) DTI tractography, (**c**) postoperative images.

your entry point and trajectory too anterior as this trajectory will make it harder to reach around the corner to get to the top of this tumor. A more posterior trajectory gives you a less steep angle into the atrium and get to the top of the tumor easier.

b) None.

c) Again, the position of the internal capsule is anterior and lateral, thus on the deep and lateral side of the tumor. The upper left panels demonstrate the safe corridor into the atrium. You do not wish to add cortical network problems into what is already a high risk case.

d) The tumor resection was excellent in this case. The key here was ensuring that we removed thalamus medially over the fornix until we entered the quadrigeminal cistern and third ventricle. The only deficit in this case was the expected field cut.

Part III

Integration

III

15 Unique Issues with Recurrent Gliomas

15.1 Introduction

This is a relatively short chapter, as there is nothing specific to the anatomy of recurrent gliomas which make the functional anatomy different than first-time surgery. But they are harder, without a doubt, and these challenges and some advice for tackling them are provided as are some examples.

15.2 Issues Unique to Recurrent Gliomas

1. Wound issues are a much bigger deal: This is especially true with a history of Avastin, but previous radiotherapy can also make this worse, and a poorly healing glioma wound can spell more of a disaster than the tumor was.
2. There was a previous surgeon: If it was someone else, they may have placed an incision in a way I would never want to be forced to reuse. If it was me, there is a good chance the tumor recurred on the margin of the resection cavity, which in my case was probably eloquent (I usually leave it for a reason).
3. The arteries may have been radiated: Radiated arteries are more prone to injury, even if you are careful.
4. The anatomy is abnormal: If the previous resection was aggressive, and involved a complete or partial lobectomy, the remaining normal anatomy probably has shifted into the cavity. For example, I expect to find the IFOF and possibly the MCA near the floor of the middle fossa if I have done an aggressive lobectomy (▶ Fig. 15.1).
5. The dura is stuck to the brain: Even if you are careful, you can injure eloquent cortices opening the dura and lose the chance to map before the case has even got started. Less obviously, if the brain is stuck to the dura, every move may transmit force to the dura and cause pain making the patient less cooperative. If I did the past surgery, it is likely that the leading edge next to the cavity was eloquent.
6. The patients are often less functional: They are often less able to map due to tumor recurrence and the long term effects of radiotherapy.
7. It is often less clear what to take out: At the first surgery, anything enhancing is probably tumor as is more of the T2 hyperintense brain. All bets are off at a repeat surgery: enhancement can be radiation necrosis or pseudoprogression and T2 change could be tumor or radiation effect, or encephalomalacia. Often it is less certain that we should be operating, let alone doing something aggressive (▶ Fig. 15.2).
8. The mandate is less clear: The data are more variable for repeat surgery, especially for GBM.
9. There is less brain than before and it's more likely that what's left is eloquent: This is more specific to those who do aggressive resections the first time.

One thing to note is that all of these rules primarily apply to true recurrence surgeries and less to cases where an inadequate first surgery is being followed with a more complete surgery, as these surgeries are more like first time cases.

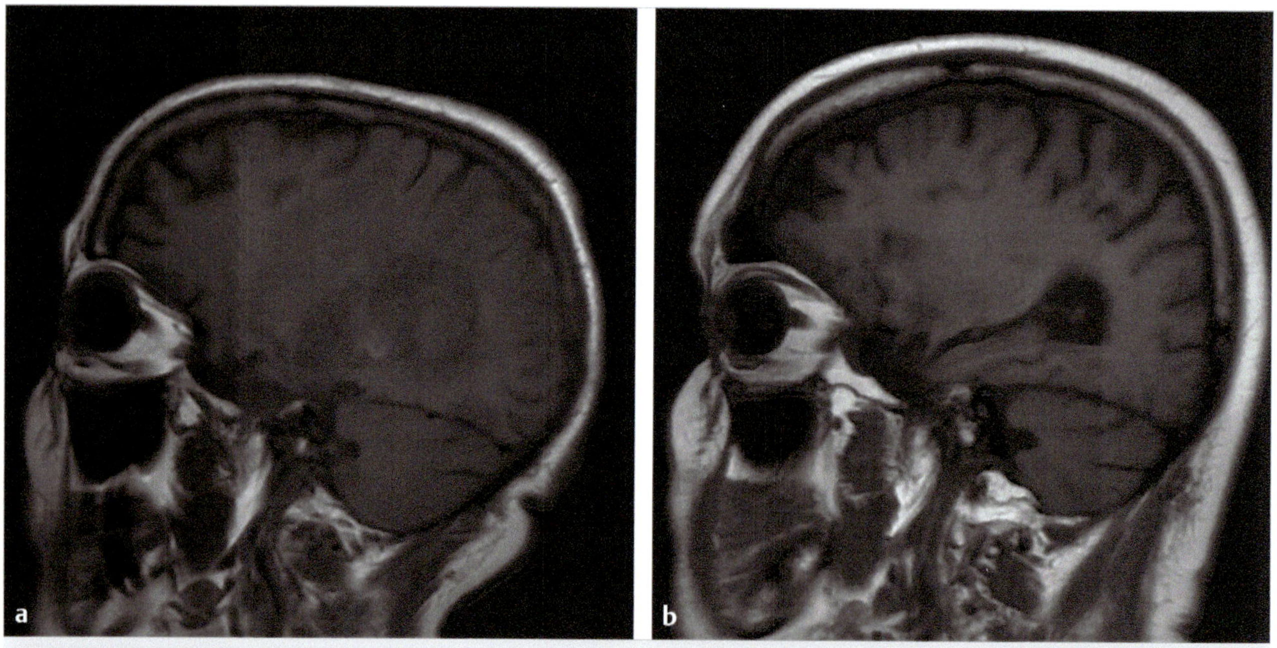

Fig. 15.1 **(a,b)** These images demonstrate cases of recurrent gliomas after temporal lobectomy. Note that while the brain roughly reaches the temporal floor, this is the insula, and not the temporal lobe touching the middle fossa floor. This is critical to note in planning these cases.

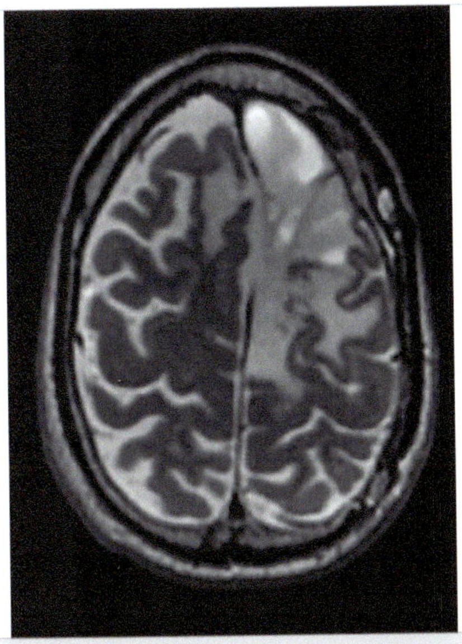

Fig. 15.2 Image depicting one of the almost infinite appearances of recurrent glioma. This image shows extensive T2 changes, and it is entirely unclear what is tumor, what radiation change is, and what is edema. This highlights the challenges of decision making in these cases, as one wants to be aggressive if you are going back in; however, it is unclear what to be aggressive with exactly with our limited imaging.

15.3 Strategies for Addressing these Problems

1. Make the surgery count: The only thing worse than operating in a radiated repeat wound for a small recurrence, is missing part of that recurrence because you were not thorough. This seems like an obvious statement, but it's quite easy to do when the anatomy is abnormal and the tumor is small.
2. Expose the minimal amount of brain possible: The less surface area of adherent dura you need to peel off of potentially eloquent brain to achieve your goal of surgery the better. Often I will plan surgery for recurrence in deeper areas of a resection cavity to only open a small area over the cavity so that no cortex is put at risk and will start subcortical mapping immediately after opening the dura (▶ Fig. 15.3, ▶ Fig. 15.4). There is no rule that one has to expose cortex in a re-do craniotomy.
3. Make functional vs oncologic trade-offs rationally: I call this the "bang-for-your-buck" rule. If removing a tumor, or part of a tumor involves a great deal of risk to a functional system to remove 1 cc of enhancement, then this is not a good trade off compared to chemotherapy alone. Alternately, removing a large amount of tumor in a nonfunctioning system or a disconnected part of the brain is a good trade off (▶ Fig. 15.5). Less intuitive is the idea that the system may be working, but unlikely to be salvaged for long. For example, a patient with a mostly paralyzed leg and a big tumor in the motor strip, is probably going to lose the leg motor function completely in the near future, and the decision to leave this tumor because "I don't want to hurt his leg function," is irrational as well-performed surgery can only improve on that natural history (▶ Fig. 15.6).

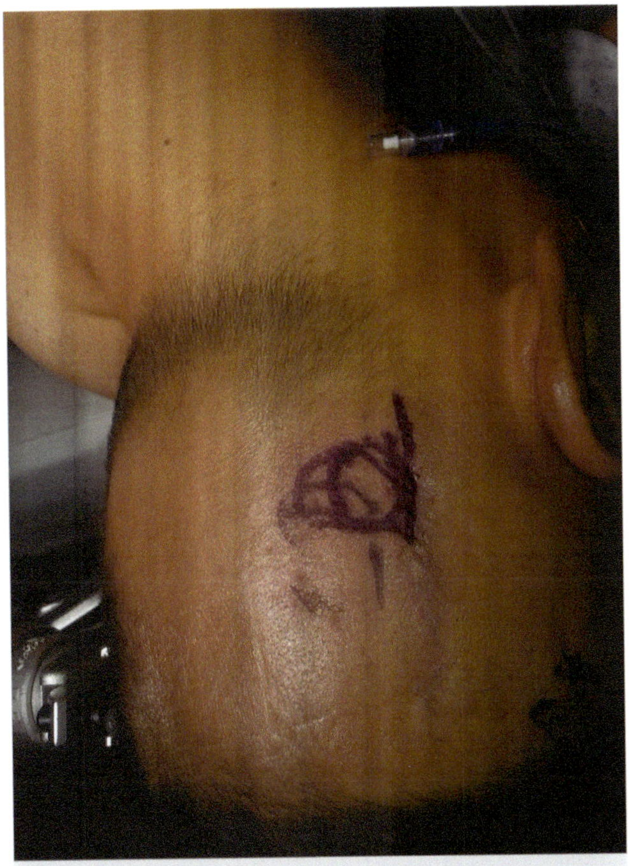

Fig. 15.3 This image demonstrates an incision planned for a recurrent glioblastoma. The previous surgery was for a larger tumor, and he presents with a small recurrence. This highlights the ability of minimally invasive techniques to reduce the threshold for going back, and reducing the need to expose large amounts of cortex scarred to dura.

4. Stay out of the old wound, if possible: The best way to avoid radiated wound problems is to not reopen it if you can avoid doing so. Often, a different cut or angle can achieve a good resection safely and stay out of the wound. Using large resection cavities can also help achieve this goal. Another trick is to use an eyebrow approach to address recurrences in the inferior frontal lobe from previously operated temporoinsular tumors (▶ Fig. 15.7). You can also decide not to open the full wound in some cases.
5. Get a running start: Sometimes a small recurrence can look deceptively easy. It looks like a lump sitting at the bottom of a resection cavity which should just pluck out. It is worth noting that to pluck it out, you generally need to cut into some brain and separate this lump from the brain. Just trying to shave off a few layers and stop will often leave some tumor in the brain, and is largely inconsistent with our understanding of gliomas. Even small tumor recurrences should be removed with a J-shaped or C-shaped cut using anatomic and/or functional boundaries to define resection goals (▶ Fig. 15.8).
6. Develop a realistic goal: Some recurrent tumors are bad, and the patient is going to lose function no matter what you do. Other times you have to try to get the patient into the best situation you can and rely on adjuvant therapy to do the rest. On the other hand, you must always remember that you are

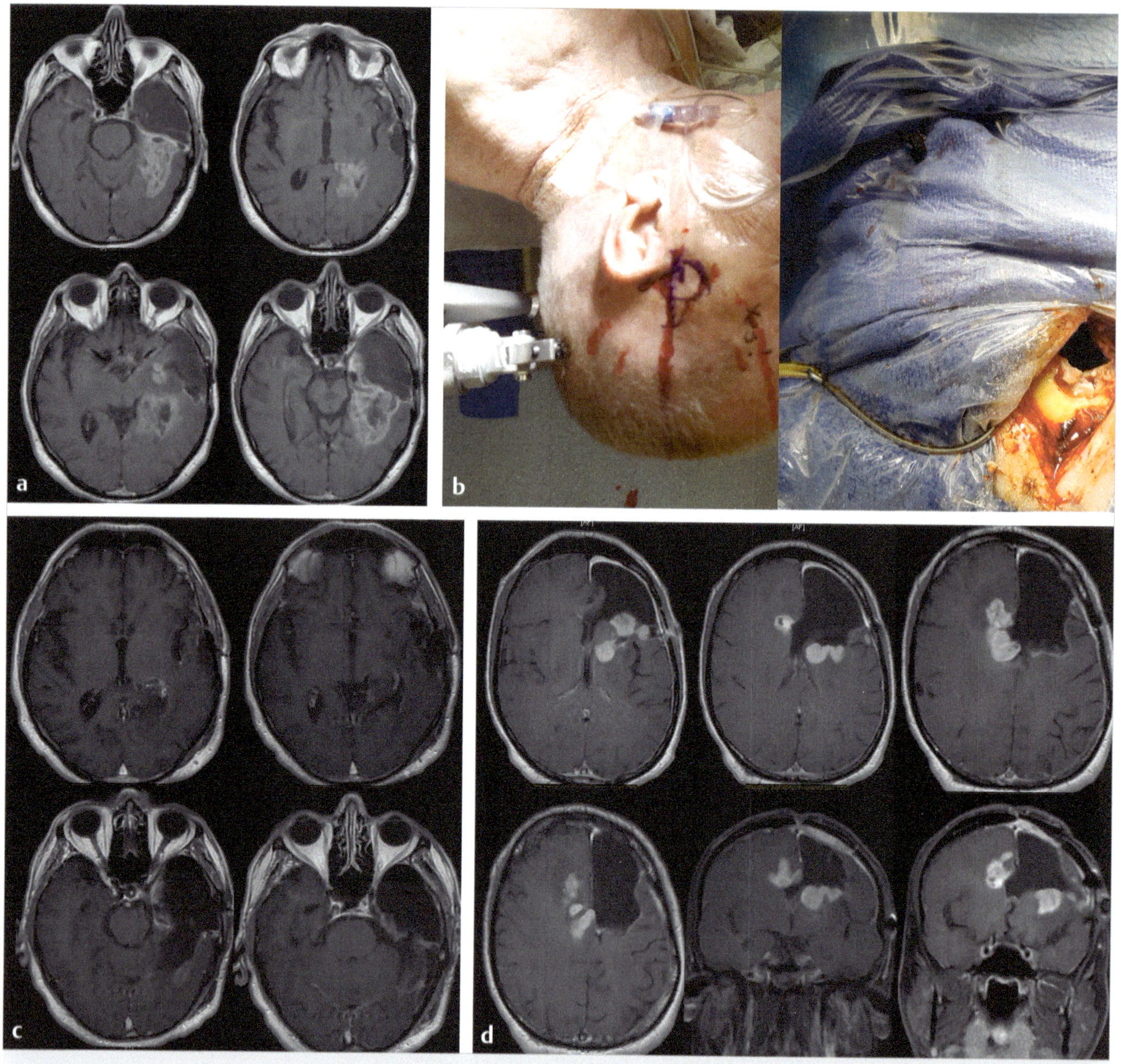

Fig. 15.4 These two cases demonstrate the technique of starting a recurrent glioma in the previous resection cavity:
Case 1: This is a recurrent hippocampal GBM. I did the previous case awake as evidenced by the typical cuts. (**a**)The tumor has recurred in the medial temporal structures, and is following the PHG and hippocampus into the fornix and into the posterior cingulate gyrus. All of these are deep structures and do not need to be exposed. The posterior cut of the lateral temporal lobe from the previous operation likely contains speech (I did the operation and I stopped my cut there for that reason) and now this is the anterior most cortex under the dura in this case. The goal here is to use subcortical mapping to try to get a lateral plane from anterior to posterior to run lateral to the enhancing area of the tumor, and to sweep this tumor out of the brain safely. I do not want to peel dura off the speech cortices as this will be stuck and may injure them. Further, I do not need to make an aggressive lateral temporal cut as this is unnecessary in this case. (**b**) The craniotomy is small and uses only enough of the incision to get into the cavity and in the cavity find an angle lateral to the tumor to disconnect the lateral border of the tumor from the lateral networks. Once this is clear, then we will put the patient to sleep and resect the medial structures. (**c**) The resection is excellent, with removal of tumor in the posterior cingulate and fornix. The speech is normal in this patient.
Case 2: These films demonstrate a case of glioblastoma which has recurred in several sites in the depths of the resection cavity. Given the lack of a need to perform cortical mapping, we limited our opening to just over the cavity, and began working in the depths. This eliminated the need to peel dura off brain that we planned on leaving. (**d**)The tumor recurrence sites are on the deep portions of the cavity, including the basal ganglia, and the contralateral cingulate. There is no role for touching the superficial cortices to make a starting "J-cut", so it's best to leave them alone. We will focus our efforts to slowly teasing tumor out of the speech networks and cingulate gyrus with subcortical mapping.

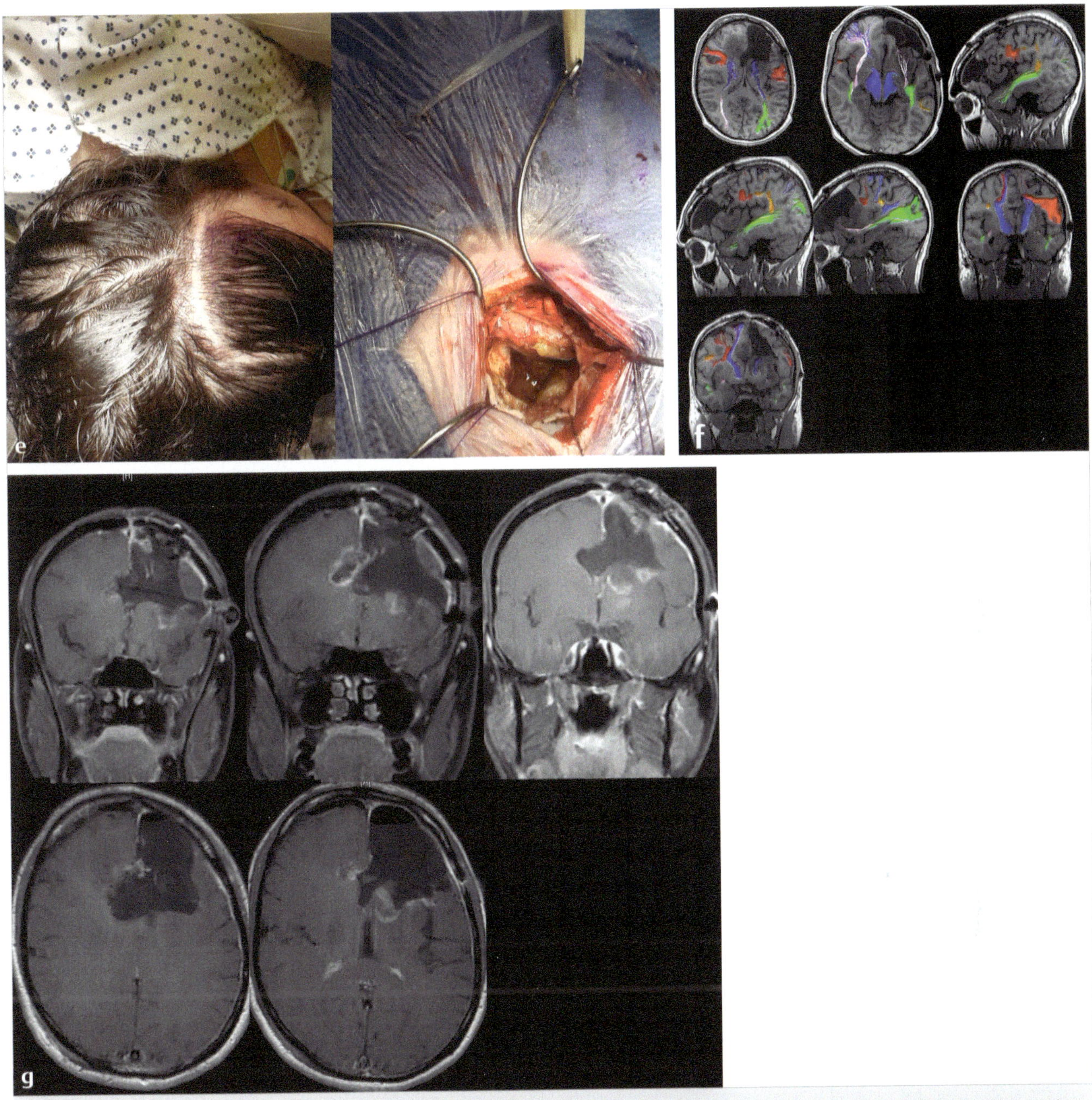

Fig 15.4 (*Continued*) (**e**) The previous incision was partially reopened and we started straight to subcortical work in this case after orienting ourselves to the cavity. (**f**)These DTIs are fascinating and informative. Review of the IFOF on the sagittal images, where the frontal lobe has been removed, shows the IFOF terminates in the caudate as the frontal rami have been cut. The patient had mostly normal speech. When working near this portion of the tumor, we had to proceed slowly as working or stimulating in these areas repeatedly caused anomias. Eventually, we got this small piece of caudate tumor out; however, this case is the best evidence I have personally seen that the target of semantic speech networks running in the IFOF is the basal ganglia and not the frontal lobe, as the IFOF in this case localized closely to language and was cut everywhere else in this case. (**g**) I have seen the situation here once before. We were able to remove the cingulate tumor in this case on the other side, despite the previous removal of the cingulate. It raises the possibility that the networks can reorganize to other areas and even both cingulate gyri might be able to remove in some cases, if they are done with a break for reorganization between resections. I would not recommend this as a general matter of course, or asleep, but in this case, it was tolerated well.

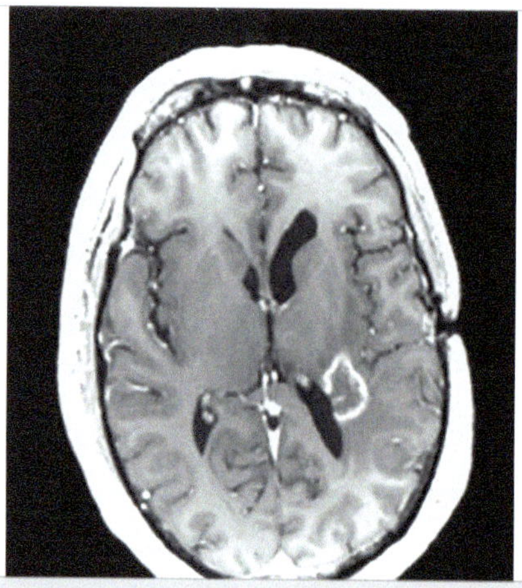

Fig. 15.5 This image demonstrates a case of a temporal glioma which has recurred in the high risk deep white matter of the TPO junction. This is a case of "low bang for your buck," by which I mean a case where great risks are necessary to get only a slight cytoreductive benefit. These are cases where I tend to seek out alternative options, such as LITT, radiosurgery, or chemotherapy alone, as opposed to going back. In contrast, a larger tumor, or one in a safer area would give you a better return on your efforts.

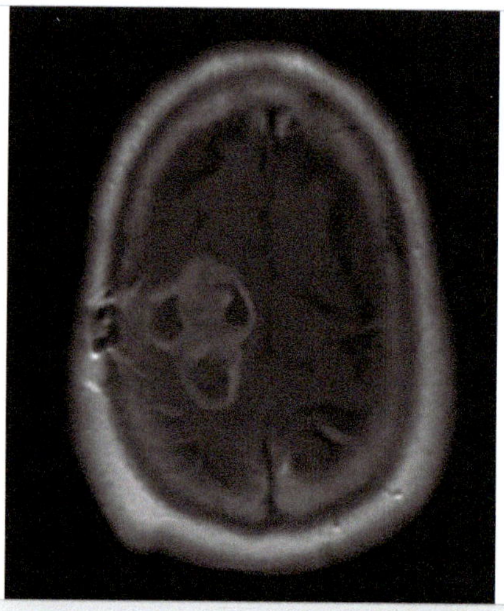

Fig. 15.6 This image depicts a GBM in the motor cortex in a patient who has become hemiplegic from this tumor. While surgery is unlikely to save the motor function, cytoreduction can be helpful in saving other functions, such as the SLF, and we should not be deterred simply because it is in a bad area, and our goals are limited.

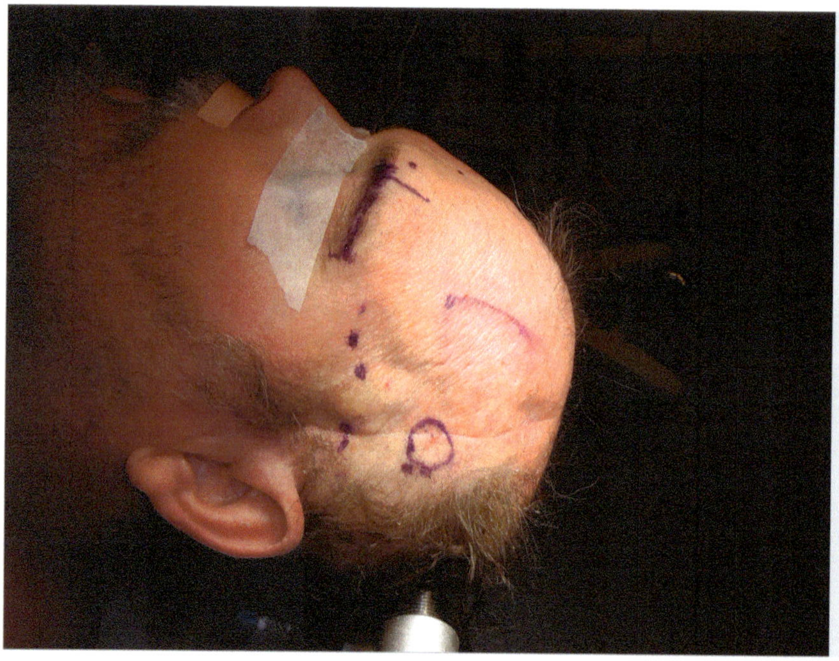

Fig. 15.7 This image depicts a patient with an extensive frontal GBM, which had been treated with two rounds of radiotherapy and Avastin. We performed a frontal lobe resection through the eyebrow to avoid this high risk wound.

treating a tumor which is highly capable of killing this patient in rapid and terrible fashion, and that you are not going to help the situation by quitting.

15.4 When Do I Not Offer Reoperation?

Sometimes, I do so because after looking at the images, it is obvious that another surgery would offer a poor "bang-for-my-buck," or in other words, that the amount of cytoreduction we would gain compared to the risk of taking it out is not likely to be worth the effort (▶ Fig. 15.7). On the other hand, a large tumor with high risk is high risk, but also a situation where the amount of cytoreduction possible may pay off.

Outside of small tumors in dangerous places, the decision to not operate is often a decision to transition towards end-of-life care. At least in theory, any chemotherapy is more likely to work on future cancer cells, and our practice is to not throw chemotherapy at an impossibly big tumor and hope for a miracle, but instead to always try to give the patient the least number of cells possible prior to chemotherapy, if this is reasonably possible.

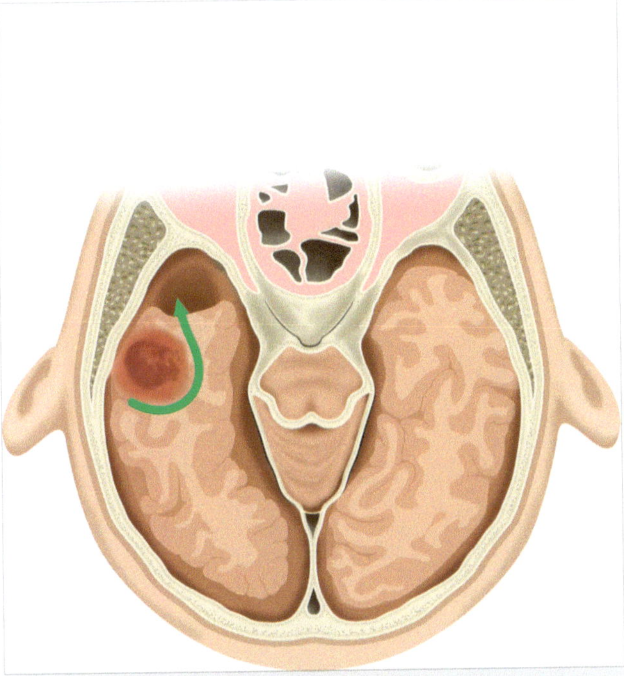

Fig. 15.8 This schematic shows the J-shaped cut helpful for small glioma recurrences. The cut begins by entering the edge of brain just behind the tumor and starts a new plane. It continues behind and eventually deep to it (thus the J-shape) landing in the resection cavity. Obviously, this cut is dictated by the mapping.

Everyone has a strong opinion about repeat glioma surgery, especially for GBM. There are all sorts of recommendations about extent of resection thresholds (i.e., if you can get out 75%, 95% etc., then don't operate, or don't re-operate). There are no consensus guidelines or class 1 evidence on this complex topic. Some centers send most patients with any recurrence home to die, even with good KPS and treatable tumors.

I personally don't use thresholds firmly in my decision making. First, it is uncommon I cannot get at least 75% of a tumor out with mapping techniques. Second, every patient needs to decide for themselves how aggressive they should be trying to extend their life, and many patients, even with bad starting points, do surprisingly well. So I have a frank discussion about their chances, and let them decide. I think the decision to go forward with more surgery and aggressive treatment often is heavily linked to preoperative functional status, and I think this is rational behavior. Life is important, and those with reasonably quality of life usually do not wish to sit there and wait to lose it. The time to quit is usually obvious to most people.

15.4.1 Glioblastoma (GBM) Checkmates

There are a few unique situations where I steer even motivated patients away from surgery. These are situations where a tumor grows in a manner where taking out the tumor truly is likely to cause problems out of any acceptable outcome. I term these GBM checkmates, as the surgical game is usually over when I see these events:

1. Growth into the brain stem (▶ Fig. 15.9): it is possible to take some tumors out of the brainstem, and it might be possible to remove a focal recurrence in the brainstem. However, the path that it has to take to get there from the supratentorial brain takes the tumor cells through so many critical areas that it seems inconceivable that surgery can offer these patients much.
2. Significant bilateral tumors (▶ Fig. 15.10): As noted previously, notably in Chapter 4, bi-anything is bad (bifrontal, bitemporal, biparietal, and bioccipital injuries) as there is no way to compensate for this. Thus, although you can follow tumor across the corpus callosum and even a little onto the other side, and although you can remove significantly asymmetric multifocal tumors, mirror image surgery is unlikely to be helpful without an improved understanding of lateral compensation and how to avoid injuring it.
3. Dense involvement of the left SLF (▶ Fig. 15.11): I personally view dense aphasia as inconsistent with quality of life in a way that dense hemiplegia is not. Preoperative aphasia can improve if the tumor is compressing the tract, but tumor following the SLF along a significant length is unlikely to be removed with improvement. It is important to be optimistic, but there are limits.
4. Invasion of the basal forebrain and hypothalamus (▶ Fig. 15.12): Even if you can remove this, as with the brainstem, the path it took to get there transgresses some critical places, which will likely thwart any benefit from a lesionectomy.

15.5 How to Deal with Bad Glioma Wounds

As my departments' glioma surgeon, I am the local expert on fixing complex cranial wound infections. Below are a few basic additions to standard wound care that are worth noting on gliomas.

1. Act fast: These are typically not good candidates for trying some minor fix and hoping it works. Usually in these cases, the factors determining wound healing are against you: poor blood supply, previous radiation, foreign body, wound under tension. You can expect getting the wound to heal to be difficult; letting things fester while you try stuff to avoid the real fix can end in more infection (including possibly intradural), loss of skin to work with later, and a sicker patient. This is true for all recurrent gliomas, but especially if Avastin has ever been used.
2. Assume there is some degree of hydrocephalus: This is one downside of routinely widely opening the ventricle (I think not injuring the basal ganglia is worth the trade of needing to put a shunt). Most of these patients develop some hydrocephalus, often low pressure. The ventricles are often not big, and they don't even always have an external subdural fluid collection or pseudomeningocele. If the wound is leaking or the patient has hydrocephalus like problems, then assume hydrocephalus is probably part of the mix.
3. Minimize delays in adjuvant therapy: If adjuvant treatment is delayed while you screw around with the wound for weeks, and the tumor grows back, you have often dished the patient a death blow. Act fast.

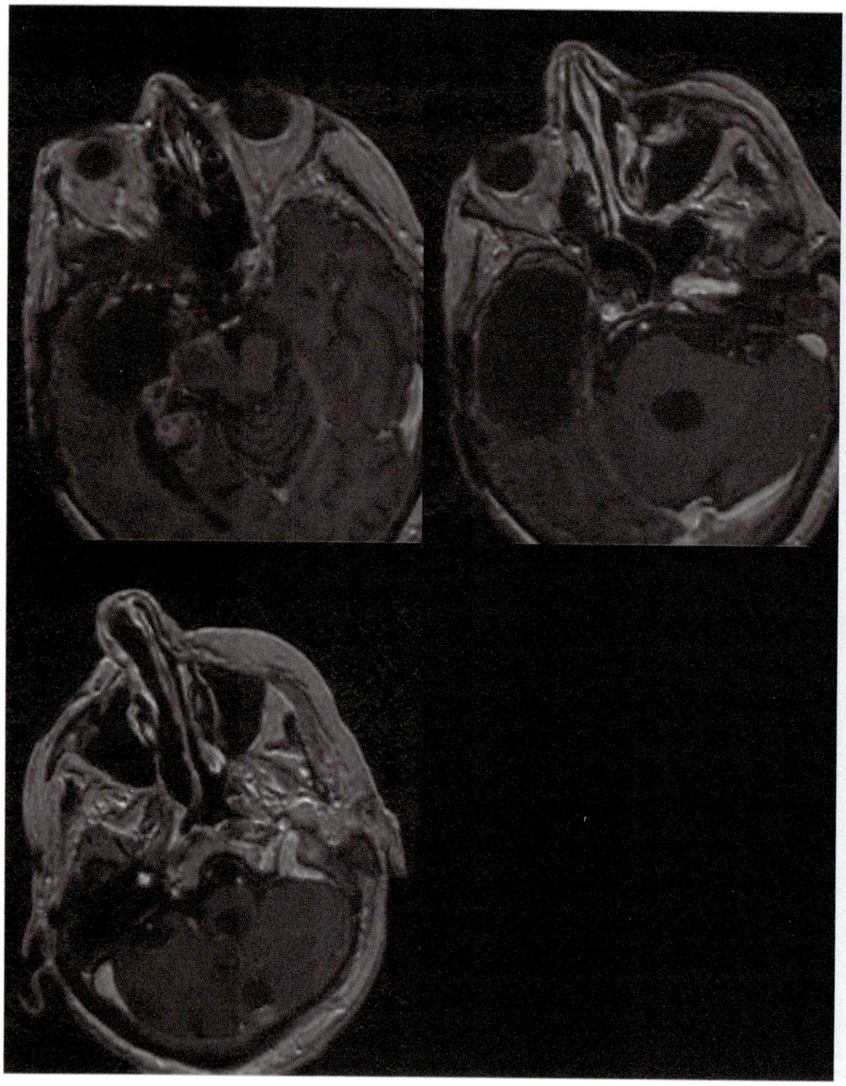

Fig. 15.9 These images depict GBM recurrence in the brainstem, a "GBM Checkmate."

4. Strongly consider throwing the bone flap out: Cosmesis is nice, but delaying adjuvant therapy in a recurrent glioblastoma because of repeat wound problems trying to save the bone flap is a bad idea. If you do small bone flaps routinely, losing a bone flap is much less of a big deal. Remember this is cancer surgery, not cosmetic surgery.
5. Get a reconstruction surgeon involved early: They often will think of wound healing ideas not obvious to you, and can help get the patient onto treatment faster. They can also get a blood supply to the area which is sorely lacking in some of these cases.

15.5.1 What about Other Laser Interstitial Thermal Therapy (LITT)?

I am a huge fan of laser interstitial thermal therapy (LITT) for recurrent glioma. It is a rare innovation in our field which enters and immediately becomes an obvious strategy for treating a disease which competes head to head with older established techniques and for which very few arguments based on experience can be made against it. In the correct patient, we have been able to treat very bad recurrences successfully, and with minimal patient problems and especially no wound problems. Deep tumors are

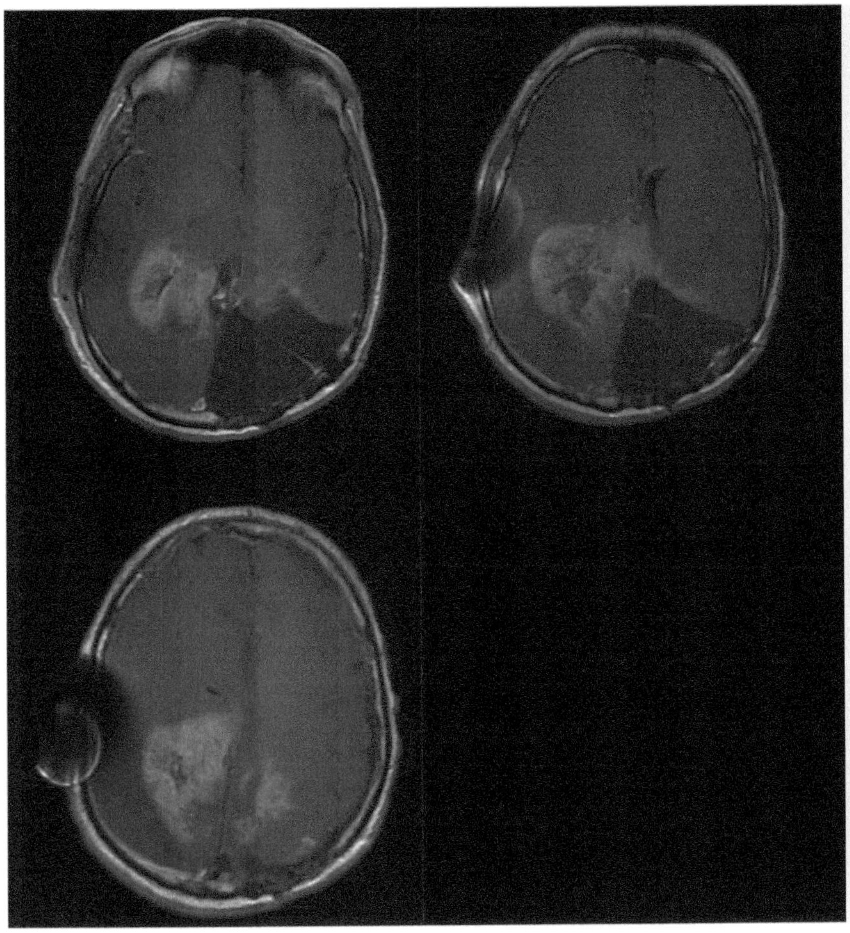

Fig. 15.10 These images depict extensive bilateral GBM recurrence, a "GBM Checkmate."

doable, treating multiple foci is reasonable, treating after Avastin or radiation is a nonissue mostly, and this does very little damage to the white matter tracts. It largely eliminates the discussion of whether something that is small, asymptomatic but enhancing is tumor or radiation necrosis as it can treat either. In the correct patient, it achieves all the benefits of cytoreduction without a lot of the costs. It has changed what we do in our practices substantially in a short time.

Having made my pitch, as with all new ideas, we need to acknowledge that LITT is a technology in evolution, and that we don't have a perfect idea who the candidates are, and who should be managed another way. Presently, I have found it best for dealing with small amounts of recurrent tumor, especially when this is deep, multifocal, or the patient has had Avastin. As this evolves, it may become increasingly able to treat worse tumors, and the techniques I describe in the rest of the book may be more foundational than practical.

Regardless, at present I see a few limitations which limit the ability of LITT to replace traditional surgery for many patients.

1. It cannot test for function. People have told me that they get around this with fMRI and DTIs, and guide the LITT treatment based on this data. This is misguided for many reasons. First, imaging does not imply essentiality, and I think this book makes manifestly obvious that we have a poor understanding of how function is organized and how it can be preserved. Many techniques such as fMRI are also highly sensitive to increased blood flow from tumors due to dependence on bold. Additionally, most present white matter imaging platforms are plagued by problems defining tracts in edematous brain, which is the nature of most glioma patients, which begs the question of how much you can trust these techniques down to the millimeter. A few millimeters can be the difference between cutting a tract, and merely causing edema in it in my experience. Finally, the present platforms

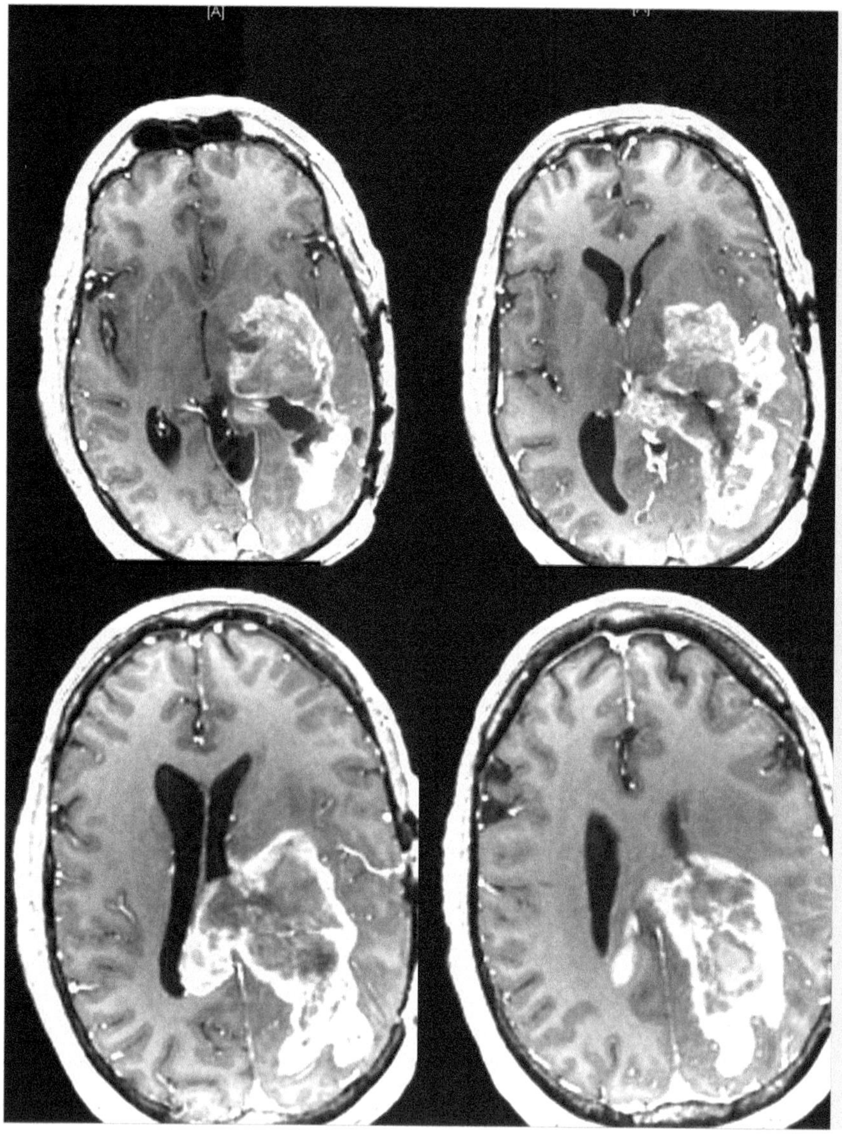

Fig. 15.11 These images depict dense recurrence in the SLF, which should make you reconsider how helpful you can be with surgery.

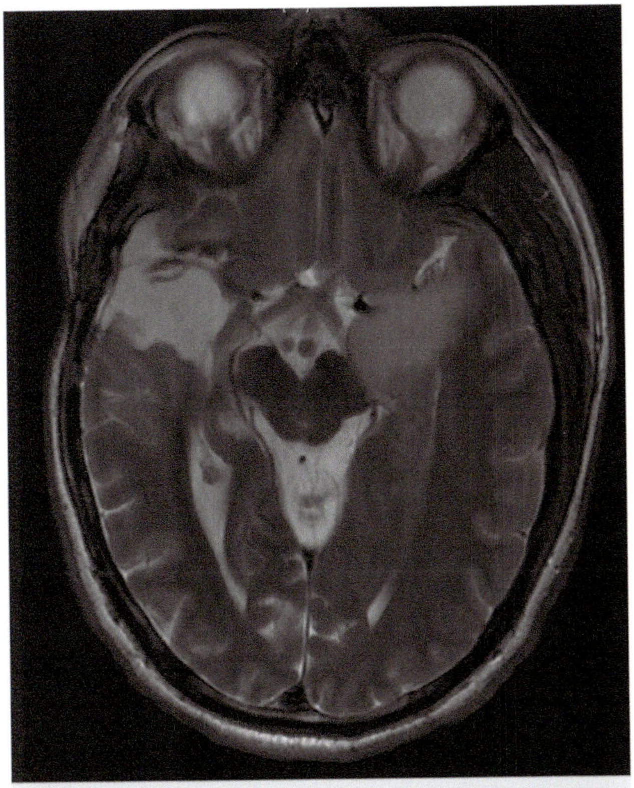

Fig. 15.12 This patient has recurred in the contralateral amygdala after a temporal lobectomy. The route for this spread is through the basal forebrain and this is unwise to resect.

for imaging during a LITT treatment show you anatomy at best in two planes, without these data available to you. I am not sure that most of us would trust our ability to talk to something with that level of accuracy.

2. The mass is burned but still there, and the edema can be intense. There is a major quality of life benefit to making room the brain to accommodate a big tumor.
3. Coverage is a key problem with existing platforms. Obtaining coverage of a large or oddly shaped tumor is the biggest challenge with the current devices, as they are only minimally able to alter their direction off their primary angle. This can be overcome with multiple lasers; however, in that case we should always ask ourselves if the multiple lasers are needed because of an odd shape, or because this tumor is too big. Also this should trigger an question of whether the patient will be able to tolerate the edema issues. I do not think the idea of adding a craniotomy to a LITT to deal with the edema as a planned procedure makes a lot of sense to me compared to performing the craniotomy. I think this may be pushing the technology beyond its sensible limits.

In short, techniques like LITT are interesting, and will slowly improve our arsenal for treating recurrent gliomas, but the core principles are the same. This book was written with the conscious idea that the techniques may be obsolete one day, and one key goal is to make a book of principles useful in any setting.

16 Large Multilobar Gliomas

16.1 Introduction

Conceptually, this chapter introduces no new information. It provides examples of techniques I have used for successfully removing very large gliomas which span more than one brain lobe. However, the previous chapters have provided all that is necessary to think through these cases and to come up with an acceptable plan to tackle these cases, and there is no way a chapter can summarize all possible combinations of spread that gliomas can obtain when they get bad.

This chapter provides some basic guidelines, and follows with some specific examples of what has worked for me in these challenging cases.

16.2 Basic Guidelines for Planning very Large Gliomas

1. Try to understand how this tumor has spread: Gliomas tend to follow white matter tracts. Smaller tumors may not clearly be following an identifiable tract, but big gliomas usually are.

Common routes of multilobar spread include:

a) ILF: The common path for tumors extending from temporal to occipital pole.
b) SLF: A bad way to spread, but unfortunately common, especially when the tumor gains access to the posterolateral temporal lobe, the MFG, IFG or the inferior parietal lobe.
c) Corpus callosum: Spread across the corpus callosum is one way we can lose control of the tumor. Remember, Bi-anything is bad
d) Cingulum: This is how tumors get from the PHG to the cingulate gyrus and back. It is a common way splenial butterfly gliomas spread.
e) Diagonal band of Broca/ventral amygdalofugal tract: This is how tumors can spread from one amygdala to the other, or from the amygdala to the hippocampus.
f) Descending tracts of the corona radiata / corticospinal tract: This is an uncommon route of spread, thankfully, because it is obviously bad.

By knowing the pathway of spread, you know what parts of the brain are probably out (especially with GBMs) and have an idea of how to tackle this tumor with the minimal amount of damage.

2. Be realistic: It is always fulfilling when our patients go home with minimal deficits. However, for patients with multilobars tumors, perfection is not a realistic goal in most cases. First, they often come in with deficits, often because the tumor has destroyed a network. Second, they have a grim natural history if you don't do something meaningful. Third, the idea that you are going to take out two lobes of the brain and nothing noticeable will occur is also misguided. The idea that someone needs to be neurologically perfect or they should be dead is overly rigid. There are meaningful lives led with some neurologic deficits. Where that line is crossed is a complex and personal question. Remember that these are bad tumors. Be realistic about what you can offer, but also be realistic about how bad the natural history of this problem is.
3. Think in terms of cuts: This is the foundation of my approach to gliomas. Large multilobar gliomas are no different; however, there are often multiple, complex and/or non-standard cuts involved. The foundation of making these kinds of decisions is grounded in the more fundamental issues described in previous chapters.
4. Plan around lobectomies/partial lobectomies: This is generally no place for dainty and tailored surgeries. A tumor of this severity needs to be thought of as the extensive cancer it is. Also, a large multilobar cut is going to leave some roads to nowhere, and you need to not leave cancer behind in disconnected nonfunctional brain.
5. Think about how to combine the cuts: Often, removing a multilobar tumor will need a long cut which is a combination of two subcuts. This does not always need a single large craniotomy along the length of the cut; it can usually be made smaller by working under the bone flap.
6. One craniotomy or two? If you choose to tackle a glioma this bad, you will be removing a lot of brain, which will make a great deal of room under the skull to work. Thus, I always strive to avoid a large hemicraniectomy type opening, as many of these cases are redo surgery, and I wish to not risk an infection of a flap this large.

There are two ways to exploit this fact. One is to make a medium-sized craniotomy in the center of the cut and to work under the skull to continue the cut in both directions. A second way is to perform two small craniotomies, to make the cut under both and then to extend them under the skull to joint them between the two craniotomies (which I call a pull-through approach). It is rarely necessary to perform a giant craniotomy.

Each case has unique needs, and there are a large number of possible options.

16.2.1 Representative Cases

It is obviously impossible to describe all possible approaches to massive gliomas, as the variability is quite significant. A few case examples are provided to provide some insight and ideas for tackling these complex cases.

▸ Fig. 16.1 demonstrates a recurrent GBM with extension from the occipital lobe, into the anterior temporal lobe. After examining the films, it seemed unlikely that this tumor could be removed while maintaining the visual input to the occipital pole, or the temporal outflow pathways, which are mostly at the back. The patient elected to undergo an occipitotemporal lobectomy.

a) The tumor is primarily located within the ILF and IFOF systems, as well as the visual system. While it is technically possible to obtain a complete resection without removing the temporal tip, it is unclear what this part of the brain would connect to in a meaningful network. The principle goal of

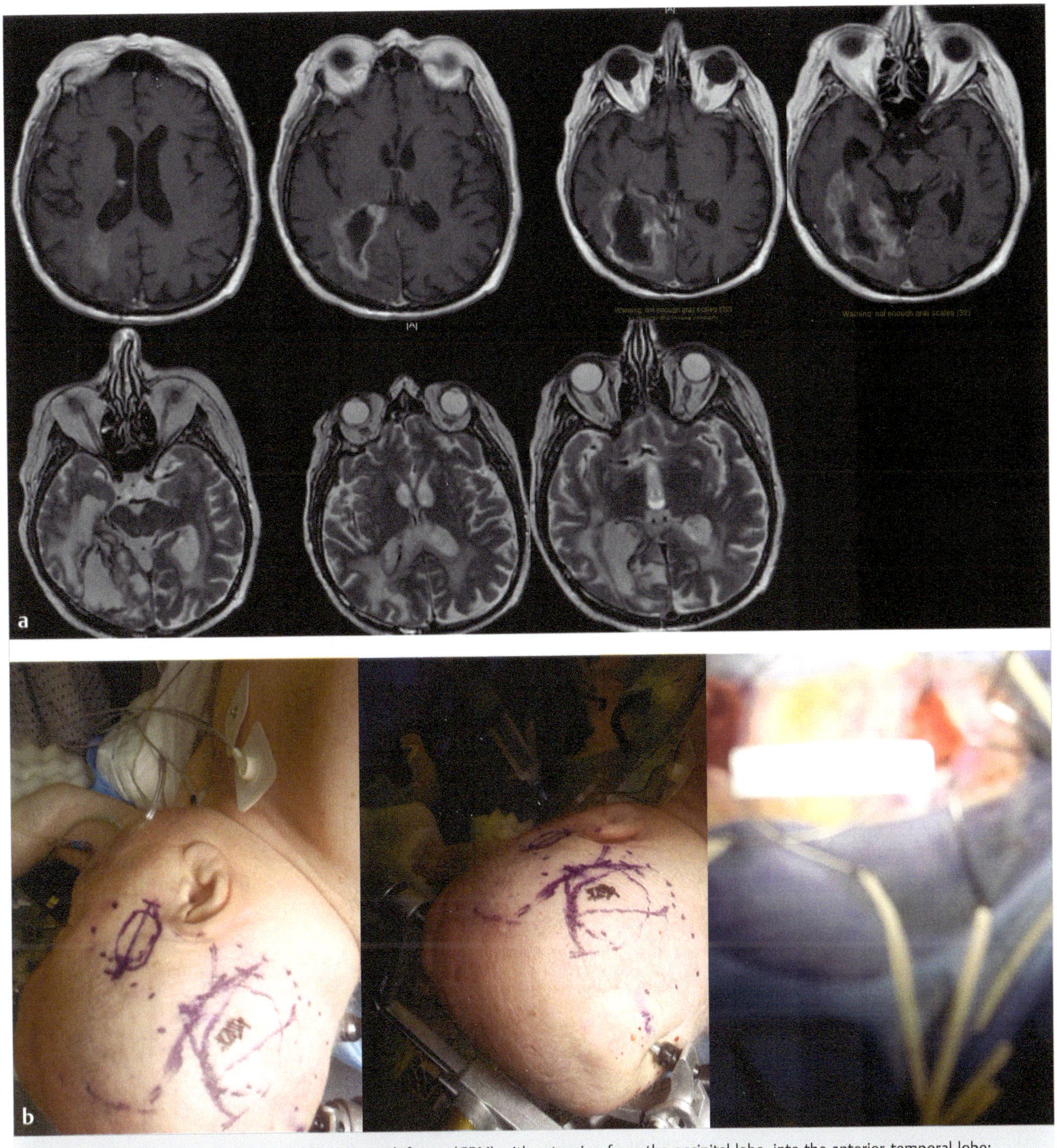

Fig. 16.1 Demonstrates a recurrent glioblastoma multiforme (GBM) with extension from the occipital lobe, into the anterior temporal lobe; (**a**) preoperative images, (**b**) images of the approach. (*Continued*)

this operation is to maintain the communication between the semantic networks and the SLF system, and ideally the crossed semantic loop. The ipsilateral visual system and IFOF is obviously not working.

b) We performed this operation via a "pull-through" technique, where occipital and temporal craniotomies were performed to make a cut extending from the posterior parietal midline heading anteriolaterally to the STG roughly paralleling the SLF and continuing into the atrium and temporal horn under the bone between the two bone flaps. After this cut was complete, we put the patient to sleep and performed occipital and temporal lobectomies and removed the intervening disconnected brain under the skull (thus the term "pull through"). This procedure did not incur any additional neurologic morbidity not previously seen preoperatively.

c) None.

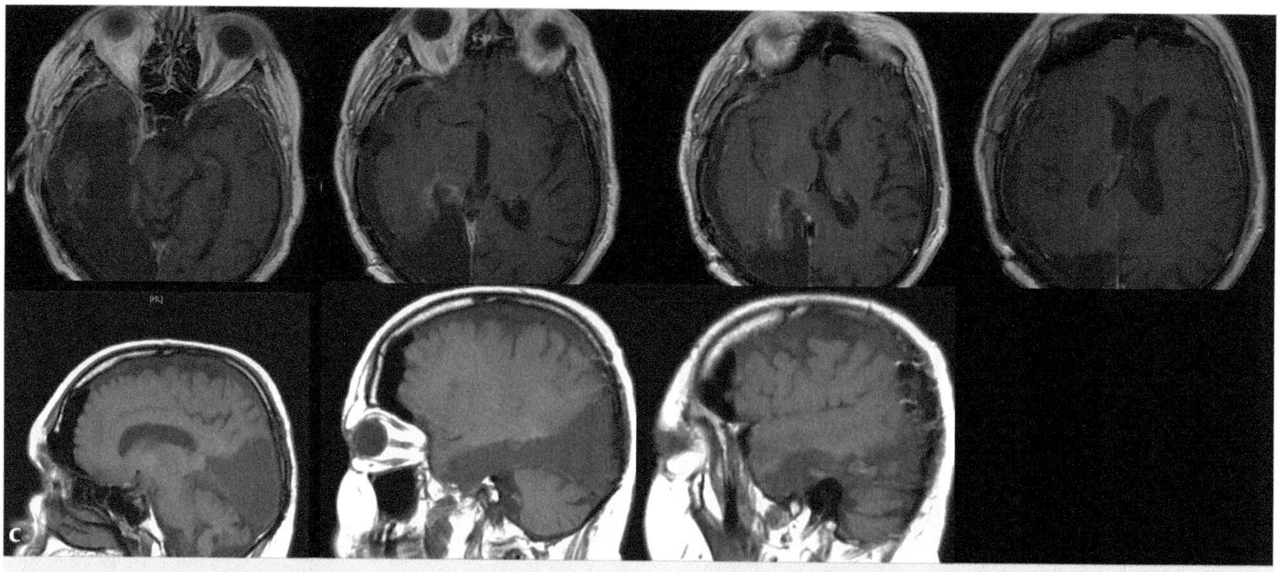

Fig 16.1 *(Continued)* **(c)** Postoperative images.

d) The resection is aggressive but complete and was well tolerated.

▶ Fig. 16.2 demonstrates a case of a patient with a dense anomia but otherwise intact fluent speech from this massive left-sided GBM.

a) This tumor is a tumor of the left-sided visual system and its extensions including the splenium. Unlike the right-sided case, we elected not to pursue as an aggressive resection involving multilobar resection, but instead elected to base our resection around an occipital lobectomy, and an anterior occipital disconnection, with the medial temporal and splenial tumor being removed through the lobectomy cavity. The primary goal was sparing the lefty SLF.
b) Given the long extension along the SLF, we performed a biportal type approach, with two small craniotomies centered over the medial parietal cut, and over the cut with the SLF. These cuts were performed awake until the SLF was clear, and then we put the patient to sleep and performed an occipital lobectomy, removed the splenium, and the medial structures.
c) None.
d) The resection is good and his speech was preserved; however, he had new problems with judgment which tempered my view of his outcome. I am not certain about why the occipital lobe and splenium play a role in judgment, but I have seen this before in two other cases.

▶ Fig. 16.3 demonstrates a complex fronto-temporo-insular GBM encasing the MCA trunk, which had undergone a minimal resection at another institution.

a) If you only look at the contrast images, this doesn't seem like an extremely extensive tumor, but the T2 is more realistically a better measure of the extent of this tumor, though admittedly some of this is edema. It is obviously not possible to completely remove all of these areas; however, temporal lobectomy and marginal resections fit better with the anatomy, but also help isolate the densely encased MCA and allow us to spare the MCA while trimming the fibrous dense enhancing tumor off the multiply encased MCA vessels to leave as little of this as possible.
b) I began this resection by completing the temporal lobectomy and performing a lateral frontal disconnection and limited frontal lobe resection. This isolated the involved MCA. Using a Doppler probe and techniques borrowed from meningioma surgery, I managed to trim this tumor to an acceptable residual which is not invading the brain (t has been separated from it).
c) None.
d) There is some enhancing tumor on the MCA vessels, which simply would not come off the arteries; however, this tumor no longer is attached to the cerebrum, and thus has less opportunity to launch tumor cells into distant white matter tracts.

▶ Fig. 16.4 demonstrates an extreme case of a left fronto-temporo-insula glioma extending into the basal forebrain. While obviously it is unlikely that we will be unable to get all of this out, especially since this patient would not cooperate with brain mapping for very long during the operation, we performed a temporal lobectomy and orbitofrontal cortex resection, and trimmed the anterior insula conservatively based on the IFOF tractography with a reasonable result.

a) Tumors like this are often termed gliomatosis cerebri because they are in multiple lobes. Obviously, this is potentially applicable in this case, but really this is not consistent with the spirit of what that disease means. This tumor is very extensive glioma of the insula which has maximized all of its routes of spread out of the insula. The temporal lobe and cingulum is densely involved, and the uncinate pathway has filled the orbitofrontal region with tumor. But there is not bilateral disease, or completely unconnected disease. This is a bad glioma in multiple lobes, but it is not really gliomatosis in my opinion.
b) The craniotomy is more extensive than other similar tumors. It needs to be somewhat anterior as we need significant

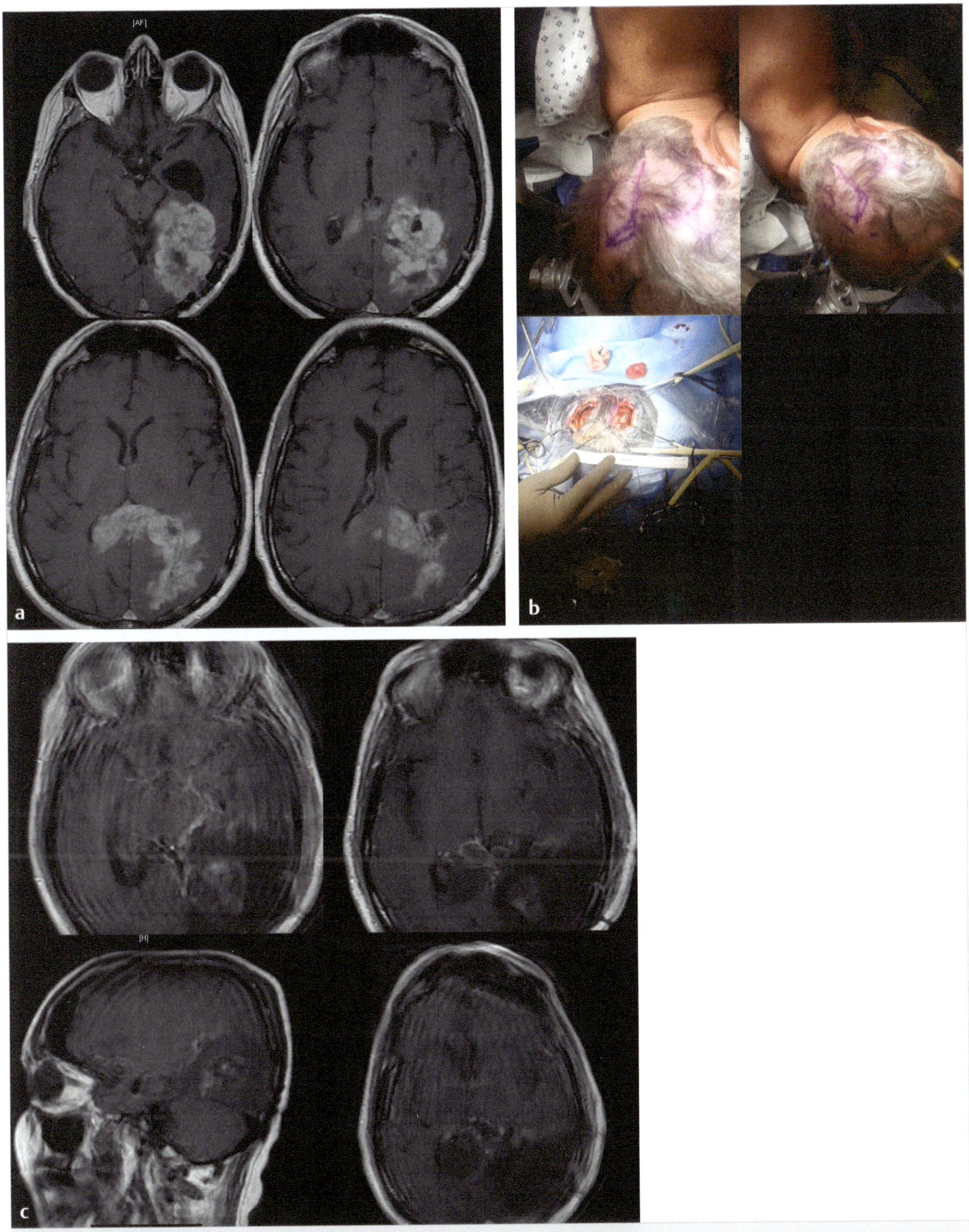

Fig. 16.2 A patient with a dense anomia but otherwise intact fluent speech from massive left-sided glioblastoma multiforme (GBM); (**a**) preoperative images, (**b**) images of the approach, (**c**) postoperative images.

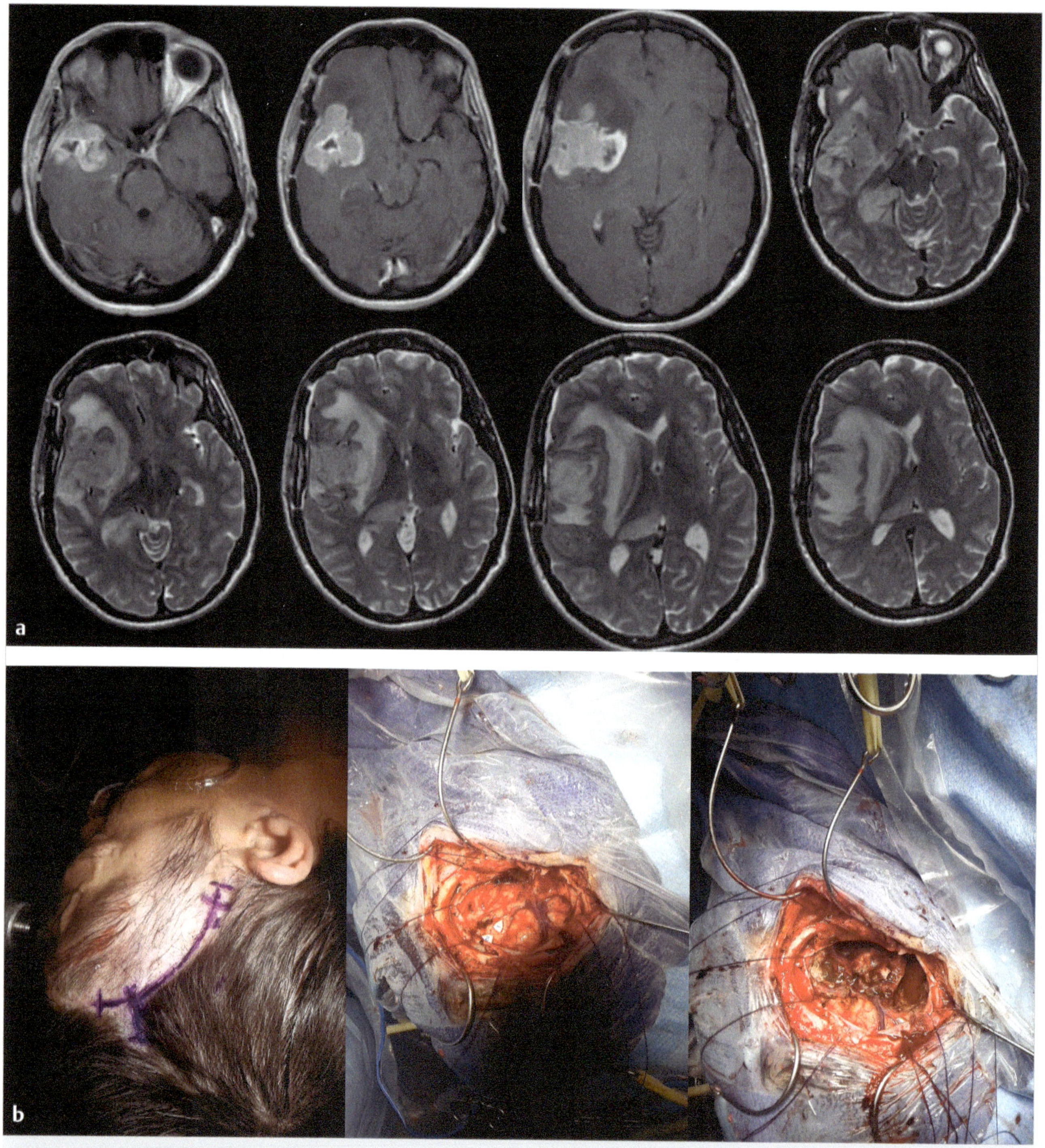

Fig. 16.3 A complex fronto-temporo-insular GBM encasing the MCA trunk, which had undergone a minimal resection at another institution; (**a**) preoperative images, (**b**) images of the approach.

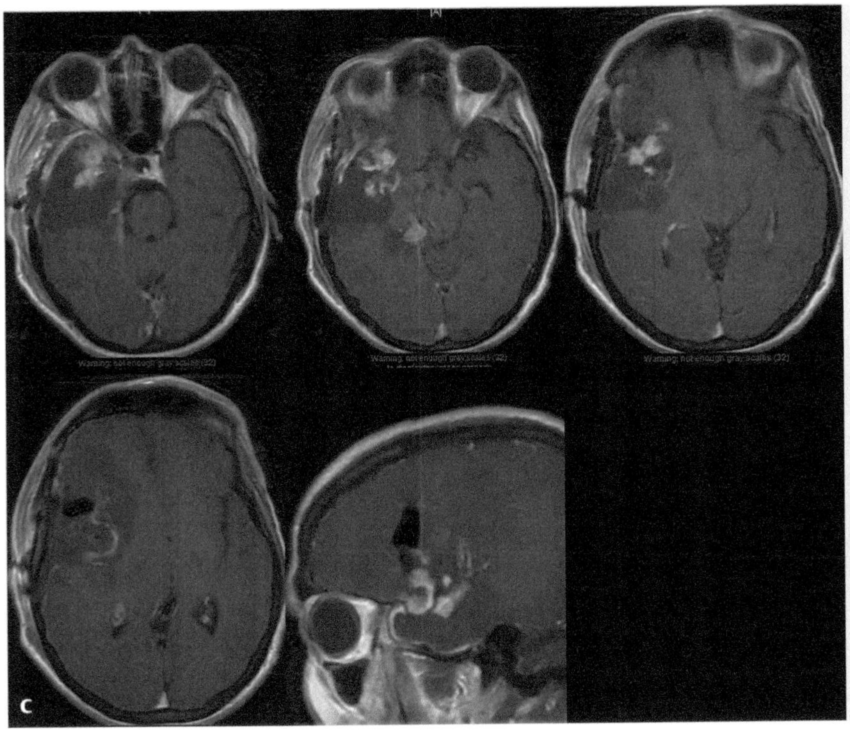

Fig 16.3 (*Continued*) (**c**) Postoperative images.

access to the supraorbital space so that we can comfortably work in the orbital frontal cortex without blind sweeping. This does not need a formal; pterional craniotomy but the spirit of the technique is the same.

The approach follows a lot of similar steps to a temporal-sided insular glioma: Temporal lobectomy, insula resection, following the curve of the uncinated forward, but eventually the pars orbitalis should be entered and a cut of the frontal lobe above the orbitofrontal component should be taken to the midline before subpializing the orbitofrontal brain up the front of M1.

a) None.

b) Despite an aggressive resection, there are a lot of things I could have done better on this early case in my experience. First, the orbitofrontal resection is not medial or posterior enough. The M1 is an excellent landmark for staying out of the basal forebrain and lenticulostriates, and since this case, is my stopping point in the coronal plane. The orbitofrontal resection should continue to the midline. There is also some temporal tumor left. Because this patient did not participate for very long during the mapping, I could not make the aggressive posterior temporal disconnection I would normally like to make.

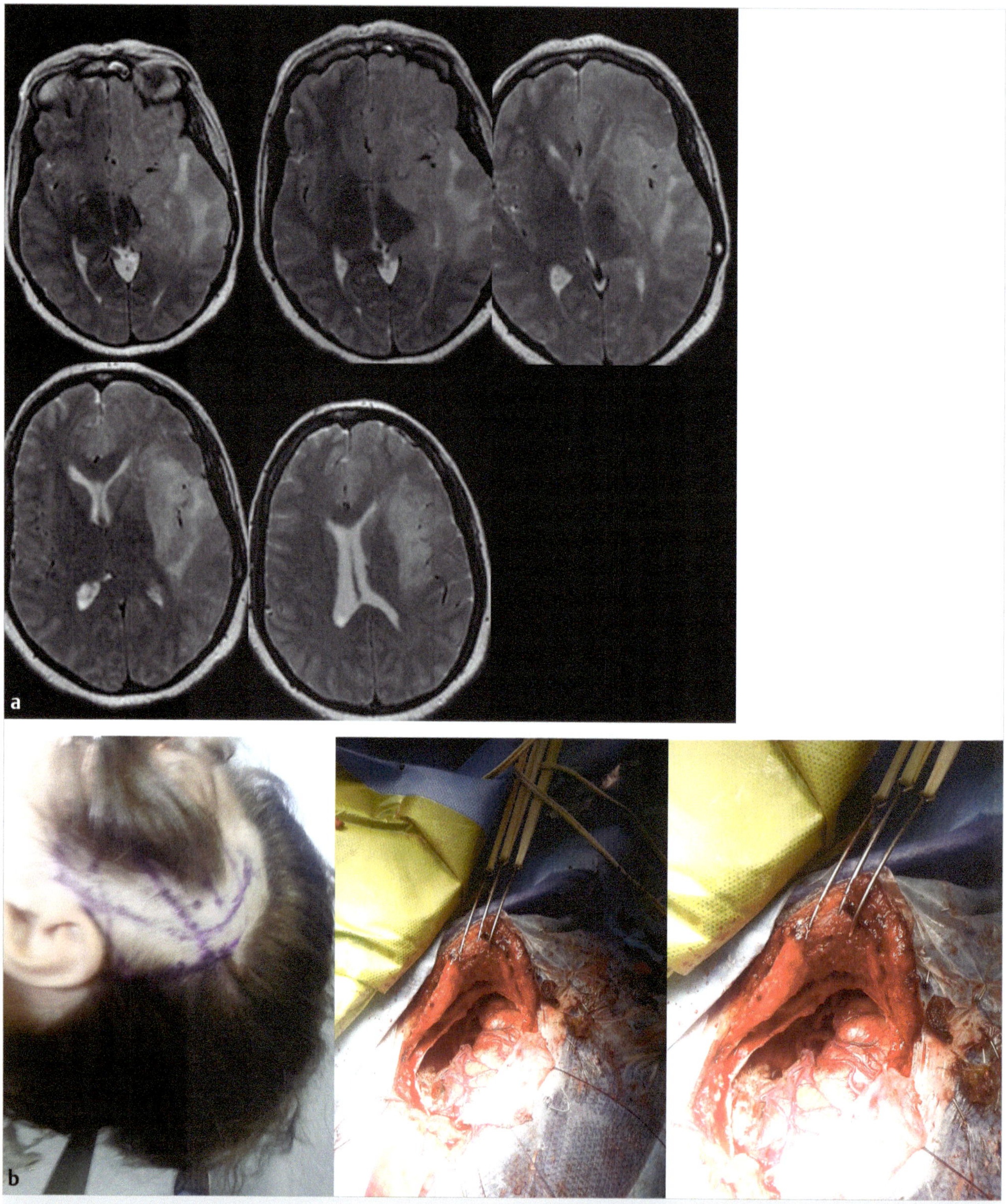

Fig. 16.4 An extreme case of a left fronto-temporo-insula glioma extending into the basal forebrain; (a) preoperative images, (b) images of the approach.

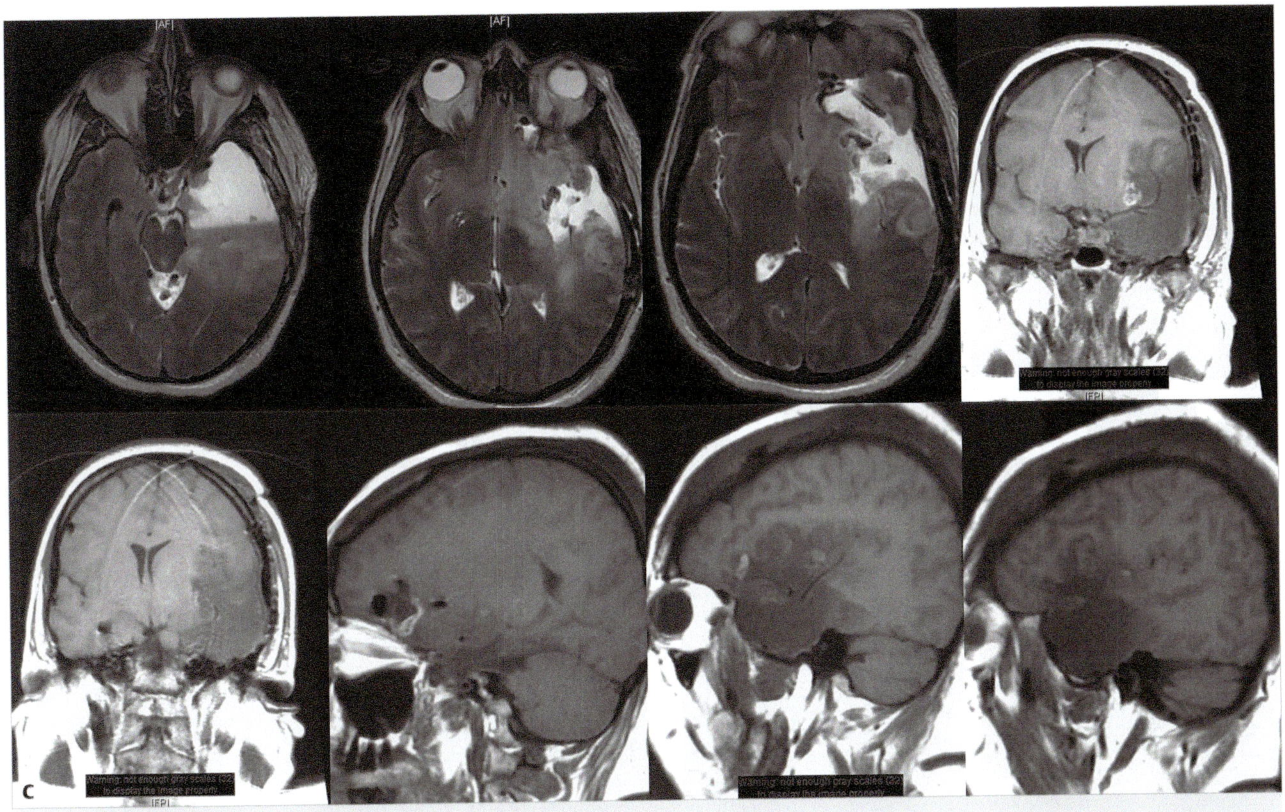

Fig 16.4 (*Continued*) (**c**) Postoperative images.

17 Cases that Taught Me Lessons

17.1 Introduction

Our field for years has had a problem with blunt full disclosure. This is not to say no one talks about complications at meetings or reports them in papers. To the contrary, "disaster sessions" are a common event. It is a common practice for people to show cases that went bad and talk about them. The issue is that in most cases, many people show themselves tackling massive or highly dangerous tumors and getting into trouble ("Oh, no kidding, you did a 9 cm intraventricular tumor and had a complication") or show cases when they did something impressive to salvage a bad mistake. Alternately, they demonstrate a complication which most people would acknowledge is hard to always avoid (i.e., a CSF leak), or something so rare that its interesting, but does not help people learn how to avoid flawed thinking and bad plans, which are at the root of a plurality of failures in neurosurgery.

It is all good and well to know that bad tumors have a lot of risk, and that master surgeons can try some impressive things to try to bail themselves out. It's just not that educational. What's often more useful are a blunt disclosure of true mistakes (i.e., real screw-ups). Cases where we often cringed looking at a post-op scan with a poor resection, or never forgot something we did that hurt a patient that we would never do again knowing what we know now. In other words, these are the real learning curve of experienced surgeons.

While the fact that tackling a 9 cm tumor or bypassing the carotid in an emergency allow people to admit that they have complications without losing face, the true screw-ups are the pearls we hang onto that keep us out of trouble. It's hard to publically show ourselves screwing up, especially if you wish to be seen as a master. Perhaps there are people who have reached the point where they do not make mistakes like that, but having worked with several outstanding surgeons, and talked to many more, and their trainees, I am highly skeptical that those people exist, or they may have a practice limited to one of two specific cases. At minimum, they probably have many mistakes that others could learn from if they were studied objectively.

At its core, I have tried to keep this book as honest as possible. While the premise of the book is that with better techniques, and a better understanding of the organization of the cerebrum we can do better glioma surgery and address tumors which we have not considered trying before, I have tried to always point out limits in my own knowledge, limits to our current techniques, and the importance of defining reasonable goals. We cannot defeat everyone's glioma, and that is not the claim of the book, just that we should try harder than we have been in the past.

I also have littered this book with my own opinions and ideas, often without a case series or citation. Evidence-based medicine is an important goal; however, in many cases it is beginning to lobotomize doctors, as not all questions can reasonably be answered by a randomized control trial, and not all randomized trials provide meaningful answers. For example, one shouldn't wait until they have a statically meaningful case series before concluding that deviating into the midbrain reticular activating system during a deep glioma resection is a bad idea. Opinions do not have the mandate.

This chapter is a frank and honest look into my learning curve told through very memorable cases. Given that many of the tumors in this book are not ones that very many surgeons that I know take on regularly, some of this learning curve involved figuring out things that were not in books, or taught at courses, or in some cases not even something you could find someone and ask for advice about. Other parts of the learning curve just involved making stupid mistakes in simple cases (that usually didn't seem stupid at the time), or finding out the hard way that the brain is more complex than I previously gave it credit for. Other parts are fascinating cases which went well, but demonstrate an idea I have never thought of prior to that case.

17.2 Lesson One (▶ Fig. 17.1)

17.2.1 My First Serious Insular Glioma and the Genesis of the Third Law

After years of thinking about how to do an insular glioma, studying the anatomy, watching cases and assisting, and preparing for my opportunity to tackle one of these, I felt prepared for the large left insular glioma which began my experience.

During the case, I felt I had done an aggressive resection. At the time I decided to stop, I was convinced I had taken out an extremely big part of the deep brain core, and was impressed how clear the cavity seemed. I also began to get concerned that I was too deep in the brain and was doing something crazy. I was happy that the patient woke up well; however, as many young tumor surgeons feel with their first serious attempt at a challenging brain tumor, my impressions of my own ability with insular tumors was smashed by the reality of the postop scan, demonstrating that I had done a glorified biopsy, and left a large part of the tumor. I always cringe when I see how little I got out.

When I see a patient who has undergone surgery elsewhere for a glioma which has left a substantial portion of the tumor, I imagine that the surgeon probably had the same impression I had in that case, that they were deep in the brain, that they had removed a large amount of brain/tumor, and that they should stop before they go too far.

When I considered the reasons I failed to do an adequate resection, the conclusion I came to, which I still base my surgeries on, were 1) we cannot expect good resections based on eyeball impressions of when it is time to stop; only when we reach anatomic landmarks, or have to stop to save function, can we be sure it is time to stop, 2) gliomas are substantially bigger tumors than we believe them to be until we have been aggressively resecting them for quite a while, and that you need to continue resecting well beyond where your instinct tells you enough is, 3) a real glioma resection should be shocking to the untrained eye.

Presently, I continue to resect the insula until I reach the circular sulcus on all sides, and have removed it down until it is flush with the temporal horn in the sagittal plane. Only the

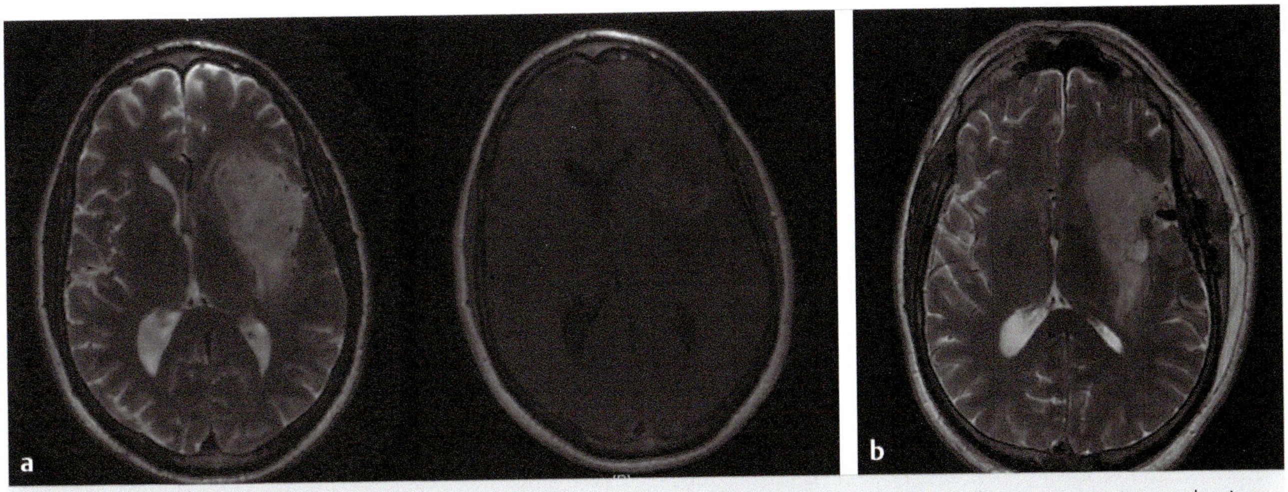

Fig. 17.1 My first serious insular glioma and the genesis of the third law case example; (**a**) preoperative images, (**b**) postoperative images showing a very subtotal resection of this tumor.

IFOF and occasionally the SLF limit this resection. My failure to do this in this case, led me to believe I had cleared out the insula when in reality I had cleared out part of a volumetrically large tumor.

17.3 Lesson Two (▶ Fig. 17.2)

17.3.1 Classic Teachings about the Anatomy of the Language System are Incomplete

For well over a century, most of us have believed that language arose from two main places in the brain, Broca's and Wernicke's areas, and as surgeons, avoidance of damaging these areas was the principle way to avoid aphasia during surgery. A careful student of neurology might note that other areas might cause speech problems of various strains, but basically, I graduated my residency with the idea that if I identified the "speech cortices" and stayed out of them, then the patient would talk afterwards. I (and I assume others in our field) didn't pay much heed to how exactly the information left these areas to cause a patient to talk, or how relevant inputs got there. I just focused on probability maps of rates of where the language sites were likely to be in glioma patients, and based my decision about awake vs asleep on those maps.

The case in ▶ Fig. 17.2 is a recurrent low grade glioma which I compared against the maps, determined that it was safe from a speech standpoint, based on the maps, and elected to resect asleep. I was stunned to find that this patient developed a dense expressive aphasia and anomia which only partially improved in long term follow-up. Perhaps others might have considered this a higher risk speech case than I did at the time; however, it did not make sense based on my understanding of how language is organized in the human brain at that time.

I unfortunately do not have preoperative tractographic data for this patient, so I can only speculate on the cause based on a large number of cases I have done since with similar features. First, the SLF can take abnormal and unpredictable courses and end fairly far posteriorly in the temporo-occipital lobe. Second, you cannot look at a brain and its gyral pattern and know what the language network looks like and where it is exactly. It is not random (i.e., the right occipital pole is not the site of language), but you cannot with confidence look at a glioma patient and know how they are wired up. Third, the brain is more complex than models made in the 1800s described it as being, and using outdated models to do brain surgery can lead to bad outcomes that we don't understand.

This case was one of the key cases which prompted my interest in network based models of brain function.

17.4 Lesson Three

17.4.1 Preserving the Left IFOF is Important for Preserving Normal Speech Function

▶ Fig. 17.3 demonstrates a left insular low-grade glioma removed awake early in my series. At the time, I was primarily interested in preservation of the SLF/arcuate and relevant language cortices as my goals of mapping. After removing the opercula and exposing the insula, I put the patient to sleep and cleared out the insula and subinsular areas down to the medial temporal structures to get a reasonable resection (▶ Fig. 17.3**b**).

The patient developed a dense anomia and partial expressive aphasia which did not make sense to me. This recovered to an extent, but never fully. I now know this is due to damage to the left IFOF by mapping the subinsular region during subcortical mapping, which will cause an anomia or speech disturbance. Interestingly, the mixed nature of the aphasia (phoenemic/semantic) raises the question of whether the IFOF carried purely semantic information, sufficed to say it is mostly semantic.

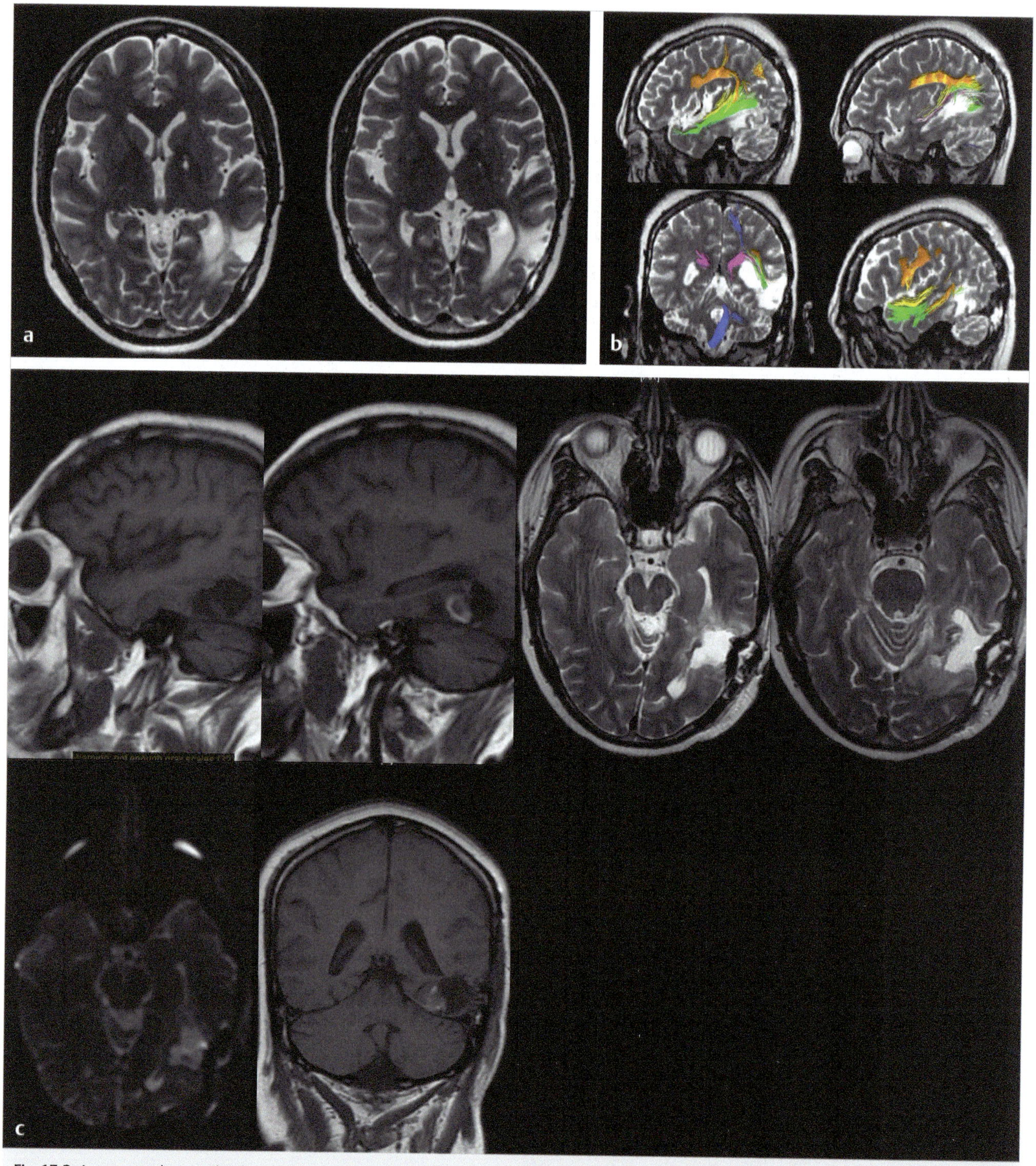

Fig. 17.2 A recurrent low-grade glioma; (a) preoperative images, (b) DTI tractography, (c) postoperative images.

17.5 Lesson Four (▶ Fig. 17.4)

17.5.1 Watch Out for Radiated High Grade Tumors in an Overgrown Uncus

This case demonstrates a GBM which was open biopsied and radiated at an outside facility. When the patient decompensated 2 months later, he was sent to us for definitive surgery. The surgery went seemingly well, and I was able to gross totally resect the enhancing portion of the tumor without problems. I recognized the enlarged uncus, and endeavored to remain subpial to remove this safely.

The patient developed an anterior choroidal infarct postoperatively, which surprised me as I had not seen the artery, nor had any significant bleeding, nor transgressed the pia to my knowledge. I am certain I am not the first person to have this problem; however, it taught me that an enlarged uncus, especially in a radiated high grade glioma, is a dangerous situation,

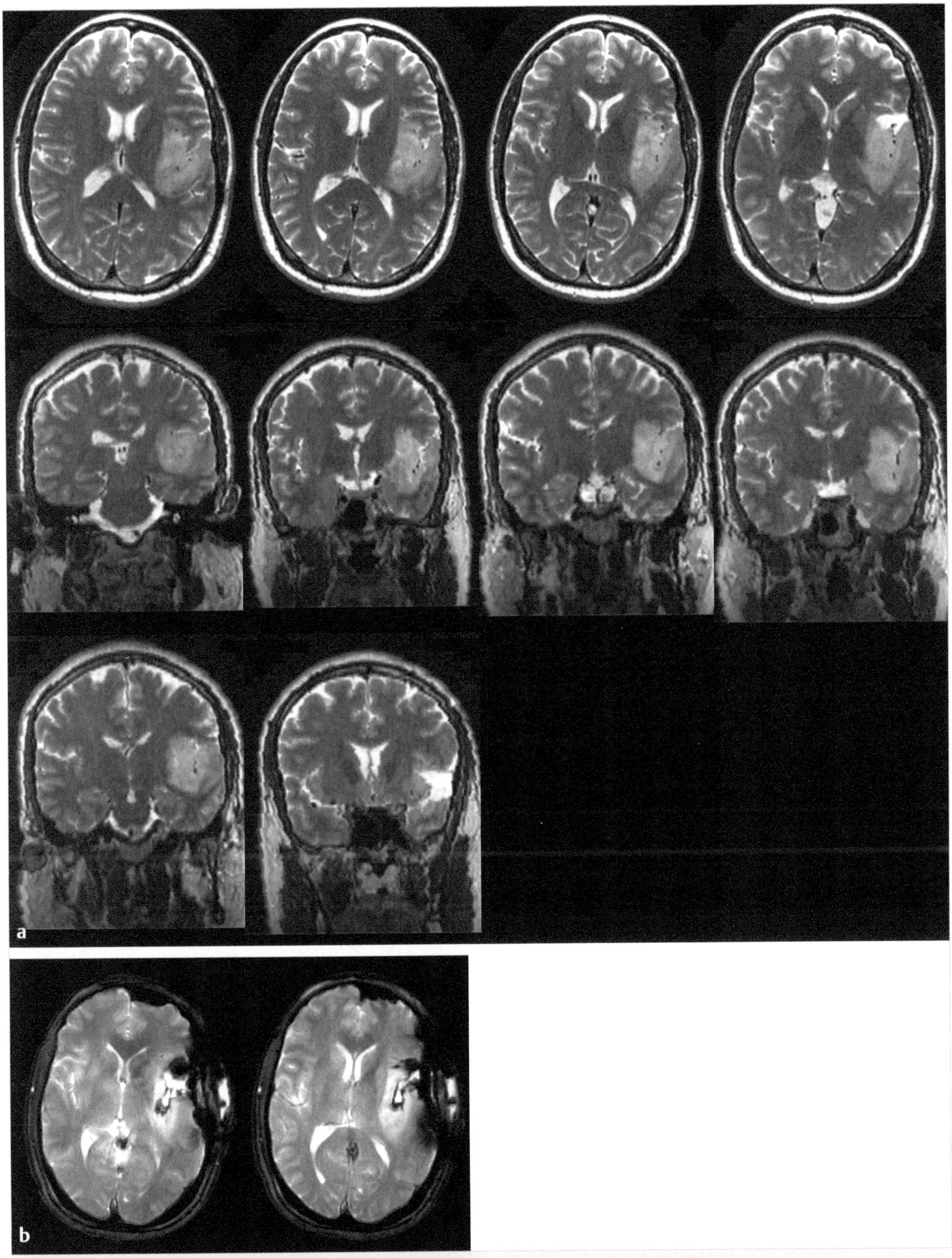

Fig. 17.3 A left insular low grade glioma removed awake; (a) preoperative images, (b) images of the approach.

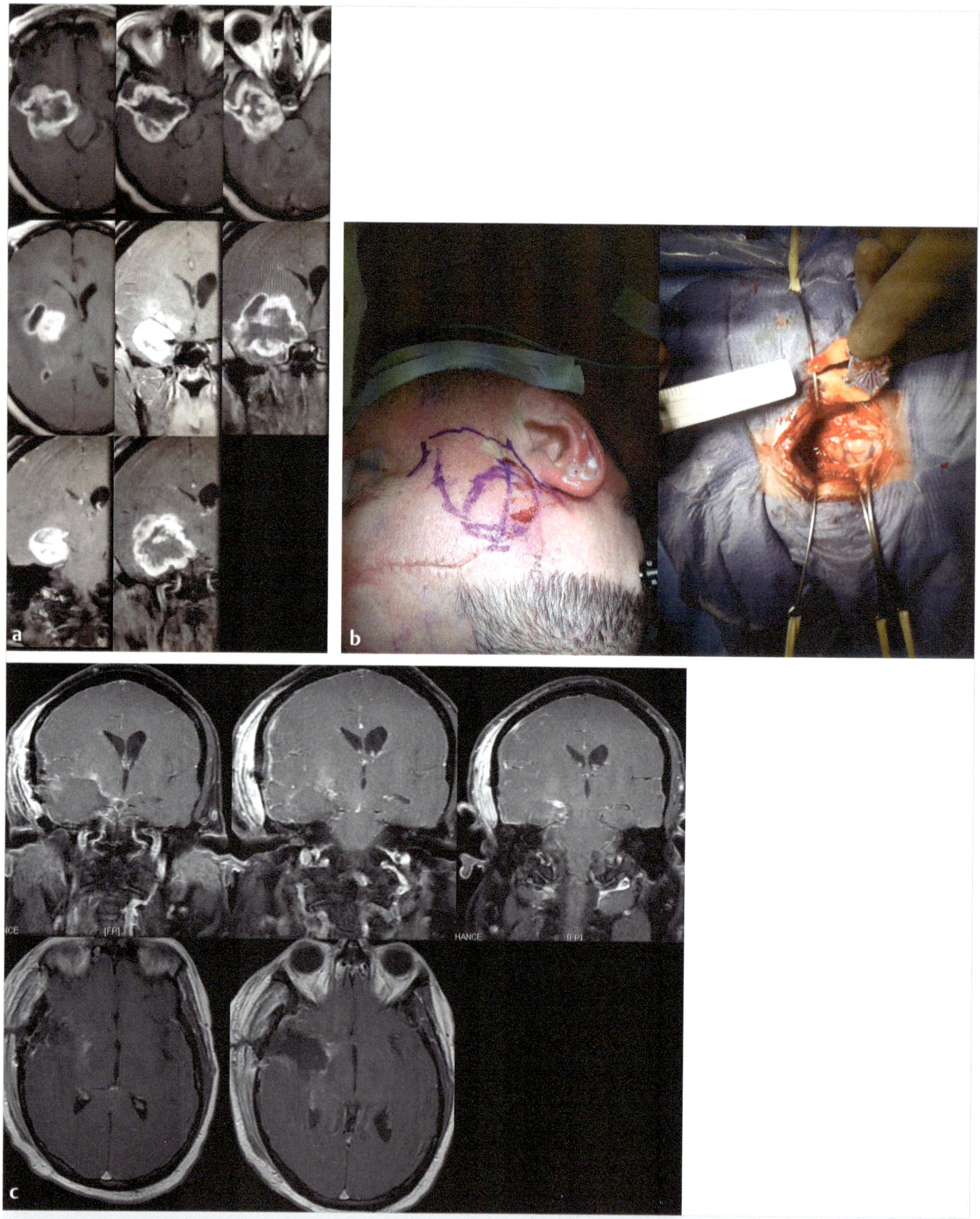

Fig. 17.4 GBM which was open biopsied and radiated at an outside facility; (**a**) preoperative images, (**b**) images of the approach, (**c**) postoperative images.

as the arteries in this area are quite tenuous, and it doesn't take much to injure them. This is true for other small arteries, such as the lenticulostriates brainstem perforators, etc.

While this patient's hemiplegia did not recover, he surprisingly lived 18 months after this surgery.

17.6 Lesson Five (▶ Fig. 17.5)

17.6.1 A Case I Can't Totally Explain, Other than that Glioma Surgery Is Dangerous

This patient initially presented with a hippocampal GBM, which we resected awake with a good outcome, followed by standard adjuvant therapy.

He did excellent for 10 months following this. He then lost most of his vision over the course of 2 days without warning or previous visual complaints. Exam demonstrated hemorrhagic papilledema and an MRI demonstrated recurrent tumor in the previous resection cavity. The best explanation for his fulminant course is that the tumor was causing increased intracranial pressure, and we repeated the surgery awake though obviously he could not participate in naming tasks due to his near blindness. His brain did not appear markedly swollen at the second surgery, and we removed all but a thin layer of tumor in the medial temporal lobe.

He did very well initially after the surgery for about a week. He then abruptly declined at rehab, and was found to have acute blood in the resection cavity, which was evacuated. At that surgery no active bleeding was noted, and no vessels were cauterized at that surgery. Follow-up scans showed a PCA infarct which developed since the initial postoperative scan. Two days later, the patient developed a dense MCA stroke as well, despite none of surgeries manipulating the MCA. Care was withdrawn.

It is unclear to me what happened either when the patient went blind, or why he began developing infarcts days after the second surgery. As always, one take home message is that what we do is always dangerous and out of our control to some extent and we must always keep this in the front of our minds and the patients decisions.

17.7 Lesson Six (▶ Fig. 17.6)

17.7.1 The SMA Syndrome Doesn't Always Get Better

The common teaching from the epilepsy (and low grade glioma literature) is that the SMA syndrome improves roughly 90% of the time in long term follow-up. This case of a GBM, which I removed from the SMA and followed the T2 changes down to the corpus callosum, was a striking example of what that 10% rate of no recovery means, as his hemiplegia, akinesias, and mutism never improved in his lifetime, and he never underwent adjuvant therapy to his exceedingly poor neurologic status. I now believe that this was due to both removal of the SMA, and severing the connection of the pre-motor areas to the other SMA via the crossed FAT, though admittedly some cases may result from a contralateral SMA which cannot carry the load for both sides. In fact, this case was the impetus for our efforts to look for the connections which allow for recovery of a limited SMA resection in the first place, as I felt I needed to understand at minimum how to not guarantee this could not recover if I were to be in this area and cause SMA syndrome again.

More saliently, it caused me to question the wisdom of entering the SMA network in the first place in glioma surgery. First, the idea that 10% of patients could be left with the SMA syndrome, which is quite severe, causes me to question whether this is worth removing a few more ccs of tumor. Second, I have observed that many of the so-called recoveries are not truly complete. Some patients recover within days (suggesting this is edema resolution and not rewiring), but many do not truly make it back to normal motor function. They are bradykinetic, they fall occasionally, and they are frequently are uncoordinated even in the long term. In other words, I am not certain "moving all four" which is usually the standard of evidence in the SMA literature, is the same as good motor function. Again I am uncertain that the additional few ccs of tumor resection makes this worth it.

Finally, glioma surgery is not epilepsy surgery, and has different goals, mandates, and logistics. Thus, while it may be worthwhile to cause SMA syndrome and wait it out for several months in a seizure patient, in a glioma patient this inevitably delays adjuvant therapy often significantly (which annihilates any benefit from high grade surgery), and can rob a patient with a limited life span of valuable quality time for a marginal improvement in extent of resection. Thus, we have begun subcortical mapping with the goal of avoiding or minimizing SMA syndrome type problems.

17.8 Lesson Seven (▶ Fig. 17.7)

17.8.1 The Anterior Cingulate Gyrus Is Important for Good Quality of Life

In this case, I approached this case with the goal of a focal lesionectomy of the involved corpus callosum and a small part of the anterior cingulate. I did these cases asleep at this point and things seemingly went well. The patient did not do well, was severely abulic to the point of being akinetic, and ultimately never pursued adjuvant radiotherapy.

While some could have said they expected this, I was long perplexed why the corpus callosum was so important for interaction and alertness. I now am relatively convinced that the key problem is disruption of the DMN and anterior cingulate networks.

17.9 Lesson Eight (▶ Fig. 17.8)

17.9.1 The Other Side Must Carry the Load

This is a case of an extensive progressive glioma of the right frontal lobe which was treated with radiotherapy alone at an outside facility. The patient progressively deteriorated with worsening balance and cognitive function and the MRI showed extensive white matter changes bilaterally.

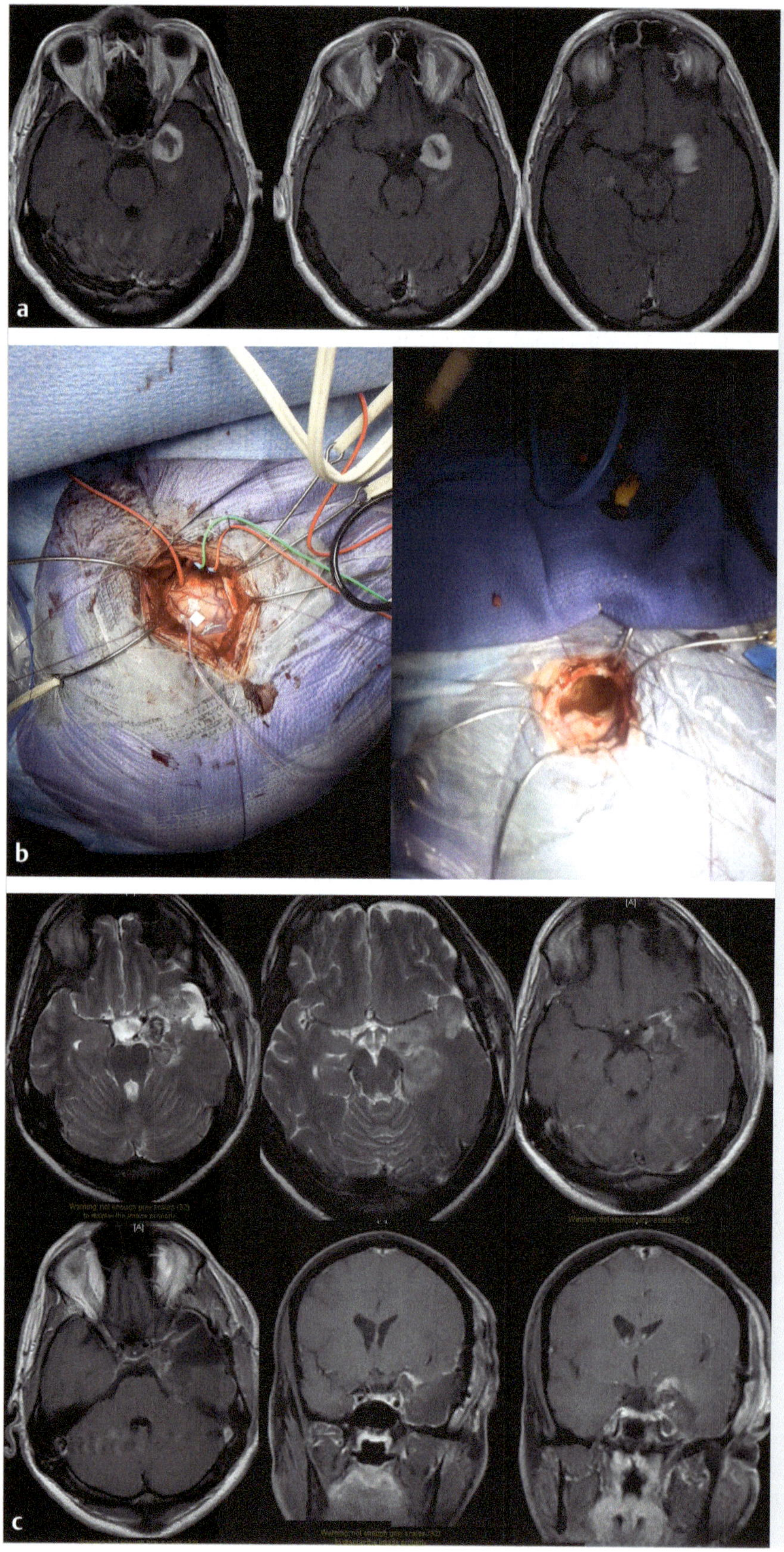

Fig. 17.5 A patient initially presented with a hippocampal GBM, which we resected awake with a good outcome, followed by standard adjuvant therapy; (**a**) preoperative images, (**b**) images of the approach, (**c**) DTI tractography.

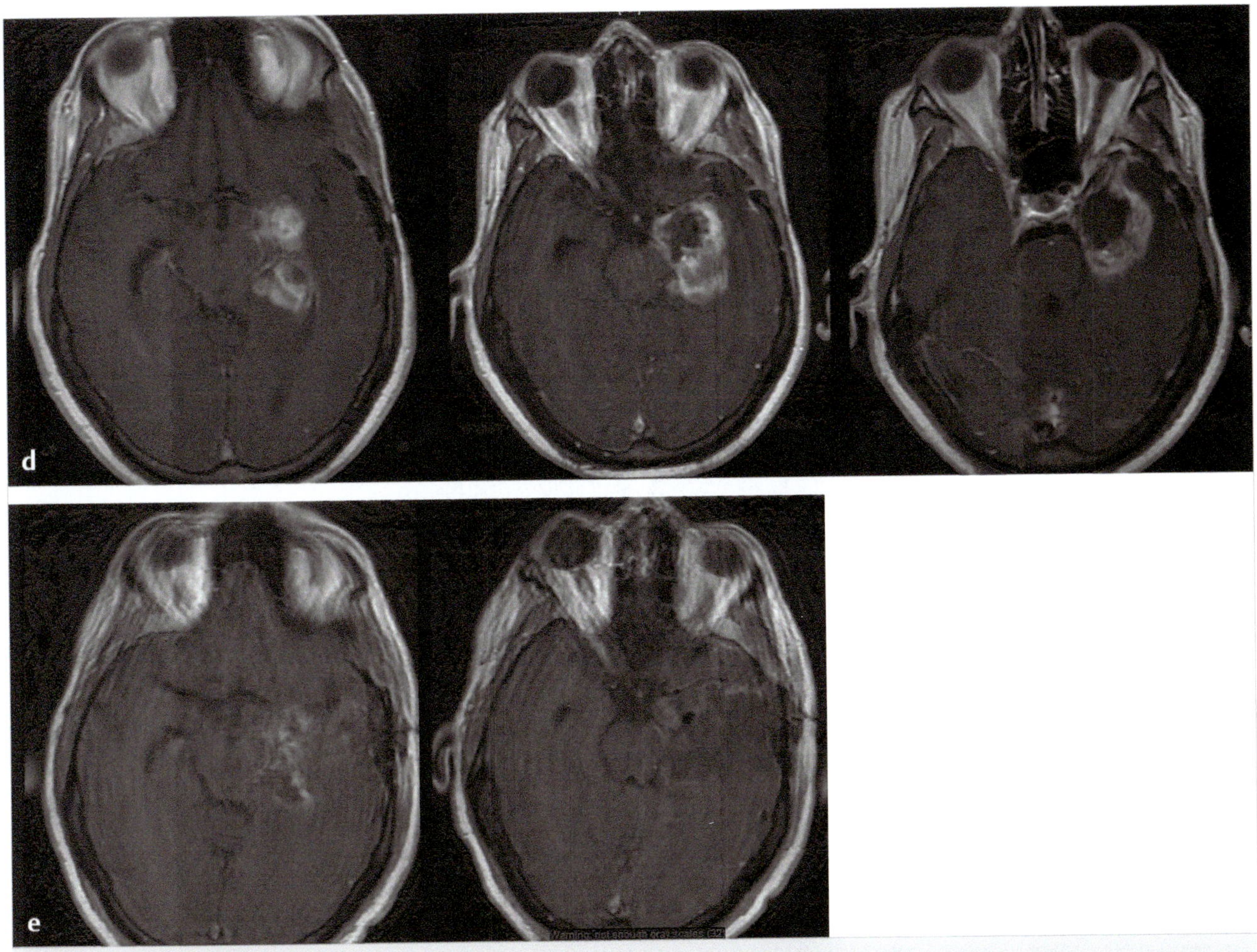

Fig 17.5 (*Continued*) (**d**) Postoperative images, (**e**) long-term follow-up images.

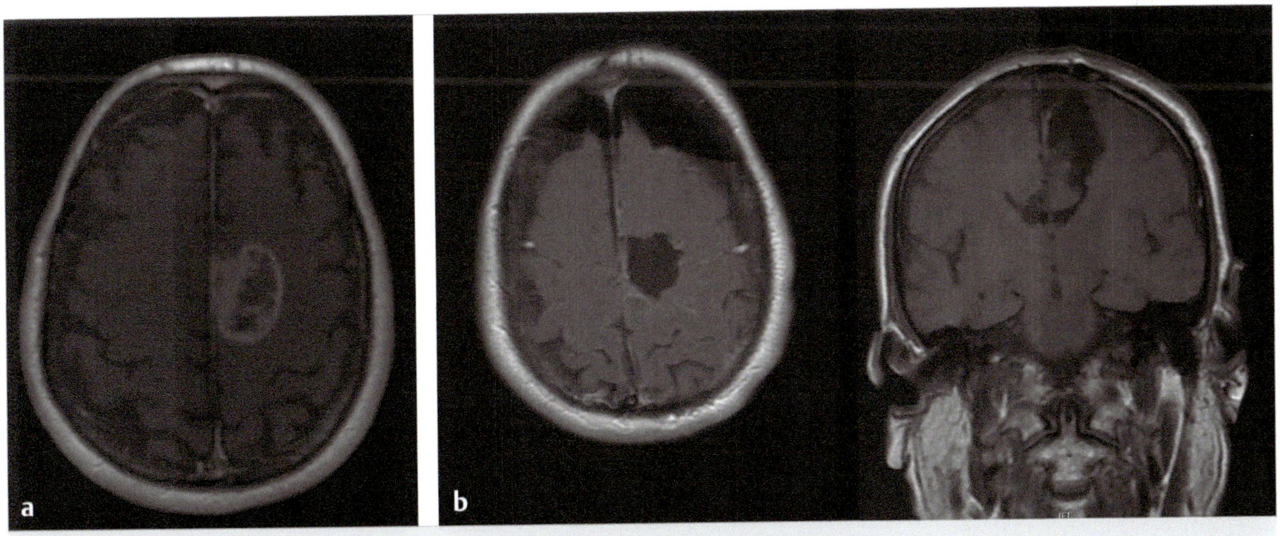

Fig. 17.6 Supplementary Motor Area (SMA); (**a**) preoperative images, (**b**) postoperative images.

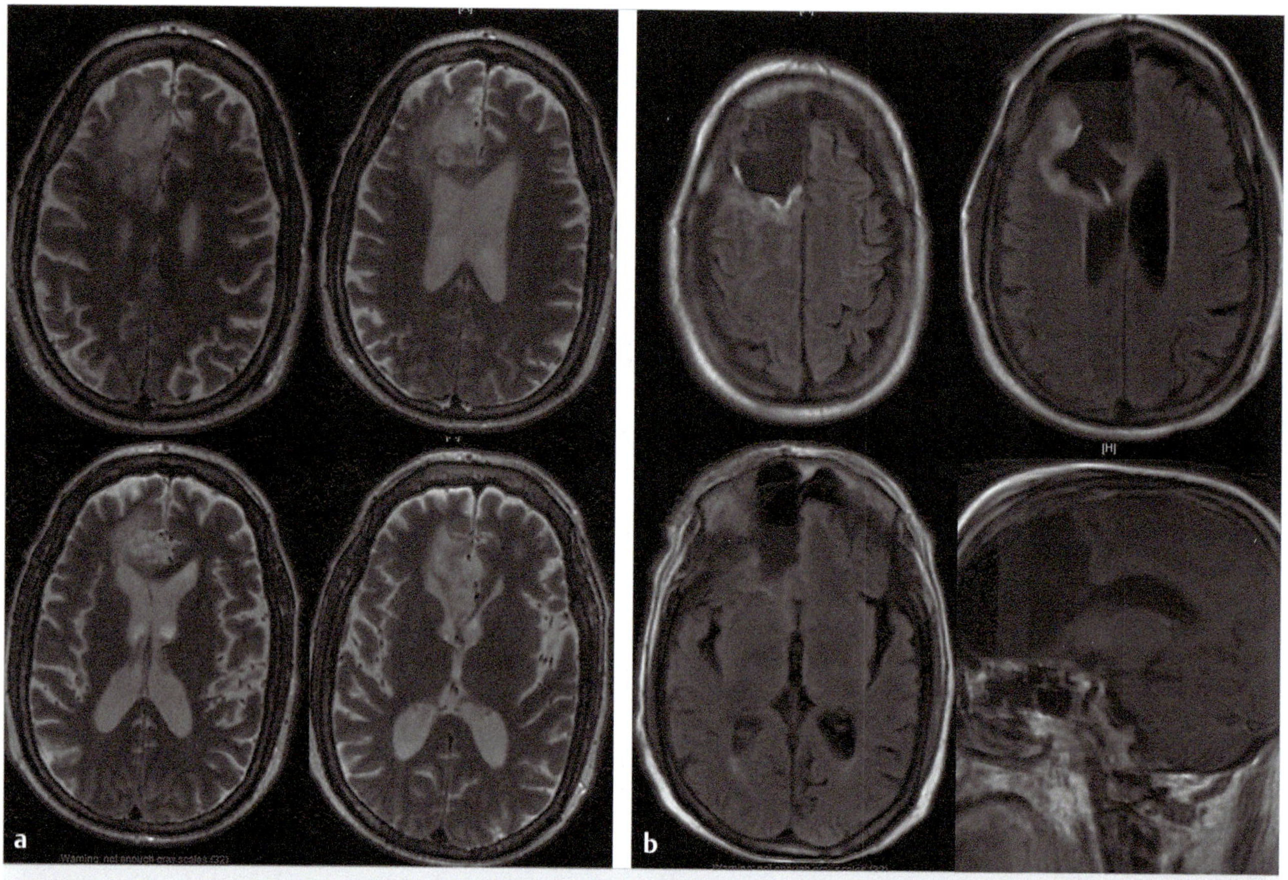

Fig. 17.7 Focal lesionectomy of the involved corpus callosum and a small part of the anterior cingulate; (**a**) preoperative images, (**b**) postoperative images.

I decided that we might be able to salvage this case by doing the surgery I would have done initially, which was an aggressive resection of the involved frontal tumor, which involved the majority of the frontal lobe prior to radiotherapy. I assumed that with the tumor and radiotherapy, this lobe likely wasn't working very well, and that we wouldn't make the situation much worse.

The resection went seemingly well. As can often happen, the patient had a markedly worse frontal syndrome. Many frontal syndromes improve with time. However, this was far worse than a normal frontal syndrome; she was very disinhibited, incontinent, and blunted, and this did not improve. While it is conceivable that some of these are from the loss of the right frontal lobe, most right frontal lobe resections do not end in a patient who requires 24-hour care, cannot walk, is incontinent, and disinhibited.

While many possible explanations could be put forward, given that this patient did not have a more type cingulate syndrome, I have interpreted this bad outcome as an indirect consequence of the extensive radiation changes on the other side, meaning that the other frontal lobe was unable to carry the work load when the right lobe, however dysfunctional it was. I have seen variations on this specific issue in other case; however, this is the most dramatic case of this type I have seen. This argues strongly that we should consider the need for other areas of the brain to compensate when we resect a brain region, and particularly assess the ability of the other side to compensate. This is especially true in cases where extensive radiotherapy has been used.

17.10 Lesson Nine (▸ Fig. 17.9)

17.10.1 Entering the Septal Area Can Have Some Dramatic Consequences

The septal nuclei are brain structure that most neurosurgeons have probably not spent a lot of time thinking about how to avoid: they are hard to find, and there are few operations which bring you close to these structures. Anterior butterfly gliomas are one of these cases.

In this case, an early case in my experience with butterfly gliomas, which was a case of a malignant transformation of a low grade glioma which recurred in the corpus callosum. We aggressively resected the involved frontal lobe and callosum. During the resection, I focused on clearing out the rostrum, which was a major focus of the tumor, and in retrospect, I entered the subcallosal area where the septal nuclei are located, extending below the inferior "tripod" of the forceps minor.

Postoperatively, the patient wasn't disinhibited, or blunted, or abulic, and he went home the next day after surgery. However, when he returned, the family told of behavioral issues such as staying up nearly all the time (even after the steroids were weaned), cooking bizarre and inedible food, making

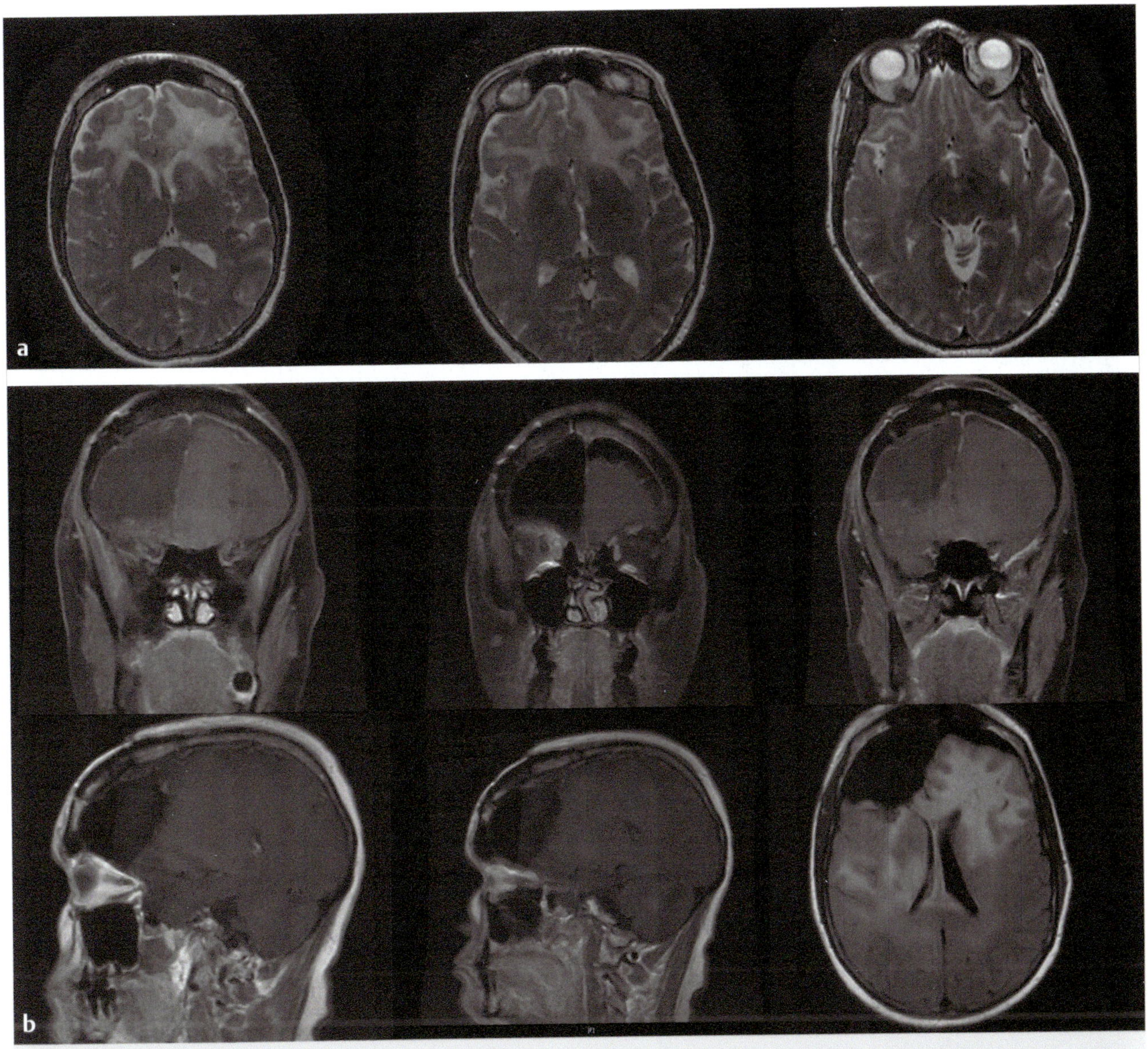

Fig. 17.8 Extensive progressive glioma of the right frontal lobe which was treated with radiotherapy alone at an outside facility; (**a**) preoperative images, (**b**) postoperative images.

phone calls at all hours to friends and family, and marked anxiety. While it's impossible to rule out that this was due to the septal nuclei and not removing the frontal lobe, this syndrome did not strike me as the usual frontal disinhibition, and when talking to the patient, much of this behavior seemed to be more a result of psychiatric problems than from poor judgment. We will never know for sure, but I have made a point of staying out of the subcallosal and septal area ever since.

17.11 Lesson Ten (▶ Fig. 17.10)

17.11.1 Respect the Artery of Death

In this case, a recurrent GBM, the patient presented with some tumor in the IFOF, but relatively normal speech. I exposed the posterior temporal lobe. The dura was stuck, so I brought the microscope in and carefully dissected the dura from the brain. The posterior temporal MCA branch was adherent to the dura and I had to dissect this free with a Rhoton #6 dissection somewhat firmly. It never bled or was kinked or twisted. However, I saw this artery begin to vasospasm in front of me, and the patient who had been talking with us, immediately developed a bad expressive aphasia. I bathed this artery in papervine and verapamil and the spasm seemed to visibly resolve, but the patient did not improve and the DWI confirmed that this was enough to cause a relevant infarct in this distribution.

In short, this artery is particularly sensitive to manipulation and not always fixable even if you are careful, and this can end a speech mapping case before it even gets started as this artery supplies the entire semantic area of the temporal lobe. It is generally wise to avoid doing anything more than absolutely necessary to this artery, as it is not as forgiving as other cortical arteries.

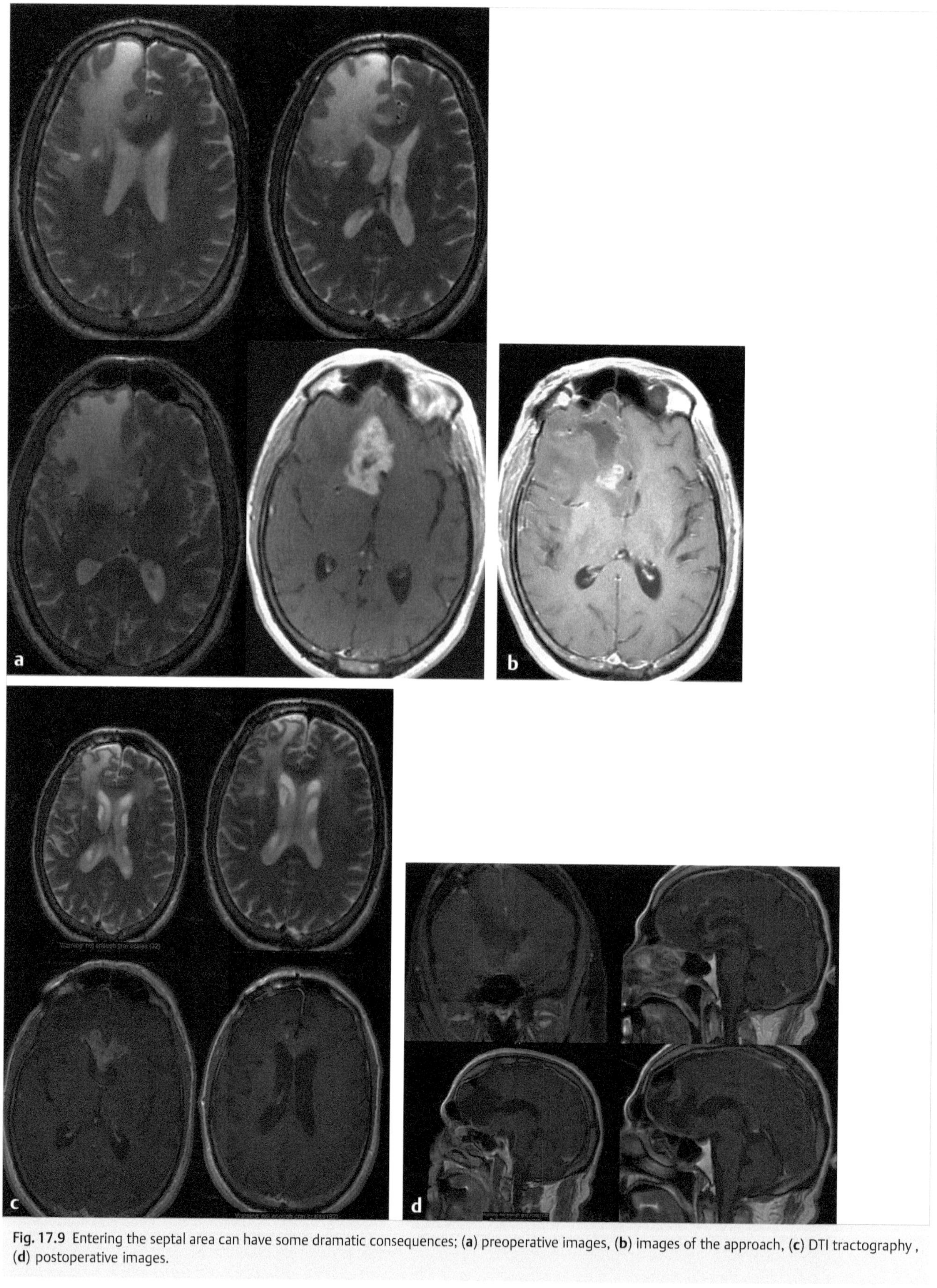

Fig. 17.9 Entering the septal area can have some dramatic consequences; (**a**) preoperative images, (**b**) images of the approach, (**c**) DTI tractography, (**d**) postoperative images.

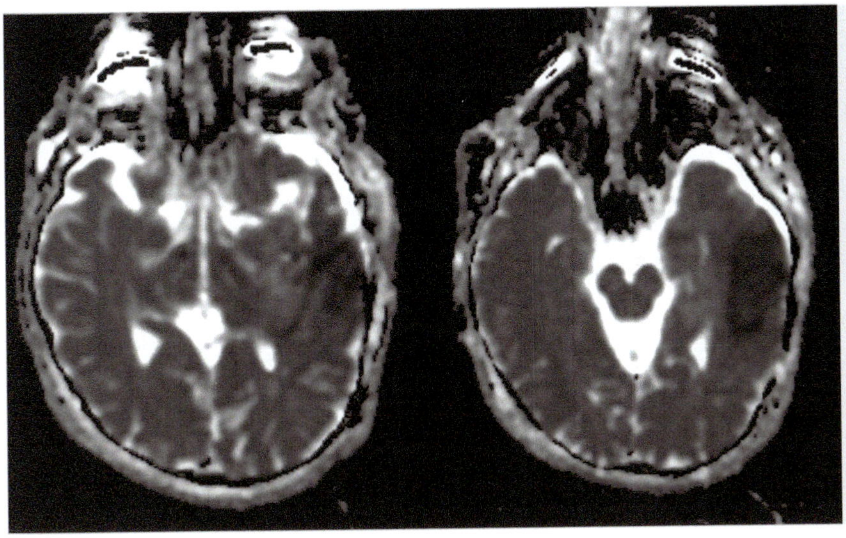

Fig. 17.10 Respect the artery of death; preoperative images.

17.12 Lesson Eleven (▶ Fig. 17.11, ▶ Fig. 17.12)

17.12.1 Don't Give Up: You Can't Predict What Will Happen

Many cases in this book are desperate attempts to turn around bad glioma cases. Not surprisingly, some of these patients do as badly as expected; however, this is not always true. In a chapter about what can go wrong in glioma surgery, I thought I'd end with two cases which show what is possible if you try, even when it looks bad.

The first case (▶ Fig. 17.11) demonstrates a case of a severe recurrence of an extensive recurrent left temporal GBM who presented with papilledema and anomia. We performed an extensive resection, and treated with avastin. At the time of this writing, the patient has been recurrence free for 4 years.

In the second case (▶ Fig. 17.12), this young patient presented with a pineal region GBM, with additional tumor in the medial temporal lobe. Despite resecting both, the patient presented in two weeks with hearing loss a massive recurrence in the pineal region. After discussing the gravity of the situation with the patient, we agreed to try our best and resected the pineal tumor, and started adjuvant therapy the next day in hopes that this fast growing tumor would respond if we could get to it fast.

The patient remained tumor free for almost two years, before eventually recurring. While this was not an indefinite cure, this allowed her to spend time with her baby which was born 2 weeks before diagnosis.

I have numerous other such stories in various forms, but these are two memorable ones. Gliomas are not curable, and we cannot always save these patients forever, but with reasonable goals and the view that we can do something positive, even in the most dire of cases, even if that is not living forever.

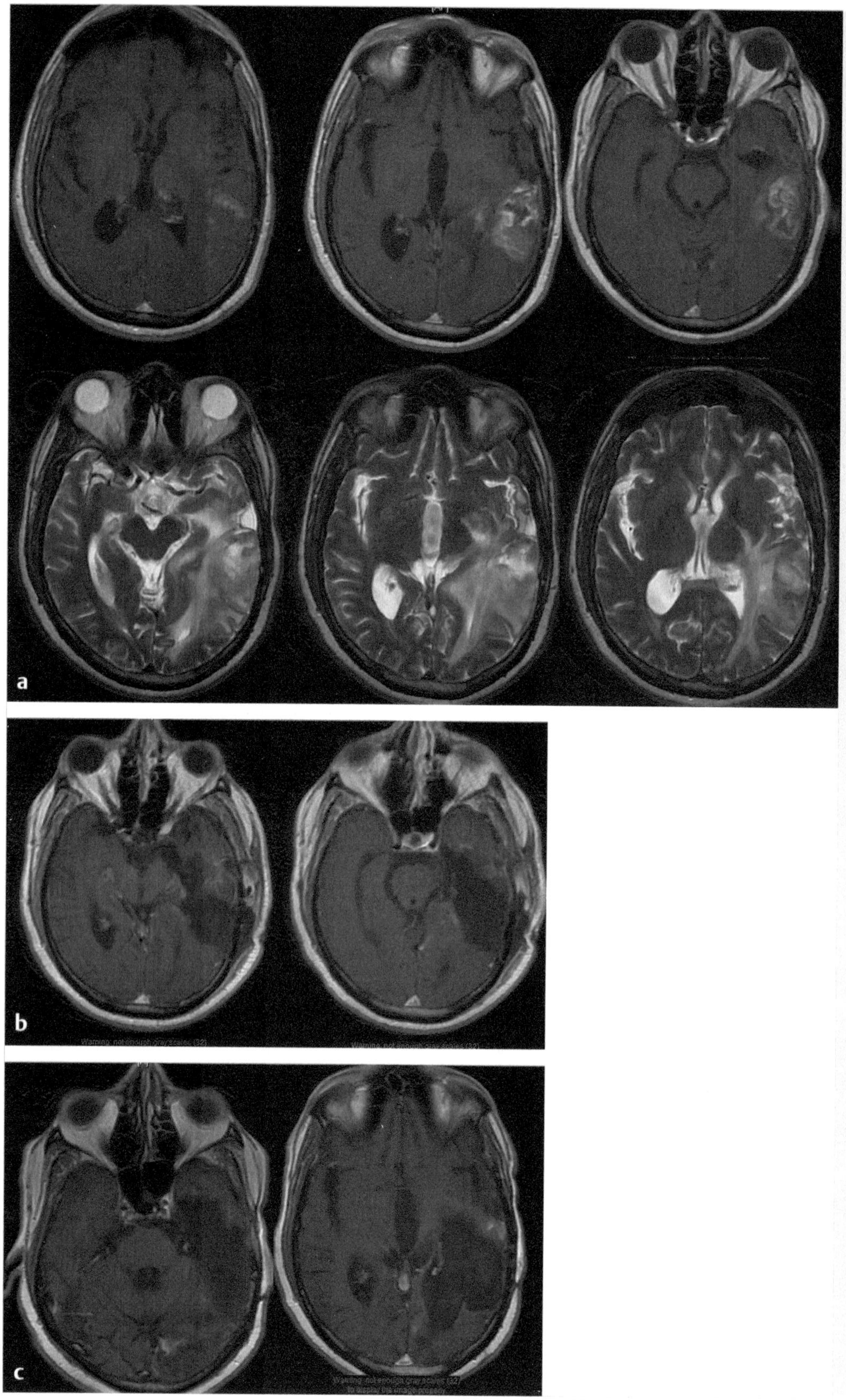

Fig. 17.11 A case of a severe recurrence of an extensive recurrent left temporal GBM who presented with papilledema and anomia; (**a**) preoperative images, (**b**) images of the approach, (**c**) DTI tractography.

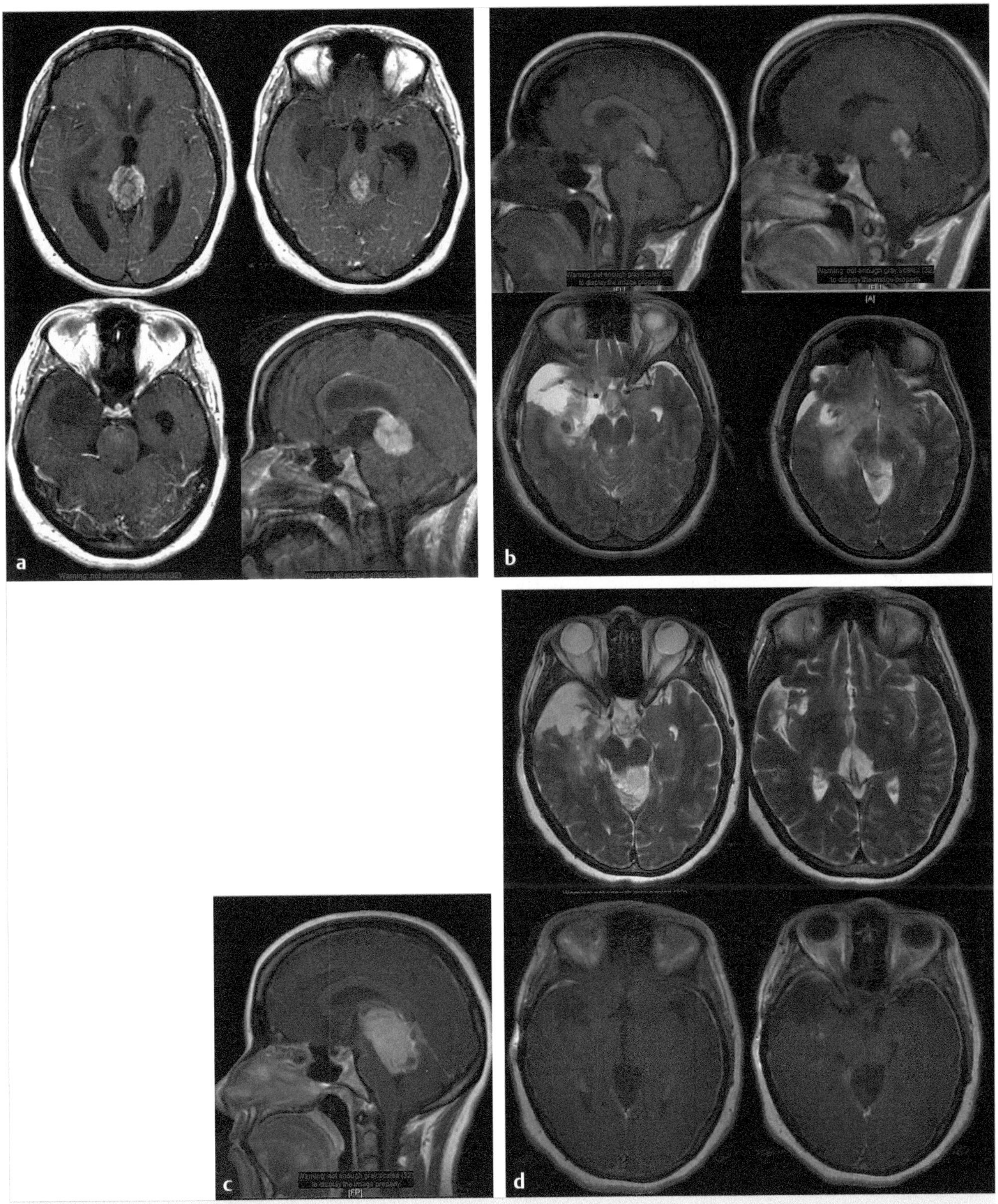

Fig. 17.12 A pineal region GBM, with additional tumor in the medial temporal lobe; (**a**) preoperative images, (**b**) images of the approach, (**c**) DTI tractography, (**d**) postoperative images.

Index

Note: Page numbers in **bold** or *italics* indicate headings or figures, respectively.

W